The Interferon System

A Current Review to 1987

The University of Texas Graduate School of Biomedical Sciences at Galveston

The University of Texas Medical Branch Series in Biomedical Science

The Interferon System

A Current Review to 1987

Edited by Samuel Baron, Ferdinando Dianzani, G. John Stanton, and W. Robert Fleischmann, Jr.

University of Texas Press, Austin

Printed in the United States of America

First Edition, 1987

For reasons of economy and speed this volume has been printed from camera-ready copy furnished by the contributors, who assume full responsibility for its contents.

LIBRARY OF CONGRESS CATALOGING-IN-PUBLICATION DATA

The Interferon system.

(The University of Texas Medical Branch series in biomedical science)
Includes bibliographies and index.
1. Interferon. I. Baron, Samuel, 1928–
II. Series. [DNLM: 1. Interferons. QW 800 I6066]
QR187.5.I5719 1987 616.07′9 87-13861
ISBN 0-292-73845-5

Contents

Foreword

The University of Texas Graduate School of Biomedical Sciences at Galveston is happy to present the fourth volume of its biomedical science series. The aim of this series is to reflect the dynamic thrust of discovery in a form that will be useful to all who work in the field. The key to the utility of each volume is the prompt editing and publishing of the latest findings and their critical review and evaluation by leading scientists. The present volume comprises a review of the status of interferon edited by Drs. Samuel Baron, Ferdinando Dianzani, G. John Stanton, and W. Robert Fleischmann, Jr. Dr. Baron is a noted research scientist in the area of interferon and has written erudite updatings of the status of interferon research which were published in *Texas Reports on Biology and Medicine*. The present volume brings that material up to the very present and it is hoped that it will be useful to workers in the field. We wish to thank our volume and section editors and their secretarial staff for their efforts in bringing the volume to press. I especially wish to thank Mrs. Theresa Copado, administrative assistant of the graduate school, who is responsible for final assembly of the completed sections. Thanks are also due to the University of Texas Press for the timely publication of these volumes.

J. PALMER SAUNDERS, PH.D.
Dean of the Graduate School
Executive Editor

Acknowledgments

The editors wish to acknowledge with gratitude the organizational ability, perseverance, and thoughtful assistance of Rhonda Peake, associate editor. We wish to thank, also, Hillary Heard and Audrey Hart for their indexing assistance. We would particularly like to thank J. Palmer Saunders, dean of the Graduate School of Biomedical Sciences at the University of Texas Medical Branch, for his leadership in maintaining the University of Texas biomedical research series.

Dedication

Peter De Somer, M.D.
1917–1985

This book is dedicated to the memory of Professor Peter De Somer, a distinguished and beloved interferon scientist, who died on June 17, 1985, at the age of 68. Dr. De Somer held an M.D. degree as well as a baccalaureate degree in Thomistic philosophy from the University of Leuven. These two areas of study in his youth shaped the personality of this remarkable man in his career as a scientist, as the founder of a prosperous pharmaceutical company, as the founder and director of the Rega Institute for Medical Microbiology, and as the rector who helped redirect the University of Leuven.

After his medical studies, he specialized in microbiology. Initially, he was productively engaged in studies of blood groups and infectious mononucleosis. In the immediate postwar years, sensing that antibiotics would become an ever-expanding field of research and development, he became actively involved in the antibiotic industry in Belgium.

His interest then turned to virology, which in the fifties was a booming scientific discipline. In the wake of breakthroughs in poliomyelitis vaccine research in the United States, Professor De Somer became one of the pioneers in the development of vaccine production on the European continent, thereby helping his small country to become the first to be completely free of poliomyelitis. Soon after the discovery of interferons in 1957, he initiated studies on the production and mode of action of these substances, and his institute soon became one of the major interferon research centers.

Over the years, Professor De Somer attracted many collaborators, whom he generously encouraged to develop their own research themes, including antiviral chemotherapeutics, medical virology and epidemiology, gnotobiology, immunopathology, and genetic engineering.

Among his fellow scientists, Peter De Somer will be remembered not only for his scientific contributions but equally for his incisive wit, his authority in matters of science management, his clairvoyance in evaluating new discoveries, his intuition for what is ethical and unethical in medical research, his authentic love for the good things of life, and the personal charm with which he could effectively voice his opinions both in private and in public.

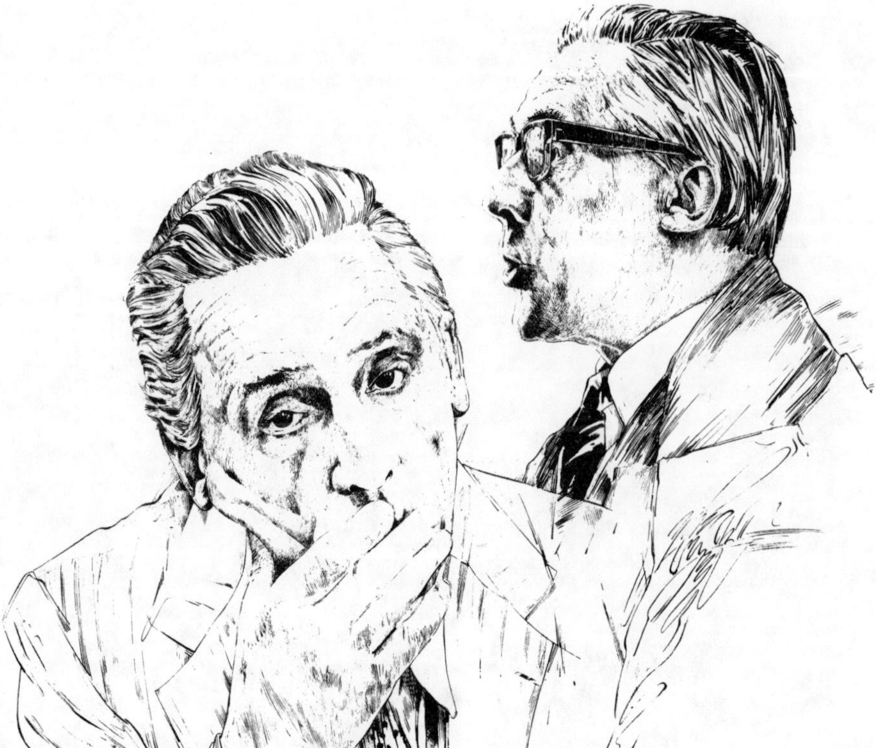

The Interferon System
A Current Review to 1987

Introduction: General Considerations of the Interferon System

Samuel Baron,[a] *G. John Stanton,*[a] *W. R. Fleischmann, Jr.,*[a] *and Ferdinando Dianzani*[b]

[a]Department of Microbiology, University of Texas Medical Branch, Galveston, TX 77550; [b]Institute of Virology, University of Rome "La Sapienza," Viale di Porta Tiburtina 28, 00185 Rome, Italy

This current review of the interferon system is the third in a series of comprehensive updatings of the field (1,2). The book is a result of a cooperative effort by many investigators throughout the world to present a current, comprehensive, authoritative, and reasonably concise historical review and current knowledge of the main areas of interferon research. When little progress has occurred in an area covered by a chapter in the first two reviews, the chapter has not been repeated. Therefore, the reader is advised to consult the first two reviews for subjects not covered here (1,2).

The purpose of this first chapter is to broadly sketch the historical developments, the fundamental mechanisms, the implications for other scientific fields, and the significance for medicine. The succeeding chapters will present the specific information and appropriate references. Since specific references for the information in this chapter are cited in the following chapters, only general references are cited for background reading (1-37).

Interferon was discovered thirty years ago by Isaacs and Lindenmann (6), who observed that fluids from virus-infected cell cultures contained a protein that could react with cells to render them resistant to infection by a wide variety of viruses. Since then much has been learned about the complex interferon system, including its applicability for treatment of disease. The field lost one of its most imaginative leaders when Alick Isaacs died in 1967, at the age of 45. Many of his original concepts continue to be borne out by subsequent studies and our intellectual debt to him is remembered on occasions such as this.

Although interferons were first recognized for their extraordinarily potent antiviral properties, it has now been established that they may profoundly affect other vital cellular and bodily functions, including cell metabolism and growth, immunity, and tumors. Thus the interferon system has been used as a model system for studying membrane changes and molecular events involved in viral replication, gene expression, cell regulation, immune regulation, and hormone production and action. Clinically, trials of interferon and its inducers during viral infections and cancer have reached the stage of controlled clinical trials and licensing for specific uses.

Overview

In the almost 30 years since interferon's discovery, the field of interferon research has progressed tremendously. We now know that the interferon of Isaacs and Lindenmann is really a family of molecules which can be divided into three species: IFN-α, IFN-β, and IFN-γ. The interferons differ in the agent which induces them and in the cell type which produces them. The interferon proteins have been purified and the interferon genes have even been cloned in bacteria. A wide variety of interferon activities including antiviral effects, antiproliferative effects, immunomodulatory effects, and hormonal effects have been described and partially characterized (Table 1). To induce these activities, interferon must activate cells to produce effector proteins.

A generalized scheme of the interferon system is presented in Figure 1. The genetic information for the interferon proteins is contained in a number of normally unexpressed genes. Production and secretion of the interferon protein(s) can be induced by foreign substances and some cytokines. Thus, in the normal state, only low to undetectable levels of interferon can be found in body tissues. Any produced interferon reacts with receptors on cells to induce effector proteins (AVP) which lead to most of the specific biochemical effects resulting in antiviral action, immunoregulation, cell regulatory activity, etc. The interferon-activated cell may transfer its activated state to adjacent cells without the continued presence of interferon.

Interferon has a very high affinity for its receptor (log Ka=10 to 11) and the interaction of interferon with its high affinity receptor is essential for the induction of new mRNA synthesis in responding cells. Findings indicate that the intracellular production or administration of interferon is not sufficient to activate an interferon response. Specifically, interferon-producing cells incubated in the presence of antisera to interferon fail to give an interferon response. Similarly, microinjection of interferon into cells failed to activate the antiviral state in the cells. There is a recent report of a possible intracellular role for the receptor/interferon complex or some derivative but further studies are needed to establish a functional role.

Induction of the Three Types of Interferon Proteins

During studies of interferon, a major advantage has been the ability to conclusively identify interferon as the active component of even impure preparations. In this way, a function of an interferon preparation can be definitively ascribed to the interferon in the preparation if the active component has the following properties: (a) is specific for the phylogenetic family in which it was produced (with a few exceptions); (b) inhibits almost all known viruses; (c) inhibits certain viruses more effectively than others; (d) requires ongoing cellular RNA synthesis for action; (e) requires ongoing protein synthesis for action; (f) is normally a repressed genetic function of the cell; (g) is prevented from acting by specific antibody to interferon; (h) induces a specific set of effector molecules; and (i) cellular activation by IFN decays over hours or days after removal of IFN. Identification can usually be accomplished by correlation of only several of these properties with the function being studied.

A number of molecules have been identified which meet these criteria. They have been divided into three families of interferons: IFN-α, IFN-β, and IFN-γ. A fourth interferon-like protein has recently described and is under active study. The assignments of interferon molecules to the three families has been based mainly on their antigenic and molecular relatedness as well as the cell type which produces them, and the agent which induces them (Figure 2).

Interferons and their Inducers

Human IFN-α is produced by lymphocytes and macrophages which have been induced with components of foreign cells and perhaps cells made foreign by transformation, infection and certain chemicals (Figure 2). Genetic sequences for at least 17 different IFN-α subtypes are encoded in human DNA. At least 8 are naturally expressed. The genes for IFN-α are all located in one region of human chromosome 9. IFN-α molecules are composed of 165-166 amino acids.

Human IFN-β is produced by fibroblast and epithelial cells which have been induced with foreign nucleic acids including those in viruses (Figure 2). Genetic sequences for at least two IFN-β subtypes are encoded in the DNA of humans. Both are expressed naturally. The gene for one of the IFN-β subtypes has been mapped. It is located in close proximity to the IFN-α genes on human chromosome 9. The mature IFN-β molecules are composed of 166 amino acids. It should be noted that in the mouse system IFNs α and β are often produced concurrently.

IFN-γ is produced by T-lymphocytes which have been stimulated with foreign antigens to which they have been previously sensitized or with mitogens which simulate this induction (Figure 2). A common site on the lymphocyte membrane may be the galactose residue, since IFN-γ can also be induced by galactose oxidase and its induction blocked by beta galactosidase. Only one genetic sequence for IFN-γ has been identified in the DNA of man. It is located on human chromosome 12. IFN-γ molecules are composed of 146 amino acids but processing may alter this number.

Relatedness of the Interferon Types

IFN-α and IFN-β share considerable homology at the nucleotide and amino acid levels. They interact with the same receptor molecule on the surface of responding cells (see below). They appear to exert their biological effects by the same mechanisms. Thus, these interferons are evolutionarily related and have probably been generated by divergent evolution from a common ancestral interferon gene.

IFN-γ does not share significant homology with IFN-α or IFN-β at either the nucleotide or the amino acid level. IFN-γ interacts with its own unique receptor molecule to activate responding cells. Further, there is some evidence to suggest that IFN-γ exerts its antiviral activity via a different mechanism than IFN-α and IFN-β.

Biologically IFN-γ has the unusual properties of: (a) exerting greater antitumor and macrophage-activating activities relative to its antiviral activity than do the other interferons, (b) exerting relatively greater immunosuppressive activity, (c) exerting relatively greater cell lytic effects, and (d) potentiating the actions of other interferons. It has recently been reported that IFNγ may exert many of its actions via the induction of the other IFNs. Even more generally, IFNγ may be a link in a complex chain of cross inductions by lymphokines and cytokines.

Biochemical Effects - Production of New Proteins

IFN-α and IFN-β induce the production of 12 new proteins in responding cells. IFN-γ induces these same proteins and an additional 12 new proteins. Some of these proteins have now been identified and some possible mechanisms of antiviral effects are shown in Figure 3. However, the precise mechanisms by which these proteins express interferon's varied activities are still unknown. Three of the best studied proteins are described below.

1. 2'-5' Oligoadenylate Synthetase

Interferon has been shown to induce the production of a novel RNA polymerizing enzyme (2'-5' oligoadenylate synthetase) which functions in the presence of double stranded RNA and synthesizes adenylate oligomers having a unique 2'-5' phosphodiester linkage between the ribose residues. The production of 2'-5' oligoadenylates by the synthetase activates a constitutively-produced ribonuclease, RNAse L, that breaks down single stranded RNA of both viral and host cell origin.

2. Protein Kinase

Interferon has been shown to specifically induce the production of a protein kinase which functions in the presence of double stranded RNA. The principal substrates for this protein kinase are itself (autophosphorylation) and the smallest subunit of initiation factor eIF-2. Phosphorylation of eIF-2 results in the inhibition of an initiation step in protein synthesis, i.e. the formation of the 40S initiation complex is inhibited.

3. The Mx Protein

Interferon has been shown to induce the synthesis (in mice) of a protein (called Mx) which blocks influenza virus replication. Influenza virus replicates in the nucleus of infected cells and the Mx protein in the nucleus inhibits the synthesis of the influenza virus mRNA.

4. mRNA Methylation Pathway

Another mechanism that has been implicated in the inhibition of viral replication involves impairment of mRNA methylation. Most eukaryotic cellular and viral mRNAs have "cap" structures at the 5' termini which influence the efficiency of translation of the mRNA under certain conditions as well as the stability of the mRNA. The impairment is due to the presence of an inhibitor of cap methylation in the extracts of IFN-treated cells.

The available information provides an emerging picture of viral inhibition by the IFN system and many studies are underway.

Comparison of the Interferon System with Other Host Defenses Against Viruses

The known defenses against viruses (Figure 4) may be divided into those which act against extracellular virus (neutralizing antibody and the phagocytic cells) and those which inhibit virus replication within cells [(a) the sensitized-lymphocyte, (b) cytolytic antibody plus complement, macrophages, or lymphocytes which can destroy infected cells, (c) fever, (d) hypoxia, (e) local acidity, and (f) interferon]. Different groups of these defenses are more effective during different viral infections.

The interferon system is the earliest-appearing of the known host defenses. It is operative within hours of infection. Figure 5 illustrates the early production of interferon in comparison with antibody during experimental infection of man with influenza virus.

The available evidence strongly supports a causal relationship between the interferon system and natural recovery from many established viral infections (Table 2). The evidence also indicates that interferon is not the sole defense that influences recovery, and in certain virus infections it may not be the most important defense. This depends on both the effectiveness of the virus as a stimulator of interferon production and on the susceptibility of the virus to the antiviral action of interferon. The interferon system appears to play its defensive role during viral infection of body surfaces, solid tissues and also during virus spread through the vascular system to target organs.

Application of Interferon for Control of Viral Diseases

Effective medical control of viral diseases has come from the application of the body's immune defenses. Thus vaccines and antibodies have brought a large number of viral diseases under control. The application of natural defenses, at least in physiological concentrations, has the advantage of relative safety. Studies of the interferon system are similarly providing increasing applications to clinical situations.

Some general principles govern the effectiveness of applied interferon. The virus must be sufficiently sensitive to the dose of interferon employed and enough interferon must reach the critical site. This factor governs the prophylactic and therapeutic use of interferon. For therapy of an ongoing viral infection, an additional determinant is the quantity and types of interferon that is produced naturally by the infected host since production of a large quantity of endogenous interferon(s) would preclude the effectiveness of lesser amounts of the same types of interferon applied from exogenous sources.

A number of viral diseases in humans have potential for application of the interferon system. These include rabies, hepatitis, respiratory virus infections, encephalitis and eye infections. Methods of application of the interferon system include administration of exogenous interferon, as well as various substances that induce body cells to produce endogenous interferon. The inducers of interferon include natural and synthetic nucleic acids, avirulent viruses, several small molecular weight compounds, and certain highly complex biologic substances such as endotoxin and microbial products.

The efficacy of interferon treatment of animal model infections has been confirmed for several human infections. In humans, interferons are clearly established to prevent rhinovirus infections (coryza), and to promote recovery from herpetic and adenovirus eye infections, papilloma virus infections (laryngeal papilloma and warts), generalized herpesvirus infections (simplex, cytomegalo and varicella-zoster) and hepatitis B.

It seems reasonable to predict that the interferon system will also be applied to help control rabies, other viral hepatitis, other respiratory virus infections, and virus encephalitis.

In addition to its role as a defense against viruses, interferon has important implications in immunology, cancer, bacterial and protozoal infections, cell genetics, regulation of protein synthesis and evolution. Some of these will be considered below.

Actions of Interferon that Effect Immunity

IFN can play a regulatory role in modulation of the immune response at several levels (Table 3). Immunoregulation by all three types of IFN has been recognized. It is of interest that IFNγ has been reported to be more active than the other types of IFN in modulating immunity relative to inhibition of virus. Several of the immunoregulatory actions of IFNs involve inhibitions of various components of the immune response, although enhancement of the immune response occurs under a few specified conditions (e.g., low dose and selective timing which may enhance by inhibiting suppressor lymphocytes). Both cell-mediated immunity and humoral immunity can be inhibited although antibody production by the fully differential plasma cell is resistant.

The interferon-activated cell may transfer the activated state to cells with which it is in contact in the absence of the continued presence of interferon. For example, human leukocytes exposed to interferon develop the activated state and effector leukocyte activities. These leukocytes are able to transfer the activated antiviral state to other cells in the body with which they may come in contact even though interferon is no longer present. Thus, immunocompetent cells, when activated by interferon, may in theory migrate through the body to target cells where they then may transfer the interferon activated state, thus providing a mechanism for distant activation of cells to influence viruses, tumors, and immune responses. Nonmigrating cells also may transfer the interferon-activated state to spread the interferon response from individual cells to surrounding tissues.

Anticellular and Antitumor Action

There is increasing evidence that interferon and inducers of interferon may function to inhibit the growth of some normal cells and some tumors. The mechanisms are not fully understood. Antitumor effects include direct inhibition of tumor cell division, direct lysis, and activation of immunocompetent cells and inhibition of oncogene expression. Other actions of interferon also may be involved (Table 4). There are now many trials with interferon in patients with different types of cancer. Interferon is therapeutically potent against hairy cell leukemia, mycosis fungoides, chronic myelogenous leukemia with the Philadelphia chromosome, ordinary warts, condyloma acuminatum and juvenile laryngeal papillomatosis. Encouraging results have been obtained with other neoplasms such as multiple myeloma, lymphomas and renal cell carcinoma but, as presently used, IFN is of unestablished efficacy against most other tumors.

Side Effects of Interferon Therapy

A number of side effects have been associated with interferon therapy. They include fever, bone marrow suppression, malaise, fatigue, nausea, and anorexia as well as some neurological effects. Originally, it was thought that these side effects were the result of contaminating proteins present in the impure interferon preparations used in the first clinical trials. The persistence of these side effects with the use of recombinant DNA-derived and purified interferons indicates that they are the result of the interferon itself. All of the effects are reversible upon cessation of interferon therapy.

Antiprotozoan and Antibacterial Activities

There is also growing evidence that IFN may play a role in natural protection against certain bacterial and protozoal infections. This evidence centers around induction of interferon during many of these infections, protection by IFN against certain of these infections, and the identification of antimicrobial mechanisms activated by IFN. For example, administration of endogenous IFN is protective in mice infected with malarial organisms. The mechanism of this protection involves leukocyte activation in addition to effects on susceptible cells.

Large Scale Production of Human Interferon

Large amounts of all three human interferons are now being produced in systems using cultured human cells or bacterial cells containing human genes. These large amounts have made possible the clinical trials that have led to governmental approval for treatment of some human diseases.

Biological Significance of Interferon

It has been pointed out that the interferon system bears a strong resemblance to some protein hormone and cytokine systems. Similarities include: (a) protein composition; (b) size range; (c) a message-carrying function between cells, tissues, and organs; (d) membrane receptors for interferon which are related to those of protein hormones; (e) cell surface activation of cells by interferon or protein hormones; and (f) genetic derepression and synthesis of new protein(s) by reacting cells, and (g) cross activation of hormonal and interferon effects by both hormones and interferon. The relatedness of IFNs, hormones, and cytokines is being studied.

Evolutionary Aspects of the Interferon System

The interferon system has been shown to be operative in animal phyla as far back as the fish. There is suggestive evidence that a mechanism analogous to the interferon system may occur in plants. These observations indicate an ancient origin for the interferon system.

As noted above, the interferon system will be considered more specifically and definitively by each of the authors in the succeeding chapters. In general, the format of each chapter is to first provide a brief background from earlier studies and then to compile recent information in each area. It is hoped that this rapid and authoritative treatment of available information will bring the reader from the beginnings to the very edge of interferon research.

SUMMARY

The purpose of this chapter is to broadly sketch the historical developments, the fundamental mechanisms, the implications for other scientific fields, and the significance for medicine. Interferon was discovered thirty years ago by Isaacs and Lindenmann who observed that fluids from virus-infected cell cultures contained a protein that could react with cells to render them resistant to infection by a wide variety of viruses. It has now been established that interferons may profoundly affect other vital cellular and bodily functions, including cell metabolism and growth, immunity, and tumors. We now know that the interferon of Isaacs and Lindenmann is really a family of molecules which can be divided into three species: interferon α, interferon β, and interferon γ. The genetic information for the interferon proteins is contained in a number of normally unexpressed genes. Production and secretion of the interferon proteins can be induced by foreign nucleic acids, foreign cells, foreign antigens, cytokines, and mitogenic stimuli. Extracellular interferon reacts with receptors on cells to induce effector proteins which lead to most of the specific biochemical effects resulting in antiviral action, immunoregulation, cell regulatory activity, etc. A number of viral diseases in humans have potential for application of the interferon system including rabies, hepatitis, respiratory virus infections, encephalitis and eye infections. The efficacy of interferon treatment of viral infections of animals has been confirmed for several human infections. In humans, interferons are clearly established to prevent rhinovirus infections (coryza), and to promote recovery from herpetic and adenovirus eye infections, papilloma virus infections (laryngeal papilloma and warts), generalized herpesvirus infections (simplex, cytomegalo and varicella-zoster) and hepatitis B. The antitumor effects of interferons include direct inhibition of tumor cell division, direct cell lysis, activation of immunocompetent cells, and inhibition of oncogene expression. Interferon is therapeutically potent against hairy cell leukemia, ordinary warts, condyloma acuminatum and juvenile laryngeal papillomatosis. Encouraging results have been obtained with other neoplasms such as multiple myeloma, nonhodgkins lymphomas, and renal cell carcinoma. A number of side effects have been associated with interferon therapy including fever, bone marrow suppression, malaise, fatigue, nausea, anorexia, and some neurological effects. All of the effects are reversible upon cessation of interferon therapy. There is also growing evidence that interferon may play a role as a natural defense against certain bacterial and protozoal infections. This evidence centers around induction of interferon during many of these infections, protection by interferon against certain of these infections, and the identification of antimicrobial mechanisms activated by interferon. Large amounts of all three human interferons are now being produced in systems using cultured human cells or microbial cells containing human genes. These large amounts have made possible clinical trials that have led to governmental approval for treatment of some human diseases. The interferon system bears a strong resemblance to some protein hormone and cytokine systems. The interferon system has been shown to be operative in animal phyla as far back as the fish and perhaps in plants. These observations indicate an ancient origin for the interferon system.

REFERENCES

1. Baron, S. and F. Dianzani: Texas Reports on Biology and Medicine, Vol. 35. The Interferon System: A Current Review to 1978, S. Baron and F. Dianzani, eds. The University of Texas Medical Branch, Galveston, TX, 1978.
2. Baron, S., F. Dianzani, and G. J. Stanton: Texas Reports on Biology and Medicine, Vol. 41. The Interferon System: A Review to 1982, S. Baron, F. Dianzani, and G.J. Stanton, eds. The University of Texas Medical Branch, Galveston, TX, 1982.
3. Baron, S.: Mechanism of recovery from viral infection. In: Advances in Virus Research, D.M. Smith and M.A. Lauffer, eds. Academic Press, Inc., New York, Vol. 10, pp. 39-60, 1963.
4. Grossberg, S.E.: The interferons and their inducers: Molecular and therapeutic considerations. N Engl J Med 287:13-19, 79-85, 122-128, 1972.

5. Isaacs, A.: Interferon. In: Advances in Virus Research, D.M. Smith and M.A. Lauffer, eds. Academic Press, Inc., New York, Vol. 10, pp. 1-35, 1963.
6. Isaacs, A. and J. Lindenmann: Virus interference. I. The Interferon. Proc R Soc Ser B, 147:258, 1957.
7. Stringfellow, D.A.: Interferon and Interferon Inducers, Marcel Dekker, New York and Basel, 1980.
8. Vilcek, J.: Interferon. In: Virology Monographs, S. Gard, C. Hallauer, and K.F. Meyer, eds. Springer-Verlag, Wien, New York, 1969.
9. Finter, N.: Interferon. Vol. 1-3, Elsevier, Amsterdam, 1984.
10. Baron, S., S.E. Grossberg, G.R. Klimpel, and P.A. Brunell: Immune and Interferon Systems. In: Antiviral Agents and Viral Diseases of Man, G.J. Galasso, T.C. Merigan, and R.A. Buchanan, eds. Raven Press, pp. 123-178, 1984.
11. Baron, S., W.R. Fleischmann, Jr., G. Klimpel, G.J. Stanton: Effects of virus induced interferons on the immune system. In: Viral Mechanisms of Immunosuppression. N. Gilmores and M.A. Wainberg, eds. Alan R. Liss, New York, pp. 225-239, 1985.
12. Stanton, G.J. and S. Baron: Interferon and viral pathogenesis. In: Concepts in Viral Pathogenesis. A.L. Notkins and M.B.A. Oldstone, eds. Springer-Verlag, New York, pp. 3-10, 1985.
13. Pestka, S.: Interferon: a decade of accomplishments, foundations of the future in research and therapy. Semin Hematol Jul: 23 (3 Suppl 1):27, 1986.
14. Borecky, L.: Current view on the perspectives of interferon therapy. Acta Virol 30(2):161, 1986.
15. Smalley, R.V. and E.C. Borden: Interferons: current status and future directions of this prototypic biological. Springer Semin Immunopathol 9(1):73, 1986.
16. Mannering, G.J. and L.B. Deloria: The pharmacology and toxicology of the interferons: an overview. Annu Rev Pharmacol Toxicol 26:455, 1986.
17. Krown, S.E.: Interferons and interferon inducers in cancer treatment. Semin Oncol 13(2):207, 1986.
18. Peters, M., G.L. Davis, J.S. Doolery, J.H. Hoofnagle: The interferon system in acute and chronic viral hepatitis. Prog Liver Dis 8:453, 1986.
19. Quesada, J.R., M. Talpaz, A. Rios, R. Kurzrock, J.U. Gutterman: Clinical toxicity of interferons in cancer patients: a review. J Clin Oncol 4(2):234, 1986.
20. Baron, S., D.A. Weigent, G.J. Stanton, and J. Peterson: The protective role of endogenous interferon in viral, bacterial, and protozoal infections. Antiviral Res 1:173, 1985.
21. Billiau, A.: The interferon system as a basis for antiviral therapy or prophylaxis. Antiviral Res 1:131, 1985.
22. Billiau, A.: The clinical application of fibroblast interferon--an overview. Med Oncol Tumor Pharmacother 1:87, 1984.
23. Bocci, V.: Evaluation of routes of administration of interferon in cancer: a review and a proposal. Cancer Drug Deliv 1(4):396, 1985.
24. Burke, D.C.: The interferons. Brit Med Bull 41(4):333, 1985.
25. DeMaeyer-Guignard, J. and E. DeMaeyer: Immunomodulation by interferons: recent developments. Interferon 6:31, 1985.
26. Rossi, G.B.: Interferons and cell differentiation. Interferon 6:31, 1985.

27. Gresser, I.: How does interferon inhibit tumor growth? Interferon 6:93, 1985.
28. Tyrrell, D.A.: Interferons and the physician. Q J Med 54(214):117, 1985.
29. Pestka, S., J.A. Langer, P.B. Fisher, I.B. Weinstein, J. Ortaldo, and R.B. Herberman: The human interferons: from the past and into the future. Symp Fundam Cancer Res 37:261, 1984.
30. Schellekens, H., A. de Reus, and P.H. v.d. Meide: The chimpanzee as a model to test the side effects of human interferons. J Med Primatol 13(5):235, 1984.
31. Forni, G., M. Bindoni, A. Santoni, M. Giovarelli, and A. Mantovani: Physiological and pathological influences of the central nervous system on the immune system: a critical appraisal. J Psychiatr Res 18(4):491, 1984.
32. Vilcek, J.: Adverse effects of interferon in virus infections, autoimmune diseases and acquired immunodeficiency. Prog Med Virol 30:62, 1984.
33. Stringfellow, D.A.: Prostaglandins and metastasis. Symp Fundam Cancer Res 55:219, 1983.
34. Baglioni, C. and T.W. Nilsen: Mechanisms of antiviral action of interferon. Interferon 5:23, 1983.
35. Friedman, R.M. and S.N. Vogel: Interferons with special emphasis on the immune system. Adv Immunol 34:97, 1983.
36. Baron, S. The interferon system. ASM News 54:358, 1979.
37. Dianzani, F. and A. Dolei: Interferon: fantasies and facts. Dev Biol Stand 60:3, 1985.

TABLE 1. Functional Effects of Interferon

Antiviral action
Antitumor action
Cell growth inhibition
Alteration of cell membranes
Immunoregulatory action
Macrophage activation
Enhancement of cytotoxicity of lymphocytes
Influence on subsequent production of IFN
Hormonal interactions

TABLE 2. Evidence that Interferons Play a Defensive Role During Viral Infections (3,5,36).

Type of Evidence	Example
Time of correlations	Interferon produced just before and during arrest of virus replication
Place correlations	Interferon produced at the site of its action
Transfer	Exogenous interferon controls viral infections
Absence	Deletion of interferon in cell culture, eggs, and animals increases severity of viral infections
Sufficiency of quantity	Concentrations of interferon produced in vivo are sufficient to account for defensive action
Specificity of probes	Definitive characterization of interferon produced during infection
Reproductibility	Confirmation in many animal species and humans

TABLE 3. Immunological Effects of Interferon

Immune Function	Most Common Effect
Antibody formation	Decrease (not always)
Cell mediated immunity	Varies
Macrophage effects	Increase
Cytotoxic T cell effects	Increase
Natural killing	Increase
Cytokines (Interleukins) production	Increase
Cell membrane components (MHC, Fc, B-2 microglobulin)	Increase

TABLE 4. Interferon's Antitumor Mechanisms

Inhibition of cell division	
Direct cell killing (mainly interferon γ)	
Indirect cell killing by activation of:	sensitized T lymphocytes
	NK cells
	Macrophages
	ADCC effector cells
Inhibition of tumor viruses	
Inhibition of oncogene expression	
Changes on the surface of tumor cells (e.g., MHC)	
Modulation of the immune response	
Hormonal effects	

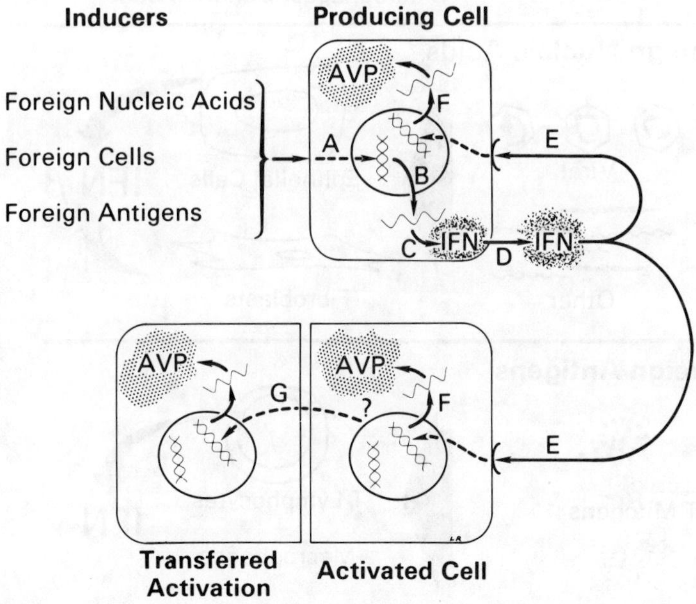

Figure 1. Induction, production and action of interferon (IFN) at the cellular level. IFN inducers react with cells to derepress the IFN gene(s) (A), leading to the production of IFN mRNA (B), that is translated into the IFN protein intracellularly (C) followed by its secretion extracellularly (D) where it reacts with the membrane receptors of cells (E). The IFN-stimulated cells derepress other genes (F) for effector proteins (AVP) that establish antiviral resistance and other cell changes (see Fig. 3). The activated cells also directly stimulate contacted cells (G) by a still unknown mechanism to produce AVP.

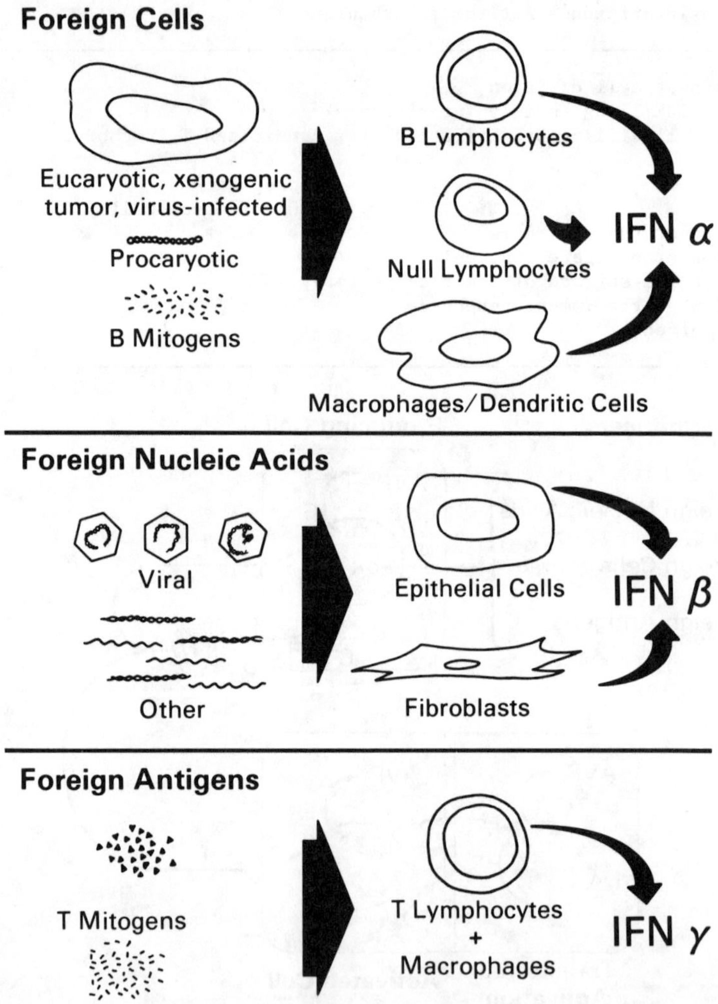

Figure 2. A general scheme for induction of human interferons α, β or γ respectively by foreign nucleic acids, foreign cells, or foreign antigens. In comparison, in the mouse system interferons α and β are usually produced together.

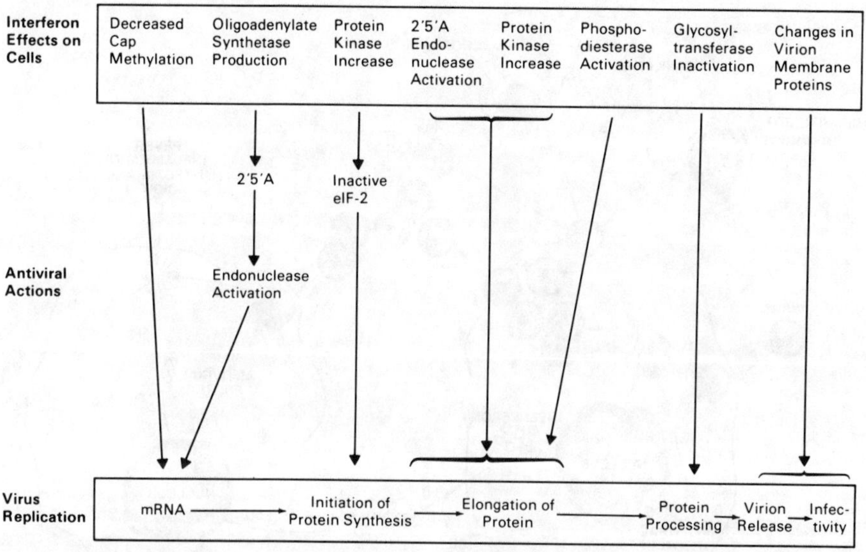

Figure 3. Some possible biochemical mechanisms of interferon's antiviral effects.

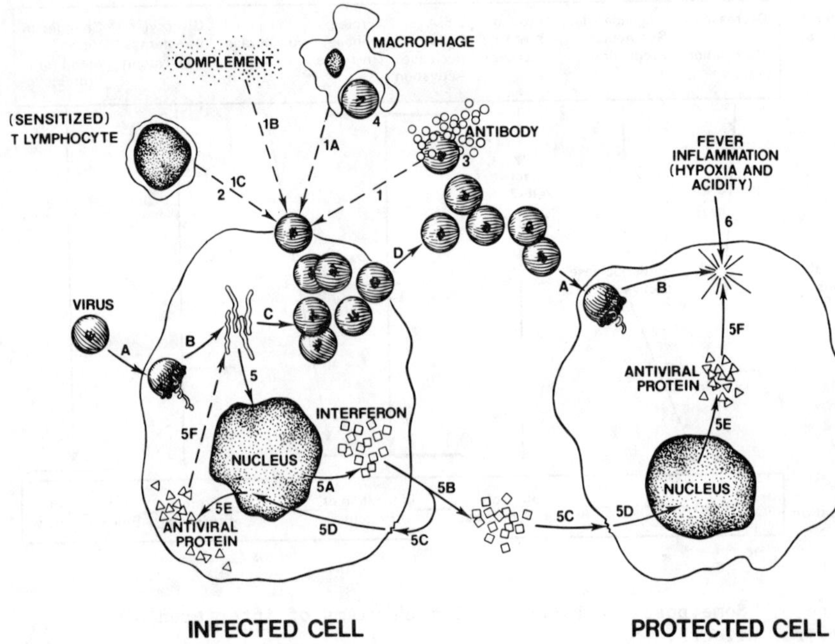

Figure 4. Host defenses against virus infection. Virus multiplication is shown in steps A - D. The extracellular defenses include antibody (3) and, to a lesser extent, the phagocytic macrophage (4) which may combine with and inactivate virus. Defenses against intracellularly replicating virus include cytolysis of virus-infected cells bearing virus surface antigens by synthesized T lymphocytes (2) acting directly or through their mediators: antibody plus macrophages (1A); antibody plus complement (1B); antibody plus T lymphocytes (1C); and antibody plus other effector leukocyte cells (not shown). Additional inhibition of intracellular viral replication (C) can be caused by the nonspecific defense mechanisms of interferon (5-5F), local acidity, local hyposia (6), and interfering virus (not shown).

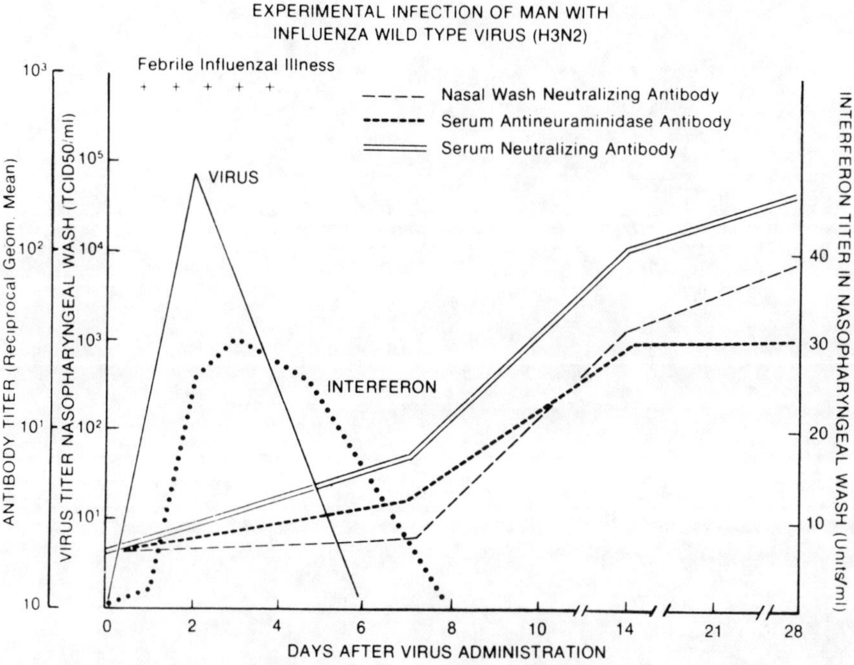

Figure 5. Production of virus, interferon, and antibody during experimental infection of humans with influenza wild-type virus (from a study by B. Murphy, E. Chalhub, S. Nusinoff, J. Kasel, C. Uhlendorf, S. Baron, and R. Chanock, National Institutes of Health).

I. Induction of Interferon

1. Mechanism of Induction of Alpha Interferon

F. Dianzani and M. R. Capobianchi

Institute of Virology, University of Rome "La Sapienza," Viale di Porta Tiburtina 28, 00185 Rome, Italy

INTRODUCTION

In 1961 it was reported that human leukocytes are capable of producing interferon (IFN) in response to viral infection (1). Since then stimulation of human white blood cells has been currently used to produce "leukocyte IFN" for clinical applications (2). The finding that human lymphoid cell-derived IFN is not neutralized by antisera raised against fibroblast-derived IFN (3) firstly suggested the eterogeneity of the IFN system, among which the "leukocyte IFN" family, now designed IFN alpha, appears to be the most complex. Evidence has been provided for a cluster of IFN alpha-related genes, many of which code for functionally active IFN, differing among each other with respect to the extent of efficacy in modulating virus growth, cell-related and immune functions (4-6).
While normal human leukocytes can produce native IFN alpha, mouse white blood cells usually produce a mixture of IFN alpha and beta. The work on the mechanism of production of IFN alpha moved from the original misleading concept of an unifying induction mechanism for all types of IFN. However, as the eterogeneity of the IFN system was subsequently established (4-6), a number of IFN inducers, completely different from molecular and biological points of view, were discovered (7), suggesting that different IFN mixtures can derive from the interaction of the various inducing agents with the appropriate target cells.
Furthermore, the availability of separation procedures and membrane markers for lymphoid cell subpopulations gave rise to a bulk of studies on the type(s) of white blood cells that are responsible for IFN alpha production.
However these studies may be complicated by the fact that, in some situations, the cooperation of different cell subpopulations is necessary for IFN production (8).

INDUCERS OF IFN ALPHA

After the initial discovery that viruses can stimulate white blood cells to produce IFN, a number of other agents have been identified as IFN alpha inducers. Namely, Svet Moldavski et al. (9) reported that tumor-derived or virus-transformed cells induce IFN in lymphoid cultures. The production of IFN, subsequently identified as alpha in the human and alpha-beta in the mouse system, was confirmed by a number of reports from other authors (10-13). Subsequent discovery that IFN alpha is induced also by mycoplasma may suggest that in some instances the observed phenomenon could be due to the presence of contaminating microorganisms in the inducing cell cultures (13).

IFN alpha production has been shown in leukocyte cultures also after exposure to a number of microorganisms (7), such as C. parvum (14) and bacterial products, like S. Aureus protein A (15) and LPS from several microrganisms (16). The latters belong to the family of B cell stimulants, most of which have been found to induce IFN alpha production in lymphocyte cultures (17).

It has to be pointed out that as early as in 1964 it was reported in vivo production of serum IFN after inoculation of chicken and mice with several bacteria, but at that time IFN subtypes were not yet identified (18).

Lastly, a number of chemical compounds, such as synthetic polyanions (19) and the low molecular weight substance 10-carboxymethyl-9-acridanone have been found capable of inducing IFN alpha in vivo and in leukocyte cultures (20, 21).

TYPES OF CELLS INVOLVED IN IFN ALPHA PRODUCTION

Since its discovery, IFN alpha has been produced for years in bulk cultures of buffy coat cells that contain a variety of cell types. The attempts to identify the white blood cell responsible for IFN alpha production have been encouraged by the availability of several separation tecniques, but often some difficulties, arising from the inability to obtain absolutely pure cell populations and to clarify the accessory cell requirements, made the study technically difficult and sometime confusing.

The results arising from the experiments based either on cell depletion, or on positive selection, as well as from studies performed on leukemia B or T cell lines, are not clear-cut, as many cell types appear to be involved, to different extent, depending on the inducer or, even with the same inducer, on the experimental conditions. For instance, B lymphocytes appear to be the main cells responsible for IFN production when the inducers are B-cell mitogens, such as bacterial products (16, 17). B or null lymphocytes have been found to produce IFN following interaction with viruses and foreign cells (10, 11, 22-25). Large Granular Lymphocytes or null cells have been reported to be the main source of IFN alpha when stimulated with C. parvum and cells persistently infected with mumps or other viruses (26).

Macrophages appear to be the main target of induction by

poly I:C (19), although all B, T and null cells are reported to occasionally produce IFN in response to this inducer (27, 28). Macrophages have been reported to secrete IFN following interaction also with bacteria and bacterial products in several animal systems (29, 30), with live viruses, such as influenza A in the human system (31) and Herpes Simplex virus (HVS) in mice (32). Viruses, on the other hand, may have different target cells. Some, such as Newcastle disease virus (NDV), can induce IFN in both lymphocytes and macrophages (22, 33). Others, such as Sendai virus, preferentially stimulate lymphocytes (34). There is some report on IFN alpha production by T lymphoid cells stimulated by viruses (35), but it has to be pointed out that these experiments are dealing with tumor cell lines and therefore they may not reflect the sensitivity pattern of normal white blood cells. Nevertheless, they document that in principle T cells have the capacity of producing IFN alpha.

From the results above reviewed it is not possible to dissect between two alternative hypotheses on the putative IFN alpha-producing cells: a) IFN alpha is produced after interaction of a specialized cell with the appropriate, specific inducer. b) all the white blood cell lineages can produce different subtype of IFN, depending on the nature of the stimulus. To this respect a recent report (36) indicates that in the native IFN alpha preparations the relative amount of the various molecular species can vary according to the inducer. In this case it is not yet clarified whether a single molecular species of IFN alpha is a product of a single cell type, inducible only by a single stimulus, or whether every cell type is capable of producing several molecular species, modulating the overall composition according to the nature of the inducer.

MECHANISM OF INDUCTION

It is widely accepted that the induction of IFN beta (fibroblast-derived) requires virus internalization and exposure of nucleic acid. Viral RNA, either single or double stranded, appears to be the critical factor in triggering the induction process (37-40). On the other hand, the activation of IFN alpha production has been reported to occur following interaction of white blood cells with a number of viral and non-viral inducers as reviewed above, without the requirement of internalization of foreign genetic material. In 1979 we were able to show that virus preparations treated with lipid solvents and deprived of nucleocapsid components, completely lose IFN beta-inducing activity but maintain the ability to induce alpha IFN production, suggesting that viral envelope rather than nucleic acid triggers the induction process (Table 1) (8). These data were subsequently confirmed using UV treated viruses (41). Therefore, it appears that simple contact of the viral glycoproteins with the cell membrane is sufficient for the induction process (42-44). The lack of requirement of penetration of the inducer in the effector cell is substantiated by the finding that virus-infected cells, irradiated or fixed with glutaraldehyde, induce IFN alpha in lymphocyte cultures (45-47). In this case, the amounts of IFN alpha produced is much higher than the yields obtained by using free virus as the inducer (47) (Fig. 1). To our experience, this phenomenon occurs with all enveloped viruses tested, suggesting that the most likely event that leads to the bulk of IFN alpha production in vivo may be the interaction of leukocytes with virus-infected cells rather than with free virions. Furthermore, high lymphocyte density favours high IFN yield, suggesting that cell cooperation play some role, whereas the depletion of adherent mononuclear cells does not affect IFN production.

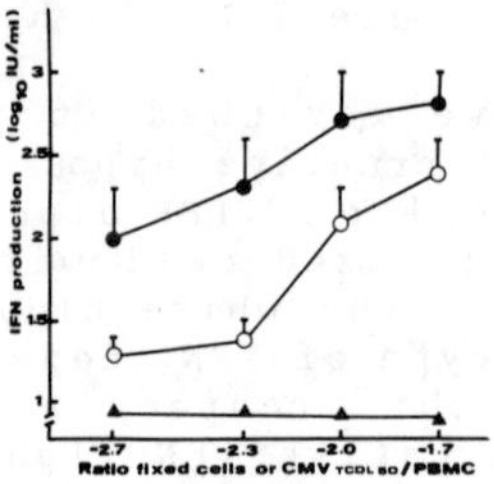

Figure 1. Interferon induction in human PBMC cultures by Cytomegalovirus (CMV) or by CMV-infected cells fixed with glutaraldehyde. PBMC were seeded at 10^6/ml and induced with live CMV (o), fibroblasts uninfected (▲) or CMV-infected (●) fixed with glutaraldehyde. Supernates were collected and titrated as described in (47).

Another system where membrane interactions seem to play a critical role is provided by mycoplasma. To avoid the possibility of any active infectious process, the inducer, Mycoplasma pneumoniae (MP), was heat killed, and cell membranes were separated from the cytosol by differential centrifugation and used as IFN inducers with peripheral blood mononuclear cells (PBMC) from human healthy donors. The results of a representative experiment are reported in Table 2, showing that the inducing ability of this microorganism resides in the membrane components, whereas the internal material appears to be irrelevant.
To identify the main cell types responsible for IFN alpha production following membrane interactions, we performed depletion experiments on PBMC by using either rosetting tecnique or filtration through nylon wool, after repeated cycles of adherence to remove the monocyte-macrophage population. The adherent cells were then collected with a rubber policemen and the various cell populations were tested with several inducers of IFN alpha, such as Newcastle disease virus (NDV) and Herpes simplex virus

(HSV), HSV-infected fibroblasts fixed with glutaraldehyde, killed MP.

The results, reported in Table 3, suggest that B lymphocytes are the best responders to virus-infected cells, while macrophages, although capable of producing IFN in response to conventional viral induction by NDV or HSV, appear completely unresponsive to virus-infected cells. T lymphocytes, as expected, are poor IFN alpha producers.

Also when the inducer was MP the main responder cells appear to belong to B lymphocyte group, while both T lymphocytes and macrophages seem not to be involved. In the case of MP involvement of NK cells is ruled out by the finding that treatment with monoclonal antibody anti Leu-7 and complement does not affect IFN yields. As for the virus-infected cells other authors reported, in a system similar to ours, that NK cells are not required for the IFN alpha production (46).

From these results it appears that, at least in the case of enveloped viruses and mycoplasma, the triggering event leading to IFN alpha production is a membrane interaction with B lymphocytes. The immune status of the donor seems to be irrelevant, since cells from immune or non immune donors or from cord blood give equal IFN yields. Stimulation of lymphocyte prolipheration does not occur during the induction both in the case of HSV-infected cells (47) and in the case of MP (Table 2).

As for the specific cell membrane components involved in the interaction with the inducer, there are several evidences that the sugar moiety of membrane glycoproteins are primarily involved in lymphocyte activation both in the case of IFN gamma (48) and alpha (49). By deletion of specific components of PBMC membrane with several glycosidases, we found that mannose residues integrity is essential for the induction of IFN alpha by virus-infected cells (Fig. 2), in agreement with the reported requirement for the presence on the responder cells of Ia antigens (50), which are rich of mannose residues in their polysaccharide moiety.

CONCLUSIONS

The data reported in this review show that IFN alpha production is activated by the interaction of several types of white blood cells with a number of viral and non viral stimuli. The triggering event seems to be a membrane interaction of the responder cells with the inducer, without the requirement of its engulfment. The interaction is facilitated by high cell density and, at least in the case of viruses, requires the integrity of sugar network on the cell membrane. Furthermore this interaction is most efficient when the lymphocytes contact virus-infected cells instead of free virions. This can provide an efficient host defense mechanism against spreading of viral infections through virus-infected cells present in the bloodstream or in endothelial layers of the blood wessels; on the other hand increasing viral resistance of these cells enhances the effectiveness of natural barriers such as blood-brain, blood lung, etc.

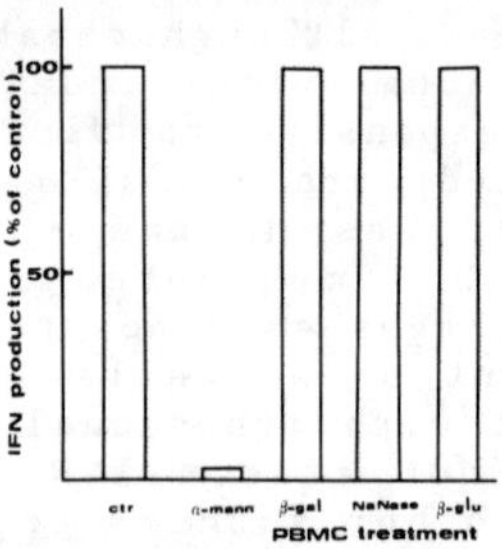

FIGURE 2. Interferon induction by HSV-infected fixed fibroblasts in human PBMC cultures after treatment with the following glycosidases: alpha-mannosidase (alpha-mann, 10 U/10 U/10^6 cells/ml, 30 m. at 25 oC), B-galactosidase (B-gal, 400 U/10^7 cells/ml 30 m. at 25 oC), Neuraminidase (NaNase 50U/10^7 cells/ml 1 h at 37 oC), B-glucosidase (B-glu, 50 U/10^7 cells/ml 30 m. at 25 oC).

ACKNOWLEDGEMENTS

This work was supported in part by a grant from CNRm P.F. Controllo Malattie da Infezione n. 85.00844.52.

REFERENCES

1. Gresser, I: Production of interferon by suspensions of human leukocytes. Proc Soc Exp Biol Med 108: 799, 1961.
2. Strander, H. and K. Cantell: Production of interferon by human leukocytes in vitro. Ann Med Exp Biol Fenn: 44: 265, 1966.
3. Duc-Goiran, P., B. Galliot and C. Chany: Studies on virus-induced interferons produced by the human amniotic membrane and white blood cells.Arch Gen Virusforsch 34:232, 1971.
4. Nagata, S., N. Mantei and C. Weissmann: Structure of one of eight or more distinct chromosomal genes for human interferon-alpha. Nature 287: 401, 1980.
5. Goeddel, D.V., D.W. Lenng, T.J. Dull, M. Gross, R.M. Lawn, R.M. Candlia, P.H. Seeburg, A. Ulrich, E. Yelverton and P.W. Gray: The structure of eight distinct human leukocyte interferon cDNAs. Nature (London) 290: 20-26, 1981.
6. Pestka, S., M. Evinger, S. Maeda, E. Rehberg, P.C. Familletti and B. Kelder. Biological properties of natural and recombinant interferons. Tex Rep Biol Med 41: 31, 1981-82.
7. Baron, S., V. Howie, M. Langford, E.M. Macdonald, G.J. Stanton, E.J. Reitmeyer and D.A. Weigent: Induction of

interferon by bacteria, protozoa and viruses: defensive role. Tex Rep Biol Med 41: 150, 1981-82.
8. Dianzani, F., T.M. Monahan, M. Zucca, C. Jordan. Disrupted virus induces interferon in lymphoid cells but not in other cultured cells. In: Kahn A., Hill NO, Dorn G. Eds. Interferon: Properties and Clinical Uses. Dallas, Texas, Wadly Inst. Mol. Med., p. 223, 1980.
9. Svet Moldavski, G.J., B.M. Nemiroskaya and T.V. Osipova. Interferogenicity and antigen recognition. Nature (London) **247**: 205, 1974.
10. Trinchieri, G., D. Santoli, R.R. Dee, B. Knowles: Antiviral activity induced by culturing lymphocytes with tumor derived or virus-transformed cells. Identification of the antiviral activity as interferon and characterization of the human effector lymphocyte subpopulation. J Exp Med 147: 1299, 1978.
11. Blalock, J.E., M.P. Langford; J. Georgiades and G.J. Stanton: Non-sensitized lymphocytes produce leukocyte interferon when cultured with foreign cells. Cell Immunol 43: 197, 1979.
12. Ronblon, L., V. Ramsted and G.V. Alm. Properties of human natural interferon-producing cells stimulated by tumor cell lines. Eur J Immunol 13: 471, 1983.
13. Birke, C., H.H. Peter, V. Langenberg, W.J.P. Muller-Hermes, J.H. Peters, J. Heiman, W. Leibold, H. Dalugge, E. Krapf and H. Kirchner: Mycoplasma contamination in human tumor cell lines: effect on interferon induction and susceptibility to natural killing. J Immunol 127: 94, 1981.
14. Vilcek, I., I.T. Sulea, F. Volvovitz and Y.K. Lip. Characteristics of interferons produced in cultures of human lymphocytes by stimulation with Corynebacterium parvum and phytohemagglutinin. In: De Weck E. ed. Biochemical Characterization of Lymphokines. Academic Press, New York, p.323, 1980.
15. Smith E.M., H.M. Johnson, J.E. Blalock: Staphylococcus aureus protein a induced the production of interferon-alpha in human lymphocytes and Interferon-alpha and beta in mouse spleen cells. J Immunol 130: 773, 1983.
16. Maehara, N. and M. Ho. Cellular origin of interferon induced by bacterial lipopolysaccharide: Infect Immun 15: 78, 1977.
17. Wietzerbin, J., S. Stephanos, R. Falcoff and E. Falcoff: Some properties of interferons induced by stimulants of T and B lymphocytes. Tex Rep Biol Med 35: 205, 1977.
18. Youngner, S. and W.H. Stinebring: Interferon production in chickens infected with Brucella abortus. Science 144: 1022, 1964.
19. Neumann, C: Mononuclear phagocytes as producers of interferon. Lymphokines 7: 165, 1982.
20. Kramer, M.J., R. Cleeland and E. Grunenberg: Antiviral activity of 10-carboxymetinyl-9-acridanone. Antimicrob Agents Chemother 9: 233, 1976.

21. Storch, E. and H. Kirchner: Induction of interferon in murine bone marrow-derived macrophage cultures by 10-carboxymetinyl-9-acridanone. Eur J Immunol 12: 793, 1982.
22. De Maeyer, E., R.M. Fauve, J. De Maeyer-Guignard: Production of interferon au niveau du macrophage. Ann Inst Pasteur 120: 438, 1971.
23. Timonen, T., E. Saksela, I. Virtanen and K. Cantell: Natural killer cells are responsible for the interferon production induced in human lymphocytes by tumor cell contatct. Eur J Immunol 10: 422, 1980.
24. Peter, H.H., H. Dalugge, R. Zawatzky, S. Euler, W. Leibold and H. Kirchner: Human peripheral cell lymphocyte. II. Producers of type 1 interferon upon stimulation with tumor cells. Eur J Immunol 10: 547, 1980.
25. Djeu, J.Y., N. Stocks, K. Zoon, G.J. Stanton, T. Timonen and R.B. Herberman: Positive self regulation of cytotoxicity in human natural killer cells by production of interferon upon exposure to influenza and herpes viruses. J Exp Med 156: 1222, 1982.
26. Minato, N., L. Reid, H. Cantor, P. Lengyel and B.R. Bloom: Mode of regulation of natural killer cell activity by interferon. J Exp Med 152: 124, 1980.
27. Wiranowska-Stewart, M. and W.E. Stewart II: Determination of human leukocyte populations involved in production of interferons alpha and gamma. J IFN Res 1: 233, 1981.
28. Herberman, R.B., J.R. Ortaldo, T. Timonen, C.W. Reynolds, J.Y. Djeu, S. Pestka and J. Stanton: Interferon and natural killer (NK) cells. Tex Rep Biol Med 41: 590, 1981-82.
29. Borecky, L., V. Lackovic and N. Fuchsberger: Comparison of interferon production in mouse leukocytes by statolon and a complexed polyribonucleotide (Poly I: Poly C). Acta Virol 14: 329, 1970.
30. Hamburg, S.J., H.B. Fleit, J.C. Unkeless and M. Rabinovitch: Mononuclear phagocytes: responders to and producers of interferons. Ann N Y Acad Sci 350: 72-90, 1980.
31. Roberts, N.J. jr, R.G. jr. Douglas, R.M. Simons and M.E. Diamond: Virus-induced interferon production by human macrophages. J Immunol 123: 365, 1979.
32. Kirchner, H., H. Engler, C.H. Schroder, R. Zawatzky and E. Storch: Herpes simplex virus type 1-induced interferon production in peritoneal exudate cells of the mouse. J gen Virol 64: 437, 1983.
33. Maehara, N., M. Ho and J.A. Armstrong: Differences in mouse interferons according to cell source and mode of induction. Infect Immun 17: 572, 1977.
34. Yamaguchi, T., K. Handa, J. Shimizu, T. Abo and K. Kumagai: Target cells for interferon production in human leukocytes stimulated by Sendai virus. J Immunol 118: 1931, 1977.
35. Cooley, M.A., M.J. Blackman and A.G. Morris: Production of type I (alpha/beta) interferon after virus infection of

cloned, alloantigen-sensitized mouse T lymphocytes. Eur J Immunol 14: 376, 1984.
36. Goren, T., D.G. Fischer, D. Novick and M. Rubinstein: Differential induction of interferon-alpha subtypes by two viruses. Antiviral Res Abstr. 1: 135, 1984.
37. Dianzani, F., A. Pugliese and S. Baron: Studies of the induction of interferon system by nonreplicating Newcastle disease virus. Proc Soc Exp Biol Med 145: 428, 1974.
38. Lockart, R.Z., N.L. Bayliss, S.T. Toy and F.H. Yin: Viral events necessary for the induction of interferon in chick embryo cells. Virology 2: 962, 1968.
39. Marcus, P.I: Interferon induction by viruses: one molecule of ds RNA as the threshold for interferon induction. In: Interferon 5, Academic Press, 115, 1983.
40. Dianzani, F., S. Gagnoni, C.E. Buckler and S. Baron: Studies on the induction of interferon system by nonreplicating Newcastle disease virus. Proc Soc Exp. Biol Med 133: 324, 1970.
41. Green, J.A., T.J. Yeh and J.C. Overall: Sequential production of IFN-alpha and immune specific IFN-gamma by human mononuclear leukocytes exposed to herpes simplex virus. J Immunol 127: 1192, 1981.
42. Ito, Y., Y. Nishiyama, K. Shimokata, I. Nagata, H. Takeyama and A. Kunii: The mechanism of interferon induction in mouse spleen cells stimulated within HVJ. Virology 88: 128, 1978.
43. Lebon, P. Inhibition of Herpes Simplex virus type-1 induced interferon synthesis by monoclonal antibodies against viral glycoprotein D and by lysosomotropic drugs. J gen Virol 66: 2781, 1985.
44. Ito, Y. and Y. Hosaka: Components of Sendai virus that can induce interferon in mouse spleen cells. Infect Immun 39: 1019, 1983.
45. Lebon, P., M.J. Commoy-Chevalier, B. Robert-Galliot and C. Chany: Different mechanisms for alpha and beta interferon induction. Virology 119: 504, 1982.
46. Reiss, C.S., L.C.M. Lin and S.L. Mowshowitz: Interferon production by cultured murine splenocytes in response to influenza virus-infected cells. J IFN Res 1: 81, 1984.
47. Capobianchi, M.R., J. Facchini, P. Di Marco, G. Antonelli and F. Dianzani: Induction of alpha interferon by membrane interaction between viral surface and peripheral blood mononuclear cells. Proc Soc Exp Biol Med 178: 551, 1985.
48 Dianzani, F., T.M. Monahan and M. Santiano: Membrane alterations responsible for the induction of gamma interferon. Infect Immun 36: 915, 1982.
49. Tsukui, K., T, Miura and E. Tokunaga: Treatment of human peripheral blood leukocytes with proteases does not affect Sendai virus-induced interferons production. Infect Immun 43: 822, 1984.
50. Hughes, T.K. and J.E. Blalock: Ia Antigen: a murine B lymphocyte receptor for trasformed cell induction of interferon alpha/beta. J Immunol 13: 1895, 1983.

TABLE 1. Effect of delipidation and RNase treatment on the inducing ability of inlfuenza virus and NDV."

Virus	Treatment	Production of IFN in the appropriate cells' (IU/ml) IFN alpha	IFN beta
Influenza	None	300	100
	Delipidation+ RNase	100	<10
NDV	None	1,000	1,000
	Delipidation+ RNase	1,000	<10

" Data partly from Dianzani F. et al. (8).
' IFN alpha in human PBMC, IFN beta in WISH cells.

TABLE 2. IFN production and ^{3}H-Thymidine incorporation in cultures of human PBMC induced with Staphylococcal enterotoxin B (SEB) whole heat-killed mycoplasma pneumoniae (MP), membrane preparations and cytosol fraction of MP.

Inducer	IFN (U/ml)	cpm
none	<3	180
SEB"	100	10,150
MP	300++	230
MP-membranes	100++	210
MP-cytosol	3	200

" 0,2 ug/ml
++ characterized as IFN gamma
++ characterized as IFN alpha

TABLE 3. IFN production by human PBMC subpopulations induced with NDV, HSV, HSV-infected, fixed fibroblasts (f-HSV) and heat-killed Mycoplasma pneumoniae (MP).

Inducer	IFN (IU/ml) PRODUCED BY PBMC	macrophages	B-lymphocytes	T-lymphocytes
None	<3	<3	<3	<3
NDV+	10,000	10,000	3,000	30
HSV++	1,000	1,000	1,000	30
f-HSV+++	30,000	30	10,000	10
MP++++	300	<3	500	20

+ 10 HA/10^6 cells/ml
++ 10^6 PFU/10^7 cells/ml
+++ 10^6 f-HSV/10^7 cells/ml
++++ 2 ug/2.5x10^6 cells/ml

2. Acid-Labile Human Interferon Alpha

Kailash C. Chadha[a] *and Maria G. Ikossi*[b]

[a]Roswell Park Memorial Institute, Buffalo, NY 14263; [b]University of Texas Cancer Center M. D. Anderson Hospital and Tumor Institute, Houston, TX 77030

INTRODUCTION

It is now well recognized that interferons (IFNs) can broadly influence various aspects of both cellular and humoral immunity and consequently may have a definite role in the development and expression of various immune disorders. Over the past several years, significant biological differences among the various species of human IFNs have become apparent. Of all types of human IFNs described to date, the acid labile interferon alpha has been the most prominently associated with disorders presumed to be the result of immune disregulation. Acid-labile alpha interferon has been detected in the sera of patients with systemic lupus erythrematosus (SLE, 1), reuhumatoid arthritis (2), acquired immune deficiency syndrome (AIDS, 3,4), homosexual men with Kaposi's sarcoma (5) and Down's syndrome (6). The presence of acid-labile alpha interferon has also been reported in children with recurrent viral infections (7), Staphylococcus aureus infection (8), patients with midgut carcinoid tumors (9) and in patients with various types of neurological disorders (10). Its identification in patients with AIDS has brought an immediate and unrestricted attention and perhaps has made a general impression that circulating acid-labile alpha interferon is an aberrant type of alpha interferon found in parallel with severe immunosuppression and opportunistic infections including HTLV-III (5). However, acid-labile alpha interferon can be produced by both immune (11) and normal lymphocytes (12-14) upon proper stimulation. Its spontaneous production by PBL has also been reported (15) and furthermore, acid-labile alpha interferon has been detected in the lymph of normal rabbits (16). As such, it probably represents a normal physiologic component of the interferon system. Nevertheless, no significant attempt has been made to elucidate its role in cell and immune regulation. In this chapter, we will restrict ourselves to studies on acid-labile interferon produced by the normal leukocytes or their subset - polymorphonuclear (PMN) cells, in response to Sendai virus. Such interferon preparations contain both the acid-labile and acid-stable alpha interferons in varying proportions.

RESULTS

Alpha Interferon Synthesis by PBL

Buffy coats were routinely obtained from the Red Cross. Each buffy coat was tested by the Red Cross both for hepatitis and for HTLV-III antibody before releasing them for our use. RBC were removed either by ammonium chloride lysis or by sedimentation through the hydroxy ethyl starch (17). WBC were induced with Sendai virus for alpha-interferon production. The inducer virus was either removed by high speed centrifugation (40,000 x g for 3 hr) or by successive affinity chromatography steps (18). The details of interferon production procedure are described in another chapter in this book (Chadha and Sulkowski: Production and Purification of Natural Human Leukocyte Interferons). This procedure preserves both the acid-stable as well as acid-labile components of alpha interferons. For the sake of clarity in this text, the abbreviation "HuIFN-α" will refer to the interferon produced by the leukocytes according to Cantell's procedure and therefore contains only acid-stable alpha interferons. "HuIFN-α_ℓ" will be referred to interferon produced by leukocytes or PMN cells according to the procedure of Chadha and Sulkowski (18) and contains both acid-labile and acid-stable alpha interferons.

In order to determine the proportion of acid-labile interferon in our preparations, a sample is dialyzed overnight against glycine/HCl pH 2.0 buffer. On the following day, the pH is brought back gradually by dialysis against 0.02M phosphate buffer, pH 7.4. The antiviral activity of both pH^{ed} and nonpH^{ed} preparations is determined on human foreskin fibroblasts (BG-9 cells) using VSV as a challenge virus (19). The results presented in Table 1 clearly indicate that nearly 40% of interferon produced by PBL in response to Sendai virus is acid-labile. There were no differences in proportion of acid-stable and acid-labile antiviral activity whether leukocytes were prepared by ammonium chloride lysis method or by hydroxyethyl starch sedimentation procedure.

Synthesis of HuIFN-α_ℓ by Polymorphonuclear (PMN) Cells

In order to determine the physico-chemical properties of HuIFN-α_ℓ, it is important to have a preparation that is highly enriched in this component(s). This could be achieved either by developing a selective purification procedure that will separate acid-labile IFN from acid-stable IFN or alternatively by identifying the target cell(s) that may predominantly synthesize this class of IFN. Several affinity ligands (e.g., Concanavalin-A agarose, Phenyl-Sepharose CL-4B, CM Sepharose CL-6B, polynucleotide-agaroses, etc.) under a variety of chromatographic conditions were tested with limited or no success in separating acid-labile and acid-stable alpha interferons. In an attempt to identify the target cell(s) that might predominantly produce acid-labile alpha interferon, we found that nearly 90% of interferon produced by polymorphonuclear (PMN) cells is acid-labile. WBC were fractionated into PMN and mononuclear cells by the double discontinuous Ficoll-Hypaque gradient centrifugation. The purity of PMN cells in different preparations were in the range of 90-95%. It is rather important to point out here that PMN cells from the majority of normal healthy donors perhaps make very little or no alpha interferon. However, PMN from an occasional normal healthy donor will make between 400-5000 IU/ml of interferon which is largely (∿90%) acid-labile alpha type (Table 2). Interferon made by PMN cells was used for further physico-chemical and biological characterization of HuIFN-α_{ℓ}.

Physico-Chemical and Biological Properties of HuIFN-α_{ℓ}

Data summarized in Table 3 unquestionably demonstrates that acid-labile interferon produced by virally induced normal PMN cells is alpha type. Its antiviral activity can be nearly completely neutralized by the polyclonal antibody to HuIFN-α. HuIFN-α_{ℓ} cross protects bovine, feline and porcine cells to somewhat lesser degree than HuIFN-α. HuIFN-α_{ℓ} has comparable antiviral activity against VSV and is even more potent against HSV-1. HuIFN-α_{ℓ} has higher antiproliferative activity against Daudi cells and breast carcinoma cells (MDA-MB231) as compared to acid-stable alpha interferon. MDA-MB-231 cells are generally insensitive to antiviral activity of HuIFN-α.

HuIFN-α_{ℓ} loses nearly 90% of its antiviral activity when the pH of interferon preparation is dropped to 3.5. However, HuIFN-α_{ℓ} seems more thermostable than acid-stable alpha interferons.

Association of HLA-B35 Phenotype with HuIFN-α_{ℓ} Synthesis

It is known that treatment with interferon enhances expression of histocompatibility antigens on mouse lymphoid cells (21) as well as an human lymphoid cells (20). However, little or no evidence exists on relationship between HLA phenotype and the ability of PBL to synthesize alpha interferons.

Leukocyte concentrates were obtained from several healthy plasmapheresis donors at RPMI. All donors were typed for 35 HLA-A, -B, and 8DR locus antigens by Terasaki microlymphocytotoxicity techniques with UCLA reagent trays. The donors were divided into two groups based upon their HLA-B35 phenotype. Leukocytes were induced with Sendai virus for interferon production. Inducer virus in nonpH^{ed} preparations was removed effectively by high speed centrifugation. The antiviral activity of both the pH^{ed} and non-pH^{ed} preparations was determined on BG-9 cells. The results are presented in Table 4. It is evident that donors that are negative for HLA-B35 antigen gave, on an average, higher titer of alpha interferon (∿17,500 IU) as compared to donors that are positive for this antigen (∿4200 IU). However, it is even more striking that proportion of acid-labile alpha produced by donors that are positive for HLA-B35 is significantly greater than donors that lack this antigen (Table 4). There was no significantly association for other HLA antigens studied. This suggests that perhaps HLA-B35 phenotype may be a useful marker for interferon related studies (22).

Heterogeneity of Acid-Labile Interferons

Evidence for heterogeneity of acid-labile alpha interferon emerges from our HPLC work. Purified interferon alpha preparation containing both acid-labile and acid-stable interferons was chromatographed on HPLC column-DEAE 5PW (7.5 cm X 7.5 mm, Waters Associates, Milford, MA), previously equilibrated with 0.02M Tris/HCl pH 8.5 buffer. One milliliter of interferon containing $5x10^6$ units of antiviral activity was applied to this column followed by 25 ml of linear sodium chloride (0-0.5M) gradient in the equilibrating buffer followed by 5 ml of terminal buffer. The column was developed at room temperature at a flow rate of 1 ml/min and 0.5 ml fractions were collected. Fractions were pooled representing the protein peaks and assayed for antiviral activity on BG-9 cells. Retention time for each peak is shown in Fig. 1. A portion of each peak was acidified by dialyzing it against glycine/HCl pH 2.2 buffer. The pH was raised back to 7.4 by dialyzing it further against 0.02M phosphate buffer. After adjusting for any volume changes, the antiviral activity of pH^{ed} material was again determined on BG-9 cells. As shown in Fig. 1 (lower panel), interferon antiviral activity was detected in peaks 3-9. Nearly 50% of antiviral activity in peaks 5, 6 and 7 is acid-labile. Antiviral activity in peak 9 is more than 90% acid-labile, although antiviral activity in this peak is only 2% of total activity recovered from the column. Total column recovery was approximately 80% of applied interferon activity.

SUMMARY

Normal leukocytes or PMN cells induced with Sendai virus produce acid-labile interferon. This interferon is alpha type as determined by its antigenicity and cross-species antiviral activity. From the very limited studies carried out so far, it seems that HuIFN-α_ℓ is more potent than HuIFN-α in its antiviral and antiproliferative activities. HuIFN-α_ℓ is heterogeneous and there seems to be some relationship between HLA B-35 antigen and the ability of WBC to preferentially synthesize this type of interferon. HuIFN-α_ℓ has been demonstrated in the sera of patients with severely disregulated immune system. At the same time, both in vitro and in vivo studies suggest that HuIFN-α_ℓ can be produced by normal lymphocytes. It is therefore important to elucidate the nature of control of its production, effect on cellular and humoral immunity and modulation of other biological responses in order to better understand its role in immune disregulation. Also, it is important to know if HuIFN-α_ℓ produced by normal leukocytes and that produced during immunosuppression are similar or different in their immune regulatory activities.

REFERENCES

1. Preble, O.T., R.J. Black, R.M. Friedman, J.H. Klippel, and J. Vilcek: Systemic lupus erythrematosus: presence in human serum of an unusual acid-labile leukocyte interferon. Science 216:429, 1982.

2. Hooks, J.J., H.M. Moutsopoulos, S.A. Geis, N.I. Stahl, J.L. Decker, and A.L. Notkins: Immune interferon in the circulation of patients

with autoimmune disease. New Eng J Med 301:5, 1979.
3. Abb, J., M. Kochen, and F. Deinhardt: Interferon production in male homosexuals with acquired immune deficiency syndrome (AIDS) or generalized lymphadenopathy. Infection 12:240, 1984.
4. Eyster, M.E., J.J. Goedert, M.C. Poon, and O.T. Preble: Acid labile alpha interferon. A possible preclinical marker for the acquired immunodeficiency sundrome in hemophilia. New Eng J Med 309:583, 1983.
5. Destefano, E., R.M. Friedman, A.E. Friedman-Kien, J.J. Goedert, D. Heuriksen, O.T. Preble, J.A. Sonnabend, and J. Vilcek: Acid-labile human leukocyte interferon in homosexual men with Kaposi's sarcoma and lymphadenopathy. J Infect Dis 146:451, 1982.
6. Funa, K., G. Anneren, G.V. Alm, and B. Bjorksten: Abnormal interferon production in children with Down's syndrome. Clin Expt Immunol 56:493, 1984.
7. Bondestam, M., K. Funa and G.V. Alm: Defective leukocyte interferon response in children with recurrent infections accompanied by arthralgia. Acta Paediart Scand 74:219, 1985.
8. Ronnblom, L., A. Forsgren, and G.V. Alm: Characterization of interferon induced by bacteria and the interferon producing leukocytes in human peripheral blood. Infect Immun 40:126, 1983.
9. Funa, K., G.V. Alm, L. Ronnblom, and K. Oberg: Evaluation of natural killer cell-interferon system in patients with carcinoid tumors treated with leukocyte interferon. Clin Exp Immunol 53:716, 1983.
10. Dussaix, E., P. Lebon, G. Ponsot, G. Huault, G., and M. Tardieu: Intrathecal synthesis of different alpha-interferons in patients with various neurological diseases. Acta Neurol Scand 71:504, 1985.
11. Blackwill, F.R., D.B. Griffin, A. Band, and P.C.L. Beverley: Immune human lymphocytes produce an acid-labile α-interferon. J Expt Med 157:1059, 1983.
12. Chadha, K.C.: Acid-labile human leukocyte interferon. In: The Interferon System, F. Dianzani and G.B. Rossi, eds., Serono Symposia Publications, 24:35, 1985.
13. Matsuoka, H., Y. Kakui, A. Tanaka, Y. Cho, and J. Imanishi: Acid-labile interferon produced in human peripheral leukocytes by induction with Sendai virus. J Gen Virol 66:2491, 1985.
14. Wiranowska-Stewart, M., and W.E. Stewart II: Determination of leukocyte populations involved in production of interferons alpha and gamma. J Interferon Res 1:233, 1981.
15. Fischer, D.G., and M. Rubinstein: Spontaneous production of interferon-gamma and acid-labile interferon-alpha by subpopulation of human mononuclear cells. Cell Immunol 81:426, 1983.
16. Bocci, V., M. Muscettola, L. Paulesu, and G. Grasso: The physiological interferon response 2. Interferon is present in lymph but not in plasma of healthy rabbits. J Gen Virol 65:101, 1984.
17. Van Oss, C.J., P.M. Bronson, E.A. Dinolfo, and K.C. Chadha: Two methods for the removal of erythorcytes from buffy coats for the production of human leukocyte interferon. Immunol Commun 10:549, 1981.
18. Chadha, K.C., and E. Sulkowski: Method for the production and purification of human leukocyte interferon. U.S. Patent #4,485,038, Nov. 27, 1984.
19. Finter, N.B.: Dye uptake method of assessing viral cytopathogeni-

city and their application to interferon assays. J Gen Virol 5:419, 1969.

20. Heron, I., M. Hokland, and K. Berg: Enhanced expression of β-microglobulin and HLA antigens on human lymphoid cells by interferon. Proc Natl Acad Sci 75:6215, 1978.

21. Sonnenfeld, G., D. Meruelo, H.O. McDevitt, and T.C. Merigan: Effect of type I and type II interferons on murine thymocyte surface antigen expression: induction or secretion? Cell Immunol 57:427, 1981.

22. Cohen, E., U. Khurana, K.C. Chadha, and J. Fitzpatrick: HLA-B35 phenotype association with acid-labile alpha interferon. Blood 66: 97a, 1985.

TABLE 1. Proportions of Acid-Labile and Acid-Stable Antiviral Activity in Different Alpha Interferon Preparations

Interferon Preparation	Total Antiviral Activity	Acid-Stable Antiviral Activity	% of Total	Acid-Labile Antiviral Activity	% of Total
1[a]	50,000	32,500	65	17,500	35
2[a]	44,000	25,500	58	18,500	42
3[a]	66,000	41,500	63	24,500	37
4[a]	39,000	23,800	61	15,200	39
5[a]	29,000	16,300	56	12,700	44
6[b]	30,000	18,000	60	12,000	40
7[b]	44,000	24,600	56	19,400	44
8[b]	27,000	17,300	64	9,700	36
9[b]	22,000	12,750	58	9,250	42

a, RBC removed by hydroxyethyl starch sedimentation procedure.
b, RBC removed by ammonium chloride lysis.

TABLE 2. Acid-Labile and Acid-Stable Interferon Alpha Production by Polymorphonuclear and Mononuclear Cells

	Interferon Antiviral Activity					
	Mononuclear Cells[2]			Polymorphonuclear Cells[2]		
Donor[1]	Non-pH[ed]	pH[ed]	Acid Labile (IFN (%)	Non-pH[ed]	pH[ed]	Acid Labile IFN (%)
BH	21,000	14,700	30	460	45	90
ED	6,000	4,020	33	720	60	92
NW	20,000	13,000	35	3,000	150	95
KZ	14,000	9,950	29	420	45	89
LL	15,000	10,500	30	5,000	500	90

1, These donors were selected from 200 normal healthy donors. Their PMN cells produce alpha interferons.
2, Cells were obtained from the same donor; purity of each cell type varied between 90-95%.

TABLE 3. Properties[1] of Acid-Labile Alpha (HuIFN-α_ℓ) Interferon[2]

1.	pH-sensitivity	A significant portion of antiviral activity is destroyed: 30% at pH 4.0 and 75% at pH 3.5.
2.	Antigenicity	Nearly completely neutralized by HuIFN-α polyclonal antibody obtained from NIH.
3.	Cross-species activity	Protects feline, bovine and porcine cells. However, percent cross reactivity is less when compared to acid stable alpha interferon.
4.	Thermal stability	More thermostable than acid-stable interferon; nearly 55% antiviral activity is retained after 1 hr at 50°C.
5.	Antiviral activity	Significantly more active against HSV; equally effective against VSV.
6.	Antiproliferative activity	More effective against Daudi and MDA-MB-231 cells.

1, For details, see reference #12. HuIFN-α prepared according to Cantell's methodology was used for comparison.
2, HuIFN-α_ℓ obtained from PMN cells in response to Sendai virus stimulation.

TABLE 4. HLA-B35 Phenotype and Ability of Leukocytes to Synthesize Acid-Labile and Acid-Stable Alpha Interferons

Donor #	Total Antiviral Activity	Acid-Stable Antiviral Activity	Acid-Labile Antiviral Activity	% Acid-Labile Antiviral Activity
	Interferon Activity * (IU)			
	HLA B-35⁻			
1	4,500	2,500	2,000	44
2	8,700	5,300	3,400	39
3	22,000	12,000	10,000	45
4	35,000	20,000	15,000	43
5	21,000	11,750	9,250	44
6	14,500	10,000	4,500	31
	HLA B-35⁺			
1	790	220	570	72
2	2,700	500	2,200	81
3	5,500	1,250	4,250	77
4	950	360	590	62
5	4,100	2,000	2,100	51
6	12,000	4,100	7,900	66
7	3,300	1,150	2,150	65

* Average of three donations from each donor.

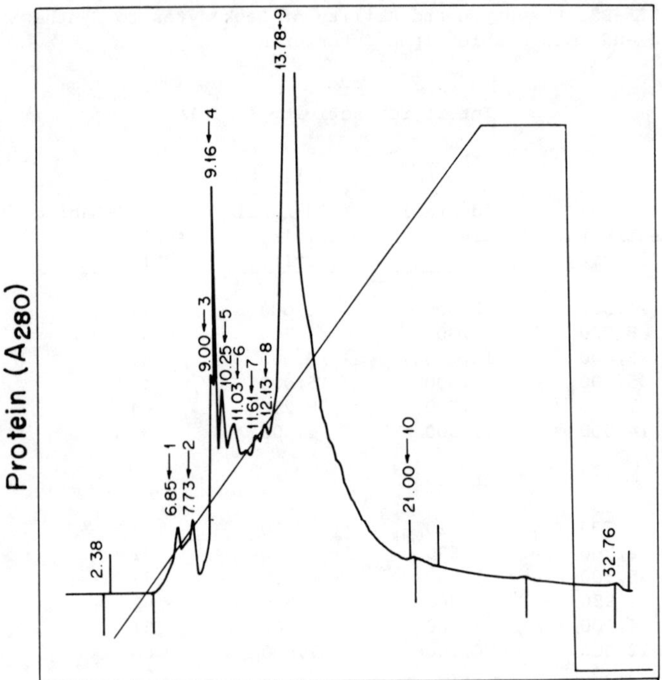

Antiviral Activity (% recovery)

Protein Peak#	Total Antiviral Activity	Acid-Stable Antiviral Activity	Acid-Labile Antiviral Activity
3	4	3.6	0.4
4	2	1.5	0.5
5	28	13.7	14.3
6	30	12.6	17.4
7	18	8.8	9.2
8	16	12.8	3.2
9	2	0.14	1.86

Protein peak # 1 and 2 had no antiviral activity. High protein concentration in peak #9 is largely due to human serum albumin contained in purified IFN preparations used for HPLC.

3. Interferon Induction, and Its Suppression, by Viruses

Philip I. Marcus

Department of Molecular and Cell Biology, U-44, University of Connecticut, Storrs, CT 06268

INTRODUCTION

In 1957 Isaacs and Lindenmann (10) discovered interferon (IFN) by infecting chick embryo cells with inactivated influenza virus. The precise nature of that inducer of IFN remains unknown, as do the molecular events that lead up to the transcription of the IFN genes. In 1967 Field and colleagues (6) discovered that double-stranded RNA (dsRNA) in the form of large molecular weight synthetic polyribonucleotides induced IFN. These seminal studies identified a molecular species capable of turning-on otherwise quiescent IFN genes, and focused attention on dsRNA as a biological response modifier of note.

In 1977 Marcus and Sekellick (19) presented evidence that a single molecule of dsRNA, when properly introduced into a cell sufficed to induce a full (quantum) yield of IFN. This remarkably low threshold provided an explanation for the induction of IFN under conditions where "no" dsRNA was detectable, and provides a unified model for the nature of the inducer molecule.

The studies on IFN induction by viruses in non-lymphoid cells reviewed in the last offering of this series (15) concerned a description and analysis of the two common types of IFN induction dose(multiplicity)-response(IFN yield) curves (18), and a definition and quantitation of virus populations in terms of their content of IFN-inducing particles (IFP). Evidence was reviewed for double-stranded(ds)RNA as the proximal molecule for IFN induction, with a threshold for induction of 1 molecule of dsRNA per cell. Other evidence suggested that dsRNA, either as a preformed molecule, or synthesized upon infection, was the IFN inducer moiety for viruses representing several different families (16). Although dsRNA of viral origin is isolable from infected cells (2,13,26,35), definitive proof is lacking for its existence in situ during induction. Little information exists to describe in molecular terms the events between entry of a single IFN-inducing particle and initiation of IFN transcription. This review will highlight recent studies from this laboratory concerned with this "black box" part of the IFN induction process.

EARLY EVENTS IN THE INTERFERON INDUCTION PROCESS

The rapidity with which virus infection can lead to IFN induction (31), dictates that formation of dsRNA and its recognition by the cell as the proximal inducer molecule occurs within minutes after virus entry. These very early events in the IFN induction process were studied by following the fate of IFN-inducing particles in cells compromised by the action of lysosomotropic agents. The simplest of these agents, NH_4Cl, functions as a lipophilic weak base that within minutes raises the pH of endosomes/lysosomes(27). This action prevents the low pH-dependent membrane fusion events required to deliver viral genomic material to the cytosol for the start of virus replication(24). Svitlik and Marcus(32) showed that a brief window of time exists in which viral inducers of IFN can interact with the cell to intitiate the induction process. If the inducer molecule is not recognized by the cell within this critical time-frame then its capacity to function as an inducer is either irrevocably lost or significantly compromised. Within 3 to 5 minutes about one-half of the IFN-inducing (and plaque-forming) particles of Sindbis and vesicular stomatitis virus (VSV) have escaped the inhibitory action of NH_4Cl. These studies indicate that processing of viruses through endocytic vesicles and low-pH dependent systems represents the critical step in controlling the efficiency of infection and IFN induction. Unless the viral genome escapes endocytic or low pH-dependent membranes within a few minutes it seems doomed to an abortive infection or induction attempt. Furthermore, successful escape from endosomal/lysosomal vacuoles may occur with higher efficiency for viral inducers that require only partial expression of the genome. The plaquing efficiency of VSV, requiring 100% expression of the genome, is lost at an exponential rate as a function of NH_4Cl concentration: there is a 100-fold decrease at 50 mM NH_4Cl(32). The IFP activity of VSV-T1026R1, requiring expression of about 10 percent of its genome(20), scores virtually all of the particles as inducers, but the quantum yields of IFN decreased with increasing concentrations of NH_4Cl(32).

IFP that do escape into the cytosol of NH_4Cl-treated cells do not function as effectively as in untreated cells--the quantum yield of IFN is reduced. The lowered efficiency of IFN production can be relegated to some very early step during virus entry. Conceivably, the inducer molecule never attains its full "strength" as a signal for induction. In this context the signal may be related to the length of the dsRNA that escapes or accumulates in the cytosol where it can react with the cell's putative recognition system for dsRNA (IFN induction receptors[17]). The length of the dsRNA and the length of time that that dsRNA remains exposed to the postulated IFN induction receptors may dictate the magnitude of a signal sent to the nucleus to initiate transcription of the IFN gene(s), and hence the absolute value of the IFN quantum.

INTERFERON INDUCTION-SUPPRESSING PARTICLES (ISP)

Although most viruses can induce IFN under appropriate conditions, many can not. Those that fail to induce IFN invariably display another attribute-- they suppress the IFN-inducing activity of viruses otherwise capable of induction. The suppression of IFN induction might reflect a generalized inhibition of cellular macromolecular synthesis, or in the other extreme, a special action directed at the IFN genes. An assay was developed to detect and quantitate this property of viruses with a view toward addressing this problem. The assay measured the capacity of a virus to suppress the yield of IFN from a cell simultaneously infected with that virus and an IFN-inducing particle. This IFN yield-reduction assay defined virus populations in terms of a newly quantifiable attribute--IFN induction-suppressing particle (ISP). IFN induction-suppressing particles need not be infectious to be detected, they need only suppress IFN induction by a coinfecting IFN-inducing particle(21).

Characteristics of IFN Induction-suppressing Particles

IFN induction-suppressing particles can express activity in both homologous and heterologous systems: wildtype VSV can function equally well as ISP when VSV[±]DI-011 particles are used as IFP (homologous), or when avian reovirus is the inducing particle(heterologous). Heterologous systems eliminate possible interactions of homologous viral components as contributors to any general mechanism for ISP action, and suggest that the capacity to suppress IFN induction is intrinsic to the virus and directed toward the cell. The expression of ISP activity can be affected by the cell: in mouse L(Y) cells the entire genome of wildtype VSV-Orsay must be expressed for it to function as an ISP. In aged primary chick embryo cells, the VSV genome could be subjected to 100 lethal hits of UV radiation(254nm) and sustain only a modest reduction (2-fold) in ISP titer. Thus, neither virus replication or amplified synthesis of viral RNA was required for ISP activity--in chick embryo cells(22).

When increasingly higher doses of UV radiation were delivered to VSV-tsO5, an RNA^- mutant, it lost its capacity to function as an ISP, in a dose-dependent manner. If the action of UV radiation is restricted to the genomic RNA, the calculated UV target for ISP activity is about 57 nucleotides. This UV target is consistent with, but not proof of, a requirement for transcription of the leader RNA sequence located at the 3' most proximal end of the VSV genome. The 47-base product of leader RNA, termed plus-strand leader RNA, has been shown to inhibit the action of cellular polymerase II in an in vitro transcribing system(8). Stocks of VSVtsO5 (UV=100 hits) --a presumed source of plus-strand leader RNA, also inhibited plaque formation by pseudorabies virus(PSRV) in a multiplicity-dependent manner in chick embryo cells(22). Herpesviruses require cellular polymerase II to initiate transcription of the immediate early genes(3) making it attractive to speculate that plus-strand leader RNA might be responsible for blocking a very early step in PSRV replication. The plaquing efficiency of Influenza virus, another virus that depends on cell polymerase II for replication(9) was also reduced significantly in cells coinfected with UV-tsO5. Replication of VSV, a virus with no dependence on the nucleus for replication(7), was reduced less than 2-fold.

The situation may be more complicated. VSV-T1026R1 does not function as an ISP even though it shares the same leader RNA sequence as its parent, VSV-HR(5). In fact, T1026R1 is an excellent inducer of IFN (28,30). Either plus-strand leader RNA is not the sole mediator of ISP action in chick cells, or some other virion-associated molecule(s) regulates its action.

UV radiation may be inactivating ISP through another target, namely the poly(rA) polymerase activity resident in the virion L-protein. This mode of action is attractive because (i) poly(A) appears to preferentially inhibit the translation of cellular mRNAs compared to a viral mRNA tested in vitro(1), and (ii) the large size of the virion-associated L-protein with its high content of cystyl and trytophanyl residues make it vulnerable to inactivation by 254nm UV (14) in the dose range used to inactivate ISP activity. At very high doses of UV radiation inactivation may also involve covalent bond formation between protein and genomic RNA(25). Preliminary results with poly(rA) in vivo support this model for ISP action. In view of the unusual sensitivity of IFN induction in chick embryo cells to inhibitors of protein synthesis, poly(A) may act by blocking the translation of a critical short-lived protein required for IFN induction, and not renewable in the aged chick cell(33)(see below).

One attribute of the ISP action of UV-inactivated VSV in chick cells is worth emphasizing: at multiplicities less than 20 or 30 ISP, sufficient to reduce the IFN yield by 100- to 1000-fold, there is no cytopathic effect. Interferon action is only modestly affected by ISP, and the induction of stress proteins by heat appears unaffected(22). Thus, the action of ISP seems to be selective, being highly active in preventing IFN induction/production, and the replication of certain viruses. Different mechanisms may of course be involved in preventing IFN production and virus replication.

INHIBITION OF PROTEIN SYNTHESIS RENDERS AGED CHICK EMBRYO CELLS REFRACTORY TO IFN INDUCTION

In mouse L cells, all steps in the induction process up to and including the transcription of IFN mRNA occur in the presence of inhibitors of protein synthesis (4,33). Indeed, implicit in the use of inhibitors of protein synthesis to achieve superinduction is the fact that most mammalian cells can be induced to the point of transcribing IFN genes in the absence of protein synthesis. This implies that either proteins are not required for IFN induction, or that enough long-lived proteins exist so they are not rate limiting in the induction process. In contrast, chicken cells are rendered highly refractory to IFN induction, regardless of the inducer, if cells are exposed to inhibitors of protein synthesis for 6 hours before, or during infection(33). Although chick cells exposed to cycloheximide(CHX) (50 µg/ml, 6 hr) displayed a marked reduction in their capacity to induce IFN (10- to 100-fold)--even days after removal of the inhibitor and thorough washing, they were fully competent in plaquing and replicating viruses, including NDV. IFN action was not affected. Thus, there was no general suppression of induction processes. Early events in virus entry and processing of the viral inducer(32) are not the basis of the refractory state to IFN induction brought about by inhibitors of protein synthesis: plaque formation and virus replication are unaffected. Reactions unique to IFN induction, and not concerned with virus replication, are most likely to be involved: for example (i)formation of the proximal IFN inducer molecule, dsRNA, (ii)dsRNA interaction with the cell's putative IFN inducer receptors, (iii)generation of signals therefrom for promoting transcription of the IFN genes and their regulation, (iv)translation of IFN mRNA and its regulation, or (v)processing and export of the IFN molecule(17).

IFN INDUCTION BY NEWCASTLE DISEASE VIRUS: A MODEL

Newcastle disease virus(NDV), one of the most extensively studied inducers of IFN displays two host related features: (i)in semi- or non-permissive hosts(mammalian cells), stocks of active NDV can be excellent inducers of IFN, and (ii) in permissive hosts, like cultures of unaged chick cells, NDV is a non-inducer. However, when NDV is inactivated by various physical, chemical or biological agents it becomes a good inducer in these cells(23). Marcus et al.(23) studied IFN induction by NDV and found (i) egg-grown NDV contains non-infectious IFN-inducing particles which are excellent IFN inducers in primary chick embryo cells(CEC) aged in vitro for several days, (non-infectious IFP do not induce IFN in monolayers of young CEC); (ii) non-infectious IFP are present in about 7-fold excess over that of PFP; (iii) infectious particles (PFP) of NDV do not induce IFN, even in aged CEC, and (iv) only about one-third the number of particles scored as PFP appear to register as IFP on mouse L cells.

As noted, NDV does not induce IFN in cultures of conventional (unaged) CEC. However, upon exposure to low doses of UV radiation(254nm) stocks of NDV rapidly acquire IFN-inducing capacity until peak activity is reached at about 1000 ergs/mm^2. Exposure to larger doses of UV results in an exponential rate of loss of IFP activity. Data from several laboratories were combined to produce a strikingly uniform curve when the fraction of maximum IFN-yield was plotted as a function of the UV dose delivered to NDV. A model was developed that involved a series of nested hypotheical UV targets displayed as a percentage of the NDV genome. It identified different targets for IFP and ISP activities within the genome and produced a theoretical curve that showed a good fit to the observed data(23). The potential for both IFN induction and its suppression contained within the genome of a single virion provides for a full range of responses, and is emerging as more the rule than the exception.

DEVELOPMENT OF IFN INDUCIBILITY IN CHICK CELLS AGED IN VITRO

When chick cells from 10-day-old embryos are plated at confluency and left undisturbed they acquire with time an enhanced capacity to produce IFN upon induction(29). The development of IFN inducibility as chick cells "age" in vitro was studied by Sekellick and Marcus (29) by analyzing the IFN-induction dose-response curves generated as a function of time in culture. For the first few days little or no IFN can be induced-- regardless of the inducer. After a few days the cells gradually gain the capacity to produce IFN, with maximal levels induced in cells aged for about 9 or 10 days. Cell monolayers that produced little or no IFN shortly after seeding and reaching confluency could be induced after aging to produce $>10^5$ U per plate of 10^7 cells. If inhibitors of prostaglandin/leukotriene synthesis are added to the growth medium within 2 days of seeding and the cells aged in their presence, the cells fail to develop IFN inducibility! Indomethacin(IM) is one of the most effective inhibitors: cells treated with 10 to 100 ug/ml IM produced 100 to >1000-fold less IFN than controls. About 2 days after seeding the cells begin to escape the action of the drug. Indomethacin added at the time of induction had no effect on the yield of IFN, but inducibility was restored partially if the drug was withdrawn during the aging process. Indomethacin had no effect on the rate of total RNA or protein synthesis, nor did it prevent the induction of stress(heat shock) proteins--an inducible system responsive at all stages of in vitro aging. Cells aged in IM were 3-fold less effective in responding to the action of IFN. The combined effect of inhibiting the development of IFN inducibility and lowering the effectiveness of IFN action results in a monolayer of chick cells that are exquisitely sensitive hosts for plaquing or growing viruses that are good inducers of IFN and/or sensitive to its action, suggesting a practical way to detect primary isolates from virus infection.

The nature of the reaction(s) in the development of IFN inducibility that prostaglandins control remains to be determined. However, since the plaquing efficiency of infectious NDV remains constant throughout the aging process, it seems unlikely that any early steps in virus infection or presentation of dsRNA to the cell are involved.

CHICKEN INTERFERON: HOW MANY TYPES?

Primary chick embryo cells aged in vitro have proved to be an excellent experimental host for studying the cells' response to viral inducers of IFN, and to the development of IFN inducibility(op cit). But what types of IFN are these cells producing? Early reports indicated a single electrophoretic band of IFN with a molecular weight of about 30KD(12). Kohase et al(11) recently saught to further characterize viral-induced chicken IFN. Using UV-NDV as the inducer, and aged chick cells as hosts, IFN was obtained with a specific activity of 2.4×10^7 (500-fold purification), and with more than 95% recovery. Two peaks of activity were observed on SDS-PAGE: a sharp peak at 18KD and a broad peak at 20-30KD. The latter was shown to represent a glycosylated form of the 18KD molecule. Polyclonal antibody from rabbits and a monoclonal antibody from mice neutralized both the 18 and 20-30KD activity. IFN induced in aged chick cells by Sindbis and Semliki forest viruses and by poly(rI.rC) were also neutralized by both antibody preparations, as was IFN induced in chicken spleen cells by NDV and from egg-derived IFN induced by Sindbis virus. These results suggest that chick cells may contain only one type of IFN.

A single type of chicken IFN would permit the simplest of interpretations for IFN induction dose-response curves generated in chick cells(18). However, a study by Thacore et al(34) indicates the situation may be more complex. They reported two types of chicken IFN based on their cellular origin and response to acid pH. It will be interesting to know whether these two types of IFN actually represent antigenically distinct proteins, and how they will respond to the antibodies described by Kohase et al(11).

SUMMARY

The molecular events that immediately follow virus infection, including presentation of the proximal IFN inducer to the cell's putative recognition system for dsRNA, represent a black box into which some light is now penetrating. Advances include:(i) identification of the mode of entry of IFP, (ii) localization of a brief window of time for the proximal inducer dsRNA to act, (iii) detection, assay and characterization of IFN induction-suppressing particles--antagonists to IFN-inducing particles, (iv) the loss of IFN inducibility in chicken (but not mammalian) cells upon exposure to inhibitors of protein synthesis, (v) a model that involves regulated expression of IFP and ISP activities to account for UV-NDV as an IFN-inducer in unaged chick cells (vi) the first demonstration that the cellular development of IFN inducibility can be regulated, and (vii) evidence that viruses may only induce a single type of IFN in aged chick cells. IFN induction dose-response curve analysis has served as an important quantitative biological tool permitting an explanation in molecular terms of how viruses induce cells to produce IFN.

ACKNOWLEDGMENTS

These studies have been supported by a grant from NIAID (AI-18381), and benefited from use of the Cell Culture Facility supported in part by the University of Connecticut Research Foundation(35-593). I am most thankful to Dr. Margaret J. Sekellick for her critical reading of this review, thoughtful suggestions and her uncanny ability to remove about one-half of the words from the original version without appearing to alter its meaning an iota.

REFERENCES

1. Bablanian, R. & Banerjee, A.K.: Poly(riboadenylic acid) preferentially inhibits in vitro translation of cellular mRNAs compared with vaccinia virus mRNAs: possible role in vaccinia virus cytopathology. Proc Natl Acad Sci USA 83:1290-1294, 1986.
2. Colby, C. and Duesberg, P.M.: Double-stranded RNA in vaccinia virus-infected cells. Nature 222:940-944, 1969.
3. Costanzo, F., Campadelli-Fuime, G., Foa-Tomasi, L. & Cassai, E.: Evidence that herpes simplex virus DNA is transcribed by cellular RNA polymerase B. J Virology 21:996-1001, 1977.
4. Dianzani, F., Gagnoni, R., Buckler, C.E. & Baron, S.: Studies of the induction of IFN system by nonreplicating NDV. Proc Soc Exp Biol Med 133:324-328, 1970.
5. Dunigan, D.D., Baird, S. & Lucas-Lenard, J.: Lack of correlation between the accumulation of plus-strand leader RNA and the inhibition of protein and RNA synthesis in VSV infected mouse L cells. Virology 150:231-246, 1986.
6. Field, A.K., Tytell, A.A., Lampson, G.P. & Hilleman, M.R.: Inducers of interferon and host resistance. II. Multi-stranded synthetic polynucleotide complexes. Proc Natl Acad Sci USA 58:1004-1009, 1967.
7. Follett, E.A.C., Pringle, C.R., Wunner, W.H. & Skehel, J.J.: Virus replication in enucleate cells: VSV and influenza virus. J Virol 13:394-399, 1974.

8. Grinnell, B.W. & Wagner, R.R.: Nucleotide sequence and secondary structure of VSV leader RNA and homologous DNA involved in inhibition of DNA-dependent transcription. Cell 36:533-543, 1984.
9. Herz, C., Stavnezer, E., Krug, R.M. & Gurney, T.: Influenza virus, and RNA virus synthesizes its nRNA in the nucleus. Cell 26:391-400, 1981.
10. Isaacs, A. & Lindenmann, J.: Virus interference. I. The interferon. Proc Royal Soc B 147:258-267, 1957.
11. Kohase, M., Moriya, H., Sato, T.A., Kohno, S. & Yamazaki, S.: Purification and characterization of chick IFN induced by viruses. J gen Virol 67:215-218, 1986.
12. Lampson, D.P., Tytell, A.A., Nemes, M.M. & Hilleman, M.R.: Characterization of chick embryo interferon induced by a DNA virus. Proc Soc Exp Biol Med 118:441-448, 1965.
13. Lucas, J.J. & Ginsberg, H.S.: Identification of double-stranded virus-specific RNA in KB cells infected with type 2 adenovirus. Biochem Biophys Res Commun 49:39-44, 1972.
14. Luse, R.A. & McLaren, A.D.: Mechanism of enzyme inactivation by ultraviolet light and the photochemistry of amino acids (at 2537 A). Photochem & Photobiol 2:343-360, 1963.
15. Marcus, P.I.: The interferon inducer moiety of viruses: A single molecule of dsRNA. Texas Rep on Biol & Med 41:70-75, 1981-1982.
16. Marcus, P.I.: Interferon induction by viruses: One molecule of dsRNA as the threshold for interferon induction. In "Interferon 5", I. Gresser, ed., Academic Press, pp.115-180, 1983.
17. Marcus, P.I.: Interferon induction by viruses: Double-stranded ribonucleic acid as the common proximal inducer molecule. In "Interferon: Mechanisms of Production and Action", Vol. 3, R.M. Friedman, ed., Elsevier Biomedical Press, Chapt. 5, pp. 113-175, 1984.
18. Marcus, P.I.: Interferon induction dose-response curves. In "Methods in Enzymology", Interferons, Part C, S. Pestka, ed., Academic Press, 119:106-114, 1986.
19. Marcus, P.I. & Sekellick, M.J.: Defective-interfering particles with covalently-linked [±]RNA induce interferon. Nature (London) 266: 815-819, 1977.
20. Marcus, P.I. & Sekellick, M.J.: Interferon induction by viruses. III. Vesicular stomatitis virus: Interferon-inducing particle activity requires partial transcription of Gene N. J gen Virol 47:89-96, 1980.
21. Marcus, P.I. & Sekellick, M.J.: Interferon induction by viruses. XII. Detection and assay of interferon induction-suppressing particles. Virology 142:411-415, 1985.
22. Marcus, P.I. & Sekellick, M.J.: Interferon induction is suppressed by the action of VSV plus-strand leader RNA. In "The Biology of the Interferon System, 1985", H. Schellekens & W.E. Stewart, II, eds., Elsevier Scientific Publishers, In press, 1986.
23. Marcus, P.I., Svitlik, C. & Sekellick, M.J.: Interferon induction by viruses. X. A model for interferon induction by Newcastle disease virus. J gen Virol 64:2419-2431, 1983.
24. Matlin, K.S., Reggio, H., Helenius, A. & Simons, K.: Pathway of VSV entry leading to infection. J Mol Biol 156:609-631, 1982.

25. Miller, R.L. & Plagemann, P.G.W.: Effect of ultraviolet light on mengovirus. Formation of uracil dimers, instability and degradation of capsid and covalent linkage of protein to viral RNA. J Virol 13:729-739, 1974.
26. Nilsen, T.W., Wood, D.L. & Baglioni, C.: Cross-linking of viral RNA by 4'-aminomethyl-4,5'-8-trimethylpsoralen in HeLa cells infected with encephalomyocardititis virus and the tsG114 mutant of vesicular stomatitis virus. Virology 109:82-93, 1981.
27. Ohkuma, S. & Poole, B.: Fluorescence probe measurements of the intralysosomal pH in living cells and the perturbation of pH by various agents. Proc Natl Acad Sci USA 75:3327-3331, 1978.
28. Sekellick, M.J. & Marcus, P.I.: Persistent Infection. II. Interferon-inducing temperature-sensitive mutants as mediators of cell sparing: Possible role in persistent infection by vesicular stomatitis virus. Virology 95:36-47, 1979.
29. Sekellick, M.J. & Marcus, P.I.: Interferon induction by viruses. XIV. Development of Interferon Inducibility and its inhibition in chick embryo cells "aged" in vitro. J IFN Res 5:651-667, 1985.
30. Stanners, C.P., Francoeur, A.M. & Lam, T.: Analysis of VSV mutant with attenuated cytopathogenicity: Mutation in viral function, P, for inhibition of protein synthesis. Cell 11:273-281, 1977.
31. Stewart, W.E., II: "The Interferon System", 2nd ed., Springer-Verlag, pp. 64-67, 1984.
32. Svitlik, C. & Marcus, P.I.: Interferon induction by viruses. XI. Early events in the induction process. J IFN Res 4:585-602, 1984.
33. Svitlik, C. & Marcus, P.I.: Interferon induction by viruses. XII. Inhibition of protein synthesis renders aged chick embryo cells refractory to interferon induction. J gen Virol 66:883-886, 1985.
34. Thacore, H.R., Kibler, P.K., Gregorio, C.C., Pollina, C.M. & Hudecki, M.S.: Characterization of lymphocyte IFNs with different species specificities from normal and genetically dystrophic chickens. J IFN Res 5:279-288, 1985.
35. Thomas, J.R. & Wagner, R.R.: Evidence that vesicular stomatitis virus produces double-stranded RNA that inhibits protein synthesis in a reticulocyte lysate. J Virol 44:189-198, 1982.

4. Mechanism of Induction of Gamma Interferon

F. Dianzani and G. Antonelli

Institute of Virology, University of Rome "La Sapienza," Viale di Porta Tiburtina 28, 00185 Rome, Italy

INTRODUCTION

Production of interferon (IFN) gamma by leukocytes in response to mitogens (53) and specific antigens (25, 56) was first reported several years ago. However, until recently not much work was done to identify the mechanisms of IFN gamma production.

Since the beginning it was clear that IFN gamma production is triggered by mechanisms different from those which occur for induction of IFN beta. In fact it is well established that IFN gamma production requires cooperation between different cell types and it may be triggered by inducers which do not penetrate the cellular membrane. On the other hand, IFN gamma inducers are the same agents that activate T cell compartment of the immune system, in a clonal or polyclonal manner, demonstrating that the early events leading to IFN gamma production are strictly correlated with the mechanisms of lymphocyte activation.

IFN GAMMA INDUCERS AND PRODUCING CELLS

Since the discovery of PHA induced-IFN gamma, many other substances have been described as inducers of this type of IFN. So far these include: antigens in specifically sensitized peripheral blood mononuclear cells (PBMC) (27, 28, 37, 57); T-cell mitogens (23, 31, 48, 52); oxidizing agents (13); calcium ionophores (14); alloantigens (26); anti-lymphocytic serum (24) or monoclonal antibodies recognizing T cells (10, 54). Rather low amounts of IFN gamma may be induced in human PBMC also by TPA and related diterpene esters (51, 55) and by some B-cell mitogens, such as LPS (8).

While it has been clearly established that in most cases the inducers require the presence of accessory cells, still debated is the nature of the producing cell(s). In fact while most investigators agree that T lymphocytes are the

IFN gamma-secreting cells, only exceptions being occasional production by NK cells (32, 39) and by B cells (20), the T-cell subtype chiefly involved in the production is still discussed. Most authors showed that human $OKT4^+$ cells (helper/inducer T cells), in the presence of accessory cells, are the producers of IFN gamma. However others reported that other cell types ($OKT4^-$ and $OKT8^-$, (41); $OKT4^+$ and $OKT8^+$, (1); a eterogenous subset of T lymphocytes, (22); cytotoxic T lymphocytes, (33)) are involved in the production of IFN gamma. At the present time one can conclude that helper T cell, recognized by OKT4 monoclonal antibodies, are the main cell type responsible for IFN gamma production although the finding do not rule out the possibility that, under certain conditions, other types of T cell may be induced to IFN gamma production. It is also possible that treatment with conventional mitogens may unnaturally induce more than one cell type.

MECHANISM OF INDUCTION

a) Mitogenic induction

Since all IFN gamma inducers share their ability to induce T-cell activation, it appears that IFN gamma production may occur through a common mechanism.
For this reason, in the past, most of studies have been conducted using conventional mitogens rather than other inducers because under experimental conditions they are easier to handle in a reproducible and standardized fashion. The mechanism of IFN gamma production has been approached by analyzing the nature of signal(s) required for activation of the cells involved in the process. Current models of mitogen triggered production of IFN gamma propose that T lymphocytes, as IFN producing cells, require the presence of accessory cells. This role is played mainly by macrophages (6, 19, 21) although lymphocyte activation leading to lymphoproliferation, antibody production, etc. may be sometimes mediated also by endothelial cells, fibroblasts and dendritic cells. It is still to be fully defined the exact nature of the necessary macrophage signal(s). It also remains uncertain whether an intact macrophage is required for T cell-production, or, alternatively, whether accessory cell signals are mediated solely by soluble factors. On this respect it has been proposed that the macrophage product interleukin 1 (IL-1) is implicated as one of signals required for activation of T cell by antigens and mitogenic lectins (7, 43, 50). In addition it has been proposed that the major and perhaps only role of macrophages and IL-1 under these circumstances is to induce interleukin 2 (IL-2) production (38, 45, 46), which in turn could induce IFN gamma in T lymphocytes (8, 42, 49).
Recent studies in our laboratory were undertaken using, as

a mitogen, the enzyme galactose oxidase (GO), that allows more reliable termination of the mitogen pulse, to dissect the macrophage influence involved in triggering resting T cells to IFN gamma production. In fact GO is a well characterized enzyme that, oxidating galactose residues on the membrane glycoproteins, induces strong proliferative response (40) and production of IFN gamma (13) in PBMC.
The precise mechanism for the activation is not known but we found that removal of terminal galactose residues with Beta-galactosidase (Table 1) inhibits the production of IFN gamma by PBMC induced by antigens, mitogens and other oxidizing agents (15, 17), suggesting that the oxidation of galactose residues represents a general feature of IFN gamma production.
Depletion of macrophages from PBMC causes a marked decrease of GO-induced IFN gamma production (5).
Reconstitution of such depleted cultures with GO-treated macrophages, but not lymphocytes, restored IFN gamma levels to those of control unfractionated PBMC. Studies with Boyden chambers (table 2) have shown that GO-treated macrophages release a soluble factors which stimulates T lymphocyte to production of IFN gamma (5).
Based on these findings, it appears that the oxidation of terminal galactose residues on the surface of macrophages leads to the induction and trasmission of a soluble signal for lymphocyte production of IFN gamma. Further studies have shown that this new macrophage-derived IFN gamma inducer is different from IL-1 because it is not able to stimulate thymocyte proliferation in the presence of suboptimal doses of PHA and because, unlike IL-1, stimulates T lymphocytes to proliferate in the absence of any other inducers. Additionally IL-1 is not able alone to induce IFN gamma production while GO-induced mediator does. Since preliminary results show that supernatants from macrophage treated with mitogens different from GO possess the same IFN gamma inducing activity, it appears that activated macrophage produce IL-1 and another soluble mediator which, unlike IL-1, directly induce the lymphocyte to proliferation and IFN gamma production. It remains to be established whether this mitogen-induced mediator participates also to IFN gamma induction by antigens.

b) Antigenic induction

Although it is quite well established that macrophages present the antigen to sensitized T lymphocytes, the mechanism of antigen presentation needed for IFN gamma induction is not completely elucidated.
Current models of lymphocyte activation propose that antigen must be presented by accessory cell to T lymphocyte in a restricted manner (44) while mitogen may be "presented" by a mismatched population (35). Consequently, T lymphocyte to be activated by antigens must recognize on the macrophage membrane the complex antigen and MHC

product. As regard to IFN gamma production this model has been recently confirmed by the findings that: anti-Ia antisera inhibits murine IFN gamma production (29); anti HLA-DR monoclonal antibodies inhibit human IFN gamma production in PBMC induced by Mycoplasma arthriditids (11); monoclonal anti-Ia antibodies inhibit lymphocyte activation and IFN gamma production in primary and secondary MLR (34); monoclonal antibodies to D-region antigens inhibit the HSV-antigens stimulated production of IFN gamma in reconstituted macrophage-T lymphocyte culture (12); finally, antibodies to HLA (class I and II) inhibit IFN gamma production induced by microbial antigen (manuscript in preparation).
Taken together these findings confirmed that, as well as in the lymphocyte activation, HLA antigens are important for IFN gamma production and suggest that D-region (Ia) antigens play an essential role in the cellular interactions leading to this phenomenon, probably through macrophage presentation of antigen. As IFN gamma increases DR antigen expression on monocytes (3, 47), a positive feedback on IFN production might be postulated.
Interestingly preliminary results from our laboratory show that antibodies against HLA class I molecules, recognizing the light chains (β_2 microglobulin), inhibit IFN gamma production by GO. This observation indicates that either β_2 microglobulin is the site of action of the GO or, alternatively, it is necessary to the process without being directly involved. Since the oxidation of galactose residues is a general feature of the mechanism of IFN gamma induction (17), it appears that β_2 microglobulin is involved, in some fashion, in such mechanism whichever is the inducer.
In an attempt to develop systems to analyze the interaction between antigen specific T lymphocytes and macrophages, recently we studied antigenic induction of IFN gamma in different combinations of cells from immunized or unimmunized animals. Therefore we have investigated the ability of macrophages from immunized animals to induce IFN gamma by T lymphocytes in the presence of the respective antigen at low doses. These experiments demonstrated that immunized macrophages are much more efficient than macrophages from unimmunized animals at presenting antigen to T cells (Table 3) and that immunoglobulins bound to the macrophage membrane via their Fc receptor may be critically involved in this effective form of macrophages and T lymphocytes interaction at least for IFN gamma induction (18).

c) Role of calcium

Although the aforementioned results could clarify some of cooperating functions of macrophages, the intracellular events, leading to IFN gamma gene expression are largely unknown.

However, several lines of evidence suggest that increased cytosolic calcium concentration delivers mitogenic signals to lymphoid (36) and non lymphoid cells (9).

A direct role of calcium in IFN gamma production is suggested by the finding that: i) calcium ionophore (A23187) induces strong production of IFN gamma in PBMC cultures (14); ii) antigens and mitogens do not stimulate IFN gamma in the presence of the chelating agent EGTA (15); iii) specific calcium entry blockers inhibit IFN gamma induction by mitogens (16) and by antigens (in preparation). These observations strongly suggest not only that a calcium flux through the cellular membrane is a necessary step for IFN gamma production but also that such flux can mimic the effects of antigens or mitogens for lymphocyte activation and subsequent production of IFN gamma. That lymphocyte are the cells in which the calcium flux leading to IFN gamma production occurs is demonstrated by the finding shown in table 4.

It can be seen that while the yield of IFN gamma induced by GO and other mitogens is considerably diminished when the macrophages are eliminated from the PBMC population, calcium ionophores induce an IFN gamma production whose yield is not affected by depletion of macrophages (4). The data clearly show that ionophores act a level that is independent and subsequent to the event involving the macrophages and suggest that an increase in cytosolic calcium concentration directly triggers T lymphocyte activation. These findings are in keeping with other observations showing that A23187 can induce lymphoproliferation in pure OKT4 positive cells (2) and that OKT3 monoclonal antibody can activate Jurkat T cell line through induction of an increase of the cytoplasmic free calcium concentration (30).

SUMMARY AND CONCLUSION

This review offers a partial explanation to some of the questions about the mechanism of IFN gamma production. The data reported indicated that IFN gamma is produced by T lymphocytes probably following a calcium influx through the membrane and that, for mitogenic and antigenic induction, macrophages are critically needed. However mitogens activate macrophages non specifically leading to production of soluble mediator(s) which are capable, alone, to induce IFN gamma production in lymphocytes. In contrast antigens activate optimally only macrophages from specifically immunized individual and, although a calcium flux in lymphocyte is still needed, it has not been established whether IFN inducing soluble mediator are required. Taking together these findings strongly suggest the hypothetical pathway for IFN gamma production shown in Fig. 1.

In the presence of T cell mitogen or oxidizing agents macrophages elaborate, along with IL-1, which alone is not capable to induce IFN, other soluble factor(s), that may trigger a calcium influx through lymphocyte membrane. This latter event leads to lymphocyte differentiation and production of IL-2 and IFN gamma, clearly involved in the modulation of immune response. On the other hand, as shown in the figure, calcium ionophores can bypass the macrophage requirement since they act directly on T lymphocyte. It remains to be established whether also specific antigens lead to production of IFN gamma through a similar sequence of events. However, since they need specifically sensitized macrophages and lymphocytes, their induction in unprimed individual may occur at later stages.

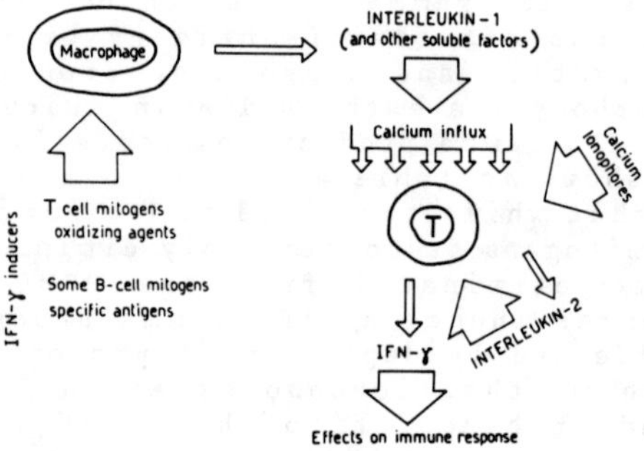

Figure 1.

One can then envisage two different pathways leading under natural conditions to IFN gamma production: one, activated by mitogenic stimuli (bacterial, viral, phagocytic, etc.), which occurs within a few hours from stimulation and one, activated by antigens in specifically sensitized lymphocytes, which requires a much longer lag. The early appearing IFN gamma could play a role on the potentiation of non specific immunity reactions, such as phagocytosis, while the other could be involved in modulation of specific immune responses.

ACKNOWLEDGEMENTS
This work was supported by a grant from CNR (P.F. "Controllo Malattie da Infezione") n. 85.00844.52.

REFERENCES

1) Abb, J., H. Abb and F. Deinhard. Characterization of human interferon gamma-producing leukocytes with monoclonal antileukocytes antibodies. Med Microbiol Immunol 171: 215, 1983.
2) Akerman, K. E.O. and L.C. Andersson. Direct mitogenic effect of ionophore A23187 on isolated human T helper lymphocytes. Eur J Immunol 14: 286, 1984.
3) Ameglio, F., M.R. Capobianchi, A. Dolei, R. Tosi. Differential effects of gamma interferon on expression of

HLA class II molecules controlled by the DR and DC loci. Infect Immun 42: 122, 1983.
4) Antonelli, G. and F. Dianzani. Induction of human interferon-gamma by calcium ionophores: lack of macrophage requirement. IRCS Med Sci 13: 59, 1985.
5) Antonelli, G., J.E. Blalock and F. Dianzani. Generation of a soluble IFN-γ inducer by oxidation of galactose residues on macrophages. Cell Immunol 94: 440, 1985.
6) Arbeit, R.D., P.L. Leary and M.J. Levin. Gamma interferon production by combinations of human peripheral blood lymphocytes, monocytes and cultured macrophages. Infect Immun 35: 383, 1982.
7) Bendtzen, K. and J. Petersen. Role of monocytes/macrophage and interleukin-1 in antigen-induced human lymphokine production. Cell Immunol 83: 101, 1984.
8) Blanchard, D.K., J.Y. Djeu, T.W. Klein, H. Friedman and W.E. Stewart. Interferon gamma induction by lipopolysaccharide: dependence on interleukin 2 and macrophages. J Immunol 136: 963, 1986.
9) Chafouleas, J.G., W.E. Bolton, H. Hidaka, A.E. Boyd and A.R. Merans. Calmoduline and the cell cycle: involvement in regulation of cell-cycle progression. Cell 28: 41, 1982.
10) Chang, T.W., D. Testa, P.C. Kung, L. Perry, H.J. Dreskin and G. Goldstein. Cellular origin and interactions involved in gamma-interferon production induced by OKT3 monoclonal antibody. J Immunol 128: 585, 1982.
11) Cole, B.C. and R.N. Thorpe. Induction of human gamma interferons by a mitogen derived from mycoplasma arthritidis and by phytoemagglutinin: differential inhibition with monoclonal anti-HLA.DR antibodies. J Immunol 131: 2392, 1983.
12) Cunningham, A.L., T.Y. Basham, M.F. Para and T.C. Merigan. Role of macrophage D-region antigens and T-lymphocyte differentiation antigens in induction of gamma interferon. J Interferon Research 5: 477, 1985.
13) Dianzani, F., T.M. Monahan, A. Scupham and M. Zucca. Enzymatic induction of interferon production by galactose oxidase treatment of human lymphoid cells. Infect Immun 26: 979, 1979.
14) Dianzani, F., T.M. Monahan, J. Georgiades and J.B. Alperin. Human immune interferon: induction in lymphoid cells by a calcium ionophore. Infect Immun 29: 561, 1980.
15) Dianzani, F., T.M. Monahan and M. Santiano. Membrane alteration responsible for the induction of gamma interferon. Infect Immun 36: 915, 1982.
16) Dianzani, F., M.R. Capobianchi and J. Facchini. Role of calcium in gamma interferon induction: inhibition by calcium entry blockers. J Virol 50: 964, 1984.
17) Dianzani, F., M. Santiano, U. Ramenghi, M.R. Capobianchi, G. Antonelli. Membrane events leading to interferon-γ induction by antigens. Proc Soc Exp Biol Med 178: 139, 1985.
18) Dianzani, F. and G. Antonelli. Macrophage-T lymphocyte cooperation for induction of gamma interferon. J Cell

Biochem 10c: 237, 1986.
19) Epstein, L.B., M.J. Cline and T.C. Merigan. The interaction of human macrophages and lymphocytes in the phytohemagglutinin-stimulated production of interferon. J Clin Invest 50: 744, 1971.
20) Epstein, L.B., H.W. Kreth and L.A. Herzenberg. Fluorescence activated cell sorting of human T and B lymphocytes. II. Identification of the cell type responsible for interferon production and cell proliferation in response to mitogens. Cell Immunol 12: 407, 1974.
21) Epstein, L.B. The ability of macrophages to augment in vitro mitogen and antigen stimulated production of interferon and others mediators of cellular immunity by lymphocytes. In "Immunobiology of the macrophage" (D.S. Nelson, ed.). Academic Press, New York, 201, 1976.
22) Epstein, L.B. and S. Gupta. Human T-lymphocyte subset production of immune (gamma) interferon. J Clin Immunol 1: 186, 1981.
23) Falcoff, R. Some properties of virus and immune-induced human lymphocyte interferon. J Gen Virol 16: 251, 1972.
24) Falcoff, R., R. Oriol and S. Isacki. Lymphocyte stimulation and interferon induction by 7S anti-human lymphocyte globulin and their uni- and divalent fragments. Eur J Immunol 2: 476, 1972.
25) Friedman, R.M. and H.I. Cooper. Stimulation of interferon production in human lymphocytes by mitogens. Proc Soc Exp Biol Med 125: 901, 1967.
26) Gifford, G.E., A. Tibor and D.L. Peavy. Interferon production in mixed lymphocyte cell cultures. Infect Immun 3: 164, 1971.
27) Green, J.A., S.R. Cooperband and S. Kibrick. Immune specific induction of interferon production in cultures of human lymphocytes. Science 164: 1415, 1969.
28) Green, J.A., S.R. Cooperband, L.F. Kleinman and S. Kibrick. Immune stimulation of interferon in human leucocyte cultures by non viral antigens. Ann N Y Acad Sci 173: 736, 1970.
29) Hecht, T.T., D.L. Longo and L.A. Matis. The relationship between immune interferon production and proliferation in antigen-specific, MHC-restricted T cell lines and clones. J Immunol 131: 1049, 1983.
30) Imboden, J.B., A. Weiss and J.D. Stobo. The antigen receptor on a human T cell line initiates activation by increasing cytoplasmic free calcium. J Immunol 134: 663, 1985.
31) Johnson, H.M., G.J. Stanton and S. Baron. Relative ability of mitogens to stimulate production of interferon by lymphoid cells and to induce suppression of the in vitro immune response. Proc Soc Exp Biol Med 154: 138, 1977.
32) Kasahara, T., J.Y. Djeu, S. F. Dogherty and J.J. Oppenheim. Capacity of human large granular lymphocytes (LGL) to produce multiple lymphokines: interleukin 2, interferon, and colony stimulating factor. J Immunol 131:

2379, 1983.
33) Klein, J.R., M.S. Pasternak and M.J. Bevatess. Activation requirements for antigen- and mitogen-induced interferon-gamma release from cytotoxic T lymphocytes. J Immunol 134: 2456, 1985.
34) Landolfo S. and H. Kirchner. Comparison with monoclonal anti-Ia antibodies of antigenic determinants inducing lymphocyte proliferation and immune interferon production in primary and secondary murine mixed lymphocyte reactions. Eur J Immunol 13: 78, 1983.
35) McCombs, C., J.P. Michalski and N. Talal. Cellular interactions in lymphocyte proliferation: effect of syngeneic and xenogeneic macrophages. Cell Immunol 23: 283, 1976.
36) Metcalfe, J.C., T. Pozzan, G.A. Smith and T.R. Esketh. A calcium hypothesis for the control of cell growth. Biochem Soc Symp 45: 1, 1980.
37) Milstone, L.M. and B.H. Waksman. Release of virus inhibitor from tuberculin-sensitized peritoneal cells stimulate by antigen. J Immunol 105: 1068, 1970.
38) Mizel, S.B. Interleukin 1 and T cell activation. Immunol Rev 63: 51, 1982.
39) Munakata, T., U. Semba, Y. Shibuya, K. Kuwano, M. Akagi and S. Arai. Induction of interferon-gamma production by human natural killer cells stimulated by hydrogen peroxide. J Immunol 134: 1, 1985.
40) Novogrodski, A. and E. Katchalski. Induction of lymphocyte transformation by sequential treatment with neuraminidase and galactose oxidase. Proc Nat Acad Sci 70: 1824, 1973.
41) O'Malley, J.A., A. Nussbaum-Blumenson, D. Sheedy, B.J. Grossmayer and H. Ozer. Identification of the T cell subset that produces human interferon. J Immunol 128: 2522, 1982.
42) Pearlstein, K.T., M.A. Palladino, K. Welte and J. Vilcek. Purified human interleukin-2 enhance induction of immune interferon. Cell Immunol 80: 1, 1983.
43) Rosenstreich, D.L. and S.B. Mizel. The participation of macrophages and macrophage cell line in the activation of T lymphocytes by mitogens. Immunol Rev 40: 102, 1978.
44) Rosenthal, A.S. and E.M. Shevach. Function of macrophages in antigen recognition by Guinea pig T lymphocytes. J Exp Med 138: 1194, 1973.
45) Smith, K.A., K.J. Gilbridge and M.F. Favata. Lymphocyte activating factor promotes T-cell growth factor production by cloned murine lymphoma cells. Nature 287: 853, 1980.
46) Smith, K.A. T-cell growth factor. Immunol Rev 51: 337, 1980.
47) Steeg, P.S., R.N. Moore, H.M. Johnson and J.J. Oppenheim. Regulation of murine macrophage Ia antigen expression by a lymphokine with immune interferon activity. J Exp Med 156: 1780, 1982.
48) Stobo, J., F. Green, L. Jackson and S. Baron. Identification of mouse lymphoid cells required for

interferon production following stimulation with mitogens. J Immunol 112: 1589, 1974.
49) Torres, B.A., W.L. Farrar and H.M. Johnson. Interleukin 2 regulates immune interferon (γ-IFN) production by normal and suppressor cell cultures. J Immunol 128: 2217, 1982.
50) Unanue, E.R. The regulatory role of macrophages in antigenic stimulation. II. Symbiotic relationship between lymphocytes macrophages. Adv Immunol 31: 3, 1981.
51) Vilcek, J., Y.K. Yip, D.S. Stone-Wolf and R.H.L. Pang. Stimulation of gamma interferon production by TPA and related diterpene esters. In "The Interferon System-a review to 1982" ed. by S. Baron, F. Dianzani and G.H. Stanton pag. 108.
52) Wallen, W.C., J.H. Dean and D.O. Lucas. Interferon and the cellular immune response: separation of interferon producing cells from DNA synthetic cells. Cell Immunol 6: 110, 1973.
53) Wheelock, E.F. Interferon-like virus inhibitor induced in human leukocytes by phytohemagglutinin. Science 169: 310, 1965.
54) von Wussow, P., C.D. Platsoucas, M. Wiranowska-Stewart and W.E. Stewart II. Human gamma interferon production by leukocytes induced with monoclonal antibodies recognizing T cells. J Immunol 127: 6, 1981.
55) Yip, Y.K., R.H.L. Pang, J.D. Oppenheim, M.S. Nachbar, D. Henriksen, I. Zerebeckyj-Eckhardt and J. Vilcek. Stimulation of human gamma interferon production by diterpene esters. Infect Immun 34: 131, 1981.
56) Youngner, J.S. Interferon production by nonviral stimuli of microbial origin. J Gen Physiol 56: 25, 1970.
57. Youngner, J.S. and S.B. Salvin. Production and properties of migration inhibitory factor and interferon in the circulation of mice with delayed hypersensitivity. J. Immunol 111: 1914, 1973.

TABLE 1. MITOGENIC AND ANTIGENIC INDUCTION OF IFN GAMMA IN PBMC TREATED WITH BETA-GALACTOSIDASE[a].

	IFN GAMMA PRODUCTION (Log_{10}) BY CELLS TREATED WITH:	
Inducer	None	Beta-galactosidase
None	<1.0	<1.0
Galactose oxidase	3.0	1.0
Con-A	2.5	1.0
PHA	2.2	<1.0
SEA	2.5	<1.0
Sodium periodate	1.8	<1.0
PPD[b]	2.0	<1.0
Tetanus toxoid[b]	1.7	<1.0

a. Experimental details in (15).
b. Specifically sensitized PBMC were used.

TABLE 2. IFN GAMMA PRODUCTION IN THE BOYDEN CHAMBER[a].

Cells in the Upper chamber	Cells in the Lower chamber	IFN IU/ml in the lower chamber
GO-treated macrophages	PBMC	1000
non-treated macrophages	PBMC	<3
GO-treated macrophages	lymphocytes	1000

a. Experimental details in (5).

TABLE 3. IFN GAMMA INDUCTION BY CULTURE COMBINATION OF LYMPHOCYTES AND MACROPHAGES FROM BCG-IMMUNIZED MICE AND MACROPHAGES FROM UNIMMUNIZED ANIMALS.

	IFN yield (IU/ml) after addition of sensitized lymphocytes on macrophages derived from:	
PPD (µg/ml) concentration	Unimmunized animals	Immunized animals
none	<4	<4
0.01	<4	<4
0.1	<4	8
1	<4	32±8
10	<4	64±16
100	64±16	128±32
1000	64±16	128±32

TABLE 4. IFN GAMMA PRODUCTION BY CONTROL AND MACROPHAGE-DEPLETED PBMC[a].

IFN inducers	IFN GAMMA IU/ml in: control	macrophage-depleted
Ionomycin	300	300
Calcium ionophore A23187	300	300
Galactose Oxidase	1000	10
Staphylococcal enterotoxin	1000	10
Concanavalin A	300	10

a. Experimental details in (4).

5. Nonviral Microbial Inducers of Interferon

Douglas A. Weigent,[a] G. John Stanton,[b] and Samuel Baron[b]

[a]Department of Physiology and Biophysics, University of Alabama at Birmingham, Birmingham, AL 35216; [b]Department of Microbiology, University of Texas Medical Branch, Galveston, TX 77550

INTRODUCTION

Interferon is well established as a natural defense against viruses. Although originally described as an antiviral activity, the possibility that IFN may serve to protect the host against bacterial and protozoal infections has also recently been strongly supported. The present review summarizes some of the evidence supporting a role for IFN in the defense against bacteria, mycoplasma, chlamydia, rickettsia, and protozoa. The main support comes from both the ability of these nonviral agents to induce IFN and also the fact that they are sensitive to the effects of IFNs in experimental animal models.

INDUCTION OF IFN BY NONVIRAL AGENTS

IFN is induced by a large number of bacteria, both gram positives and gram negatives, by chlamydia, mycoplasma, rickettsia, and by protozoa. Many of these agents have been shown to induce IFNs in animals and in cell cultures (reviewed in detail in 1,2). More recent evidence has added to the list of the number of bacteria that induce IFN as well as identified several inducer molecules. Our interest in IFN as a possible defense against bacteria began with the observation that several hundred units could be detected in middle ear fluids during acute otitis media from which no virus could be isolated but from which pathogenic bacteria (e.g., pneumococci, hemophilus, streptococci, staphylococci) could be isolated (3). In other studies and because streptococci were good IFN inducers, we decided to examine the ability of subcellular fractions including the M protein to induce IFN. The results showed that structurally defined peptide fragments of M proteins rapidly induced gamma IFN (4). Additional reports show that a wide range of bacteria can induce IFN (5,6). More specifically, streptococcal extracts such as OK-432 (7) and TH-69 (8,9) can induce IFN. Similarly, IFN gamma can be induced in peripheral blood leukocytes stimulated with mycoplasma (10,11) and rickettsia (12).

There is also growing evidence that IFN may play a role in the natural protection against certain protozoal infections. There are a number of reports that IFN is produced in reasonable quantities during infections by malaria organisms (13-17), toxoplasma (18-21), trypanasomes (22-24), and leischmania (25). It is not yet clear whether the inducer in these infections is derived from the organism or whether the IFN is a result of the immune response.

POSSIBLE PROTECTION BY IFN AGAINST NONVIRAL AGENTS

Additional evidence that IFN may play a natural role in the defense against nonviral agents are the observations that: (1) IFN can be protective against infection, and (2) the identification of antibacterial mechanisms that may be activated by IFN. The studies by Degre and his colleagues (26-29) have shown that under certain conditions, IFN can induce protection against bacterial infection. We have extended such studies using a lethality model in mice challenged with S. pneumoniae (see below) (30). In one study of IFN-inhibited multiplication of Shigella organisms, it has been shown that pretreatment of human cells with human alpha IFN protected against Salmonella organisms but not against Shigella organisms (29). Under other conditions, S. flexneri-infected HeLa cells can be recognized and destroyed by peripheral blood leukocytes which have NK cell activity (32). Similarly, there are reports of IFN inhibition of histoplasma capsulatum (33), Chlamydia psittaci (34,35), Rickettsia prowazekii (12), and E. coli (27). Transfer of endogenous IFN has also been shown to be protective in mice infected with malarial organisms (14). Taken together, the available and growing evidence indicates that a large number of bacteria can induce IFN during infection, that some of the bacterial infections can be controlled by the IFN, and that effector leukocytes, activated by IFN, often play an important role in this protection.

POSSIBLE PROTECTION BY IFN AGAINST STREPTOCOCCUS PNEUMONIAE

Our previous in vitro studies showed that treatment of mouse spleen cells with M+ protein strains resulted predominately in the induction of IFNγ whereas treatment with M- protein bacteria resulted in no IFN induction (4). The antiviral activity stimulated in mice treated with S. pyogenes M+ or M- bacteria, however, was partially neutralized by antiserum to IFNα/β and IFNγ and was neutralized to undetectable levels by a combination of the antisera (30). To determine whether pretreatment with heat-killed IFN-inducing M protein positive S. pyogenes strains significantly protects against pneumococcal infection in vivo, we injected mice with various M+ or M- organisms and 5 hours later challenged them with S. pneumoniae type 25. The results using different paired strains of bacteria showed that the M+ strain treated groups consistently showed a greater percent survival than their M- counterparts (30). Thus, M+ S. pyogenes, but not M- organisms, contribute to protection against pneumococcus and the protection correlated with the induction of IFN. In additional experiments (data not shown), we have observed that heat-killed pneumococci protect against challenge by the homologous organism. To further study the role of IFN during pneumococcal infections, we tested the effect of IFN deletion by treatment with antibodies to IFN on the survival of mice against pneumococcal challenge (i.e., without any M protein treatment). Groups of mice were treated with either an antibody to IFNα/β or a monospecific antibody developed to a synthetic N terminal peptide of IFNγ; at the same time, heat-killed M+ organisms were injected into these mice. Table 1 shows that antibodies (500 units) to IFNα/β and monospecific antibodies to IFNγ abrogate the protection provided by heat-killed M+ bacteria. To demonstrate the importance of IFN alone in the protection against pneumococcal disease, the mortality for mice given IFNγ or IFNα/β and then challenged 5 hr later with pneumococci was compared to mice given pneumococci only. Table 2 shows that treatment with 1,000 units of IFNγ or 10,000 units of IFNα/β per animal resulted in a delay of mortality compared with controls. After 7 days, 63-80% out of 30 mice were alive in either IFN group for either outbred ICR or inbred Balb/c mice, whereas in the control group no mice survived ($p < 0.05$). Levels of IFNγ and IFNα/β as low as 100 units per mouse per single treatment were effective in providing protection (data not shown). Taken together, the data strongly support a role for IFN either directly or indirectly in protection against pneumococcal infections.

MECHANISMS OF IFN-MEDIATED PROTECTION AGAINST NONVIRAL AGENTS

The mechanisms by which bacteria can be inhibited by IFN are incompletely understood. Under some conditions, the IFN may activate phagocytes such as macrophages to confer protection against bacterial and protozoal infection (13-15, 33,35,36). IFN may also act by activating natural cytotoxic cells (37,38). Our studies (38) have shown that cell-mediated cytotoxicity against normal human fibroblasts was dependent on treatment of the fibroblasts with *Streptococcus pneumoniae*. Both spontaneous and IFN-enhanced lymphocytes killed human foreskin (HFS) or skin muscle cells cocultured with *S. pneumoniae* five- to eightfold more than control nontreated cells. The human IFN produced from mixtures of HFS cells, lymphocytes, and *S. pneumonia* was a mixture of IFNα and IFNγ and in an amount 500 times greater than that observed with lymphocytes on HFS cells alone, and it was in an amount 12 times greater than when lymphocytes and bacteria were cultured together. A mixture of antibodies to IFNα and γ added to cocultures of fibroblasts and bacteria blocked the killing of fibroblast targets by lymphocytes (47 versus 13%). Thus, endogenously produced IFN was essential for the effective killing of the fibroblasts. The observation that normal diploid cells exposed to bacteria can be killed by lymphocytes suggests that natural cytotoxic cells are active at the site of bacterial infection and conceivably play roles in defense or pathogenesis. Administration of IFN to mice with staphylococcal infection promoted elimination of the bacteria from their organs and increased the phagocytic activity of the peritoneal macrophages against the staphylococci. Addition of IFNα to antibiotic therapy of patients with purulent septic infections of staphylococcal etiology markedly increased its efficiency (39). Peritoneal exudate cells and splenic cells of mice infected with *Listeria monocytogenes* show increased production of IFNγ after antigen or mitogen stimulation. The results indicate that IFNγ production is required for the in vivo generation of activated macrophages and the clearance of bacteria during *Listeria* infection (40). Furthermore, T cell dependent elimination of bacteria during the late stages of infection has been implicated as an IFN mechanism during infection with Listeria monocytogenes (41). Most of these antibacterial mechanisms seem to be mediated by effector leukocytes, but it remains to be determined whether a more direct antibacterial action of the IFN can also occur (31).

The mechanism of protection of mice from malarial organisms (14), as well as that against T. cruzi (42-48) and Leishmania (44-48), involve macrophage and perhaps NK cell activation. In mice and rats infected with sporozoites of Plasmodium berghei, mouse and rat IFNγ's strongly inhibited the development of the exoerythrocytic forms in the liver cells of the hosts, but not the development of the erythrocytic stages. Human IFNγ also diminished the parasitemia in chimpanzees infected with sporozoites of the human malaria parasite Plasmodium vivax. The target of IFNγ activity may be the infected hepatocytes themselves, as shown by in vitro experiments in which small doses of the human lymphokines inhibited the development of exoerythrocytic forms of Plasmodium berghei in a human hepatoma cell line (49). Perhaps other effector cells may be involved in the IFN-induced protection. Interestingly, synergistic protection by specific antibodies and IFN against T. cruzi infection has been reported in an in vitro situation (50).

CONCLUSIONS

The available evidence strongly supports a role for endogenous IFN in protection against nonviral infections. The evidence centers around induction of IFN during the infections, protection by IFN against certain of these infections, and the identification of mechanisms activated by IFN. The mechanisms of protection against nonviral agents are thought to be mediated by phagocytic cells, especially macrophages and more recently natural killer lymphocytes.

To prove whether IFN has any biological role in nonviral infections, more data are needed on the chemistry of nonviral IFN inducer molecules, the phenotype of IFN producer cells, and the identification of other cells that nonviral agents may interact to influence the outcome of these infections.

REFERENCES

1. Baron, S., V. Howie, M. Langford, E.M. Macdonald, G.J. Stanton, and D.A. Weigent: Induction of the interferon protein by bacteria. Tex Rep Biol Med 41:150, 1982.
2. Stewart, W.E. II.: III. Interferon inducers. In: The Interferon System, eds. Springer Verlag, pp. 27-57, 1979.
3. Howie, V., R.B. Pollard, K. Kleyn, B. Lawrence, T. Peskuric, K. Paucker, and S. Baron: Presence of IFN during bacterial otitis media. J Infec Dis 145:811, 1982.
4. Weigent, D.A., E.H. Beachey, T. Huff, J.W. Peterson, G.J. Stanton, and S. Baron: Induction of human gamma interferon by structurally defined polypeptide fragments of Group A streptococcal M protein. Infect Immun 43:122, 1984.

5. Gore, M.M., N. Kedarnath, A.C. Banerjia, S.V. Ranbhor, and S.N. Ghosh: Interferon induction by formalinized Staphylococcus aureus (Cowen x) in human mononuclear leukocytes. Indian J Med Res 77:770, 1983.
6. Ronnblom, L., A. Forsgren, and G.V. Alm: Characterization of interferons induced by bacteria and interferon producing leukocytes in peripheral blood. Infect Immun 40:126, 1983.
7. Kaneto, E., H. Sasaki, I. Tamura, O. Kurimura, and T. Kurimura: Interferon-alpha in serum and carcinomatous pleural effusion after repeated intrapleural injections of antitumor agents. Biken Journal 26:99, 1983.
8. Saito, M., T. Ebina, M. Koi, T. Yamaguchi, Y. Kawade, and N. Ishida: Inductions of interferon gamma in mouse spleen cells by OK-432, a preparation of Streptococcus pyogenes. Cell Immunol 68:187, 1982.
9. Yamaguchi, T., Y. Kuroda, M. Saito, T. Ebina, F. Hoshino, and N. Ishida: Immune interferon production by TH69, a lypholized preparation of treptococcus frecalis, in murine spleen cell cultures. Microbiol Immunol 28:601, 1984.
10. Cole, B.C. and R.N. Thorpe: Induction of human gamma interferons by a mitogen derived from mycoplasma arthritidis and by phytohemagluttinin: Differential inhibition with monoclonal anti-HLA.Dr antibodies. J Immunol 131:2392, 1983.
11. Moritz, T., D. Giebler, E. Gunther, W. Nicklas, and H. Kirchner: Lymphoproliferative responses of spleen cells of inbred rat strains to mycoplasma arthritidis mitogen. Scand J Immunol 20:365, 1984.
12. Turco, J. and H.H. Winkler: Cloned mouse interferon gamma inhibits the growth of Rickettsia prowazekii in cultured mouse fibroblasts. J Exp Med 158:2159, 1983.
13. Jahiel, R.I., J. Vilcek, R. Nussenzweig, and J. Vanderberg: Interferon inducers protect mice against Plasmodium berghei malaria. Science 161:802, 1968.
14. Huang, K.: Effect of interferon on phagocytosis. Tex Rep Biol Med 35:350, 1977.
15. Schultz, W.W., K. Huang, and F.B. Gordon: Role of interferon in experimental mouse malaria. Nature 220:709, 1968.
16. Druilhe, P., A. Rhodes-Feuillette, M. Canivet, P. Boulland, J. Pieries, and M. Gentilini: Production of circulating interferon in human malaria. Bull Soc Pathol Exot Filiales 76:34, 1983.
17. Ockenhouse, C.F., S. Schulman, and H.L. Shear: Induction of crises forms in the human malaria parasite Plasmodium falciparum by gamma interferon activated, monocyte derived macrophages. J Immunol 133:1601, 1984.
18. Remington, J.S. and T.C. Merigan: Interferon: Protection of cells infected with an intracellular protozoan (Toxoplasma gondii). Science 161:804, 1968.
19. Degre, M.: Interferon production and prevention of viral infections in mice by components of a mixed bacterial vaccine. Acta Path Microbiol Scand B80:478, 1972.
20. Omata, Y., K. Yagami, H. Sakurai, A. Saito, and N. Suzuki: Interferon production in Toxoplasma gondii infected mice. Zentralbe Bakteriol Mikrobiol Hyg 255:392, 1983.

21. Omata, Y., K.K. Sethi, and H. Brandis: Analysis of the roles of immune interferon and colony stimulating factor(s) in the induction of macrophage anti-toxoplasma activity. Immunobiology 166:146, 1984.
22. Schmunis, G.A. and A. Szarfman: Congenital Chagas' disease. Medicina 37:47, 1977.
23. Schmunis, G., M. Weissenbacher, E. Chowchuvech, L. Sawicki, M.A. Galin, and S. Baron: Growth of Toxoplasma gondii in various tissue cultures treated with In.Cn or interferon. Proc Soc Exp Biol Med 143:1153, 1973.
24. Rytel, M.W. and P.D. Marsden: Induction of an interferon-like inhibitor by Trypanosoma cruzi infection in mice. J Trop Med Hyg 19:929, 1970.
25. Herman, R. and S. Baron: Effects of interferon inducers on the intracellular growth of the protozoan parasite, Leishmani donovani. Nature 226:168, 1970.
26. Degre, M. and H. Rollag, Jr.: Effect of murine interferon on phagocytosis in vitro and in vivo. Ann NY Acad Sci 350:582, 1980.
27. Degre, M., G. Sonnenfeld, H. Rollag, and B. Morland: Effect of gamma interferon preparations on in vitro phagocytosis and degradation of Escherichia coli by mouse peritoneal macrophages. J IFN Res 1:505, 1981.
28. Melby, K., T. Midtvedt, and M. Degre: Effect of human leukocyte interferon on phagocytic activity of polymorphonuclear leukocytes. Acta Path Microbiol Scand B90:181, 1982.
29. Buckholm, G. and M. Degre: Effect of human leukocyte interferon on invasiveness of Salmonella species in Hep-2 cell cultures. Infect Immun 42:1198, 1983.
30. Weigent, D.A., T.L. Huff, J.W. Peterson, G.J. Stanton, and S. Baron: Role of IFN during streptococcal infection. Microbial Path in press.
31. Gober, L.L., A.E. Friedman-Kien, E.A. Havell, and J. Vilcek: Suppression of the intracellular growth of Shigella flexneri in cell cultures by interferon preparations and polyinosinic-polycytidylic acid. Infect Immun 5:370, 1972.
32. Niesel, D., G. Klimpel, and K. Klimpel: Natural cytotoxic activity against bacteria-infected cells. J Immunol 136:1081, 1986.
33. Wu-Hsieh, B., A. Zlotnik, and D.H. Howard: T cell hybridoma produced lymphokine that activates macrophages to suppress intracellular growth of histoplasma capsulatum. Infect Immun 43:380, 1984.
34. Byrne, G.I. and D.A. Krueger: Lymphokine-mediated inhibition of chlamydia replication in mouse fibroblasts is neutralized by anti-gamma interferon immunoglobulin. Infect Immun 42:1152, 1983.
35. Rothermel, C.D., B.Y. Rubin, and H.W. Murray: Gamma interferon is the factor in lymphokine that activates human macrophages to inhibit intracellular Chlamydia psittaci replication. J Immunol 131:2542, 1983.
36. Kaufman, S.H. and V. Brinkmann: Attempts to characterize the T cell population and lymphokine involved in the activation of macrophage oxygen metabolism in murine listeriosis. Cell Immunol 88:545, 1984.
37. Yanagawa, E., A. Uchida, E.M. Kokoschka, and M. Mickosche: Natural cytotoxicity of lymphocytes and monocytes and its augmentation by OK432 in melanoma patients. Cancer Immunol Immunother 16:131, 1984.

38. Weigent, D.A., S. Baron, and G.J. Stanton: Streptococcus pneumoniae cocultured with fibroblasts enhances both interferon production and cytotoxic activity by lymphocytes. Infect Immun 49:593, 1985.
39. Zueva, V.S., V.P. Kuznetsov, and N.I. Spivak: Interferon inhibition of the development of a staphylococcal infection. Antibiot Med Biotekhnol 11:863, 1985.
40. Buchneier, N.A. and R.D. Schreiber: Requirement of endogenous interferon-gamma production for resolution of Listeria monocytogenes infection. Proc Natl Acad Sci USA 21:7404, 1985.
41. NaKane, A. and T. Minagawa: The significance of alpha/beta interferons and gamma interferon produced in mice infected with Listeria monocytogenes. Cell Immunol 88:29, 1984.
42. Quan, P.-C., B. Rager-Ziman, M. Wittner, and H.B. Tanowitz: Interferon and natural killer cells in murine Chagas disease. J Parasit 69:1164, 1983.
43. Kierszenbaum, F. and G. Sonnenfeld: Beta interferon inhibits cell infection by Trypanosoma cruzi. J Immunol 132:905, 1984.
44. Murray, H.W., B.Y. Rubin, S. Carriero, and A.M. Acosta: Reversible defect in antigen-induced lymphokine and gamma interferon generation in cutaneous leishmaniasis. J Immunol 133:2250, 1984.
45. Titus, R.G., A. Kelso, and J.A. Louis: Intracellular destruction of Leishmania tropica by macrophages activated with macrophage activating factor/interferon. Clin Exp Immunol 55:157, 1984.
46. Murray, H.W., B.Y. Rubin, and C.D. Rothermel: Killing of intracellular Leishmania donovani by lymphokine stimulated human mononuclear phagocytes. J Clin Invest 72:1506, 1983.
47. Weinstein, M.J., J.A. Waitz, and P.E. Came: Induction of resistance to bacterial infections of mice with Poly I.poly C. Nature 226:170, 1970.
48. Kirkpatrick, C.E. and J.P. Farrell: Mechanisms of depression of splenic natural killer cell function in C57BL/6 mice infected with Leishmania donovani. Cell Immunol 87:601, 1984.
49. Ferreira, A., L. Schofield, V. Enea, H. Schellekens, P. Van der Meide, W. E. Collins, R.S. Nussenzweig, and V. Nussenzweig: Inhibition of development of exoerythrocytic forms of malaria parasites by γ-interferon. Science 232:881, 1986.
50. Plata, F., J. Wietzerbin, F.G. Pono, E. Falcoff, and H. Eisen: Synergistic protection by specific antibodies and interferon against infection by Trypanosoma cruzi in vitro. Eur J Immunol 14:930, 1984.

TABLE 1. Effect of antibodies to IFN on the survival of mice injected with M positive containing S. pyogenes prior to challenge with S. pneumoniae

S. pyogenes Strain designation	Treatment[a]	Challenge	% survival Exp. 1	% survival Exp. 2
T28/150A	-	+	72	86
T28/150/A	anti-IFNγ	+	0	0
T28/150/A	anti-IFNα/β	+	0	0
-	anti-IFNα/β	+	0	0
-	anti-IFNγ	+	0	0
-	-	+	0	0

[a]Animals were injected i.p. with a total of 0.5 ml of heat-killed M+ organisms (klett = 200) and/or anti-IFN (500 units). Five hours later, 0.5 ml of S. pneumoniae type 25 was injected i.p. (10 LD_{50}) and the animals observed for seven days. Control normal rabbit serum did not alter the percent survival of challenged nontreated mice (0%) or mice treated with heat-killed M+ (80%) organisms. In all cases, nonchallenged controls either nontreated or treated with normal rabbit serum or anti-IFN serum and/or M+ organisms had 100% survival. For the 20 animals tested per group per experiment, the data are significant at a <0.05 level by the Chi-squared method (total of 40 animals per group tested).

TABLE 2. Protection of mice infected with S. pneumoniae by IFN[a]

Treatment	% survival ICR	% survival Balb/c
None	0	0
IFNγ	80	68
IFNα/β	72	63

[a]Fifteen animals per group ICR or Balb/c were injected intraperitoneally with a total of 0.5 ml of mouse IFNγ (1,000 units) or mouse IFNα/β (10,000 units). Five hours later, 0.5 ml of S. pneumoniae type 25 was injected intraperitoneally (10 LD_{50}) and the animals scored for seven days. Control inducer diluent (phosphate buffered saline) and/or mock IFN-treated and challenged animals had 0% survival. Control IFN and/or inducer alone treated and all unchallenged animals had 100% survival. The data shown are the average of two experiments for each type of mouse for a total of 30 animals used per group per mouse.

6. Chemical and Polyribonucleotide Induction of Interferons

S. E. Grossberg and J. L. Taylor

Department of Microbiology, Medical College of Wisconsin, Milwaukee, WI 53226

A variety of chemicals (reviewed in reference 1) can induce interferon (IFN) in animals and cultured cells of the reticuloendothelial system. These observations provide the basis for the expectation that highly soluble, relatively nontoxic, small-molecular-weight chemical IFN inducers even after oral administration will become available for human use. This review attempts to describe recent developments with chemical inducers, such as pyrimidinones or acridines (see Table 1), as well as discuss some recent observations with synthetic RNA polymers.

Carboxymethylacridanone. 10-Carboxymethyl-9-acridanone (CMA) is an exceptionally potent IFN inducer in mice and hamsters (1,2). Although CMA fails to induce detectable IFN in murine fibroblastic cell lines, such as L cells, it can induce IFN production in cultures of murine bone marrow-derived macrophages (3) as well as in murine T lymphocytes (4). Although resting splenic T-cells depleted of macrophages did not produce IFN after CMA treatment, interleukin 2 (IL2)-dependent T-cell lines, originally derived from concanavalin A (conA)-stimulated splenocytes, did produce IFN in response to CMA by producing only IFN-β. These T-cell lines produced either IFN-γ following induction by conA or a mixture of IFN-α and -β when infected by Newcastle disease virus (NDV) but failed to produce detectable IFN after treatment with poly(I).poly(C). Unfractionated splenocyte cultures produced IFN with all these inducers. Both Lyt $1^+ 2^-$ and Lyt $1^- 2^+$ cell lines produced IFN following CMA treatment. With prolonged culture (>16 weeks) one T-cell line lost the ability to produce IFN after treatment with conA; however, this cell line was still capable of producing detectable IFN after cells had lost their responsiveness to conA, although the response to CMA diminished with time in culture. The appearance of IFN in mouse peritoneal fluid after CMA as well as other inducers (poly(I).poly(C) and herpes simplex virus) was enhanced ≥4-fold by prior intraperitoneal (i.p.) injection of Corynebacterium parvum (5). Of interest are the observations that certain analogs of CMA, which are themselves weak or inactive inducers, when given i.p. or orally to mice before or together with CMA, enhanced serum levels 10- to

60-fold (6). Such enhancement was also demonstrated in murine bone marrow-derived macrophage cultures (7).

Teleocidin. Although IFN-γ has been shown to be produced primarily by T-cells induced by mitogenic or antigenic stimuli, it appears that other cells can also produce IFN-γ. Teleocidin, an indole alkaloid, was reported to induce IFN-γ production in one of 25 B-cell lymphoblastoid lines (8) derived from EBV-transformed lymphocytes from infectious mononucleosis patients as well as those obtained from undifferentiated lymphomas of both the Burkitt and non-Burkitt types; the single responding line was EBV-positive. Peak IFN production was approximately 100 U/ml 3 to 4 days after stimulation. Teleocidin concurrently enhanced IL-1 secretion 10-fold over levels in unstimulated cells and increased B-cell growth factor production 3-fold. Neither cell surface antigens nor production of cytoplasmic or surface immunoglobulins were altered by teleocidin. Although IL-2 was induced by teleocidin treatment of some B-cell lines, the line that produced IFN-γ failed to secrete IL-2. Thus, IFN production in B-cells does not necessarily result from IL-2 stimulation, as has been reported for T cells. Teleocidin shares some activities with another tumor promoter 12-O-tetradecanoylphorbol-13-acetate (TPA) and with the structurally unrelated, polyacetate, marine algae toxins, aplysiatoxin and debromoaplysiatoxin. In human peripheral blood lymphocytes all these compounds induced IFN-γ and lymphotoxin simultaneously (9). Stimulation of lymphocytes by phytohemagglutinin (PHA) in concert with any of these IFN inducers resulted in enhanced lymphokine production, with yields of IFN of 300-500 U/ml increasing to 5,000-8,000 U/ml in the presence of PHA stimulation. Maximum yields of IFN were achieved in 24 to 48 hours after addition of teleocidin, TPA, or the two toxins.

Dipyridamole. Dipyridamole (2,6-bis(diethanolamino)-4,8-dipiperidino-pyrimido-[5,4d]-pyrimidine) is a vasodilator and antiaggregant which has been shown to induce IFN in cells in culture. In mice injected i.p. or given oral dipyridamole, IFN is detected in serum as early as 6 hrs. Peak production of 256 IU/ml occurred 24 to 48 hrs after treatment. Higher titers of IFN were detected after oral administration of a dose of 12.5 mg/kg than following i.p. injection in doses up to 16.7 mg/kg (10). Dipyridamole has been given orally to human volunteers in 10 mg doses, and the IFN induced (about 1,000 IU/ml serum in 24-28 hrs) was neutralized by anti-HuIFN-α antibody. A hyporeactive state following oral administration persisted for 4-6 days after treatment during which time a second dose of agent induced less than 15% of the IFN detected after the initial administration (11).

Pyrimidinones. The pyrimidinone, 2-amino-5-bromo-6-methyl-4(3H)-pyrimidinone (ABMP) has IFN-inducing activity (12,13). Modification of the basic structure of this compound has led to the development of a series of related compounds which vary in their IFN inducing activity and their antiviral activity in mice. Skulnick et al. (14) synthesized 119 different 2-amino-5-halo-6-aryl-4(3H)-pyrimidinones and analyzed their IFN-inducing activity as well as their effectiveness against Semliki Forest virus (SFV) and herpes simplex virus (HSV) infections in mice; although antiviral activities against SFV and HSV correlated well, the correlation between anti-SFV activity and IFN-inducing activity was poor. Thus, the compounds may act through some antiviral mechanism that is effective against SFV and HSV infections other than IFN. Three related compounds were examined for their effect in assays of natural killer (NK) cell activity in mice. Enhanced NK cell activity was found in peritoneal exudate cells as early as 6 hrs after i.p. administration. Like the earlier studies of antiviral activity, no direct correlation was found between augmented NK activity and IFN-inducing activity (15).

The pyrimidinones appear to have a variety of effects in animals. Anthony et al. (16) found the administration of these compounds increased the survival of mice infected with <u>Listeria monocytogenes</u>, although, as in the previously cited studies, this activity did not depend upon IFN production. One pyrimidinone, 2-amino-5-bromo-6-phenyl-4-pyrimidinone, has been shown to reduce the size of athrosclerotic lesions which develop on the aortic intima of rabbits with hypercholesterolemia. A second IFN inducer, poly(I).poly(C), had similar activity, but a correlation with IFN production has not been made (17).

<u>Lectins</u>. Numerous lectins, used to induce IFN-γ in leukocyte cultures, are included here because the nature of their carbohydrate substituents affect the IFN response. Ito et al. (18) systematically examined 22 plant lectins for their IFN-inducing ability in mouse spleen cells. The lectins were divided into four subgroups based upon the ability of specific monosaccharides to inhibit lectin-associated hemagglutination. The majority of those eleven lectins inducing IFN production were members of two subgroups inhibited by D-mannose and D-glucose or N-acetyl-D-glucosamine. None of nine lectins whose cell binding was inhibited by D-galactose and N-acetyl-D-galactosamine was capable of IFN induction. Only one lectin whose binding was inhibited by fucose induced low levels of IFN. Kinetics of IFN production in response to lectins followed three patterns. Four of the lectins induced early IFN production with a peak 6 hrs after treatment. Two inducers showed biphasic induction with peaks at 6 and 48 hrs. A third group consisting of three lectins induced IFN throughout the three-day incubation period, at the end of which maximum titers were detected. The two groups of lectins which stimulated maximal IFN production by 6 hrs induced IFN of the β type. The third group of inducers induced with slower kinetics predominantly IFN-γ, with only a small α/β component. This latter group of inducers are those which have been frequently used for IFN-γ induction, namely pokeweed mitogen, <u>Lens culinaris</u> type A, and succinylated concanavalin-A. Those lectins inducing IFN-γ are also mitogenic for mouse spleen cell cultures, while those inducing IFN-β are not. The lectins whose cell binding was inhibited by D-mannose and D-glucose were mitogenic and induced IFN-γ production. In a similar study, Naruho et al. (19) examined the IFN-inducing ability of plant lectins in human leukocytes. Lectins were separated into two major groups based upon type of linkage between the carbohydrate chain and polypeptide to which the lectin binds. Seven of 17 lectins examined induced IFN-γ; six of these had carbohydrate chains bound by glycosylamine linkage of N-acetylglucosamine to

asparagine residues on polypeptides. IFN responses to lectins by mouse splenocytes and human leukocytes may differ; for example, wheat germ agglutinin induced IFN-β in mouse cell cultures but induced IFN-γ in human leukocyte cultures.

A lectin derived from the hemolymph of injured flesh-fly larvae (Sarcophaga peregrina) was also noted to stimulate the production of IFN-γ production in human leukocytes. IFN activity was detected in control cell cultures, but after two days of treatment, titers were over 2-fold higher in cultures treated with this lectin. Higher titers were found when T-cell-enriched cultures were used (20).

Little is known about the mechanisms by which IFN-γ is induced by lectins or mitogens. The addition of mezerein to an IFN-γ inducer (21,22) results in increased IFN-γ production, reflecting an increase in IFN-γ mRNA production. Treatment with inhibitors of protein synthesis, cycloheximide and puromycin, did not affect IFN-γ mRNA levels in human leukocytes or T cells induced with staphylococcal enterotoxin A. This enhancement was eliminated by cycloheximide, suggesting that some second protein may mediate this effect (22).

Polyribonucleotides. Like the IFNs, the polyribonucleotides modulate immunologic responses and alter cellular macromolecular processes, although their inhibition of cell growth seems to be less than that of the IFNs. While some other effects correlate with IFN induction, yet other effects do not. Some of these polyribonucleotides, especially poly(I).poly(C) and poly(A).poly(U), continue to be used in clinical trials in cancer patients (23-25). One of the major problems with polyribonucleotides (and other inducers) has been hyporesponsiveness after repeated injection. Recent observations indicate that higher plasma IFN levels as well as elevated NK-cell activity can be maintained after continuous i.p. infusion in mice (26). That the IFN mechanism is indeed involved in poly(I).poly(C)-induced effects is suggested by the observation that protein kinase and 2'5'A-synthetase activities were induced similarly after poly(I).poly(C) or IFN administration to mice bearing ascitic tumors of IFN-sensitive and resistant L1210 leukemia cells (27).

The formulation of poly(I).poly(C) preparations continues to receive attention. Although poly(I).poly(C) is known to be a potent inducer of HuIFN-β in human fibroblasts, it has not been thought to be an effective inducer in human leukocytes. However, when poly(I).poly(C) was suitably prepared by treatment with heat followed by gradual cooling, titers of HuIFN-α of 10,000-60,000 IU/ml was obtained from leukocyte cultures (28). The complex of poly(I).poly(C) with poly-L-lysine and carboxymethylcellulose (polyICLC) has been shown to be somewhat effective in some patients with advanced malignancies as well as considerably toxic. Purification of the carboxymethylcellulose by ethanol extraction significantly reduced its toxicity in mice and retained its IFN-inducing ability (29). However, carboxymethylcellulose not only is poorly degradable, but may also leave long-term irritating residues, and has been included in the NIOSH list of suspected carcinogens. Its replacement by carboxymethyldextran has resulted in a soluble complex that retains its effective IFN-inducing activity in mice and rhesus monkeys, but with reduced toxicity in mice (30). Another interesting derivative is poly(I).mercapto-poly(C), which is produced by thiolation of position 5 of some of the cytosine bases in poly(C) followed by annealing to poly(I). This poly(I)-MPC induced IFN-α in lymphocyte cultures somehwat less well than did poly(I).poly(C). Both polyribonucleotide preparations induced IFN activity, half of which was not inactivated by anti-HuIFN-α antibody but was destroyed at pH 2 and therefore thought to be IFN-γ. Poly(I)-MPC was less toxic than poly(I).poly(C) (31).

Poly ICLC could induce IFN in grivet monkeys that were immunosuppressed by drugs. The hyporesponsiveness following daily or alternate-day injections was not observed if injections were given every third day (32). A sex difference has recently been suggested in IFN responses to poly ICLC in patients and rhesus monkeys such that the levels of IFN were higher in males (33); the number of subjects, however, was small. One interesting effect of poly(I).poly(C) is the significant decrease in the number of thoracic duct lymphocytes, a phenonomen also seen with IFN and ablated with anti-IFN antibody (34). Poly(I).poly(C) also given i.v. reduced the number of T lymphocytes present in cerebrospinal fluid after vaccinia virus meningitis (35). An interesting mismatched polymer, poly(I).poly(C_{12}U) retains IFN-inducing and antiproliferative activities with reduced toxicity; its antitumor effect was enhanced by IFN (36).

Poly(A).poly(U) has received increasing attention clinically as well as experimentally (37). Despite its relatively poor IFN-inducing ability, at least in comparison with poly(I).poly(C), IFN-related enzymes, such as protein kinase and 2'5'A-synthetase, increase in patients following i.v. injection, with a subsequent increase in NK cells (38).

The technical conditions in the preparation of poly(G).poly(C) necessary for the full expression of its IFN-inducing activity have recently been described (39). This complex induced IFN in rabbits and mice and gave a more protracted response than did poly(I).poly(C). It was more resistant to degradation by serum nucleases but induced IFN to only very low levels in human, mouse, and rabbit cell cultures only with DEAE-dextran or after prolonged incubation. The IFN titers in human skin fibroblasts after treatment with poly(A).poly(U) or poly(G).poly(C), if the polyribonucleotides were pretreated with Mg^{++} or with ethidium bromide, were $>10^5$ units/ml (40).

Polyribonucleotides have begun to be combined with IFNs and drugs. Whereas poly(I).poly(C) alone induced 2',5'A-synthetase activity but had no effect on the associated activity of phosphodiesterase, the combination of either HuIFN-β or -α(A) and poly(I).poly(C) increased 2',5'A-phosphodiesterase activity in human colon carcinoma cells. However, there was no dose-response relation between the induction of 2',5'A and the cytostatic activity of IFN alone or in combination with dsRNA (41). On the other hand, HuIFN-γ and poly(I).poly(C) was synergistic, with a 70-90% reduction in colony formation observed (42). Whereas poly(I).poly(C) was antagonistic to the cell lethality produced by 5'-fluorouracil in human colon carcinoma cells *in vitro* (43), the antitumor effect against L1210 leukemia in mice was synergistic between fluoroprimidines and poly(I).poly(C) (44). Further, the combination of poly(I).poly(C) and indomethacin led to the greatest inhibition of carcinogen-induced bladder cancer in rats (45). Another approach has been to combine platinum, especially chloro-diethylene-triaminoplatinum (II) to poly(I).poly(C) such that both IFN induction and resistance to nuclease degradation were increased (46).

Studies on the mechanisms of induction of IFN have begun with polyribonucleotides as inducers. Readily inducible cells may have specific receptors for poly(I).poly(C) such that only about 30% is adsorbed specifically; nonspecific adsorption to cells lacking receptors may result in weak induction when transcriptional controls are altered by superinduction or priming (47). Superinduction with poly(I).poly(C) could be achieved (>100-fold in human cells and >40-fold in mouse and chicken cells) by treatment with cycloheximide and dihydrorifampicin (48). Inhibition of induction by poly(I).poly(C) was demonstrated in fibroblasts exposed to the carcinogen, benzo-(a)-pyrene, varying in part according to the genetic background of the mice from which the cells were taken (49). Nocodazole, an antitubulin drug, inhibited induction of IFN by poly(I).poly(C) but not by NDV (50).

Some progress is beginning to be made in the molecular biology of IFN induction by poly(I).poly(C). Mouse cells transfected with the HuIFN-β gene cDNA and herpesvirus thymidine kinase gene were induced by poly(I).poly(C) to form HuIFN-β, but the mechanism to switch off its continued synthesis appeared to be inoperative (51). The specific regulation of the HuIFN-β gene appears to depend upon the promoter region between nucleotides -144 and -186 from the mRNA initiation site, a sequence remarkably homologous with a consensus sequence found in the 5' flanking region of steroid-hormone-responsive genes (52). Poly(I).poly(C)-inducible expression of the HuIFN-β_1 gene linked to a bovine papilloma virus DNA vector maintained extrachromasomally was demonstrated in mouse cells (53). Finally, poly(I).poly(C) and NDV differ in their effects on the expression of IFN and cellular genes; MuIFN-β_1 was expressed well (and MuIFN-α to only low levels) by poly(I).poly(C) whereas both α and β genes were well expressed after NDV infection (54).

REFERENCES

1. Taylor, J.L. and Grossberg, S.E.: Chemical induction of interferon: carboxymethylacridanone and other low-molecular-weight chemicals. Tex. Rep. Biol. Med. 41:158, 1982.
2. Taylor, J.L., Schoenherr, C.K., and Grossberg, S.E.: High-yield interferon induction by 10-carboxymethyl-9-acridanone in mice and hamsters. Antimicrob. Agent. Chemother. 18:20, 1980.
3. Storch, E., and Kirchner, H.: Induction of interferon in bone marrow-derived macrophage cultures by 10-carboxymethyl-9-acridanone. Eur. J. Immunol. 12:793, 1982.
4. Storch, E., Kirchner, H., Brehm, G., Huller, K., and Marcucci, F.: Production of interferon-β by murine T-cell lines induced by

10-carboxymethyl-9-acridanone. Scand. J. Immunol. 23:195, 1986.
5. Storch, E., and Kirchner, H.: Interferon inducibility in mice treated with Corynebacterium parvum. Antiviral Res. 5:117, 1985.
6. Inglot, A.D., Mlochowski, J., Szulc, Z., Inglot, O., and Albin, M.: Induction of interferon in mice by sodium salt of 9-oxo-10-acridineacetic acid: specific enhancement by analogs. Archivum Immunologiae et Therapiae Experimentalis 33:275, 1985.
7. Szulc, B., Inglot, A.D., Szulc, Z., and Miochowski, J.: Competition of sodium salt of 9-oxo-10-acridineacetic acid with analogs during induction of interferon in the mouse bone marrow-drived macrophages. Archivum Immunologiae et Therapiae Experimentalis 33:287, 1985.
8. Benjamin, D., Hartman, D.P., Bazar, L.S., and Jacobson, R.J.: Burkitts cells can be triggered by Teleocidin to secrete interferon-γ. Am. J. Hematol. 22:169, 1985.
9. Yip, Y.K., Kelker, C., Stone-Wolff, D.S., Pearlstein, K., Urban, C. and Vilcek, J.: Stimulation of lymphokin production by teleocidin, aplysiatoxin, and debromoaplysiatoxin. Cell. Immunol. 79:389, 1983.
10. Galabov, A.S., and Mastikova, M.: Interferon-inducing activity of dipyridamole in mice. Acta Virol. 27:356-358.
11. Galabov, A.S., and Mastikova, M.: Dipyridamole induces interferon in man. Biomed. Pharmacother. 38:412, 1984.
12. Stringfellow, D.A., Vanderberg, H.C., and Weed, S.D.: Interferon induction by 5-halo-6-phenyl-pyrimidinones. J. Interferon Res. 1:1, 1980.
13. Stringfellow, D.A. 1984. Nonpolynucleotide inducers of interferon. Hndbk Expt. Pharmacol. 71:371-383.
14. Skulnick, H.I., Weed, S.D., Eidson, E.E., Renis, H.E., Wierenga, W., and Stringfellow, D.A.: Pyrimidinones. 1. 2-Amino-5-halo-6-aryl-4(3H)-pyrimidinones. Interferon-inducing antiviral agents. J. Med. Chem. 28:1864-1869.
15. Lotzova, E., Savary, C.A., and Stringfellow, D.A.: 5-Halo-6-phenyl pyrimidinones: new molecules with cancer therapeutic protential and interferon-inducing capacity are strong inducers of murine natural killer cells. J. Immunol. 130:965, 1983.
16. Anthony, L.S., Stevenson, M.M., and Skamene, E.: Enhancement of resistance to Leisteria monocytogenes infection in mice by pyrimidine analogs. Clin. Invest. Med. 7:343, 1984.
17. Kuo, P.T., Wilson, A.C., Goldstein, R.C., and Schaub, R.G.: Suppression of experimental athrosclerosis in rabbits by interferon-inducing agents. J. Am. Coll. Cardiol. 3:129, 1984.
18. Ito, Y., Tsurudome, M., Yamada, A., and Hishiyama, M.: Interferon induction in mouse spleen cells by mitogenic and nonmitogenic lectins. J. Immunol. 132:2440, 1984.
19. Naruho, K., Ichimori, Y., Koyama, M., and Tsukamoto, K.: Correlation of interferon gamma inducing ability to sugar-binding specificities of various lectins. J. Interferon Res. 4:235, 1984.
20. Tamura, M., and Natori, S.: Induction of human-γ interferon by Sarcophaga peregrina humoral lectin. FEBS Lett. 175:325, 1984.
21. Taylor, J.L., Sedmak, J.J., Jameson, P., Lin, Y-.G., and Grossberg, S.E.: Markedly enhanced production of gamma interferon in murine T-lymphocytes treated with lentil lectin and the diterpene ester, mezerein. J. Interferon Res. 4:315, 1984.
22. Siggens, K.W., Tinsley, J.M., and Morris, A.: Role of protein synthesis

in induction of interferon-γ by mitogens in human lymphocytes. Eur. J. Immunol. 15:1079, 1985.
23. Borden, E.C., Verman, A.K., and Wolberg, W.H.: Potential role of polyribonucleotid in human neoplastic diseases. J. Biol. Resp. Mod. 4:676, 1985.
24. Krown, S.E., Kerr, D., Stewart, W.E., II, Field, A.K., and Oettgen, H.F.: Phase I trials of poly(I,C) complexes in advanced cancer. J. Biol. Resp. Mod. 4:640, 1985.
25. Herberman, R.B., and Pinsky, C.M.: Polyribonucleotides for cancer therapy: summary and recommendations for further research. J. Biol. Resp. Mod. 4:680, 1985.
26. Rothmann, S.A., Paul, P., Oluic, T.J., Sturkie, K.A., and Proffitt, M.R.: Chronic induction of interferon by continuous infusion of polyriboinosinic: polyribocytidilic acid. J. Interferon Res. 5:273, 1985.
27. Riviere Y. and Hovanessian A.: Response of L-1210 tumor in mice toward treatment with interferon of poly(I)·poly(C). J. Interferon Res. 3:417, 1983.
28. Tamura M. and Sasakawa S..: Induction of human leukocyte interferon by heat-treated polyI:polyC. Biochem. Biophys. Res. Comm. 110:851, 1983.
29. Bello, J., O'Malley J., and Granados, E.: Purification of carboxymethylcellulose decreases toxicity of polyICLC in mice. J. Interferon Res. 5:429, 1985.
30. Granados, E.N., Dawidzik, J., O'Malley, J., McGarry, M., and Bello, J.: Poly ICL-M dextran: an interferon inducer of reduced toxicity. J. Interferon Res. 4:155-160.
31. Vastola, K.A., Ho, Y.-K., Bardos, T.J., Grossmayer, B.J., Fruck-Diviak, L. and O'Malley, J.A.: Poly I-mercapto poly C: antiviral, anticellular, and pharmacologic effects. Res. Comm. Chem. Path. Pharm. 45:407, 1984.
32. DeWitt, C.M. and Field, A.K.: Interferon response to poly IC/poly-L-lysine in normal and lymphocyte-suppressed primates. J. Interferon Res. 4:1, 1984.
33. Bever, C.T., Jr., McFarlin, D.E., and Levy, H.B.: A comparison of interferon responses to poly ICLC in males and females. J. Interferon Res. 5:423, 1985.
34. Korngold, R., Blank, K.J., and Murasko, D.M.: Effect of interferon on thoracic duct lymphocyte output: induction with either polyI:polyC or vaccinia virus. J. Immun. 130:2236, 1983.
35. Korngold, R., and Doherty, P.C.: Treatment of mice with polyinosinic-polycytidilic polyribonucleotide reduces T-cell involvement in a localized inflammatory response to vaccinia virus challenge. J. Virology 53:489, 1985.
36. Carter, W.A., Hubbell, H.R., Krueger, L.J., and Strayer, D.R.: Comparative studies of ampligen (mismatched double-stranded RNA) and interferons. J. Biol. Resp. Mod. 4:613, 1985.
37. Michelson, A.M., Lacour, F., and Lacour, J.: Polyadenylic·polyuridylic acid in the cotreatment of cancer (42055). Proc. Soc. Exp. Biol. Med. 179:1-8.
38. Hovanessian, A.G., Riviere, Y., Montagnier, L., Michelson, M., Lacour, J., Lacour, F.: Enhancement of interferon-mediated protein kinase in mouse and human plasma in response to treatment with polyadenylic-polyuridylic

acid (poly A:poly U). J. Interferon Resp. 2:209, 1982.
39. Torrence, P.F., and De Clercq, E.: Preparation and biological properties of a highly active poly(G)·poly(C) inducer of interferon. Antiviral Res. 4:339, 1984.
40. Jamison, J.M., Koo, P.H., and Tsai, C.-C.: Interferon induction in vitro by polyribonucleotides and intercalating drugs. In Molecular Basis of Cancer, Part B: Macromolecular Recognition, Chemotherapy, and Immunology, Alan R. Liss, Inc., pages 243, 1985.
41. Chapekar, M.S., and Glazer, R.I.: Effects of fibroblast and recombinant leukocyte interferons and double-stranded RNA on ppp(2'-5')A_n synthesis and cell proliferation in human colon carcinoma cells in vitro. Cancer Res 43:2683, 1983.
42. Chapekar, M.S., and Glazer, R.I.: Synergistic effect of human interferon and double-stranded RNA against human colon carcinoma cells in vitro. Cancer Res. 45:2539, 1985.
43. Iigo, M., and Glazer, R.K.: Antagonistic effect of polyinosinic-poly-cytidylic acid on the cell lethality produced by 5-fluorouracil in human colon carcinoma cells in vitro. Cancer Res. 45:1953, 1985.
44. Iigo, M., Chapekar, M.S., and Glazer, R.I.: Synergistic antitumor effect of fluoropyrimidines and polyinosinic-polycytidylic acid against L1210 leukemia. Cancer Res. 45:4039, 1985.
45. Droller, M.J., and Gomolka, D.: Indomethacin and poly I:C in the inhibition of carcinogen-induced bladder cancer in an experimental animal model. J. Urology 131:1212, 1984.
46. De Clercq, E., Hermann, D., and Guschlbauer, W.: Interferon induction by platinum(II)·poly(O)·poly(C) complexes. Biochimica et Biophysica Acta, 741:358-363.
47. Yoshida, I., and Azuma, M.: Adsorption of poly rI:rC on cell membrane participating and nonparticipating in interferon induction. J. Interferon Res. 5:1, 1985.
48. Kara, J., Tazulakhova, E.B., Sokolova, T.M., and Ershov, F.I.: Regulation of interferon production. Superinduction by dihydrorifampicin in human and chick embryo fibroblasts and mouse L929 cells. Acta Virol. 27: 130, 1983.
49. Golemboski, K.A., and Sonnenfeld, G.: Genetics of susceptibility of mice to inhibition of interferon induction by benzo-(a)-pyrene. J. Interferon Res. 4:329, 1984.
50. Fleit, H.B.: Nocodazole inhibits polyI:C induction of interferon by mouse macrophages. J. Interferon Res. 3:479, 1983.
51. Pitha, P.M., Ciufo, D.M., Kellum, M., Raj, N.B.K., Reyes, G.R., and Hayward, G.S.: Induction of human β-interferon synthesis with poly(rI.rC in mouse cells transfected with cloned cDNA plasmids. Proc. Natl. Acad. Sci. USA, 79:4337, 1982.
52. Tavernier, J., Gheysen, D., Duerinck, F., Van der Heyden, J., and Fiers, W.: Deletion mapping of the inducible promoter of human IFN-β gene. Nature 301:634, 1983.
53. Mitrani-Rosenbaum, S., Maroteaux, L., Mory, Y., Revel, M., and Howley, P.M.: Inducible expression of the human inerferon β_1 gene linked to a bovine papilloma virus DNA vector and maintained extrachromosomally in mouse cells. Mol. Cell. Biol. 3:233, 1983.
54. Kelley, K.A., and Pitha, P.M.: Differential effect of poly rI·rC and Newscastle disease virus on the expression of interferon and cellular genes in mouse cells. Virology 147:382, 1985.

55. Smejkal, F., Zelena, D., Krepelka, J., and Vancurova, I.: Derivatives of benzo(c)fluorene. VI. Antiviral and interferon-inducing activities of three benzo(c)fluorenone derivatives in mice. Acta virol. 29:11, 1984.
56. Munakata, T., Semba, U., Shibuya, Y., Kuwano, K., Akagi, M., and Arai, S.: Induction of interferon-γ production by human natural killer cells stimulated by hydrogen peroxide. J. Immunol. 134:2449, 1985.
57. Sakai, A., Ebina, T., and Ishida, N.: Interferon induction in mice by oral administration of K-582, a new peptide antibiotic. J. Antibiotics 3:335, 1982.
58. Miyakoshi, H., and Aoki, T.: Acting mechanisms of lentinan in human--II. Enhancement of non-specific cell-mediated cytotoxicity as an interferon inducer. Int. J. Immunopharmac. 6:373, 1984.
59. Matsuura, M., Kojima, Y., Homma, Y., Kubota, Y., Shibukawa, N., Shibata, M., Inage, M., Kusumoto, S., and Shiba, T.: Interferon-inducing, pyrogenic and proclotting enzyme of horseshoe crab activation activities of chemically synthesized lipid A analogues. Eur. J. Biochem. 137:639, 1983.
60. Stevenson, H.C., Dekaban, G.A., Miller, P.J., Benyajati, C., and Pearson, M.L.: Analysis of human blood monocyte activation at the level of gene expression: Expression of alpha interferon genes during activation of human monocytes by poly IC/LC and muramyl dipeptide. J. Exp. Med. 161:503, 1985.

TABLE 1. Chemical inducers of interferon

Inducer	Production in	IFN type	Reference
Carboxymethylacridanone	Murine T-cell lines	β	(4)
"	Murine macrophage	α/β	(3)
Benzo(c)fluorenone	Mice	?	(55)
Dipyridamole	Mice	?	(10)
"	Mice	α	(11)
Pyrimidinones	Mice	α	(14)
Teleocidin	Human peripheral blood leukocytes	γ	(9)
"	Human B cell line	γ	(8)
Hydrogen peroxide	Human NK cells	γ	(56)
K-582 septapeptide from *Metarhizium anisopliae*	Mice	α/β	(57)
Lentinan glucan from *Lentinus edodes*	Human peripheral mononuclear cells	γ	(58)
Lipid A analogues	Reticuloendothelial cell cultures	?	(59)
Muramyl dipeptide	Monocytes	α	(60)
Lectins	Murine spleen cells	γ	(18,21)
"	Murine spleen cells	γ and β	(19)

7. Regulation of Interferon Production and Hyporesponsiveness

Dale A. Stringfellow

Cancer Research, Bristol-Myers Pharmaceutical Research and Development, Wallingford, CT 06492-7660

INTRODUCTION:

Like most native biologically active proteins, cellular production of interferons is a carefully regulated process. The diverse biologic effects of interferons on cellular function, including cellular division rate, suggest that a cell would stringently regulate production of such a molecule. Such a control process has now been observed experimentally and in the clinic (1-3). When animals, including humans, are exposed to any of a variety of interferon inducing agents, they temporarily lose their ability to respond fully to the same inducing stimulus (Table 1) (2-3). Likewise, cells in culture when exposed to inducers are transiently (up to 48 hours) unresponsive to restimulation (1). This phenomena has been referred to as hyporesponsiveness and appears to be similar to tachyphylaxis which has been described for other native pharmacologically active proteins or peptides.

The precise process by which interferon synthesis is regulated is, however, not well understood. In a series of studies designed to probe this regulatory process, no differences were detected between normal and hyporeactive cells with regard to rate of protein, RNA or DNA synthesis, interferon messenger RNA turnover, inducer uptake or cellular division rate or morphology (4). The only consistent difference noted was that hyporeactive cells had lower adenylatecyclase and intracellular cAMP levels.

This observation prompted a subsequent series of studies to try to determine if agents that modulate adenylatecyclase activity and subsequent intracellular cAMP levels could modulate interferon responsiveness. Although such a correlation could not be demonstrated, the data from these studies suggested that hyporeactive cells would respond to interferon induction similarly to normal cells if the interferon inducer was administered concomitantly with any of several prostaglandins (5-6). This observation was subsequently confirmed in vivo in the intact animal (Table 2). Likewise, prostaglandins could increase the therapeutic activity of inducers in hyporeactive Friend leukemia virus infected mice suggesting a corresponding therapeutic benefit of co-administration of inducers with prostaglandins in virus infected hyporeactive mice (7-8).

The phenomena of hyporeactivity to interferon induction has also been observed in animals infected with any of several viruses or carrying L1210 or P388 leukemia (9) (Figure 1). In both virus infected and leukemic animals, a protein was detected in the serum of virus infected mice that could transfer the hyporesponsiveness observed in vitro to otherwise normal cells cultured in vitro (10). Although the exact nature of the protein has yet to be determined, this suggested that a protein is involved in regulation of the responsiveness of animals to interferon induction. The inter-relationship between this protein and prostaglandin restoration of interferon responsiveness is at present unclear.

Further evidence that a protein or polypeptide is involved in regulation of interferon synthesis is provided by studies of superinduction in fibroblast cells induced to synthesize interferon-beta. In general, the expression of interferon is stringently controlled and cells do not usually synthesize interferon in the absence of an external stimulus (11-12). Furthermore, the induction process appears to follow a single step kinetics suggesting that a mechanism is normally operational that limits interferon synthesis which is induced soon after cells are stimulated to produce interferon. By treating induced cells with a combination of actinomycin D and cycloheximide at the early stages of the induction process, cells respond by producing up to 10 times more interferon than normally induced cells (13). This phenomena has been referred to as superinduction and suggests that a protein is involved in the down regulation of interferon synthesis. This regulatory protein appears to be induced early during the induction of interferon synthesis and serves to counterbalance the induction process.

The kinetics of the interferon response and superinduction support the hypothesis that a regulatory peptide or protein is involved in down regulation of the interferon response. The hyporesponsive period that follows induction may represent the period of time needed for decay of the regulatory protein before the cells are capable of again being stimulated to produce more interferon. Whether interferon alpha or gamma are similarly regulated is unclear at present and whether this hypothesized protein is the same protein that has been isolated from the serum of hyporeactive animals is also unclear.

SUMMARY:

As with most potent physiologically active native proteins, the synthesis and production of interferons is a stringently controlled and at least for interferons is presently a poorly understood process. Cells and intact animals become temporarily unresponsive or hyporeactive to re-stimulation by the same or related inducing agents. Evidence points to the existence of a regulatory protein produced by cells early during the induction process that serves to down regulate interferon synthesis. Such a protein has been detected in the serum of virus infected hyporeactive mice, but it is presently unclear if it is the same or a related protein to the hypothesized cellular associated regulatory protein. Prostaglandins administered concomitantly with inducers can overcome hyporesponsiveness in vivo and likewise in vitro cells taken from hyporeactive animals can become responsive by exposure to prostaglandins. The inter-relationship of these observations with the hypothesized regulatory protein is not presently understood. Understanding this regulatory process is important in understanding viral pathogenesis and ways of developing and optimally utilizing interferon inducing agents clinically as antiviral and antineoplastic agents.

REFERENCES

1. Borden, E.C., E.V. Prochownik, and W.A. Carter: The interferon refractory protein. J Immun 114:752, 1975.
2. Stringfellow, D.A. and L.A. Glasgow: Tilorone hydrochloride, an oral interferon inducing agent. Antimic Ag Chemoth 2:73, 1972.
3. Krown S., H. Oettgen, W. Stewart, and H.B. Levy: Phase I trials of poly ICLC in cancer patients. In: Proceedings of Symposium on Biological Modifiers in Cancer Treatment of Cancer, M. Chrigos, ed Raven Press, NYC, 1980.
4. Stringfellow, D.A.: Interferon inducers - Theory and experimental application. In: Interferon and Interferon Inducers - Clinical Applications, D.A. Stringfellow ed. Marcel Dekker, Inc., NYC, 1980.
5. Stringfellow, D.A.: Prostaglandin restoration of the interferon response of hyporeactive animals. Science 201:376, 1978.
6. Sinzinger, H., H. Ludwig, W. Linkesch, H. Gisslinger, and R. Flener: Interaction between interferon and the prostaglandin system. ACTA Medica Austriaca 12:73, 1985.
7. Stringfellow, D.A.: Antiviral and interferon inducing properties of interferon inducers administered with prostaglandins. Antimic Ag Chemoth 17:455, 1980.
8. Zor, U., R. Bendori, I. Maoz, D. Wallach, and D. Gurarirotman: Inhibition by glucocorticosteroid hormones of interferon and prostaglandin E induction by poly I:C. J Gen Virol 63:359, 1982.
9. Stringfellow, D.A.: Murine leukemia - depressed response to interferon induction correlated with a serum hyporeactive factor. Inf Imm 13:392, 1976.
10. Stringfellow, D.A., E.R. Kern, D.K. Kelsey, and L.A. Glasgow: Suppressed interferon response in mice infected with viruses. J Inf Dis 135:540, 1977.
11. Ho, M. and J.A. Armstrong: Accentuation of production of murine interferon by metabolic inhibitors. Proc Soc Expt Biol Med 193:295, 1972.
12. Smith-Johannsen, H., Y.T. Hon, X.Y. Liu, and Y.H. Tan: Regulatory control of interferon synthesis and action. In: Interferons and Their Actions, P.E. Came and W.A. Carter, ed. Springer Verlag, NYC, pp. 101-136, 1984.
13. Havell, E.A. and J. Vilcek: Production of high titered interferon in cultures of human diploid fibroblasts. Antimic Ag Chemoth 2:47, 1974.

TABLE 1. Serum Interferon Response to Daily Doses of Inducer

	DAILY DOSE				
Inducer	1	2	3	4	5
Poly I:C	5,500*	3,500	900	300	50
Tilorone	12,000	300	<50	<50	<50
ABPP	7,500	2,000	950	50	<50
NDV	5,000	500	<50	<50	<50

* Maximum serum interferon response following daily administration of the same inducer. Poly I:C (100μg, ip), Tilorone (250mg/kg, po), ABPP (500mg/kg, po), and NDV (10^6 PFU, ip).

TABLE 2. Serum interferon response in mice infected with encephalomyocarditis (EMC) virus and injected with inducer with and without prostaglandin (1mg/kg, ip). The doses of inducers were: tilorone, (250mg/kg, po), poly I:C (100μg, ip) and ABPP (500mg/kg, po).

INDUCER		PROSTAGLANDIN			
		A_1	E_1	$F_1\alpha$	PBS
Poly I:C	(EMC infected)	3,000*	4,000	3,200	500
	(uninfected control)	5,500	3,500	3,800	2,500
Tilorone	(EMC infected)	2,000	5,500	1,000	350
	(uninfected control)	3,500	6,000	2,500	5,000
ABPP	(EMC infected)	4,000	2,100	1,500	400
	(uninfected control)	4,100	4,700	3,300	2,500
PBS	(EMC infected)	<50	<50	<50	<50
	(uninfected control)	<50	<50	<50	<50

* Serum interferon, units/ml

Figure 1. Serum interferon response and serum hyporeactive factor levels in P388 leukemic mice. Interferon titers are expressed as a percentage of levels induced in normal non-tumor bearing mice. Inducers were injected as a single dose 1 to 8 days after injection of 10^6 leukemia cells ip. (See reference 9 for details.)

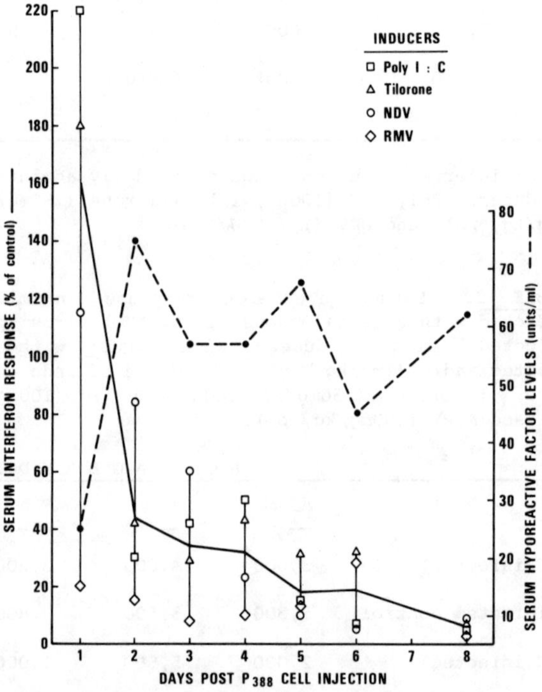

II. Large-Scale Production of Interferon

8. Production and Properties of Natural Human Leukocyte Alpha Interferon

Hanna-Leena Kauppinen[a] *and Kari Cantell*[b]

[a]Finnish Red Cross Blood Transfusion Service, 00310 Helsinki, Finland;
[b]National Public Health Institute, 00280 Helsinki, Finland

INTRODUCTION

Studies on human leukocyte interferon (IFN) have been carried out in Finland since 1963 (2). In 1971 pilot scale production was started at the Finnish Red Cross Blood Transfusion Service. In the beginning clinical studies were made with KSCN-concentrated IFN, called C-IF (22). At the same time a method was developed for the partial purification of crude IFN (4). This product, called P-IF, has been available for clinical trials since 1973. Studies to optimize production and increase IFN yield have continued (5,6,7). At present, the yield per blood unit is consistently around 7 million IU of crude IFN. After losses due to the purification and manufacturing of clinically acceptable preparations, the net yield of IFN is a little over 3 million IU (12).

Until 1978 most of the human leukocyte IFN prepared was used for antiviral studies supported by NIAID and for antitumor trials carried out by Hans Strander's group in Sweden. Then expansion of production was made possible by the decision of the American Cancer Society and the Lasker foundation to fund clinical research on leukocyte IFN with more than 2 million dollars. On account of the wide publicity caused by this decision, the production and use of IFN increased considerably. During the next few years many laboratories around the world started the preparation of human leukocyte IFN by the Finnish methods. More recently the number of producers of natural leukocyte IFN has decreased.

Successful cloning of leukocyte IFN in E. coli was reported in 1980 (16). Within a year the recombinant IFN-α2 became available for clinical trials. At about the same time large amounts of lymphoblastoid IFN produced in Namalwa cells also became available (11). Interest in clinical applications of natural leukocyte IFN appears to be declining and the clinical future of this preparation seems uncertain (3). Nevertheless, during the past few years 200 to 300 billion IU of natural leukocyte IFN have been delivered annually from Finland for clinical trials. This paper deals with the production and properties of such IFN preparations.

PRODUCTION

The method currently used for the large scale production of leukocyte IFN, embodying the latest information on its optimization, has already been described in detail (6). Therefore the method is presented here only briefly.

The main source of leukocytes is fresh donor blood, which, according to the principles of modern blood banking, is centrifuged within 6 hours to yield fresh plasma and cell concentrates. The leukocyte fraction of the blood, the buffy coat is removed to obtain a red cell concentrate with low leukocyte contamination. Routinely a 30 ml volume of the top layer of the centrifuged red cells is harvested. Fresh leukocytes, not more than one-day old, are the most potent producers of IFN. Apart from the production of IFN, there are few clinical uses for the leukocyte fraction of the blood.

At our institutes the red cells are removed from the pooled buffy coats by two successive treatments with 0.83 % NH_4Cl solution. One production batch comprises routinely 100 to 200 buffy coats. Red cells can also be removed by enhanced sedimentation (13). The leukocytes are suspended in a suitable culture medium at a concentration of 10^7 cells per ml and incubated in round bottles. The cells are primed with IFN and induced with a virus. So far the most efficient inducer found is particular "Cantell" strain of the Sendai paramyxovirus (8). Under these conditions monocytes are the main or perhaps the only producers of the IFN-α(19). After overnight incubation at 37.5°C the supernatant containing the crude IFN is separated from the cell debris by centrifugation or filtration.

Our current procedure for partial purification of crude IFN has also been published (7,14). This method with slight modifications has been used almost exclusively for the preparation of leukocyte IFN for clinical trials. Briefly, the crude IFN is precipitated at pH 3.5 with KSCN and extracted with cold 94 % ethanol. The interferons dissolve, but other proteins are denatured and removed as a precipitate. A stepwise increase of the pH leads to further precipitation of contaminating proteins, which are removed. IFN is precipitated at pH 8, dissolved, concentrated with KSCN at low pH, and finally dialyzed against phosphate buffered saline, pH 7.3. For the maximum recovery of IFN activity the purification procedure is done in batches of around 20 liters. The recovery of P-IF corresponds to 60 to 70 per cent of the crude IFN.

P-IF preparations have been purified further using NK2 monoclonal antibody (21), with a recovery of 67 % (14). This immunoadsorbent has also been used to purify crude leukocyte IFN prepurified by adsorption on controlled pore glass, with about the same recovery of activity (10).

PROPERTIES

There are at least 15 distinct, potentially functional IFN-α genes (24). Many of these genes are activated in monocytes upon induction with Sendai virus (9). When a crude leukocyte IFN preparation was purified with a series of monoclonal anti-IFN-α antibodies, 23 species of IFN-α were identified by HPLC chromatography (25). The IFN-α subtypes α1(D), α2(A) and α4 are the main components in leukocyte IFN (9), IFN-α1(D) possibly being the predominant subtype (23,9). Crude IFN also contains small amounts of IFN-β and IFN-γ as well as IL-1, IL-2 and TNF (unpublished).

It is not known how much partial purification with acid ethanol alters the composition of the IFN present in crude preparation. This step certainly inactivates the acid-labile IFN-α , that is shown to be produced in leukocytes by Sendai virus (15). Sequential purification of P-IF by monoclonal NK2 and YOK antibodies has yielded altogether 8 to 10 IFN bands in SDS-PAGE (14). Additionally, some IFN-α subtypes are not bound to these antibodies. The clinical significance of the subtype composition of IFN preparations is unclear. The subtypes have different biological activities (18,23) and they may have interactions with each other (23). It has been reported that α1 and α2 can potentiate each other's antiviral activity in human cells (17). Small modifications in the purification procedure can alter the subtype composition of the P-IF (14). This may be one of the reasons for the differences observed among P-IF preparations from different laboratories (14).

The specific activity of P-IF is about 2 million IU/mg protein. Accordingly, it contains about 1 % IFN. The impurities are mainly proteins derived from human "agamma" serum (6) added to the culture medium and from the blood cells in the culture. Minor amounts of Sendai virus and chick protein antigens are also present, but no allergic reactions towards these contaminants have been reported. There are no detectable amounts of IFN-β, IFN-γ, IL-1, IL-2 or TNF in the P-IF preparation. Lately, the possible contamination of leukocyte-derived interferons by viruses has been under special consideration. The routine screening of donor blood for HBs antigen and HTLV-III antibodies does not ensure absolute safety regarding these viruses. During the partial purification of IFN by ethanol fractionation (7) the IFN is dissolved for ca. 5 hours in about 80 % ethanol. We have demonstrated that this step effectively inactivates HTLV-III and and Sendai virus (unpublished). Extensive clinical trials with this P-IF preparation during about 15 years indicate that hepatitis B and non A - non B viruses are also inactivated during the purification procedure.

The NK2 antibody-purified IFN is a highly purified product with a specific activity of 100 to 200 million IU/mg protein. It contains about 65 % of the IFN activity in P-IF, but lacks some subtypes, which are not bound to NK2 (1). About 25 % of the nonbound activity can be further recovered using the monoclonal YOK antibody (14). The risk of virus contamination in these preparations can be totally excluded only if some inactivation procedure such as treatment with ethanol is performed. The NK2-purified IFN preparation was used in a clinical study and its side effects were indistinguishable from those of P-IF (20). However, a highly purified product would be preferable and the ideal method would be immunoaffinity purification. A monoclonal antibody that would bind all IFN-α subtypes with affinities appropriate for immunopurification would be very useful.

REFERENCES

1. Allen, G., K.H. Fantes, D.C. Burke and J. Morser. Analysis and purification of human lymphoblastoid (Namalwa) interferon using a monoclonal antibody. J Gen Virol 63:207, 1982.

2. Cantell, K. Why is interferon not in clinical use today? In: Interferon 1, Academic Press, London, ed. I Gresser, pp. 1 - 28, 1979.

3. Cantell, K. Clinical performance of natural human leukocyte interferon. Immunobiology, 1986, in press.

4. Cantell, K., S. Hirvonen, K.E. Mogensen and L. Pyhälä. Human leukocyte interferons: Production, purification, stability and animal experiments. In: In Vitro Monograph 3, Tissue Culture Association, Rockville, Maryland, ed. C. Waymouth, pp. 35 - 38, 1974.

5. Cantell, K. and S. Hirvonen. Preparation of human leukocyte interferon for clinical use. Texas Rep Biol Med 35:138, 1977.

6. Cantell, K., S. Hirvonen, H-L. Kauppinen and G. Myllylä. Production of interferon in human leukocytes from normal donors with the use of Sendai virus. Meth Enzymol 78:29, 1981.

7. Cantell, K., S. Hirvonen and V. Koistinen. Partial purification of human leukocyte interferon on a large scale. Meth Enzymol 78:499, 1981.

8. Cantell, K. and S. Hirvonen. Preparation and assay of Sendai virus. Meth Enzymol 78:299, 1981.

9. Hiscott, J., K. Cantell and C. Weissman. Differential expression of human interferon genes. Nucleic Acids Res 12:3727, 1984.

10. Horowitz, B. W.J. Swiggard, R.W. Shulman, M.E. Weibe and K.R. Woods. Abstract. Preparation of highly purified human leukocyte interferon type alpha (IFN-α). The Third International Congress for Interferon Research, Miami, FL, 1982.

11. Johnston, M.D. Sources of interferon for clinical use: -interferons from human lymphoblastoid cells. In: Interferon 4, In vivo and clinical studies, Elsevier, Amsterdam, eds. N.B. Finter and R.K. Oldham, pp. 81 - 87.

12. Kauppinen, H-L. Sources of interferon for clinical use: α-interferons from blood leukocytes. In: Interferon 4, In vivo and clinical studies, Elsevier, Amsterdam, eds. N.B. Finter and R.K. Oldham, pp. 73 - 79, 1985.

13. Kauppinen, H-L and G. Myllylä. Efficient use of blood leukocytes for interferon production. In: Interferon: Properties and Clinical Uses, Leland Fikes Foundation, Dallas, TX, Ed. A. Khan, pp. 1 - 8, 1980.

14. Kauppinen, H-L., S. Hirvonen and K. Cantell. Effect of purification procedures on the composition of human leukocyte interferon preparations. Meth Enzymol 119:27, 1986.

15. Matsuoka, H., Y. Kakui, A. Tanaka, Y. Cho and J. Imanishi. Acid-labile interferon produced in human peripheral leukocytes by induction with Sendai virus. J Gen Virol 66:2491, 1985.

16. Nagata, S. H. Taira, A. Hall, L. Johnsrud, M. Streuli, J. Ecsödi, W. Boll, K. Cantell and C. Weissmann. Synthetis in E. coli of a polypeptide with human leukocyte interferon activity. Nature (London): 284:316, 1980.

17. Orchansky, P., T. Goren and M. Rubinstein. Isolated subtypes of human interferon-α: synergistic action and affinity for the receptor. In: The Biology of the Interferon System, Elsevier, Amsterdam, eds. E. DeMaeyer and H. Schellekens, pp. 183 - 188, 1983.

18. Pestka, S., B. Kelder, E. Rehberg, J.R. Ortaldo, R.B. Herberman, E.S. Kempner, J.A. Moschera and S.J. Tarnowski. The spesific molecular

activities of interferons differ for antiviral, antiproliferative and natural killer cell activities. In: The Biology of the Interferon System, Elsevier, Amsterdam, eds. E. DeMeyer and H. Schellekens, pp. 535 - 549, 1983.
19. Saksela, E., I. Virtanen, T. Hovi, D.S. Secher and K. Cantell. Monocyte is the main producer of human leukocyte alpha interferons following Sendai induction. Progr Med Virol 30:78, 1984.
20. Scott, G.M., D.S. Secher, D. Flowers, J. Bate, K. Cantell and D.A.J. Tyrrell. Toxicity of interferon. Brit Med J 282:1345, 1981.
21. Secher, D.S. and D.C. Burke. A monoclonal antibody for large scale purification of human leukocyte interferon. Nature (London) 285: 446, 1980.
22. Strander, H., K. Cantell, G. Carlström and P. Jakobsson. Systemic administration of potent interferon to man. J Natl Cancer Inst 51:733, 1973.
23. Weck, P.K., S. Apperson, L. May and N. Stebbing. Comparison of the antiviral activities of various cloned human interferon-α subtypes in mammalian cell cultures. J Gen Virol 57:233, 1981.
24. Weissmann, C. and H. Weber. The interferon genes. Progr Nucl Acid Res, 1986, in press.
25. Zoon, K.C, R-Q. Hu, D. Zur Nedden, J. Enterline, J. Bekisz and N.Y. Nguyen. Abstract. Purification and characterization of human interferon alphas derived from Sendai virus-induced Namalwa cells and peripheral blood lymphocytes. The 1985 TNO-ISIR meeting on the Interferon System, Clearwater, FL, 1985.

9. The Production and Purity of a Mixed Human Alpha Interferon Preparation (Wellferon) Derived from Lymphoblastoid Cells

W. G. Lewis and N. B. Finter

Wellcome Biotech, Langley Court, Beckenham, Kent, BR3 3BS, England

Previously in this series of Reports (1) we described the use of the transformed human B lymphoblastoid cell line, Namalwa, as a source of a mixture of alpha interferons. We outlined the studies used to demonstrate that the final product is acceptable for use in man, and the method of production on a 1,000 litre scale. Since that time, the scale of production has been very greatly increased, and the final product, Wellferon™, has been licensed for certain clinical uses, so far in the United Kingdom and Canada.

Production of Wellferon at our plants in the United Kingdom and Spain has progressively increased from the use of a single 1,000 litre cell culture tank to the use of 2,000, 3,000, 8,000 and 10,000 litre tanks, with several harvests a week. In 1986, our staff successfully commissioned in Japan what is currently the largest facility in the world for mammalian cell culture, an interferon production plant designed for the Sumitomo Chemical Company.

Although the scale has greatly increased, significant modifications to the original production and purification systems have not been required. The multistep purification and concentration process routinely applied to each primary production batch, or pool of two or three such batches, yields a very highly purified product which is subjected to quality control tests. When these have been completed, ten or more purified batches are blended, and a final purification step is applied. A sample is retained for analytical purposes, and human serum albumin is added to the remainder to a final concentration of 1.5 mg/ml: this further improves the excellent stability of the purified material. The biological potency of the blend in International Units, in terms of the International Reference Preparation of human lymphoblastoid interferon, is accurately determined to agreed statistical limits on the basis of at least six replicate assays. From this result, the blend is further diluted with tris-glycine buffer to give the required final concentration of interferon. After a final filtration through a sterilising membrane filter, the product is filled into the final containers. Further analytical checks are made at this stage before the vials are released for clinical use.

The purity of each filling lot is determined by application of sodium dodecyl sulphate polyacrylamide gel electrophoresis (SDS-PAGE) to 30 microgram samples of highly concentrated interferon taken from the blend before the addition of the albumin stabiliser. The gels are stained with Coomassie blue and analysed by densitometry. A stained gel and the corresponding densitometry trace are shown in figure 1. As might be expected in view of the content of many different alpha interferon subtypes, multiple protein bands are obtained on SDS-PAGE. To identify the nature of these bands, Western blotting has been carried out with antisera raised against all the contaminating proteins that might conceivably be present in the final preparation, namely Sendai virus, allantoic fluid protein, bovine serum and Namalwa cell proteins; also with a mixture of two monoclonal antibodies HC33 and HC46, each of which reacts with a number of human alpha interferon subtypes (2). The bands identified as 'h', 1, 2, 3 and 4 in figure 1 all contain alpha interferons as shown by the fact that each reacts with both HC33 and HC 46. The protein in band 'h' is of relatively high molecular weight, and presumably represents a complex of interferon proteins such as form in highly concentrated interferon preparations. This band also contains a protein reacting with monoclonal antibody to human beta interferon. This is hardly surprising, since Namalwa cells are known to produce substantial quantities of beta interferon, and Billiau (personal communication, 1984) using specific high titre antisera to human alpha and beta interferons, has estimated that Wellferon preparations contain 0.5 - 1% of beta interferon. The band, 's', in figure 1 reacts only with an antiserum raised against a preparation of Sendai virus harvested from fertile hens' eggs. The amount of protein in this band corresponds to about 1% of the total protein present, equivalent to about 50 ng per mega unit of interferon. None of the bands react with the antisera to bovine protein and Namalwa cell protein. The purity of the interferon preparation can be assessed in terms of the proportion of protein in the bands staining as alpha interferons, expressed as a percentage of the total protein on the trace. The average purity exceeds 97%, and a minimum purity of 95% with respect to protein is required for material to be released for clinical purposes.

Figure 2 illustrates the effectiveness of the purification scheme: SDS-PAGE was applied to 30 microgram samples of crude interferon (lane A); the product from the first stage of purification (lane B); the product from the third stage of purification (lane C); and the purified product (lane D). It will be seen that the bands corresponding to purified interferon (lane D) cannot be visualised in the crude preparation, but after each stage of purification, as the protein impurities are progressively eliminated during purification, these bands become visible.

Wellferon has been used in extensive clinical trials in many countries to treat patients with various forms of cancer or virus infection, and has been licensed in the United Kingdom and Canada for the treatment of hairy cell leukaemia. From the results which have been obtained in a number of other clinical conditions, regulatory approvals for its use in other conditions are expected in the near future: these conditions include wart virus infections (juvenile laryngeal papillomatosis, condyloma acuminata and cutaneous warts); chronic infectious hepatitis B; renal cancer, non-Hodgkin's lymphoma, chronic myelogenous leukaemia and Kaposi's sarcoma. Superficially, the clinical results obtained with this polyvalent product appears similar to those obtained with monovalent preparations of recombinant alpha 2 interferon, derived from bacteria by recombinant DNA techniques. There is a need for comparison of the two types of product under controlled conditions to see whether the theoretical advantages of the polyvalent product will be realised in practice. In any event, our plants have sufficient capacity to produce hundreds of grams of interferon a year, should such amounts be needed, so that this mixture of interferons is a viable long term alternative to recombinant interferons in terms of cost, of purity and availability.

ACKNOWLEDGEMENT

The photographs in this article are reproduced with the kind permission of the Cold Spring Harbour Laboratory.

REFERENCES

1. Finter, N.B.: Large scale production of human inteferon from lymphoblastoid cells. Tex Rep Biol Med 41:175, 1982.

2. Lewis, W.G., K.H. Fantes, G. Allen and J. Ivanyi: The specificity of monoclonal antibodies raised against human alpha interferons. Antiviral Research, ABSTR 1, No.2: P58, 1983.

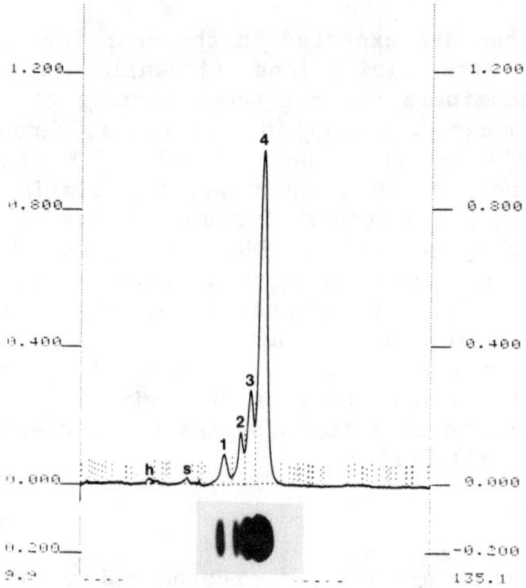

Fig 1: SDS-PAGE and densitometry of a sample of Wellferon before the addition of stabilizing protein. The identity of labelled peaks is described in the text.

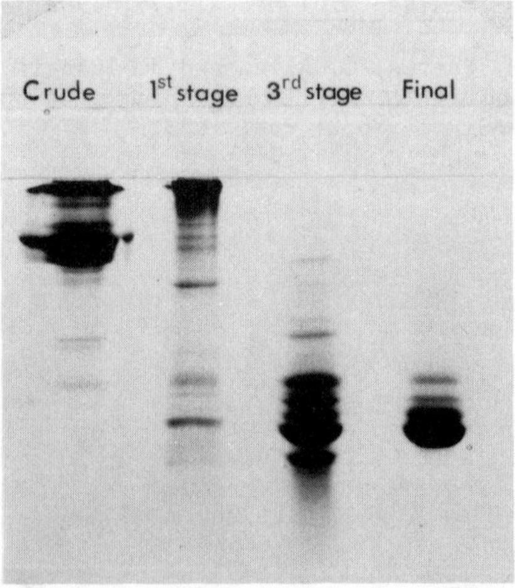

Fig 2: SDS-PAGE of samples taken at various stages in the purification of Wellferon.

10. Production of Natural Interferon Gamma

J. Georgiades and M. Kruzel

Immuno Modulators Laboratories, Inc., 10521 Corporate Drive, Stafford, TX 77477

INTRODUCTION

In the late 70's there was a great hope that interferon could be an effective tool in the treatment of different diseases of viral and neoplastic origin. This hope was further substantiated by the application of genetic engineering methods for the production of large quantities of inexpensive interferons. However, with a few notable exceptions, clinical results have been below expectation. Results of studies using recombinant interferons were generally less impressive than those using natural preparations (1). This discrepancy between recombinant and natural interferons and their therapeutical efficacy once again renewed interest in the use of natural interferons.

The increased demand for natural interferons creates a need for a reevaluation of the existing methods of production and purification and for the development of new and more efficient ones. Due to space limitations, references will often be the review articles.

PRODUCTION

Sources of Cells

Peripheral white blood cells (PWBC) are most frequently used as the source for large scale production of interferon alpha and interferon gamma. However, both interferons can also be produced using established cell lines (2,3,4). Other sources are represented by lymphocytes obtainable from normal spleens removed during emergency operations (5) or from the thoracic duct (6). However, the scarcity of these sources makes them inadequate for large scale production. Patients with chronic myelogenous leukemia, although representing a very rich source of cells, obviously cannot be utilized in the production of interferon alpha and interferon gamma for clinical use (7). In addition, their cells are very poor producers of interferon gamma (Georgiades, unpublished observation).

Problems Associated With Large Scale Production of Natural Interferons

As the total number of buffy coats for production of interferons increases so does the possible contamination with microorganisms. Contamination of the WBCs with viruses which may derive from apparently healthy individuals who donate blood at the time of subclinical viral infection is of greatest concern. Infection with hepatitis A is a good example. However, cells can also be contaminated by other DNA and RNA viruses known to infect man. Since viremia or viruria cannot be assessed routinely by blood banks, there is a risk factor when the natural product derived from donated blood is used. Much more serious contaminants are the viruses responsible for chronic infections which are present in the blood for prolonged periods of time. Cytomegalo and Epstein Barr viruses, members of the herpes virus family, may serve as examples of this. More recently retroviruses of the Lentivirinae subfamily (Human Immunodeficiency Virus [HIV], previously known as LAV-I/HTLV-III), have created a serious problem as a source of WBC contamination. Members of this subfamily are the etiologic agents of Acquired Immuno Deficiency Syndrome (AIDS) which is characterized by a prolonged viremic state. The U.S. Food and Drug Administration (FDA) regulations require that leukocytes must come from blood which is negative for hepatitis B surface antigen and does not show antibodies to HTLV-III virus. However, these precautions may not be sufficient. There are cases where viremia occurs without the presence of antibodies (8). Furthermore, Montagnier et al (9) recently have found a new AIDS virus with an antigenic structure so different from the prototype that "classical" antigens did not react with antibodies to the new virus and, antibodies against the "classical" strain of the HIV viruses did not recognize the antigens of the new isolate. Discovery of new members of the HIV family was confirmed and extended by other groups of investigators who isolated similar HIV viruses more closely related to simian lymphotropic virus, but not identical to those isolated by Montagnier (10). In addition, considerable antigenic variations occur inside "classical" HIV viruses and these may lead to false negative results (11). In other words, some of the viruses from the retrovirus family may escape detection at screening, thus they may contaminate batches of starting WBCs.

Moreover, the assumption that interferon may inhibit multiplication of a contaminant virus is erroneous. In hepatitis B infected leukocytes this virus grew in the presence of newly induced interferon gamma (Georgiades, unpublished observation) and HIV viruses multiplied in the presence of high concentrations of interferon gamma (Yamamoto et al) (12).

During interferon gamma production, several other lymphokines are synthesized. One of these is interleukin 2 (IL-2). There are reports that IL-2 can activate the production of viruses present in leukocytes in their latent form (13).

Since virus contamination may cause problems for the production of natural interferons and of other lymphokines and blood products, development of methods for its elimination are of the highest priority.

Selection of The Proper Population of Cells for Interferon Production:

Another problem facing the producer of natural interferons is selection of cells for its production.

There are established cell lines (mostly from the lymphoblastoid series) which will spontaneously produce significant amounts of interferon. Their cultivation is generally tedious (4); and while they may be a good source for the induction of interferon alpha, they rarely are for interferon gamma. Recently, several excellent review articles have covered this subject (14), which emphasize the difficulties facing those who choose this route. Today, very few people are using cell lines, the majority still use buffy coats as a source of interferons.

When considering the large scale production of interferon from buffy coats, it is necessary to select the proper cell population and purification methods. Generally there are five major methods of preparing lymphocytes: (a) use of an enriched lymphocyte fraction directly from donated blood (plateletpheresis residue) (15), (b) purification of lymphocytes by an ammonium chloride method (16,17,18,19), (c) separation of lymphocytes by accelerated sedimentation of red cell in starch (20), (d) recovery of lymphocytes from Ficoll-Hypaque gradient, and (e) separation of white blood cells from erythrocytes by differential sedimentation.

None of the above mentioned methods is ideal. Each has its own limitations. For example, the least damaging is the separation of the lymphocytes by differential centrifugation; however, this procedure is laborious, tedious and almost impossible to apply to large scale production where hundreds of buffy coats must be processed simultaneously.

The Ficoll-Hypaque method gives excellent separation but is not adaptable to large scale production because it is costly. Thus, it remains as an analytical laboratory procedure. The starch method is very gentle, simple, and gives relatively high recovery of lymphocytes. The polymorphonuclear leukocytes preserved during starch sedimentation apparently play an important role in the synthesis of a pH labile form of interferon alpha (Chadha in this issue); however, they do not seem to be of advantage for interferon gamma production.

Ammonium chloride purification, generally used for the lysis of red cells in laboratories producing large quantities of interferon alpha and interferon gamma, may be adapted well for separating lymphocytes. However, overexposure of the cells to ammonium chloride might easily damage the lymphocyte membranes to such an extent that the cells will form large clumps and may loose the capability to produce interferons efficiently. Another limitation of the lysis method is that a large amount of different proteases are released. This can cause loss or modification of interferons at the very beginning of the production.

Using lymphocytes mixed with RBC for interferon production results in extensive lysis of the RBC. Released hemoglobin is degraded by enzymes released to the medium from activated lymphocytes and these degradation products co-purify with interferon.

Depending upon the method selected for cell separation, certain isospecies of interferon alpha may be present in different proportions in crude preparations of interferon. In IML, we routinely produce interferon alpha and interferon gamma from lymphocytes purified with an ammonium chloride method (19).

INDUCTION

Induction of interferon, particularly interferon gamma, is highly dependent upon the quality of cells. Removal of lymphocytes adhering to nylon wool normally increase interferon gamma yields (21). It is also possible to obtain large quantities of interferon gamma from PWBC free of B-cell population by treating the PWBC cells with double stranded RNA normally used for interferon beta production (22).

In spite of considerable attention to detail and standardization of the induction process, the yield of interferon has varied from batch-to-batch. This variation has occurred both when the cell lines were employed (14) or when PWBC were used. In addition, over several years, we have demonstrated a seasonal variation in the yield of interferon gamma (23). This phenomenon has also been observed by others (Langford, personal communication); but all the attempts to identify the causative factors have failed thus far.

Influence of Volume on Interferon Yield:

The volume in which the induction is carried out influences the final yield of interferon. This can be seen with cultures of the lymphoblastoid cell lines as well as with PWBC primary cultures. For instance, when interferon alpha or interferon gamma was induced in relatively small vessels (1-2 ml), a considerably higher yield was obtained compared with large volume induction (14). This phenomenon is particularly evident with interferon gamma (Georgiades, unpublished observation).

The production of interferon alpha has been standardized by Cantell and co-workers. Routinely, induction is carried out in five liter round bottom flasks filled with 2.5 liters of cell suspension. During the incubation period, the cells are agitated by an egg-shaped stirring bar. Any deviation from the conditions described by Cantell generally give lower interferon alpha yield. This method, however, is not applicable to the induction of interferon gamma. In our laboratory, we have found that 2 liter plastic flasks containing 0.5-1.0 liters of cell suspension incubated under stationary conditions at 37° C for three days give the best yield.

Influence of Media on Interferon Yield:

Laboratories producing interferon alpha from lymphoblastoid cells lines have preferentially used RPMI-1640 medium, although other types of media adapted for cells grown in suspension can also be used. Some laboratories use RPMI-1640, MEM, or modified MEM (14,17,18). At IML, we use the Wadley Institute modification of MEM medium. This medium is supplied by K.C. Biologicals, Inc., Lenexa, Kansas. Selection of media for interferon gamma production is even less stringent. In our hands, basic medium RPMI-1640, MEM or modified MEM alone is equally suitable for the synthesis of interferon gamma.

Use of Proteins To Supplement The Basic Medium:

In the past, casein, albumin, and tryptic broth were used as a source of protein for interferon alpha production, but they give very poor results where interferon gamma induction is concerned. The best source of protein has been fetal calf serum. Supplementation of the basic medium to 10% of this serum always gives the highest titer of interferon gamma. A diminishing serum concentration below 6% or substitution with human or other types of serum gives less satisfactory results. However, Kauppinen et al (18) have reported the successful application of silicic acid-adsorbed human agamma serum for production of human interferon gamma.

<u>Factors Influencing Interferon Gamma Production</u>:

There are different drugs, hormones, and other biologically active molecules which negatively influence interferon gamma production. Prostaglandins, cortisone, ACTH, cyclic AMP, and certain inhibitors of lipoxygenase metabolism are a few examples of very effective inhibitors of interferon gamma synthesis (24). Furthermore, viruses that cause herpes, hepatitis, or AIDS are also efficient inhibitors of interferon gamma production. In addition, cells from patients with other immuno deficiencies or with certain connective tissue disorders such as lupus erythematous or arthritis have diminished capabilities to produce interferon gamma. This might partially be due to increased production of prostaglandins.

There are other factors which positively influence interferon gamma production. For example, peptide hormones such as oxitocine or arginine vasopressin (AVP) and the tumor-promoter phorbol-12-myristic-13-acetate (PMA) can replace IL-2 in the production of interferon gamma. There is evidence that many mitogens induce monocytes by acting on galactose residue on the cell membrane (25). Excellent reviews on this subject have been published (26,27).

It is generally believed that induction of interferon gamma is mediated by two signals: mitogen or antigen and IL-2. Following stimulation of PWBC by mitogen, a cascade reaction occurs. As a result of the interaction between mitogen and macrophages, IL-1 is released. It becomes a signal for the stimulation of helper cells which, when exposed to mitogen and IL-1, provide IL-2 to the system. This mediator, in cooperation again with mitogen, activates interferon gamma-producing cells. Release of interferon gamma may further stimulate helper cells to produce more IL-2. This dynamic interaction between helper cells and interferon gamma-producing cells is controlled by suppressor cells which may sequester IL-2 and interrupt the synthesis of interferon gamma. Dianzani, et al, suggest an alternative activation mechanism for interferon gamma production. Macrophages treated with mitogens release a "non IL-1" lymphokine which directly stimulates lymphocytes for the production of interferon gamma (28).

Studies conducted by many investigators show that IL-2 activates a guanylate cyclase which increases the level of cyclic guanosine monophosphate (cGMP) inside the cells. The IL-2 signal can be replaced by neuroendocrine hormones arginine vasopressin (AVP), oxytocin, acetylcholine, and other factors (26). Bacterial protein (29) is also capable of increasing the level of cGMP in the cells. Leukotrines, intermediates of the arachidonic acid metabolism, also have the ability to replace the IL-2 requirement in interferon gamma production. All these substances apparently activate guanylate cyclase, thus increasing the level of cGMP in the cells. Increased level of intracellular cGMP may induce the influx of calcium into interferon gamma-producing cells with the subsequent activation of phospholipase and release of arachidonic acid from membrane phospolipids. Arachidonic acid is degradated to leukotrine which may increase further the cellular level of cGMP with amplification of interferon gamma production. The influx of calcium into the cell may be considered as a general activation signal, not only affecting interferon gamma synthesis but also that of other lymphokines. Thus the simultaneous nonspecific activation of many lymphokines suggests their close collaboration in the modulation of immunological responses.

The complexity of the "classical" mechanisms of interferon gamma production may explain the long period of incubation before interferon gamma is synthesized. Activation of cells with beta galactosidase or calcium ionophore (25) or another stimulator of the guanyl cyclase shortens the time necessary for interferon gamma synthesis (26). Secondary factors such as leukotrines prolong interferon production thus permitting the design of rational large-scale production.

The above considerations on the mechanism of interferon gamma induction have a practical aspect. There are two strategies for the induction of interferon gamma. In the first, interferon gamma-producing cells are activated by treatment with mitogens: Crude interferon is harvested three to four days later (18,19). In the second strategy, the cells are either treated simultaneously with mitogens and a second signal such as IL-2, tumor promoter PMA, or with calcium ionophore alone (30). In this situation interferon gamma is produced within 24 hours in relatively large quantities.

At IML, we selected an intermediary route and performed a double induction. As mentioned earlier, production of interferon gamma is prolonged and may last for several days. Initially, we induce cells with staphylococcal enterotoxin B (SEB) and allow cells to respond in slow fashion. After three days of incubation, the first portion of interferon gamma is collected and the cells are resuspended in a fresh incubation medium containing phytohemagglutinin (PHA) and the cells are grown for the next 36 hours. Using this strategy, we have doubled the interferon gamma yield and made the production less expensive.

Under dissociating conditions, highly purified interferon gamma exists in two forms: 20,000 and 25,000 daltons. However, Pestka (Cyt. from 20) showed that native molecules exist in tetrameric form. Fish et al showed that interferon gamma may exist in two molecular forms having different biological and physico-chemical properties (31). It is possible to assume that these basic units may polymerize, form-

ing three types of dimers: for example, 20,000 + 20,000, 25,000 + 25,000 and 20,000 + 25,000 daltons. As we have shown earlier, these dimers or tetramers show different properties (32).
The formation of different forms of interferon gamma seems to have a direct impact on its biological activity: especially the antiviral titer. Depending on the form of interferon gamma existing in solution, a four fold difference may be seen in its titer. This problem is particularly evident during the purification process, when a sudden drop or increase in activity may be observed.

Another element influencing the initial titer is the interaction of interferon gamma with inhibitors. This factor may also affect the immunoregulatory functions of interferon gamma (32) In summary, the measurable interferon activity present in the crude preparation is the result of many different factors. For this reason, evaluation of the purification procedure in terms of percent recovery may be misleading.

PURIFICATION

There are many methods for interferon gamma purification, such as a combination of several classical chromotography methods, monoclonal antibodies immobilized on gel matrixes, high performance liquid chromotography (HPLC), etc. By using different techniques, different degrees of purity may be achieved. The investigator has ample choice of methods to be used.

Classical chromotographic procedures carried out under gentle conditions cause limited denaturation of proteins. However, these methods generally are not very efficient. The use of monoclonal antibodies or HPLC methods generally requires more severe conditions which might effect the tertiary or quaternary structure of the molecules. Kauppinen et al have proposed a gentle procedure in which interferon gamma is chromotographed successfully on CM Sepharose and on Phenyl-Sepharose 4B columns. The eluate is equilibrated with PBS and stored at -70° C for eventual further purification (18).

In another method described by Novick et al (cyt. from 19), interferon gamma was partially purified and concentrated on controlled pore glass (CPG) beads, then further purified on HPLC column. The same authors also described conditions for purificaiton of interferon gamma on monoclonal antibodies. In IML, interferon gamma is purified by CM Sepharose, Zn++ chelate chromotography followed by chromotography on Con A Sepharose (19). There are many other methods of purification where the authors claim to obtain excellent results (19, cyt. from 32).

CONCLUSIONS

Only three of the above mentioned methods were used for preparation of interferon gamma for clinical trials (18,19,33). Early clinical trials have not indicated a clear advantage of IFN-G over other IFNs; however, more trials are needed. The possible presence of an IFN inhibitor in interferon gamma preparations must be excluded and synergistic interactions of IFNs warrent study.

BIBLIOGRAPHY

1. Strander, H.: The interferon system in antitumor therapy; some personal views. In: The Biology of Interferon System 1984, H. Kirschner and H. Shellekens, eds. Elsevier, p. 489, 1985.

2. Cellis, E., W. Miller, T. J. Wiktor, B. Dietzschold, and H. Koprowski: Isolation and characterization of human T cell lines and clones reactive to rabies virus: Antigen specificity and production of interferon gamma. J of Immunol, 136:692, 1986.

3. Strander, H., K.E. Mogensen, K. Cantell: Production of human lymphoblastoid interferon. J Clin Microbiol, 1: 1:116, 1975.

4. Golde, D.W. and S.G. Quan: Unique T-lymphocyte line and products derived therefrom. U.S.A. Patent No. 4.438.032, March 20, 1984.

5. Fouconnier, B.: Large scale production of human interferon form human spleens. J of Interferon Res, 1:15, 1980.

6. Langford, M.P., D.A. Weigent, G. J. Stanton, R.B. Pollard, J.C. Fish, M.W. Flye: Rapid production of high levels of gamma interferon by human thoracic duct leukocytes stimulated with staphylococcal enterotoxin A. In: Human Lymphokines, A. Kahn, ed. Academic Press, p. 155, 1982.

7. Hersberg, R.D., E.G. Guciora, P.C. Famillieti, S. Rubinstein, C. A. Rose and S. Pestka: Induction and production of human interferon with human leukemic cells. In: Methods in Enzymology, Interferons, Part B, S. Pestka, ed. Academic Press, 78:45, 1981.

8. Asjo, B.: In vitro properties of AIDS virus isolated from infected individuals; possible clinical correlation. Proc. 1st Intl Meeting of AVIS, AIDS, Naples, Italy, December 1985 (in press).

9. Clavel, F., Brun-Vezinet, D. Guetard, S. Chamaret, A. Laurent, C. Rouzioux, M. Rey, C. Katlama, F. Rey, J.L. Champelinaud, J.S. Nina, K. Mansinho, M.O. Santos-Ferreira, D. Klatzmann and L. Montagnier: Virology - LAV type II: a second retrovirus associated with AIDS in West-Africa. C.R. Acad. Sc. Paris, t. 302, Serie III, n° 13, 1986.

10. Kanki, P.J., F. Barin, S. M'Boup, J.S. Allen, J.L. Romet-Lemonne, R. Marlink, M.F. McLane, T.H. Lee, B. Arbeille, F. Denis, and M. Essex: New human T-lymphotropic virus type III (STLV-III Agm). Science, 232:238, 1986.

11. Hahn, B.H., G.M. Shaw, M.E. Taylor, R.R. Redfield, F.D. Markham, S.Z. Salahuddin, F. Wong-Stahl, R.C. Gallo, E.S. Parks, and W.P. Parks: Genetic variation in HTLV-III/LAV over time in patients with AIDS or at risk for AIDS. Science, 232:1548, 1986.

12. Yamamoto, J.K., F. Barre-Sinoussi, V. Bolton, N.C. Pedersen, and M.B. Gardner: Human alpha and beta interferon but not gamma suppresses the in vitro replication of LAV, HTLV-III and ARV-2. J Interferon Res, 6:143, 1986.

13. Milstein, J.B., M.J. Klutch, B. Bhatia, and C.J. Lucas: Effect of interferon and interleukin-2 on measles virus infection. In: The Biology of the Interferon System, E. de Maeyer and H. Schellekens, eds. Elsevier, p. 275, 1983.

14. Finter, N.B. and K.H. Fantes: Lymphoblastoid interferon: Production and characterization in interferons and their applications. In: Handbook of Expl Pharmacology: Interferons and Their Applications, P.E. Came and W.A. Carter, eds. Springer-Verlag, 71:271, 1984.

15. Pang, R.H.L., Y.K. Yip, J. Vilcek: Immune interferon induction by monoclonal antibody specific to human T cells. Cellular Immunol, 64:304, 1981.

16. Cantell, K., S. Hirvonen, K. Mogensen, L. Pyhala: Human leukocyte interferon: Production, purification, stability and animal experiments. In: In Vitro [Monograph 3], 35:38, 1974.

17. Hill, N.O.: Production and characterization of human leukocyte interferon. In: Handbook of Exp. Pharmacology: Interferons and Their Applications, P.E. Came and W.A. Carter, eds. Handbook of Experimental Pharmacology, Springer-Verlag, 71:259, 1984.

18. Kauppinen, H.L., B. Bang, J. Eronen, R. Majuri, G. Myllyla, H. Tolo, S. Hironen, K. Cantell: Preparation of natural human gamma interferon for clinical use. In: The Biology of The Interferon System. Elsevier, 1985 (in press).

19. Georgiades, J.: Large scale production, concentration, and partial purification of human immune interferon. In: Methods in Enzymology: Interferons, S. Pestka, ed. Academic Press, 119:83, 1986.

20. Van Oss, C.J., P.M. Bronson, E.A. Dinolfo and K.C. Chadha: Two methods for the removal of erythrocytes from buffy coats for the production of human leukocyte interferon. Immunological Commun., 10:549, 1981.

21. Weck, P.K., L. May, C.J. Weck: Gamma interferon production by different population of human splenic lymphocytes. J Interferon Res, 3:121, 1983.

22. Tamura, M., S. Saito, S. Sasakawa: Induction of human interferon gamma in nylon-column nonadherent human lymphocyte cells by heat-treated poly I:poly C. J Interferon Res, 5:77, 1985.

23. Georgiades, J.A., J. Gumulka, B. Cain, M. Haywood, T. Marks, D.S. Wong: Seasonal variations in human gamma production by cells induced with SEB and PHA. In: The Biology of The Interferon System, E. de Maeyers and H. Schellekens, eds. Elsevier, p. 401, 1983.

24. Johnson, H.M.: Cyclic AMP regulation of mitogen-induced interferon production and mitogen suppression of immune response. Nature, 265:154, 1977.

25. Dianzani, F., T. Monahan, and M. Santiano: Mechanism of induction of gamma interferon. In: Texas Reports on Biology and Medicine, 41:99, 1982.

26. Johnson, H.M.: Neuroendocrine hormones and immune system. In: Biological Response Modifiers, P.F. Torrence, ed. Academic Press, p. 245, 1985.

27. Johnson, H.M.: Mechanism of interferon gamma production and assessment of immunoregulatory properties. Lymphokines, 11:33, 1985.

28. Dianzani F., G. Antonelli: In: The Interferon System, F. Dianzani and G. B. Rossi, eds. Serono Symposa Publications, May 8-11, 1985, Rome, Italy.

29. Weigent, D.A., Beachey, E.M., T. Huff, J.W. Peterson, G.J. Stanton, S. Baron: Induction of human interferon gamma by structurally defined polypeptide fragments of

group A streptococcal M. proteins. J Immun, 43:122, 1984.

30. Dianzani, F., T.M. Monahan, J.A. Georgiades, J.B. Alperin: Human immune interferon: Induction in lymphoid cells by a calcium inophore. Infectious Immunol, 29:561, 1980.

31. Fish, E.N., K. Banerje, T. Arakawa, N.K. Alton, N. Stebbing: Biological characterization of the two structurally distinct forms of recombinant gamma interferon. The 1985 TNO-ISIR Meeting on the Interferon System, Clearwater Beach, Florida, 13-18 October 1985.

32. Georgiades, J.A., S. Baron, W.R. Fleischmann Jr., M. Langford, D.A. Weigent and G. J. Stanton: Immune interferon. In: Handbook of Expl Pharmacology: Interferons and Their Applications, P.E. Came and W.A. Carter, eds. Springer Verlag, 71:305, 1984.

11. Production of Animal Interferons

H. Schellekens and P. H. v. d. Meide

TNO Primate Center, P.O. Box 5815, 2280 HV Rijswijk, The Netherlands

INTRODUCTION

Animal studies are not only important to elucidate the biology of the interferon system but also to provide data on the efficient use of interferon in man. The number of interferon studies in animals is, however, limited (1). Because of the species specificity, interferons to be used in animals have to be produced specifically. Initially animal interferons could only be produced from cell cultures. During the seventies large scale cell culture systems were set up that not only provided material for a limited number of animal studies but also for purification. The introduction of recombinant DNA technology provided a revolution. In principle, a number of animal interferons can now be produced in unlimited amounts. In this review we will restrict ourselves to the rodent interferons that are being produced in amounts which make animal studies on a routine basis possible.

I. MOUSE INTERFERONS

A large number of papers have been published about the production, purification and characterization of murine interferons. Within the scope of this review it is not possible to acknowledge all the excellent contributions. We refer to other reviews for a more comprehensive discussion (2-3).

The Large Scale Production of Mouse Interferon α/β

In 1964 Finter described mouse brain tissue infected with West Nile virus as a rich source of mouse interferon (4). The disadvantages of such a production system are obvious. In 1971 Stewart II and coworkers reported on a large scale production unit based on L cells cultured in roller bottles (5). After priming and induction with the MM strain of encephalomyocarditis virus approx. 10^4 units/ml culture medium were produced. This sytem was boosted up to a tenfold increase by Knight et al. (6) using multisurface glass roller bottles. Tovey and coworkers, elaborating on the finding of Oie et al. that C-243-3 cells (MSV-transformed 3T3 cells) were excellent producers (7), developed a suspension culture system with these cells (8). Using NDV as inducer in a superinduction scheme with cycloheximide and actinomycine-D he was able to produce > 10^5 U (ml supernatant). Taira et al. (9) used Erhlich ascites cells grown in roller bottles. These cells were grown in CM-Sephadex-fractioned-serum-proteins, induced with NDV and treated with 6mM theophyline and produced > 10^6 U/ml supernatant.

Purification and Characterization of Murine Interferon α/β

All published purification schemes for murine interferon α/β start with concentration of the culture medium to workable volume by precipitation, ultrafiltration or CPG adsorption, followed by different forms of gel chromatography. Very important has been the introduction of affinity chromatography. Using antibodies as a ligand, Sipe et al. (10) reported 2000 fold purification in a single step. Ogburn et al. (11) using more purified antibodies purified mouse interferon α/β to a specific activity of 3×10^8 U/mg protein. Important was the affinity of mouse interferon α/β to poly nucleotides reported by DeMaeyer-Guignard (12). Using affinity columns with antiserum and poly U, she was able to purify up to 8×10^9 U/mg protein, the highest purity achieved (13).

In 1974 Stewart II et al. reported that SDS-PAAGE analysis of mouse interferon α/β showed two peaks of activity (14). 90% of the activity could be found at 38K and 10% at 22K. In 1980 Yamamoto and colleagues (15) found that the two peaks were antigenically different. In the same year Taira et al. reported on the partial amino acid sequence of the three size classes, A: 35-40K, B: 26-33K, and C: 20K, produced by NDV induced Ehrlich ascites cells (16). The A and B peak showed homology with human beta interferon and the C peak with human alpha interferon. This directly linked the human interferon system to the mouse interferon system, which was definitely proven by the cloning of the murine interferon genes.

The Cloning of Murine Interferon α/β

In 1983 Shaw et al. (17) reported on the structure and expression of cloned murine IFN-α genes. He reported that like the human system the murine α family consists of at least 4 and likely more than 10 members. A chromosomal murine α1 gene and a cDNA of the murine α2 gene were expressed in COS cells and in E.coli. In COS a transient expression of up to 13,000 U/ml culture medium was achieved. In the extracts of E.coli about 1000 units/ml of cell culture could be found. To be an efficient source of murine alpha interferon, the expression in E.coli has to be extensively enhanced, but also other attempts to reach high expression of murine alpha interferons in E.coli have failed (18). As an alternative recombinant human hybrid alpha interferon (r-IFNα A/D) which has antiviral activity in vitro and in vivo in mice has been used (19). However, the use of heterologous interferon should be avoided as much as possible. Efficient expression of murine alpha has been achieved by Zwarthoff and others

(20) in CHO cells. These cells consecutively secreted up to 100,000 units per ml in 24 h.

In 1983 Higashi and others (21) reported on the cloning of mouse interferon beta. The gene was identified by screening a c-DNA library prepared from m-RNA from NDV induced L cells. Introduced into COS cells with the proper vector a transient expression of 9000 units/ml was achieved. Recently Kobayashi reported on the cloning of this murine beta gene in E.coli. High levels of expression up to $4x10^6$ U/ml culture were achieved allowing crystallization of this interferon (22).

Production, Purification and Cloning of Murine Interferon Gamma

Wietzerbin was the first to report on the large scale production of murine interferon gamma in 1978 (23). She used spleen cells from 8-15 weeks old normal or nude mice. The cells were induced with PHA and the supernatant harvested after 24 hours. The supernatant contained 200-300 U/ml. 100 spleens yielded about $0.5\text{-}1x10^6$ units. By ammonium-sulphate precipitation and affinity chromatography the immune interferon was purified to a specific activity of $2x10^5$ units/mg protein. This material showed consistently two peaks of activity when analysed by different chromatographic methods (24).

In 1979 Osborne (25) reported on the induction of mouse immune interferon in cells from spleen of C57BL/6 mice cultured in roller bottles. The cells were induced by SEA in the presence of 10^{-5}M 2-mercaptoethanol. The supernatant was harvested after 3 days and contained about 1000 units/ml. After concentration of this material by ammoniumsulphate precipitation, ultrafiltration or CPG adsorption, the material was purified by affinity chromatography with BSA as ligand and gel filtration on ultragel Aca-34 resulting in a specific activity of 500,000 U/mg protein. This material was reported to contain 2 peaks at 40K and 80K.

Heremans and others (26) reported on the use of S. aureus lysate induced interferon. The supernatant of the spleen cells cultured on 24-well plates in a density of $3x10^6$ cells/ml contained about 5000 units. This material was purified by silicic acid adsorption and elution followed by Aca44 gel chromatography to about $10^{4.5}$ units/mg protein. This purified material contained a single peak of 50K. A problem of natural immune interferon is that induction of spleen cells by mitogens leads to the production of a variety of lymphokines known to interact strongly. Effects can therefore never be explained completely by the presence of gamma interferon. And of course the need of a constant supply of fresh cells from sacrificed animals is a disadvantage.

Both problems were solved by the cloning and expression of mouse immune interferon gene by Gray and Goeddel in 1983 (27). The gene was isolated from a mouse gene library and transiently expressed in COS cells using a SV40 based expression vector resulting in 6000 units/ml. With the genomic gene a cDNA gene was isolated and introduced in E.coli in an expression plasmid resulting in approx. 50,000 units per ml culture medium. Others have published on the constituent expression of murine gamma in CHO cells, transformed by an expression vector containing a cDNA of murine immune interferon mRNA under control of the SV40 early promotor (28). Production up to 10^5 units/ml medium per 24 hours have been achieved, consituting an efficient source of lymphokine-free mouse immune interferon.

II. RAT INTERFERON

It is important to realize that international standards for rat interferons are not yet available, which obscures the direct comparison of results obtained in different laboratories. Also the international nomenclature committee has not yet given the different interferon (sub)types their names. But the similarities between the rat interferons on one hand and the murine and human interferons on the other hand are so great that we can safely adopt the nomenclature for the latter.

The Production and Purification of Natural Rat Interferon α/β (rat IFNα/β)

The production of this type of interferon was pioneered by Schonne some 20 years ago (29). In his paper published in 1966, he described the use of DE7R rat tumor cells and induction with Sinbis virus. In 1978 Coupin and others (30) reported several methods of interferon induction in vitro and in vivo. The most efficient production system proved to be rat embryo fibroblasts or C6 glial cells induced with NDV. The supernatant contained about 256 units/ml. He also noted crossreactivity of murine and rat interferon and partial neutralization of rat interferon by mouse interferon antiserum.

In the early eighties the groups of Abreu, Murasko and our group reported on large scale production methods (31,32,33). The similarities among these methods are striking. All three laboratories found a cell line spontaneously transformed during subcultivation of rat embryo cells the best source and NDV and/or Sendai the best inducers. All three noticed the lack of induction by poly I-C even employing 'superinduction' schedules, which was also reported by Coupin in 1978. Abreu et al. named their cell line RFA-1. Induction with NDV and treatment with theophyline resulted in titers of $10^{4.5}$ units/ml medium. The CD cell line established by Murasko's group produced about $10^{4.3}$ units/ml when induced with Sendai virus. They compared their line with the Ratec cell line that was developed by our group and found similar production by the two lines. In our laboratory we use commercially obtained Sendai virus and obtain some what lower interferon titer in the order of $10^{3.7}$ units/ml.

Purification of Natural Rat Interferon α/β

The same three groups mentioned above have been employed in the development of purification methods and characterization of rat interferon α/β.

Kaplan and Abreu reported the nearly complete purification of interferon produced in RFA-1 cells by employing absorption and elution from controlled pore glass and phenyl-agarose chromatography (34). Their purification results in a specific activity of 3.7×10^8 U/mg protein. SDS-PAAGE of this preparation revealed two major bands of 26K and 22.5K and a minor band at 18.5K. Murasko and her coworkers (35) used antibody affinity chromatography with antiserum to human alpha interferon or mouse L cell interferon to purify rat interferon from CD cells. This resulted in preparations with a specific activity of $5\text{-}8 \times 10^7$ U/mg protein. Their interferon preparation analysed in SDS-PAAGE contained three species at around 30-33K, 25-27K and 17-23K. The antibody binding profile suggested that the majority of their preparation was of the alpha type.

We are able to purify the Sendai induced Ratec cell interferon to a specific activity of 10^7 U/mg protein by precipitation with ammonium sulphate, Aca44-gel-filtration and monoQ-anion-exchange-chromatography utilizing a FPLC-system. SDS-PAAGE of the material in the presence of β-mercaptoethanol resulted in two distinct classes of molecules of 40K en 20K both consisting of a continuous gradient of molecules varying in size. An antiserum raised to HuIFNα2 bound about 15% of the Ratec cell derived interferon indicating the presence of alpha type like interferon and homology with human alpha interferon (36).

Cloning of Rat Alpha-1 Interferon

In our Ratec cell/Sendai virus interferon production system the total year production is about 100 μg. For this amount we have to culture about 100 m^2 of cells in 1200 roller bottles. The production costs for these 100 μg is 50.000 US dollars. Recombinant DNA technology was therefore an attractive alternative to us. c-DNA made from rat interferon m-RNA isolated from Sendai induced Ratec cells was cloned in E.coli. A c-DNA fragment identified by hybridization with the mouse α-2 gene was used to screen a rat gene library. A 2.5 kb fragment encoding for the rat IFN α1 gene was isolated and introduced in E.coli in a pMBL 604 plasmid. The E.coli strain carrying this plasmid made biologically active interferon. As with the mouse alpha interferons the expression of rat alpha is disappointingly low either because of the low transcription of the m-RNA or because of the instability of rodent interferons in E.coli cells. Anyway, the expression is still too low to provide material for in vivo experiments.

Production of Recombinant Rat Gamma Interferon

There are no methods published for the production of rat gamma interferon from T-cells. We, however, have developed an efficient source by cloning the rat interferon gamma gene in CHO cells (38). The rat interferon gamma gene was identified by use of hybridization with the human interferon gamma gene. The gene was expressed in $DHFR^-$ CHO cells under control of a SV40 promotor after cotransformation with the murine DHFR gene. Initially the CHO cells produced about 10,000 units/ml. By gene amplification by progressively increasing the amount of methotrexate in the culture medium the production was boosted to 50,000-100,000 units/ml.

Concentration by freeze drying and antibody affinity chromatography using a monoclonal antibody directed to rat interferon gamma, this purification leads to a pure interferon preparation with a specific activity of $4x10^6$ U/mg protein. SDS-PAAGE of this material shows at least seven molecular forms with Mr values ranging between 14 and 25K with a relative abundant 18K protein. The rat gamma interferon shows a 87% homology with the mouse gamma and a 39% homology with human gamma concerning protein sequence. At the moment we produce about $200x10^6$ units of this material per week.

III. OTHER ANIMAL INTERFERONS

Interferon induction and physicochemical characterization have been performed for a large number of species including extraordinary ones as trout and turtles. The results have been reviewed extensively elsewhere (1,2). None of these interferons have been produced for regular in vivo testing except the bovine interferons that have been cloned mainly for commercial reasons (39). They were therefore not included in this review.

A part of our work mentioned in this review was made possible by generous support from the Dutch Cancer League (KWF). Among many others we especially thank Charles Weissmann for the generous gift of different probes and his constant advice and help.

SUMMARY

Because of the introduction of recombinant DNA technology a number of animal interferons can now be produced in unlimited amounts: murine IFN-α, β and γ, rat IFNγ and bovine IFNα, β and γ.

REFERENCES

1. Schellekens, H., and P.H. v.d. Meide: Animal studies with interferon. In: The Biology of the Interferon System 1983, E. DeMaeyer, and H. Schellekens, eds. Elsevier Science Publishers, p. 409, 1983.
2. Stewart II, W.: The interferon system, Springer Verlag, 1979.
3. Pestka, S.: In: Methods in Enzymology, Volume 79, part A/B, Interferons, Academic Press, 1981.
4. Finter, N.B.: A rich source of mouse interferon. Nature 204:1114, 1964.
5. Stewart II, W., L. Gosser, and Lockart, R.: Priming: a non-antiviral function of interferon. J Virol 7:792, 1971.
6. Knight, E.: A multisurface glass roller bottle for growth of animal cells in culture. Appl Environ Microbiol 33:666, 1977.
7. Oie, H.K., A.F. Gadzar, C.E. Buckler, and S. Baron: High interferon producing line of transformed murine cells. J Gen Virol 17:107, 1972.

8. Toey, M.G., Begon-Lours, J., and I. Gresser: A method for the large-scale production of potent interferon preparations. Proc Soc Exp Biol Med 146:809, 1974.
9. Taira, H., R.J. Broeze, E. Slattery, and P. Lengyel: Large scale production of mouse interferons from monolayers of Ehrlich ascites tumour cells. J gen Virol 49:231, 1980.
10. Sipe, J.D., J. De Maeyer-Guignard, B. Fauconnier, and E. De Maeyer: Purification of mouse interferon by affinity chromatography on a solid-phase immunoadsorbent. Proc Nat Acad Sci USA 70,4:1037, 1973.
11. Ogburn, C.A., K. Berg, and K. Paucker: Purification of mouse interferon by affinity chromatography on anti-interferon globulin-Sepharose. J of Immunol 111,4:1206, 1973.
12. De Maeyer-Guignard, J., M. Nguy Thang, and E. De Maeyer: Binding of mouse interferon to polynucleotides. Proc Natl Acad Sci USA 74,9:3787, 1977.
13. De Maeyer-Guignard, J., M.G. Tovey, I. Gresser, and E. De Maeyer: Purification of mouse interferon by sequential affinity chromatography on poly U and antibody-agarose columns. Nature 271:622, 1978.
14. Stewart II, W.E.: Distinct molecular species of interferons. Virology 61:80, 1974.
15. Yamamoto, Y., and Y. Kawade: Antigenicity of mouse interferons: distinct antigenicity of the two L cell interferon species. Virology 103:80, 1980.
16. Taira, H., R.J. Broeze, B.M. Jayaram, P. Lengyel, M.W. Hunkapiller, and L.E. Hood: Mouse interferons: amino terminal amino acid sequences of various species. Science 207,1:528, 1980.
17. Shaw, G.D., W. Boll, H. Taira, N. Mantei, P. Lengyel, and C. Weissmann: Structure and expression of cloned murine IFN-α genes. IRL Press Ltd., pp. 555, 1983.
18. Daugherty, B., D. Martin-Zanca, B. Kelder, K. Collier, T. Craig Seamans, K. Hotta, and S. Pestka: Isolation and bacterial expression of a murine alpha leukocyte interferon gene. J of Interferon Research 4:635, 1984.
19. Rehberg, E., B. Kelder, E.G. Hoal, and S. Pestka: Specific molecular activities of recombinant and hybrid leukocyte interferons. J Biol Chem 257:11497, 1982.
20. Zwarthoff, E.C., I.J. Bosveld, W.P. Vonk, and J. Trapman: Constitutive expression of a murine interferon alpha gene in hamster cells and characterization of its protein product. J gen Virol 66:685, 1985.
21. Higashi, Y. Sokawa, Y. Watanabe, Y. Kawade, S. Ohno, C. Takaoka, and T. Taniguchi: Structure and expression of a cloned cDNA for mouse interferon-β. J of Biol Chemistry 258,15:9522, 1983.
22. Tanaka, T., S. Hatsuda, G. Kawano, and T. Kobayashi: Production, purification and crystallization of recombinant murine interferon beta. In: The Biology of the Interferon System 1985, W. Stewart, and H. Schellekens, eds., Elsevier Publishers, Amsterdam, p. 65, 1986.
23. Wietzerbin, J., S. Stefanos, R. Falcoff, M. Lucero, L. Catinot, and E. Falcoff: Immune interferon induced by phytohemagglutin in nude mouse spleen cells. Inf and Imm 21:966, 1978.

24. Wietzerbin, J., S. Stefanos, M. Lucero, E. Falcoff, J.A. O'Malley, and E. Sulkowski: Physico-chemical characterization and partial purification of mouse immune interferon. J gen Virol 44:773, 1979.
25. Osborne, L.C., J.A. Georgiades, and H.M. Johnson: Large-scale production and partial purification of mouse immune interferon. Infection and Immunity 23,1:80, 1979.
26. Heremans, H., M. De Ley, A. Billiau, and P. De Somer: Mouse immune interferon: production and partial purification. In: The Biology of the Interferon System, E. De Maeyer, G. Galasso, and H. Schellekens, eds. Elsevier Biomedical Press, p. 295, 1981.
27. Gray, P.W., and Goeddel, D.V.: Cloning and expression of murine immune interferon cDNA. Proc Natl Acad Sci USA 80:5842, 1983.
28. Dijkmans, R., G. Volckaert, J. van Damme, M. De Ley, A. Billiau, and P. De Somer: Molecular cloning of murine interferon gamma (MuIFN-γ) cDNA and its expression in heterologous mammalian cells. J of Interferon Research 5:511, 1985.
29. Schonne, E.: Properties of rat-tumor interferon. Biochim Biophys Acta 115:429, 1966.
30. Coupin, G., D. Illinger, P. Poindron, and B. Fauconnier: L'interféron de Rat. Induction in vivo et in vitro. Étude de quelques propriétés biologiques. Annales pharmaceutiques francaises 36,9-10:431, 1978.
31. Abreu, S.L., and P. Kaplan: Rat fibroblast-derived interferon: Production in serum-free medium and enhancement by theophylline. J. Interferon Research 4,2:161, 1984.
32. Davis, C.T., M. Rusckowski, D.A. Goldstein, and D.M. Murasko: Production and partial purification of rat fibroblast-derived interferon induced in a newly established cell line. J. of Interferon Research 4,3:365, 1984.
33. Schellekens, H., G.A. de Wilde, and W. Weimar: Production and initial characterization of rat interferon. J gen Virol 46:243, 1980.
34. Kaplan, P., and S.L. Abreu: A high-yield chromatographic method for the purification of rat fibroblast interferon to a high specific activity. J. of Interferon Research 5:415, 1985.
35. C.T. Davis, M. Rusckowski, and D.M. Murasko: Biological similarities of rat fibroblast interferon to human and mouse alpha interferons. J gen Virol 66:1961, 1985.
36. Meide, P.H. v.d., J. Wubben, K. Vijverberg, and H. Schellekens: Production, purification and characterization of rat interferon from transformed rat cells. Methods in Enzymology, 1986.
37. Meide, P.H. v.d., R. Dijkema, M. Caspers, K. Vijverberg, and H. Schellekens: Cloning, expression and purification of rat IFN-α_1. Methods in Enzymology, 1986.
38. Dijkema, R., P.H. v.d. Meide, M. Dubbeld, M. Caspers, J. Wubben, and H. Schellekens: Cloning, expression and purification of rat IFN-γ. Methods in Enzymology, 1986.
39. Leung, D.W., D.J. Capon, and D.V. Goeddel: The structure and bacterial expression of three distinct bovine interferon-β genes. Biotechnology May:44, 1984.

III. Purification and Characterization

12. Production and Purification of Natural Human Leukocyte Interferons

Kailash C. Chadha and Eugene Sulkowski

Department of Molecular and Cellular Biology, Roswell Park Memorial Institute, Buffalo, NY 14263

INTRODUCTION

The purification of natural and recombinant human interferons is the subject of several recent reviews (1-6). The large scale purification of natural human leukocyte interferons, nHuIFN-α(s), has been accomplished by classical work of Kari Cantell and his colleagues (7). Recent refinements in their purification procedure brought the purity of nHuIFN-α(s) into the range from 2.5×10^6 to 1.25×10^7 IU per mg protein (2). Our present procedure provides for comparable purity of nHuIFN-α(s).

By and large, all available purification procedures (2) are quite complex and employ experimental conditions that are not compatible with the preservation of the tertiary structure of an interferon molecule (6,8,9). Presently, there is no detailed study available on the relationship between biological properties of individual members of the human family of leukocyte interferons and their exposure to harsh sorbent/solvent conditions (reverse phase media, low pH, chaotropes). Not precluding any possible outcome of such a study, it seems prudent for the time being to invest an effort in the elaboration of mild purification schemes. This purification procedure constitutes such an attempt. The resulting purified nHuIFN-α(s) preparation has the specific activity ca 6×10^6 per mg protein and contains both acid-stable and acid-labile interferon activities.

RESULTS

A. Preparation of Crude nHuIFN-α(s)

1. Preparation of leukocytes. In preparation of leukocytes, one usually uses ammonium chloride (NH_4Cl) to lyse red blood cells (RBC). However, in our earlier studies, we had shown that granulocytes were heavily damaged by NH_4Cl even though the cell viability, as expressed by trypan blue dye exclusion test, remained very high (10). These damaged granulocytes could release proteolytic enzymes with an ensuing

inactivation of interferon activity. Therefore, we opted for the removal of RBCs by agglomeration and sedimentation with the help of hydroxyethyl starch (HES). Penford Gum-260 (PG-260, Penick & Ford Ltd., Cedar Rapids, MI) was found to be the most effective and the least expensive source of HES. Briefly, leukocytes were separated from contaminating RBCs by mixing the buffy coat cells with equal volume of sterile PG-260 solution (6% solution in 0.9% sodium chloride) and allowing the cells to settle by gravity sedimentation at room temperature for 45-60 min. Nearly all RBCs (∿95%) usually sediment to the bottom of the cylinder. The top layer containing leukocytes was collected, the cells were washed twice with sterile phosphate buffered physiological saline to ensure complete removal of HES and they were resuspended in interferon induction media.

2. Preparation of a-gamma serum. Human a-gamma serum used during interferon production was routinely processed to remove certain proteins that are not essential for maximal interferon yield. It was sequentially chromatographed on Controlled-Pore Glass (CPG) and Phenyl-Sepharose CL-4B under the same chromatographic conditions that were employed for interferon purification. Nearly 70% of a-gamma serum proteins appeared in the breakthrough after sequential chromatography on these two sorbents. These proteins were routinely used for interferon production. This approach of prepurifying a reagent to be used in the interferon production eliminates those nonessential proteins which otherwise would bind and coelute with interferon.

3. Induction of interferon. Interferon induction medium consisted of 199 medium (Gibco, Grand Island, NY) containing 4% human a-gamma serum, 150 HAU of Sendai virus and 30 mg/L of neomycin. Leukocytes were resuspended in the induction medium in a round bottom flask at density of $1x10^7$ cells/mL and incubated at 37°C and 5% CO_2 for 20 hr. Cells were gently stirred using an egg shaped magnetic bar. At the end of the induction period, leukocytes were removed by centrifugation (2000 xg for 10 min). The supernatant was further clarified by centrifugation at 10,000 x g for 20 min. The clear supernatant is designated as crude nHuIFN-α(s).

4. Removal of inducer virus. In case of a small batch of crude nHuIFN-α(s) (100-200 ml), the inducer (Sendai virus) was effectively removed by high speed centrifugation (30,000 x g for 3 hr). However, in case of large batch of crude nHuIFN-α(s) (5-15 L), the majority of Sendai virus was removed by filtration through 100,000 MW cut-off hollow fiber filter (Amicon, Lexington, MA). This step removes nearly 80-90% of the virus based upon its titer in the retentate fraction at the end of filtration. The remaining Sendai virus was readily removed (12) when crude nHuIFN-α(s) was chromatographed on Controlled-Pore Glass (CPG) and Phenyl-Sepharose CL-4B; the steps employed for the purification of interferon. In a pilot experiment, Sendai virus (150 HAU/mL) was filtered through 100,000 MW cut-off hollow fiber filter and the filtrate sequentially chromatographed on CPG and Phenyl-Sepharose CL-4B under conditions identical to those employed for interferon purification. The final eluate from the column failed to show the

presence of any trace of infectious Sendai virus even after three successive passages through fertilized eggs. This ensures that inducer virus can be effectively removed without an acidification step which otherwise is the integral operation in the other methods of nHuIFN-α(s) production.

5. Interferon assay. Interferon antiviral activity was assayed on human foreskin fibroblasts (BG-9) by the dye uptake method of Finter (11) using VSV as a challenge virus. All titers are expressed as reference international units (IU).

The results presented in Table 1 show that yield of leukocytes per buffy coat is approximately 25% lower after treatment with HES than with NH_4Cl. However, interferon yield per $1x10^7$ leukocytes is on an average 3 times higher from leukocytes obtained after HES treatment than from those treated with NH_4Cl. No significant differences were seen in the proportion of lymphocytes to granulocytes between HES and NH_4Cl treatment. An important merit of using HES for obtaining leukocytes over NH_4Cl is that nHuIFN-α(s) produced is very stable: no significant loss in antiviral activity occurred when crude nHuIFN-α(s) was stored for two and a half years at -70°C.

6. Large scale preparation of crude nHuIFN-α(s). In order to process large numbers of buffy coats (>100) each day, it is convenient that induction process is being carried out in large round bottom flasks, in a waterbath at 37°C (without any supply of CO_2 gas). In that case, however, the major concern was to maintain the pH value of 7.4-7.6 throughout the interferon production period. This was achieved by adding 3 g/L of tricine and by increasing sodium bicarbonate concentration in the medium by 10%. The remaining conditions for the isolation of leukocytes and interferon induction remained unchanged.

B. Purification of nHuIFN-α(s)

Purification of crude nHuIFN-α(s) was achieved by a simple three step procedure which employs essentially non-overlapping chromatographic principles. Sequential chromatography of crude nHuIFN-α(s) was performed on (a) Controlled-Pore Glass (CPG)/Silicic acid, (b) CM-Sepharose CL-6B and (c) Phenyl-Sepharose CL-4B. Sendai virus used for interferon induction was effectively removed during these chromatographic steps and therefore the need for its inactivation at low pH was eliminated. As a result, the interferon purified by the present procedure has both the "acid-stable" and "acid-labile" antiviral activities. This procedure is also amenable to a scale-up for the processing of large volumes of crude nHuIFN-α(s).

1. Controlled-Pore Glass. CPG (350) was obtained from Electro-Nucleonics Inc., Fairfield, NJ. A CPG column (0.9 x 15 cm) was equilibrated with 0.01 M potassium phosphate, pH 7.4. A 100 ml of crude nHuIFN-α(s) containing 25,000 units of activity and 1.2 mg protein/mL, dialyzed overnight against column equilibrating buffer, was applied on the column. The column was washed with 50 ml of 0.01 M potassium

phosphate, pH 7.4 and then equilibrated with 0.1 M Tris·HCl, pH 8.0. Interferon activity was then displaced from the column with 0.3 M tetramethylammonium chloride (TMAC) in 0.1 M Tris·HCl, pH 8.0. The interferon eluate contained 2.4×10^6 IU and 7.5 mg protein. This represents 16-fold purification and interferon yield of ca 96%. Other details are described elsewhere (12).

Silicic acid from a variety of commercial sources, i.e., Fluka, Sigma and Mallinkrodt, can be used instead of CPG under similar chromatographic conditions. However, it is important that fine particles of Silicic acid are carefully removed before column is packed.

2. CM-Sepharose CL-6B. The pH of interferon eluate obtained from CPG/Silicic acid column was adjusted to 4.5 with 1 N HCl and applied to a CM-Sepharose CL-6B column (0.9 x 5 cm) equilibrated with 0.05 M sodium acetate, pH 4.5. The column was developed with 1) 30 mL of column equilibrating buffer, 2) 30 mL of 0.02 M sodium phosphate, pH 7.4 and finally 3) with 30 mL of 0.5 M NaCl in 0.02 M sodium phosphate, pH 7.4. The last eluate contained 2.04×10^6 IU of interferon and 1.5 mg of protein. This represents an additional 5-five fold purification and interferon recovery of 85%.

3. Phenyl-Sepharose CL-4B. The eluate from the previous step was directly (in tandem) transferred on Phenyl-Sepharose CL-4B column (0.9 x 5 cm) previously equilibrated with 0.02 M sodium phosphate, pH 7.4, containing 0.5 M NaCl. This direct transfer of interferon from one column onto another was possible because the elution conditions of interferon from CM-Sepharose CL-6B column were compatible with the adsorption conditions of interferon on Phenyl-Sepharose CL-4B sorbent. On occasion, not more than 5% of interferon appeared in the break-through fraction. After washing the column with the equilibrating buffer, the bound interferon was displaced from the column with 0.02 M phosphate buffer, pH 7.4, containing 50% ethylene glycol. A total of 1.83×10^6 IU of interferon and 0.14 mg of protein was recovered. This represents 90% interferon recovery and an additional 10-fold purification. The specific activity of interferon purified after all these three steps was 1.3×10^7 IU/mg protein.

C. Large Scale Purification of nHuIFN-α(s)

Twenty to thirty liter batches of crude nHuIFN-α(s) were processed to demonstrate the feasibility of our procedure for a large scale purification. Interferon preparations used contained 25,000 to 40,000 IU and 1.2 to 1.5 mg protein/mL. A crude interferon preparation was first subjected to molecular filtration, sequentially through 100,000 and 10,000 MW cut off hollow fiber filters (Amicon, Lexington, MA). This filtration eliminates the majority of inducer virus (80-90%) and high molecular weight proteins and at the same time reduces the volume to nearly 10% of the starting crude nHuIFN-α(s). The protein content at the end of two step filtration process is usually between 3.5 to 7.5 mg/mL and interferon titer of 200,000 to 500,000 IU/mL. It is essential that each filter is primed with 5 mg/mL of human serum albumin to minimize interferon losses.

The concentrated crude nHuIFN-α(s) was mixed with either CPG (20 g/L) or Silicic acid (50 g/L). Prior to mixing, both CPG and Silicic acid were equilibrated with 0.01 M potassium phosphate, pH 7.4. The mixture was stirred gently using suspended propeller for 60-90 min. During that time, 95% of the interferon was taken up by the sorbent. The sedimented CPG or Silicic acid was then poured into a column. The sequence of eluants used to develop such a column remains essentially the same as described above. The interferon recovery is usually 90-95%. The pH of the interferon solution was adjusted to 4.5 with 1 N HCl and mixed in a plastic roller bottle with CM-Sepharose CL-6B (1 mL of gravity packed gel for 10 mL of interferon solution) previously equilibrated with 0.1 M sodium acetate, pH 4.5. The mixture was allowed to rotate gently on a roller bottle apparatus so that the gel remained in suspension. At the end of 90 min at 4°C, the gel was allowed to sediment. Supernatant contained about 5% of interferon, and it was discarded. The CM-Sepharose CL-6B gel was then packed into a column and washed with the equlibration buffer. The bound interferon was eluted with 0.02 M phosphate, pH 7.4 containing 0.5 M NaCl. In this step, usually 80-85% of interferon activity is recovered with the additional 5-fold purification. Interferon recovered from CM-Sepharose CL-6B column was transferred onto a Phenyl-Sepharose CL-4B column. The chromatographic conditions were identical to those described for analytical runs described above and those described elsewhere (12).

The results of four separate large scale purification runs are shown in Table 2. The overall recovery at the end of the large scale purification procedure varies between 63-77% and specific activity of $3x10^6$ to $7.2x10^6$ IU/mg protein.

D. The Content of Acid-Labile Activity in Purified nHuIFN-α(s)

We have earlier shown that nearly 40% of antiviral activity of crude nHuIFN-α(s) produced by leukocytes, induced with Sendai virus, is sensitive to pH 2.0 inactivation (13, Chadha and Ikossi, in this issue). The proportion of acid-labile to acid-stable activity in crude material and purified preparations remains the same. Therefore, there is no selective loss of a putative acid-labile component(s) during the purification procedure itself.

DISCUSSION

Two issues deserve some discussion: (i) our purification procedure itself, and (ii) the origin of "low pH sensitive" interferon activity recovered from crude interferon preparations.

(i) The purification procedure, as delineated above, is rather simple and should be readily reproducible in other laboratories. Critical factor for its reproducibility, assuming standard technical skills, is the quality (read stability) of crude interferon preparations. Inasmuch as the procedure avoids low pH conditions, the presence of proteolytic enzymes (not inactivated by low pH) may render it impractical. Therefore, the preservation of mild conditions during the isolation of human leukocytes (no NH_4Cl treatment) ought to be considered as a precondition for successful purification.

The use of CPG/Silicic acid, as the first purification step, seems to be firmly in place. However, additional optimization of desorption conditions of nHuIFN-α(s) is still feasible. The residence of interferon on glass surface should be kept to a minimum to avoid losses of activity: proteins tend to crawl on glass surface and undergo denaturation.

Adsorption of nHuIFN-α(s) on CM-Sepharose CL-6B has been successfully performed at relatively low pH 4.5 due to the presence of TMAC. It should be noted, however, that prolonged exposure of interferon preparation at this pH results in the loss of activity. Dialysis seems like a simple remedy but in itself, it is an ackward exercise. Clearly, CM-Sepharose CL-4B step ought to be preceeded by a new sorbent which will adsorb interferon from a preparation obtained after glass (TMAC) and will also allow its elution at pH higher than 4.5 but low enough (pH 5.5?) to allow subsequent adsorption on CM-sorbent. The search for such a sorbent is now underway.

(ii) The origin of "low pH-sensitive" fraction of nHuIFN-α(s) activity is of considerable interest. A priori, it is not clear whether a new subspecies of leukocyte interferon has been discovered which is labile, in contrast to the other subspecies which are low pH treatment insensitive. Perhaps, a subset of leukocyte interferons is "low pH sensitive"? Perhaps all leukocyte interferons are, in principle, vulnerable to low pH inactivation and they differ among themselves only by the extent of this property? The isolation of individual members of leukocyte family of interferons, under mild purification conditions, and detailed characterization of their vulnerability to low pH treatment is very much warranted.

REFERENCES

1. Knight, E.: Purification and characterization of interferons. In: Interferon 2, I. Gresser, ed. Academic Press, 1, 1980.
2. Pestka, S., ed.: Interferons, Part A. Meth Enzymol 78: 1981.
3. Rubinstein, M.: The structure of human interferons. Biochim Biophys Acta 695:5, 1982.
4. Sulkowski, E.: Purification and characterization of interferons. Tex Rep Biol Med 41:234, 1982.
5. Lewis, W.G., and K.H. Fantes: The purification of interferons: recent developments. In: Interferon 1, N.B. Finter, ed. Elsevier, 251, 1984.
6. Dembinski, W.E., K.C. Chadha, and E. Sulkowski: Purification of interferons: an ongoing endeavor. In: The Interferon System, F. Dianzani and G.B. Rossi, eds. Serono Symposia Publications, Raven Press, 24:1, 1985.
7. Cantell, K., and S. Hirvonen: Preparation of human leukocyte interferon for clinical use. Tex Rep Biol Med 35:138, 1977.

8. Bewley, T.A., H.L. Levine, and R. Wetzel: Structural features of human leukocyte interferon A as determined by circular dichroism spectroscopy. Int J Peptide Protein Res 20:93, 1982.
9. Utsumi, J., S. Yamazaki, K. Hosoi, H. Shimizu, K. Kawaguchi, and F. Inagaki: Conformations of fibroblast and E. coli-derived recombinant human interferon-βs as studied by nuclear magnetic resonance and circular dichroism. J Biochem 99:1533, 1986.
10. Van Oss, C.J., P.M. Bronson, E.A. Dinolfo, and K.C. Chadha: Two methods for the removal of erythrocytes from buffy coats for the production of human leukocyte interferon. Immunological Commun 10:549, 1981.
11. Finter, N.B.: Dye uptake method of assessing viral cytopathogenicity and their application to interferon assays. J gen Virol 5: 419, 1969.
12. Chadha, K.C., and E. Sulkowski: Method for production and purification of human leukocyte interferon. U.S. Patent #4,485,038, 1984.
13. Chadha, K.C.: Acid-labile human leukocyte interferon. In: The Interferon System, F. Dianzani and G.B. Rossi, eds. Serono Symposia Publications, 24:35, 1985.

Table 1. Comparison of Two Methods of RBCs Removal: NH_4Cl Lysis and HES Agglomeration and Sedimentation

Exper. #	Leukocyte Yield*		Granulocyte/ Lymphocyte Ratio		Interferon Yield ($IU/10^7$ cells)	
	NH_4Cl	PG-260	NH_4Cl	PG-260	NH_4Cl	PG-260
1	$6.0x10^8$	$4.5x10^8$	1.65	1.50	10,000	31,000
2	$6.5x10^8$	$3.9x10^8$	1.30	1.25	12,500	40,000
3	$8.0x10^8$	$6.4x10^8$	2.10	1.85	17,200	44,500
4	$7.2x10^8$	$5.5x10^8$	1.40	1.65	8,000	17,000
5	$5.5x10^8$	$4.2x10^8$	1.55	1.60	14,500	50,000
6	$7.0x10^8$	$5.6x10^8$	1.45	1.35	18,000	45,000

*Each buffy coat was divided into two halves - one half used for NH_4Cl and the other for PG-260 treatment.

Table 2. The Recovery of nHuIFN-α(s) Activity During Its Large Scale Purification

Prep.#	Crude Interferon	Molecular Filtration	CPG/Silicic Acid	CM-Sepharose CL-6B	Phenyl-Sepharose CL-4B	Cumulative Recovery %	Specific Activity IU/mg Protein*
1	$6.0x10^8$	$5.52x10^8$	$5.24x10^8$	$4.45x10^8$	$4.00x10^8$	67	$5.70x10^6$
2	$1.0x10^9$	$9.50x10^8$	$8.74x10^8$	$7.69x10^8$	$7.30x10^8$	73	$3.00x10^6$
3	$7.0x10^8$	$6.30x10^8$	$5.67x10^8$	$4.53x10^8$	$4.43x10^8$	63	$7.25x10^6$
4	$7.5x10^8$	$7.12x10^8$	$6.76x10^8$	$6.08x10^8$	$5.77x10^8$	77	$6.00x10^6$

* IU, interferon activity.

13. Monoclonal Antibodies to Interferons: Their Use in Purification and in Analysis of Biological Activity

S. Landolfo,[a] M. Prat,[b] F. Cofano,[a] A. Fassio,[a] M. Simon,[c] and G. Cavallo[a]

[a]Institute of Microbiology and [b]Department of Biomedical Sciences, University of Torino, Torino, Italy; [c]Max-Planck-Institut für Immunobiologie, Freiburg, Federal Republic of Germany

INTRODUCTION

At least three classes of interferons (IFN-α, -β, -γ) have been distinguished on the basis of their antigenic properties, mode of induction by producing cells and mode of action on target cells (1). In vitro, interferons modulate cell activity by activating genes coding for a number of enzymes, as yet poorly characterized, and also by enhancing the synthesis of cell surface components. In vivo, interferons have been shown to participate in host defence against infecting agents, modulate allograft rejection, enhance natural killer activity and inhibit tumor cell growth (1). All these results have been achieved either by the use of recombinant material obtained by the DNA technology or by the in vitro establishment of hybridomas secreting monoclonal antibodies (MoAb) against human and murine IFN's.

MONOCLONAL ANTIBODIES TO INTERFERONS

Characterization and purification of various molecules by antibodies is of great value. Conventional antibodies, however, being polyclonal, are heterogeneous in their affinity and therefore do not meet the required criteria (2). The introduction of the cell fusion technique by Kohler and Milstein (3) has overcome this obstacle. In fact the advantage of this method is that it allows the production of specific antibodies in unlimited amounts to unpurified antigens. Moreover by using suitable screening methods it is possible to isolate rare hybrids producing antibodies of the desired specificity against antigens present in the immunizing material at concentrations as low as 0.1-1% of the total protein injected.

Based on this premise, Secher and Burke (4) were able to establish a monoclonal antibody anti-human IFN-α in vitro at the beginning of 1980 by immunizing mice with human leukocyte IFN present at a concentration of 0.1-1% of the total protein injected and using the inhibition of nucleic acid synthesis assay for screening the positive hybrids. The radiolabelled HuIFN-α, purified by an immunoadsorbent column made with this MoAb, displayed in SDS-PAGE a mol. wt. of about 18,000. Following this study, other laboratories using either recombinant or natural IFN's purified by different techniques, have produced MoAb to the known human IFN species (-α, -β, -γ) (5-7). In particular, Hochkeppel et al. (5), by immunizing BALB/c mice with purified blue Sepharose-adsorbed HuIFN-β, set up in vitro a MoAb neutralizing and immunoprecipitating the HuIFN-β with a mol. wt. of about 19,000, as shown in SDS-PAGE. Yet Novick et al.(6), immunizing mice with highly purified HuIFN-γ, obtained a series of hybridomas that neutralized the antiviral activity of HuIFN-γ. Immunoprecipitation of radiolabelled HuIFN- showed two proteins bands of 26,000 and 21,000 d. In the mouse system, Bosveld et al. (8), immunized Wistar rats with total crude poly(I).poly(C)-induced mouse L cell interferon, to estabhlish a MoAb to the MuIFN-β. SDS-PAGE of the material purified by an immunoadsorbent column showed that L cell interferon contains a MuIFN-β species with a mol. wt. of 32,000 to 34,000.

We have recently established in vitro a murine T-cell lymphoma producing huge amounts of homogeneous IFN-γ apparently not contaminated by other known lymphokines on stimulation with phorbol myristic acetate (PMA) (9). By immunizing Wistar rats with MuIFN-γ produced by the PMA-stimulated L12-R4 cells, we set up in vitro a hybridoma, AN-18, producing a monoclonal antibody against the MuIFN-γ (10). An immunoadsorbent column was prepared with the AN-18 MoAb and used for purification of MuIFN-γ produced in different mouse systems: a) PMA-stimulated L12-R4 cells; b) Con A-stimulated normal T lymphocytes; c) recombinant MuIFN-γ produced in E. coli(11). As shown in Table 1, the products from L12-R4 cells and normal T lymphocytes were quite heterogeneous being made up of least two molecular species with Mr of 16,500 and 17,500 and of 20,600 and 21,800 respectively. By contrast the recombinant MuIFN-γ displayed only one molecular species with a Mr of about 15,500.To analyze the origin of the molecular heterogeneity of the natural product, biosynthesis studies of MuIFN-γ were performed taking advantage of our AN-18 MoAb (12). Metabolic labeling of the intracellular and secreted forms followed by immunoprecipitation with anti-IFN-γ MoAb revealed that MuIFN-γ is synthetized as a single peptide of Mr=17,500 and undergoes proteolytic cleavage during or after secretion. Peptide mapping indeed showed that the profile of both species is very similar, suggesting a high degree of homology in the primary structure. Altogether these results demonstrate that the molecular heterogeneity of the MuIFN-γ is probably caused by different degrees of glycosylation of the two molecular species and also by a proteolytic processing during or after secretion.

Table 1. Molecular characteristics of MuIFN-γ from different sources.

Source	Molecular species	Mol. wt.
Con A stimulated T lymphocytes	2	20.6 21.8
PMA-stimulated T lymphoma	2	16.5 17.5
Recombinant MuIFN-γ	1	15.5

To analyze the origin of the molecular heterogeneity of the natural product, biosynthesis studies of MuIFN-γ were performed taking advantage of our AN-18 MoAb (12). Metabolic labeling of the intracellular and secreted forms followed by immunoprecipitation with anti-IFN-γ MoAb revealed that MuIFN-γ is synthetized as a single peptide of Mr=17,500 and undergoes proteolytic cleavage during or after secretion. Peptide mapping indeed showed that the profile of both species is very similar, suggesting a high degree of homology in the primary structure. Altogether these results demonstrate that the molecular heterogeneity of the MuIFN-γ is probably caused by different degrees of glycosylation of the two molecular species and also by a proteolytic processing during or after secretion.

ANALYSIS OF IFN ACTIVITY BY MONOCLONAL ANTIBODIES.

Establishment in our laboratory of MoAb against MuIFN-γ has provided a new tool for the analysis of the role of IFN-γ in the immune response. For this purpose two main approaches have been adopted: 1) Addition of MoAb anti-IFN-γ to in vitro systems;2) Administration of anti-IFN-γ MoAb to mice grafted with allogeneic tumor transplants.

As far as activation of T-lymphocytes is concerned, Simon et al.(3) have recently demonstrated that interleukin-2 induces IFN-gamma production by alloantigen- or mitogen-activated T lymphocytes and that an anti-IFN-gamma antiserum inhibits both proliferative and cytotoxic responses of T lymphocytes in mixed lymphocyte cultures (MLC) . Our establishment of the anti-IFN-γ monoclonal antibody, AN-18, has provided a new tool for analyzing the role of IFN-γ in antigen recognition by T lymphocytes. When AN-18 MoAb was added at the beginning of the MLC, recognition of histocompatibility antigens by T lymphocytes was completely suppressed. By contrast, addition 48-96 h later had only a slight or nil effect on T-cell activation (14). In the next set of experiments, selected Lyt-2‡ T lymphocytes were stimulated with Concanavalin A or alloantigens and increasing concentrations of exogenous recombinant interleukin-2, in either the presence or absence of anti-IFN-γ MoAb. Addition of anti-IFN-γ antibody completely abrogated IL-2 dependent proliferation and induction of cytotoxic T-lymphocytes (15). We also extended our investigations to explore the ability of anti-IFN-γ MoAb to recognize alloantigens in vivo, using chemically-induced tumors as allografts. As expected, subcutaneous injection of tumor cells in allogeneic mice resulted in quick and total rejection in recipients which differ from the tumor allograft both in major as well as in minor histocompatibility antigens. By contast, tumor outgrowth and death took place when subcutaneous injections of anti-IFN-γ MoAb were also given at the challenge site (14). These data allow one to conclude that IFN-γ plays a crucial role in vivo by regulating the recognition of alloantigens by effector T lymphocytes. Using the AN-18 MoAb we have analyzed the involvement of IFN-γ in other in vitro immune reactivities (16). As shown in Table 2, IFN-γ seems to be capable to activate tumoricidal macrophage activity and to boost natural killer cell cytotoxicity.

Table 2. Immune reactivities inhibited by anti-IFN-γ MoAb.

Alloantigen-induced T cell proliferation.
Generation of cytotoxic T lymphocytes against alloantigens.
In vivo allograft rejection.
Tumoricidal macrophage activation.
Boosting of natural killer cell cytotoxicity.

CONCLUSIONS

The advent of MoAb, which are monospecific and homogeneous in their affinity, has allowed the achievment of those goals previously unreachable with polyclonal antibodies. By using immunoadsorbents made of monoclonal antibodies, purification degrees of about 5,000 fold in a single step have been frequently described. This has indeed greatly facilitated IFN molecular studies and provided the opportunity to use highly-purified material for in vitro and in vivo experiments. Anti-IFN MoAb have also been employed to develop radioimmunoassays useful for monitoring interferons during purification and for their analysis in biological fluids and in cell cultures. Finally the in vivo use of anti-IFN monoclonal antibodies specifically neutralizing these molecules has provided definitive evidence for a natural biological role of interferons in modulating host resistance to infectious agents.

ACKNOWLEDGEMENTS

This work was supported by grants from the CNR, PF 'CMI' (N. 85.00860) and PF 'Oncologia' (N. 85.02164.44).

REFERENCES

1. Baron, S., F. Dianzani, and G.J. Stanton: The Interferon System. Tex Rep Biol Med 41: 1982.
2. Paul, W.E., ed.: Fundamental Immunology. Raven Press, 1984.
3. Kohler, G., and C. Milstein: Continuous cultures of fused cells secreting antibody of predefined specificity. Nature 256: 495,1975.
4. Secher, D.S., and D.C. Burke: A monoclonal antibody for large-scale purification of human leukocyte interferon. Nature 285: 446,1980
5. Hochkeppel, H.K., U. Menge, and J. Collins: Monoclonal antibodies against human fibroblast interferon. Nature 291:500, 1981.
6. Novick, D., Z. Eshhar, D.G. Fischer, J. Friedlander and M. Rubinstein: Monoclonal antibodies to human interferon-γ : production, affinity purification and radioimmunoassay. EMBO J 2:1527, 1983.
7. Chang, T.W., S. McKinney, V. Liu, P.C. Kung, J. Vilcek, and J. Le: Use of monoclonal antibodies as sensitive and specific probes for biologically active human γ-interferon. Proc Natl Acad Sci USA 81:5219, 1984.
8. Bosveld, I.J., W.P. Vonk, R.A.C.P. Hekman, P.W. van Vliet, P. de Jonge, W. van Ewijk, and J. Trapman: Preparation and properties of monoclonal antibodies against murine interferon-β . Virology 120:235, 1982.
9. Landolfo, S., B. Arnold, and M. Suzan: Immune interferon production by murine T cell lymphomas. J Immunol 128: 2807, 1982.
10. Prat, M., G. Gribaudo, P.M. Comoglio, G. Cavallo, and S. Landolfo: Monoclonal antibodies against murine IFN-γ . Proc Natl Acad Sci USA 81: 4515, 1984.
11. Gribaudo, G., F. Cofano, M. Prat, and S. Landolfo: Monoclonal antibodies to murine interferon-γ : affinity purification and molecular characterization of murine interferon-γ. J Interferon Res

5: 194, 1985.
12. Gribaudo, G., F. Cofano, M. Prat, C. Baiocchi, G. Cavallo, and S. Landolfo: Natural murine interferon-γ. Evidence for post-translational proteolytic processing. J biol Chem 260: 9936, 1985.
13. Simon, P.L., J.J. Farrar, and P.D. Kind: Biochemical relationship between murine immune interferon and a killer cell helper factor. J Immunol 122: 127, 1979.
14. Landolfo, S., F. Cofano, M. Giovarelli, M. Prat, G. Cavallo, and G. Forni: The inhibition of interferon-γ suppresses allograft reactivity by T-lymphocytes both in vitro and in vivo. Science 229: 176, 1985.
15. Simon, M.M., U. Hochgeschwender, U. Brugger, and S. Landolfo: Murine cytolytic T cells are induced from their lectin or antigen reactive precursor cells by recombinant interleukin 2 in collaboration with endogenous interferon-γ. J Immunol, 1986 in press.
16. Landolfo, S., F. Cofano, L. Gandino, G. Gribaudo, and M. Prat: Monoclonal antibodies against mouse interferon-γ inhibit tumoricidal macrophage activaton by T lymphocytes. Exp Cell Biol 53: 265, 1985.

14. Interferon Genes

P. P. Trotta and S. K. Narula

Schering-Plough Corporation, Bloomfield, NJ 07003

INTRODUCTION

It is well established from the isolation and characterization of interferon (IFN) cDNA's and genomic clones that the IFN genes from both human and animal sources represent a complex multigene family. Three classes of IFN genes have been identified that encode the three groups of IFN proteins that can be distinguished by antigenic, biological and biochemical characteristics; namely, α (leukocyte or type I), β (fibroblast or type I) and γ (immune or type II) IFNs. High homology exists between various members of the IFN-α gene family (85%-98%), moderate homology between IFN-α and -β genes (e.g., 45% between IFN-α1 and -β_1) and negligible homology between genes encoding for type I and type II IFNs. The heterogeneity that has been described in both the structure and function of the IFN proteins appears to be derived, at least in part, from the multiplicity of distinct IFN genes and allelic variants.

In this paper we will attempt to review and update progress on selected topics in this rapidly expanding, complex field of investigation. The majority of the data will relate to the human IFN-α gene system, for which the most information is available, although related aspects of bovine and murine genes will also be discussed.

STRUCTURE OF THE IFN GENES

Weissmann and colleagues (1,2) originally cloned and characterized two forms of IFN-α cDNA prepared from 12 S polyadenylated RNA. The IFNs produced by these clones were designated α1 and α2. The multiplicity of the IFN gene family was further supported by the studies of Goeddel and colleagues, who utilized cloned cDNA to identify 10 IFN-α genes in the human genome as well as 8 distinct cDNA clones prepared from a myeloblastoid cell line (3). Henco et al (4) have recently reported the isolation and characterization of additional human IFN-α sequences. In conjunction with DNA sequences published in other laboratories, these authors have described 7 linkage groups containing 23 loci for IFN-α. The sequence of 15 of these genes suggests that they are likely to encode potentially functional IFNs, while 6 are apparently non-functional pseudogenes. The remaining two loci were uncategorized with respect to function since they were not sequenced. None of the IFN-α genes contain introns in their coding regions (4). By employing specific oligonucleotide probes, it has recently been demonstrated that nucleotide sequences corresponding to both IFN-αA and -α2 exist in human genomic DNAs (5). These results imply that these two IFNs, which differ at only one amino acid position, represent products of closely related but distinct loci. Two genes with identical nucleotide sequences in their coding region (i.e., IFN-α13 and -α1) are, in fact, non-allelic.

These IFN-α genes have been referred to as class I or IFN-α_I subfamily (6). They are localized to the short arm and the proximal 10% of the long arm of chromosome 9 (7). Members of this class generally encode mature polypeptides with either 165 or 166 amino acids. By screening a human genomic library with a human IFN-α cDNA probe, Capon et al (6) have identified an IFN-α gene that belongs to a second family (class II or IFN-α_{II} subfamily) that encodes a mature protein of 172 amino acids in length. The human class II IFN-α gene subfamily may contain as many as 6-7 members. Low stringency hybridization with a human IFN-α cDNA probe has identified two distinct classes of bovine IFN, I and II, analogous to the two classes observed in the human genome (6). Southern blot analyses indicated that the bovine IFN-α gene class I subfamily consists of 10-12 members, and the bovine IFN-α class II subfamily has 15-20 members. Interestingly, both bovine class I and class II genes demonstrate in their coding regions more homology with the respective human class I and class II than to each other. Both bovine and human class II genes expressed in _E. coli_ were demonstrated to encode proteins with antiviral activity.

A single species of human IFN-β cDNA, termed IFN-β_1, derived from double-stranded RNA-induced diploid human fibroblasts has been cloned and characterized (8,9). The screening of human genomic libraries with IFN-β_1 cDNA has resulted in the isolation of a single IFN-β gene that does not contain introns (10,11). Several lines of evidence, however, suggest the possibility of multiple IFN-β genes. IFN-β mRNA that does not readily cross-hybridize with an IFN-β_1 cDNA probe has been detected in poly(I): poly(C)-induced human fibroblasts (12,13). Analysis of human-rodent hybrids has demonstrated the production of IFN-β when any of three human chromosomes (i.e., chromosome 2, 5 or 9) is present (14,15). In addition, two novel, distinct non-allelic genomic DNA clones have been isolated from a human fetal DNA library that hybridize to IFN-β_1 cDNA and that can be distingushed from the classical IFN-β_1 gene (16). Since it has been shown that human IFN-β nucleotide sequences can hybridize with class II IFN-α genes (6), cross-hybridization with IFN-β_1 probes may not be indicative of an IFN-β gene family. Recent data have indicated that in some individuals there does appear to be duplication of the IFN-β gene (17). However, the scientific community remains divided on the existence of multiple human IFN-β genes. Only one or two IFN-β genes have been detected in most other mammalian species so far tested, although the same species demonstrate complex IFN-α multi-gene families (18). The claim for multiple murine IFN-β genes appears to be controversial since the original report (19) was not found to be reproducible (20).

The coding region of the human IFN-γ gene has been shown to consist of a unique single copy DNA by both southern hybridization of a human genomic DNA and *in situ* hybridization of chromosome preparations with cDNA probes (7). An analysis of the genomic clone has revealed 3 introns. These introns begin with a GT dinucleotide and end with an AG dinucleotide, sequences essential for correct splicing. Introns 1, 2 and 3 are 1238, 95 and 2422 base pairs long, respectively. The four exons contain 38, 23, 61 and 44 amino acids, respectively. The first intron also contains a repetitive sequence that is distinct from the repetitive human Alu family sequences (21). The IFN-γ gene has been assigned to a specific subband in chromosome 12 (22).

The human IFN-α gene cluster and the IFN-β gene are closely linked. At least 5 restriction fragment length polymorphisms have been identified with an IFN-α probe and two with an IFN-β probe in the α/β IFN region of the human genome (17). The IFN-γ gene does not show any evidence for the existence of restriction fragment length polymorphism (21).

REGULATION OF IFN GENES

Human IFN-α and -β genes are expressed in response to a variety of viral and non-viral inducers. This induction is due, in part, to an effect of the IFN gene promoters on the level of transcription. The 5' flanking regions of IFN-β and several IFN-α genes have been found to share extensive homology. The Hogness box (TATA) is found in all three classes of IFN at approximately -25 base pairs from the mRNA start. Regions upstream of the TATA box are involved in the inducible expression of these genes (22,23). In the case of the IFN-α1 gene promoter, it has recently been demonstrated by use of deletion mutants that a 46 nucleotide segment is sufficient to confer inducibility on unrelated promoters (24). This segment is derived from the region -109 to -64 upstream of the promotor fragment and has two sets of repeats: a perfect pentameric repeat and an imperfect octameric repeat. This fragment is equally effective in either orientation. Insertion of two or three such units was shown to increase inducibility. This region is conserved to various degrees in the IFN-α gene family and IFN-β genes.

In the case of the IFN-β gene promoter, two functionally distinct sequences that mediate transcriptional control have been demonstrated (25). The sequence encompassing -77 to -55 is a constitutive promoter element that is necessary and sufficient for the inducible expression of IFN-β. However, a cis acting element that is located in the region between -65 and -30 acts as a negative transcriptional regulator (26). Footprinting experiments have provided clear evidence for repressor molecules (proteins I and II) that bind to the -94 to -167 and -68 to -38 regions, respectively, of the IFN-β promoter and are released on induction (25). An IFN transcriptional factor that binds to a region located within -77 to -64 was observed concomitant with the initiation of transcription.

The expression of IFN-γ is highly cell-specific (27). The promoter region contains a number of palindromes and repeat sequences that are probably recognized by specific proteins (21). A DNAse I hypersensitive region could be detected in the first intervening sequence of IFN-γ, which is 83% homologous to a hypersensitive site that lies 300 base pairs upstream of the interleukin 2 promoter (28). DNAse I hypersensitivity is usually an indication of the unique conformation of the regulatory regions of the genes. Preliminary data from the same laboratory support the presence of several control regions that may respond in an inducer-specific manner. Since the genes for both interleukin 2 and IFN-γ appear to be coordinately expressed (28), it is possible that they share potential regulatory elements. The concept of shared regulatory circuits is appealing in the context of the regulation of the expression of multiple cytokines.

EVOLUTIONARY AND FUNCTIONAL SIGNIFICANCE OF IFN GENES

An evolutionary tree for IFN-α genes can be constructed

based on homologies in the nucleotide sequences. The evolution of the system can be understood in terms of the duplication of an ancestral IFN gene ca 4-5 hundred million years ago to give rise to the primordial precursors of the IFN-α and -β gene families. However, based on an average mutation rate of 0.1% per million years for a single-copy DNA, the IFN-α genes were amplified relatively recently (i.e., 50-75 million years ago). It is not known whether the IFN-γ gene diverged earlier in evolution or was of independent origin. Several mechanisms appear to be involved in the generation of the IFN-α multi-gene family. In most of the IFN-α genes, divergence is attributable to insertions or deletions of either single nucleotides or short stretches of nucleotides that give rise to short frame-shifted regions. Both gene amplification (6) and gene conversion (29) have also been implicated.

Application of a mathematical method termed "metric analysis" by using the Sellers TT algorithim has indicated that both the IFN-α1 and -β_1 genes are internally duplicated (30). Based on a partial consensus nucleotide sequence of all four repeats contained within these two genes, Erickson et al (30) have proposed that the IFN-α1 and -β_1 genes may have evolved from a single "half-gene" segment. Important confirmation of this concept would be the preparation of fragments derived from the amino and carboxyl terminals that retain either biological activity or the ability to bind to the type I IFN receptor. It may be relevent that a 110-amino acid amino-terminal fragment of IFN-α2 has been reported to demonstrate antiviral activity (31).

The functional significance of the existence of a variety of IFN-α and -β genes remains speculative. It has been observed that the ratio of IFN-α to IFN-β transcripts (32) as well as the proportion of distinct IFN-α proteins (33, 34) is dependent on the cell type. The precise ratio of subtypes that are expressed may have profound consequences on both the level of antiviral activity and the viral specificity. Thus, the specific antiviral activities of purified recombinant human IFN-α subtypes have been observed to vary by 1-2 orders of magnitude (Table 1). IFN-α1 expresses the lowest specific antiviral activity (7.1×10^6 IU/mg) among the naturally occurring IFN-α subtypes, while IFN-α2 is the most potent antiviral agent (2×10^8 IU/mg) among this group. An even wider range of specific activities was observed when antiproliferative activity was assayed (Table 1), suggesting that antitumor effects may also be dependent on the ratios of subtypes. Other experiments support that the natural killer cell activity of these purified IFN-α subtypes is also highly variable (35).

IFN STRUCTURE-FUNCTION RELATIONS

The construction of genes encoding novel IFN variants and hybrids of naturally occurring subtypes has been utilized to provide important insights into IFN structure-function relations. By utilizing common restriction sites, a series of human IFN-α2/α1 and -α1/α2 hybrids have been constructed and analyzed for biological activity. The activity profiles have identified a sequence of amino acids potentially important for augmentation of natural killer cell activity (36) and have indicated the existence of two distinct receptor binding sites located in the amino- and carboxyl-terminal regions, respectively (37). The fact that all cloned leukocyte IFNs share in common 4 cysteine residues (4), which at least in one IFN-α subtype have been demonstrated to exist as two disulfide linkages (38), indicates that the conformational integrity of either or both of these domains may depend on disulfide bonds. However, as noted in Table 1, two IFN-α variants (i.e., Δ4α1 and Δ4α2/α1) that lack the disulfide linkage in which Cys_1 participates are active as antiviral agents, suggesting that it is the Cys_{29}-Cys_{138} disulfide linkage that is critical for maintaining the biologically active conformation (39).

Site-directed mutagenesis has also been employed to elucidate the functional importance of evolutionarily conserved amino acid positions. Site-directed point mutations introduced into codons 48 and 49 of the human IFN-α2 gene, positions that are strictly conserved in human IFN-β_1, did not significantly alter the specific antiviral activity (40). Similarly, substitution of lysine for the glutamic acid residue at position 62 in IFN-α2, a residue conserved in all known human, murine and bovine type I IFNs, did not affect antiviral activity. In distinction, Camble et al (41) have recently utilized synthetic gene technology to demonstrate that changes in the arginine residue at position 33 of IFN-α2, which is strictly conserved in human type I IFNs, resulted in large decreases in both antiviral and antiproliferative activity.

Since studies on natural human IFN-γ imply that the Cys-Tyr-Cys residues are removed from the amino terminus during secretion (42), gene modification has been employed to assess the importance of these residues for the expression of biological activity. Human IFN-γ analogs lacking this sequence were produced by gene synthesis methods and were found to exhibit similar antiviral activity in comparison to the full-length molecule (43). Parallel studies have been conducted in our laboratory (44) to investigate the importance of these residues through genetic engineering of variants of murine IFN-γ (Table 2). The specific antiviral activity of murine IFN-γD, which lacks these three residues, was 10-fold higher than that of murine IFN-γA. Removal of the 6 carboxyl-terminal amino acids from nIFN-γD, resulting in the formation of variant IFN-γD', did not change the specific antiviral activity, while removal of 4 additional carboxyl-terminal amino acid residues appeared to depress activity by several-fold. Thus, none of the three Cys residues (positions 1, 3 and 136) in the full-length murine IFN-γ is essential for antiviral activity.

CONCLUSIONS

The data summarized here demonstrate the current rapid progress and expansion of information on the IFN gene family as well as on the use of genetic engineering for elucidating the structure-activity relations of the encoded proteins. The cloning and expression of both type I and II human IFNs in E. coli has enabled sufficient quantities of material to be produced for world-wide clinical trials. It is anticipated that future studies on the structure-activity relations within the IFN gene family will provide a basis for the design of second generation IFNs that may exhibit greater clinical efficacy with fewer toxicities.

Acknowledgements

The authors wish to thank Dr. Jerome Schwartz and his staff for performance of the antiviral and antiproliferative assays.

REFERENCES

1. Nagata, T., N. Mantei, and C. Weissmann: The structure of one of the eight or more distinct chromosomal genes for human interferon-α. Nature 287:401, 1980.
2. Streuli, M. S. Nagata and C. Weissmann: At least three human type α interferons: structure of α2. Science 209:1343, 1980.
3. Goeddel, D.V., D.W. Leung, T.J. Dull, M. Gross, R.M. Lawn, R. McCandliss, P.H. Seeburg, A. Ullrich, E. Yelverton and P.W Gray: The structure of eight distinct cloned human leukocyte interferon cDNAs. Nature 290:20, 1981.
4. Henco, K., J. Brosius, A. Fujisawa, J.I. Fujisawa, J.R. Haynes, J. Hochstadt, J. Kovacic, M. Pasek, A. Schambock, J. Schmid, K. Todokoro, M. Walchli, S. Nagata and C. Weissmann: Structural relationship of human interferon alpha genes and pseudogenes. J Mol Biol 185:227, 1985.
5. Pestka, S., K. Hotta, J. Monahan and K.J. Collier: Detection of human leukocyte interferon αA and α2 genes in genomic DNAs by the use of deoxyoctadecyloligonucleotide probes. Abstracts of 1985 TNO-ISIR Meeting, Clearwater Beach, Florida, p. 5, 1985.

6. Capon, D.J., H.M. Shepard and D.V. Goeddel: Two distinct families of human and bovine interferon-α genes are coordinately expressed and encode functional polypeptides. Mol Cell Biol 5:768, 1985.
7. Trent, J.M., S. Olson and R.M. Lawn: Chromosomal localization of human leukocyte, fibroblast, and immune interferon genes by means of in situ hybridization. Proc Natl Acad Sci USA 79:7809, 1982.
8. Taniguchi, T., S. Ohno, Y. Fuji-Kuriyama and M. Muramatsu: The nucleotide sequence of human fibroblast interferon cDNA. Gene 10:11, 1980.
9. Derynck, R., J. Content, E. DeClercq, G. Volckaert, J. Tavernier, R. Devos, and W. Fiers; Isolation and structure of a human fibroblast interferon gene. Nature 285:542, 1980.
10. Houghton, M., I.J. Jackson, A.J. Porter, S.M. Doel, G.H. Catlin, C. Barber and N.H. Carey: The absence of introns within a human fibroblast gene. Nucl Acids Res 9:247, 1981.
11. Tavernier, J., R. Derynck and W. Fiers: Evidence for a unique human fibroblast interferon (IFN β_1) chromosomal gene devoid of intervening sequences. Nucl Acids Res 9:461, 1981.
12. Sehgal, P.B. and A.D. Sagar: Heterogeneity of poly(I). poly(C)-induced human fibroblast interferon mRNA species Nature 287:95, 1980.
13. Weissenbach, J., Y. Chernajowsky, M. Zeevi, L. Shulman, H. Soreq, U. Nir, D. Wallach, M. Perricaudet, P. Tiollais and M. Revel: Two interferon mRNAs in human fibroblasts: in vitro translation and Escherichia coli cloning studies. Proc Natl Acad Sci USA 77:7152, 1980.
14. Tan, Y.H. R.P. Creagan and F.H. Ruddle: The somatic cell genetics of human interferon: assignment of human interferon loci to chromosomes 2 and 5. Proc Natl Acad Sci USA 71:2251, 1974.
15. Meager, A. H. Graves, D.C. Burke, and D.M. Swallow: Involvement of a gene on chromosome 9 in human fibroblast interferon production. Nature 290:493, 1979.
16. Sehgal, P.B., L.T. May, A.D. Sagar, K.S. LaForge and M. Inouye: Isolation of novel human genomic DNA clones related to human interferon-β_1 cDNA. Proc Natl Acad Sci USA 80:3632, 1983.
17. Ohlsson, M., J. Feder, L.L. Cavalli-Sforza and A.V. Gabain: Close linkage of α and β interferons and infrequent duplication of β interferon in humans. Proc Natl Acad Sci USA 82:4473, 1985.
18. Wilson, V., A.J. Jeffreys, P.A. Barrie, P.G. Boseley, P.M. Slocombe, A. Easton and D.C. Burke: A comparison of vertebrate interferon gene families detected by hybridization with human interferon DNA. J Mol Biol 166:457, 1983.
19. Skup, D., J.D. Windass, F. Sor, H. George, R.G. Williams, H. Fukuhara, J. De Maeyer-Guignard and E. De Maeyer: Molecular cloning of partial cDNA copies of two distinct mouse IFN-beta mRNAs. Nucl Acids Res 10: 3069, 1982.

20. Higashi, Y., Y. Sokawa, Y. Watanabe, Y. Kawade, S. Ohno, C. Takaoka and T. Taniguchi: Structure and expression of a cloned cDNA for mouse interferon-β. J Biol Chem 258:9522, 1983.
21. Taya, Y., R. Devos, J. Tavernier, H. Cheroutre, G. Engler and W. Fiers: Cloning and structure of the human immune interferon-γ gene. Embo J 1:953, 1982.
22. Naylor, S.L., A.Y. Sakaguchi, T.B. Shows, M.L. Law, D.V. Goeddel and P.W. Gray: Human immune interferon is located on chromosome 12. J Exp Med 57:1020, 1983.
22. Weidle, O. and C. Weissmann: The 5' flanking region of a human IFN-α gene mediates viral induction of transcription. Nature 303:442, 1983.
23. Zinn, K.D., DiMaio, and T. Maniatis: Identification of two distinct regulatory regions adjacent to the human β-interferon gene. Cell 34:865, 1983.
24. Ryals, J., P. Dirks, H. Ragg and C. Weissmann: A 46 nucleotide promoter segment from an IFN-α gene renders an unrelated promoter inducible by virus. Cell 47:497, 1986.
25. Zinn, K. and T. Maniatis: Detection of factors that interact with the human β-interferon regulatory region in vivo by DNAse I footprinting. Cell 45:611, 1986.
26. Goodburn, S., H. Burstein and T. Maniatis: The human β-interferon gene is under negative control. Cell 45:601, 1986.
27. Young, H., L. Varesio and P. Hwu: Posttranscriptional control of human gamma interferon gene expression in transfected mouse fibroblasts. Mol and Cell Biol 6:2253, 1986.
28. Hardy, K.J., B.M. Peterlin, R.E. Atchison and J.D. Stobo: Regulation of expression of the human interferon γ gene. Proc Natl Acad Sci USA 82:8173, 1985.
29. Todokora, A., D. Kioussia and C. Weissmann: Two non-allelic human interferon alpha genes with identical coding regions. Embo J 3:1809, 1984.
30. Erickson, B.W., L.T. May and P.B. Sehgal: Internal duplication in human α1 and $β_1$ interferons. Proc Natl Acad Sci USA 81:7171, 1984.
31. Ackerman, S.K., D. Zur Nedden, M. Heintzelman, M. Hunkapiller and K.C. Zoon: Biologic activity in a fragment of recombinant human interferon-α. Proc Natl Acad Sci USA 81:1045, 1984.
32. Hiscott, J., J. Ryals, P. Dierks, V. Hofmann and C. Weissmann: The expression of human alpha genes. Phil Trans R Soc Lond B 307:217, 1984.
33. Allen, G. and K.H. Fantes: A family of structural genes for human lymphoblastoid (leukocyte-type) interferon. Nature 287:408, 1980.
34. Levy, W.P., M. Rubinstein, J. Shively, U. Del Valle, C.Y. Lai, J. Moschera, L. Brink, L. Gerber, S. Stein and S. Pestka: Amino acid sequence of a human leukocyte interferon. Proc Natl Acad Sci USA 78:6186, 1981.

35. Platsoucas, C.D., M. Galinski, J. Higgins, J. Keen, H.-J. Feichert and P.P. Trotta: Regulation of natural killer cytotoxicity and of proliferative responses of human leukocytes by recombinant alpha interferons. Antiviral Res Abstr 1, No. 3, p. 74, 1984.
36. Herberman, R.: Interferon and cytotoxic effector cells. In: Interferons and the Immune System, J. Vilcek and E. DeMaeyer, eds. Elsevier Science Publishers, pp. 61-99, 1984.
37. Streuli, M. A., Hall, W. Boll, W.E. Stewart III, S. Nagata and C. Weissmann: Target cell specificity of two species of human interferon-α produced in Escherichia coli and of hybrid molecules derived from them. Proc Natl Acad Sci USA 78:2848, 1981.
38. Wetzel, R.: Assignment of the disulphide bonds of leukocyte interferon. Nature 289:606, 1981.
39. Lydon, N.B., C. Favre, S. Bove, O. Neyret, S. Benureau, A.M. Levine, G.F. Seelig, T.L. Nagabhushan and P.P. Trotta: Immunochemical mapping of α-2 interferon. Biochem 24:4131, 1985.
40. Valenzuela, D.,H. Weber and C. Weissmann: Is sequence conservation in interferons due to selection for functional proteins? Nature 313:698, 1985.
41. Camble R., N.N. Petter, P. Trueman, C.R. Newton, F.J. Carr, R.C. Hockney, V.E. Moore, A.R. Greene, D. Holland and M.D. Edge: Functionally important conserved amino-acids in interferon-α_2 identified with analogues produced from synthetic genes. Biochem Biophys Res Commun 134:1404, 1986.
42. Rinderknecht, E., B.H. O'Connor and H. Rodriguez: Natural human interferon-γ. J Biol Chem 259:6790, 1984.
43. Alton, K., Y. Stabinsky, R. Richards, B. Ferguson, L. Goldstein, B. Altrock, L. Miller and N. Stebbing: Production, characterization and biological effects of recombinant DNA derived human IFN-α and IFN-γ analogs. In: The Biology of the Interferon System 1983, E. De Maeyer and H. Schellekens, eds. Elsevier Science Publishers, pp. 119-128, 1983.
44. Le, H.V., C.A., Mays, R. Syto, T.L. Nagabhushan and P.P. Trotta: Structure-function relations in recombinant murine gamma interferon. In: The Biology of the Interferon System-1985, W.E. Stewart III and H. Schellekens, eds. Elsevier Science Publishing Co., 1985, in press.

Table 1. Specific Antiviral and Antiproliferative Activities Of Purified Recombinant Human IFN-α Subtypes[a]

IFN Subtype	Specific Activities: Antiviral (IU/mg)	Specific Activities: Antiproliferative (ng/ml)
α1	7.1×10^6	125.0
Δ4α1	2.8×10^6	N.D.[b]
α2	2.0×10^8	6.0
Δ4α2/α1	1.0×10^8	15.0
α4	1.0×10^8	0.12
α5	8.0×10^7	0.6
α7	2.0×10^7	1.3

[a] Antiviral activity was determined by the cytopathic effect-inhibition assay employing encephalomyocarditis virus and human foreskin cells. Antiproliferative assays were performed on the WISH cell line. The data are expressed as the minimum concentration required to inhibit cellular proliferation. The IFN preparations were greater than 95% pure. Δ4 refers to a deletion of the first 4 amino acids from the amino terminus.

[b] N.D. = Not determined.

Table 2. Specific Antiviral Activity of Purified Recombinant Murine IFN-γ Subtypes[a]

IFN Subtype	Antiviral Activity (Units/mg)
γA	2×10^6
γD	2×10^7
γD'	2×10^7
γD"	4×10^6

[a] Antiviral activity was determined by the cytopathic effect-inhibition assay employing encephalomyocarditis virus and L929 cells. Based on the numbering of the amino acid sequence in murine IFN-γA, the IFN-γ variants, as defined by Le et al (44), are: γA (1-136), γD (4-136), γD' (4-130), and γD" (4-126).

15. Interferons: Protein Structure

Abbas Rashidbaigi and Sidney Pestka

Roche Institute of Molecular Biology, Roche Research Center, Nutley, NJ 07110

INTRODUCTION

Interferons are proteins expressed in cells upon viral infection and by induction with other nonviral substances. They are involved in regulatory activities such as cellular differentiation and immune modulation in addition to protecting cells from virus infection. Interferons are classified into three major groups: leukocyte (IFN-α), fibroblast (IFN-β), and immune (IFN-γ) (1). The amino acid sequences of many of them have been determined by sequencing the proteins or from the DNA sequence of their corresponding genes. Many of the interferons have been expressed in bacteria or heterologous hosts, and have been purified to homogeneity. Although crude interferons have been used therapeutically, purified interferons have been used in recent clinical trials on patients with various diseases. They have also been used for biological and biochemical studies in order to understand the molecular mechanism of their action. The aim of this review is to summarize the structural information currently available on interferons. For related aspects of interferon genetics, structure, function, and production, readers are referred to other relevant reviews in this volume and elsewhere (2-10).

The properties of various types of interferons are summarized in Table I. There are more than fifteen highly related Hu-IFN-α species (3,21,22). Hu-IFN-β and -γ are single protein species. However, it has already been shown that the pattern of heterogeneity may be quite different from species to species (23) and that bovine IFN-β consists of three distinct proteins (24).

Primary Structure of Leukocyte Interferons (IFN-α)

Various chromatographic techniques and SDS-polyacrylamide gel electrophoresis demonstrated that natural IFN-α's were heterogeneous (25-29). Their size ranged from 17.5 kd to 23 kd. The source of heterogeneity is the result of different primary sequences (30-32). Hu-IFN-α species are somewhat acidic with isoelectric points of 5.7-7.0 (4,26,33). Partial and complete amino acid sequences were derived from several natural Hu-IFN-α species (34,35). Additional sequences of Hu-IFN-α's were obtained from DNA sequencing of cDNA or genomic clones (36-43). The sequences of Hu-IFN-α species derived from DNA sequences are listed in Figure 1. In Figure 2 the sequence of Hu-IFN-α is compared to the sequences of IFN-α's derived from DNA sequencing of murine, rat, and monkey species. These Hu-IFN-α's have about 165 or 166 amino acids with about 80% sequence homology (7-10,22,36). The Mu-IFN-α species are 78% homologous to each other, and the Ra-IFN-α's are 81% homologous to Mu-IFN-α1 (48). Monkey IFNα-D (Fig.2) shows 94% sequence homology to Hu-IFN-αD (49). Recently, some distinct families of IFN-α-related genes were characterized (22,51-53). In Figure 3, the amino acid sequence of Hu-IFN-α is compared to the sequences of these human and bovine IFN-α-like species. Both bovine and human IFN-α-like genes encode for a mature polypeptide of 172 amino acids. The secondary structure of Hu-IFN-α's was also predicted experimentally with circular dichroism and by computer analysis (56-58). These analyses showed 55-70% α-helix content with less than 16% β-sheet.

Two of the natural Hu-IFN-α's which were sequenced contained only 155 amino acids lacking 10 carboxy-terminal amino acids predicted from the coding sequence of the corresponding genes (34). This truncation may be due to processing during biosynthesis, production or purification. The biological activity of these truncated interferons is comparable to the specific activity of the corresponding cloned intact interferons. This indicates that the 10 carboxy-terminal amino acids are not required for biological activity.

All of the Hu-IFN-α's except IFN-αD have four cysteine residues at positions 1, 29, 99 and 139 (in IFN-αB the third cysteine is at position 98). IFN-αD has a fifth cysteine at position 86. Like Hu-IFN-α's, Bo-IFN-α spcies contain four cysteine residues at identical positions (55). The murine sequences so far reported contain five cysteine residues, four of which are at the same positions as in the human counterparts (positions 1, 29, 99, 139). The fifth cysteine is at position 86 which is the same position as the fifth cysteine of human IFN-αD. Ra-IFN-α, like Mu-IFN-α, has also a fifth cysteine at position 86. For Hu-IFN-αA, two disulfide bonds have been assigned, connecting cysteines 1 to 99, and 29 to 138 (or cysteines 29 to 139 in other Hu-IFN-α's) (59). The importance of the 29-138 disulfide bond in retention of biological activity and conformational stability of IFN-α's has been demonstrated (60).

Hu-IFN-αH has two potential *N*-linked glycosylation sites (Asn-X-Ser/Thr) at positions 2 and 78. Hu-IFN-α-like sequences also contain a potential glycosylation site at position 78 (51-53). Other Hu-IFN-α's do not contain *N*-linked glycosylation sites. However, several natural IFN-α species have been shown to contain significant amounts of glucosamine and galactosamine residues which suggests the presence of *O*-linked carbohydrates (61). There is one potential *N*--linked glycosylation site in Mu-IFN-α1 and Mu-IFN-α2 at position 78, but not in Mu-IFN-αA, and one in Ra-IFN-α at position 167.

<u>Primary Structure of Fibroblast Interferons (IFN-β)</u>

The characteristics of fibroblast interferon (IFN-β) are summarized in Table I. Hu-IFN-β has been purified from induced fibroblasts by various chromatographic techniques (62-68). Natural Hu-IFN-β is a glycoprotein with a molecular weight of about 23,000 (68,69) and isoelectric point of 6.8-7.8 (70). Although Hu-IFN-β has 29% structural homology to Hu-IFN-α (39,71), and shares common receptors with IFN-α's (72,73), it is antigenically distinct (74) and its protein is coded by an entirely different gene (75).

Mu-IFN-β has also been purified from various cultured mouse cells (76-81). Mu-IFN-β, in contrast to its human counterpart, was shown to be heterogeneous. It is composed of two size classes, a species with a molecular size in the range of 26-33 kd and a species with a molecular size of 35-40 kd. Partial amino acid sequencing of the *N*-termini of human (64,65,68) and mouse (50) IFN-β has been reported and it appears that both, in contrast to the IFN-α families, are single species. The entire amino acid sequences of human, murine, and bovine IFN-β's were deduced from sequencing the cDNA or genomic clones (24,38,39,82-86). The structures of these proteins are shown in Figure 4. The Hu-IFN-β is encoded by a single gene which contains no intervening sequences (39,87) and maps to chromosome 9 (14,15). It is composed of 166 amino acids; a 21 amino acid signal peptide is removed during secretion from cells. The Mu-IFN-β gene codes for a protein of 182 amino acids, the first 21 of which represent the signal peptide. The mature mouse protein of 161 amino acids has a predicted molecular size of 19.7 kd. Mu-IFN-β shows 48% amino acid homology to Hu-IFN-β (86). Each of the three bovine genes codes for a protein containing 165 amino acids, plus a 21 residue signal peptide, that have about 83-95% homology to each other (10,24). Computer analysis has also been used to predict the secondary structure of IFN-β (58).

Hu-IFN-β contains cysteine residues at positions 17, 31, and 141. The cysteine at position 17 is not essential for biological activity. When cysteine 17 was substituted with a serine by site-directed mutagenesis, the resultant interferon was fully active (88). However, when cysteine at position 141 was converted to tyrosine, the biological activity of interferon was lost (89). Like Hu-IFN-β, Bo-IFN-β species contain three cysteines at identical positions (17, 31, and 141). Mu-IFN-β has only a single cysteine residue at position 17.

Hu-IFN-β has a single potential *N*-linked glycosylation site at position 80. However, glycosylation is not required for its biological activity, since *Escherichia coli*-derived recombinant IFN-β, which does not contain a sugar moiety, has full activity. Mu-IFN-β contains three potential *N*-linked glycosylation sites at positions 29, 69, and 76. The heterogeneity of Mu-IFN-β is believed to be due to various degrees of glycosylation (50). Bo-IFN-β sequences contain two potential *N*--linked glycosylation sites at positions 110 and 153.

Primary Structure of Immune Interferons (IFN-γ)

Human immune (IFN-γ) was first described by Wheelock in 1965 (90). It was distinguished from other interferons by its instability to acid treatment (91). The loss of biological activity of Hu-IFN-γ at low pH was shown to be the result of changes in the structure of the protein (92). IFN-γ has some role in immune regulation (reviewed in 93). It is identical to the protein, macrophage activating factor (94). Hu-IFN-γ has been purified by various chromatographic techniques (95-98). The protein is heterogeneous and has molecular sizes of 20 kd and 25 kd upon SDS-polyacrylamide gel electrophoresis (95,98-100). The functional unit of Hu-IFN-γ is a tetramer or trimer (101). Natural Hu-IFN-γ is a highly basic protein with an isoelectric point of 8.6-8.7 (91).

Natural Mu-IFN-γ has also been purified from various sources (102-104). Heterogeneity for the mouse protein has also been observed. T-cell-derived Mu-IFN-γ consisted of two proteins of 17.5 kd and 16.5 kd under denaturing conditions (105). Both of these species are glycosylated. Pulse-chase experiments showed that the smaller peptide is derived from the 17.5 kd peptide.

The amino acid sequence of Hu-IFN-γ was derived from the DNA sequence (106-108). It is composed of 143 amino acids with a molecular weight calculated to be 16,757. The coding sequence is preceeded by a 23 residue signal sequence. There are two clusters of basic amino acid residues at positions 89-92 and 131-134. The Hu-IFN-γ gene shows only 11% amino acid homology to IFN-α or IFN-β (109). Analysis of the protein has shown that the amino terminus is pyroglutamate (98). The natural Hu-IFN-γ lacks between 9 to 16 carboxy terminal amino acid residues depending on the source of production (98). Recombinant Hu-IFN-γ is also processed after purification if it is not stored properly (J.A. Langer, F.R. Khan and A. Rashidbaigi, unpublished observation). It is not known whether this processing is spontaneous or whether it is due to a protease contamination in purified protein.

The amino acid sequences for mouse (110), bovine (111,112) and rat (113) IFN-γ have been predicted from their respective DNA sequences (Figure 5). The mature mouse protein is composed of 136 amino acid residues corresponding to a molecular weight of about 15,800 and has 40% amino acid homology to the human protein. The bovine sequence has the same length as the human protein and shares 61% amino acid homology with Hu-IFN-γ. The small sequence homology between various IFN-γ species may explain the high species specificity of these proteins (20).

There are two potential sites for *N*-linked glycosylation in human (residues 28 and 100) and mouse (residues 19 and 71) IFN-γ's. It has been shown that the 20 kd human species was glycosylated at Asn 28, while 25 kd species was glycosylated at both Asn 28 and 100 (98). Therefore, the basis of heterogeneity in natural human protein seems to be due to the differential glycosylation.

Both human and murine IFN-γ species have been phosphorylated at serine residues with retention of biological activity (114-116). These phosphorylated IFN-γ's are useful for receptor binding studies (116,117). The serine residues 132 and 142 were identified as the sites of phosphorylation for the recombinant Hu-IFN-γ (118).

CONCLUSION

Interferons are potent bioactive proteins. They modulate the immune system, protect cells from virus infection, affect cellular proliferation and differentiation, and exhibit many other activities. Understanding the structure of these proteins may help to unravel their molecular mechanism of action. In the exciting past decade, development of new biochemical techniques such as high performance liquid chromatography of proteins, amino acid sequencing at the picomole level, monoclonal antibodies and recombinant DNA technology have been important tools in extending our knowledge of the primary structure of these molecules. The secondary structure of interferons have been predicted from the available amino acid sequences. Despite reports of the crystallization of Hu-IFN-αA (119), no crystal structure has been reported to date. Nevertheless, detailed secondary and tertiary structural analysis, will depend on X-ray crystallography. These studies will be of great importance in the development of new structurally related molecules and in understanding how these proteins function.

REFERENCES

1. Pestka, S. and S. Baron: Definition and classification of the interferons. *Meth. Enzymol.* **28**:3, 1981.
2. Berg, K.: Purification and characterization of murine and human interferons; A review of the literature of the 1970s. *Acta Path. Microbiol. Scand. C, Supplement* **279**:1, 1982.
3. Pestka, S.: Interferon from 1981 to 1986. *Meth. Enzymol.* **119**:3, 1986.
4. Zoon, K.: Purification, sequencing and properties of human lymphoblastoid and leukocyte interferons. in: *The Biology of the Interferon System*, E. De Maeyer, G. Galasso, and H. Schellekens, eds., Elsevier/North-Holland, Amsterdam, pp. 47, 1981.
5. Dziewanoska, Z.E., and S. Pestka: The human interferons. *Med. Res. Rev.* **2**:325, 1982.
6. Weissmann, C.: The alpha interferons: Some answers and many questions. *The Harvey Lectures, Ser. 77*, Academic Press, New York pp. 129, 1981-1982.
7. Pestka, S.: The human interferons - from protein purification and sequence to cloning and expression in bacteria: Before, between, and beyond. *Arch. Biochem. Biophys.* **221**:1, 1983.
8. Pestka, S.: The purification and manufacture of human interferons. *Sci. Am.* **249**(2):37, 1983.
9. Langer, J.A., and S. Pestka: Purification, bacterial expression and biological activities of the human interferons. *J. Invest. Dermatol.* **83**:128, 1984.
10. Langer, J.A., and S. Pestka: Structure of interferons. *Pharm. Ther.* **27**:371, 1985.

11. DeStefano, E., R.M. Friedman, A.E. Friedman-Kien, J.J. Goedert, D. Henriksen, O.T. Preble, J.A. Sonnabend, and J. Vilcek: Acid-labile human leukocyte interferon in homosexual men with Kaposi's sarcoma and lymphadenopathy. *J. Infect. Dis.* **146**:451, 1982.
12. Preble, O.T., R.J. Black, R.M. Friedman, J.H. Klippel, and J. Vilcek: Systemic lupus erythrematosis: Presence in human serum of an unusual acid-labile leukocyte interferon. *Science* **216**:429, 1982.
13. Revel, M.: Genetic and functional diversity of interferon in man. in: *Interferon 5*, I. Gresser, ed., Academic Press, New York, pp. 205, 1983.
14. Owerbach, D., W.J. Rutter, T.B. Shows, P. Gray, D.V. Goeddel, and R.M. Lawn: Leukocyte and fibroblast interferon genes are located on human chromosome 9. *Proc. Natl. Acad. Sci. USA* **78**:3123, 1981.
15. Trent, J., S. Olson, and R.M. Lawn: Chromosomal location of human leukocyte fibroblast, and immune interferon genes by means of *in situ* hybridization. *Proc. Natl. Acad. Sci. USA* **79**:7809, 1982.
16. Naylor, S.L., A.Y. Sakaguchi, T.B. Shows, M.L. Law, D.V. Goeddel, and P.W. Gray: Human immune interferon gene is located on chromosome 12. *J. Exp. Med.* **57**:1020, 1983.
17. Tan, Y.H., J. Tischfield, and F.H. Ruddle: The linkage of genes for the human interferon induced antiviral protein and indolphenol oxidase-B traits to chromosome G-21. *J. Exp. Med.* **137**:317, 1973.
18. Slate, D.L., L. Shulman, J.B. Lawrence, M. Revel, and F.H. Ruddle: Presence of human chromosome 21 alone is sufficient for hybrid cell sensitivity to human interferon. *J. Virol.* **25**:319, 1978.
19. Raziuddin, A., F.H. Sarkar, R. Dutkowski, L. Shulman, F.H. Ruddle, and S.L. Gupta: Receptors for human α and β interferon but not γ interferon are specified by human chromosome 21. *Proc. Natl. Acad. Sci. USA* **81**:5504, 1984.
20. Rashidbaigi, A., J.A. Langer, V. Jung, C. Jones, H.G. Morse, J.A. Tischfield, J.J. Trill, H.-F. Kung, and S. Pestka: The gene for the human interferon receptor is located on chromosome 6. *Proc. Natl. Acad. Sci. USA* **83**:384, 1986.
21. Golding, G.B., and B.W. Glickman: Sequence-directed mutagenesis: evidence from a phylogenetic history of human α interferon genes. *Proc. Natl. Acad. Sci. USA* **82**:8577, 1985.
22. Henco, K., J. Brosius, A. Fujisawa, J.-I. Fujisawa, J.R. Haynes, J. Hochstadt, T. Kovacic, M. Pasek, A. Schambock, J. Schmid, K. Todokorro, M. Walchi, S. Nagata, and C. Weissmann: Structural relationship of human interferon alpha genes and pseudogenes. *J. Mol. Biol.* **185**:227, 1985.
23. Wilson, V., A.J. Jeffreys, P.A. Barrie, P.G. Boseley, P.M. Slocombe, A. Eaton, and D.C. Burke: A comparison of vertebrate interferon gene families detected by hybridization with human DNA. *J. Mol. Biol.* **166**:457, 1983.
24. Leung, D.W., D.J. Capon, and D.V. Goeddel: The structure and expression of three distinct bovine interferon-β genes. *Biotech.* **2**:458, 1984.
25. Chen, J.K., W.J. Jankowski, J.A. O'Malley, E. Sulkowski, and W. Carter: Nature of the molecular heterogeneity of human leukocyte interferon. *J. Virol.* **19**:425, 1976.

26. Stewart, W.E.,II, L.S. Lin, M. Wiranowska-Stewart, and K. Cantell: Elimination of size and charge heterogeneities of human leukocyte interferons by chemical cleavage. *Proc. Natl. Acad. Sci. USA* **74**:4200, 1977.
27. Rubinstein, M., S. Rubinstein, P.C. Familletti, M.S. Gross, R.S. Miller, A.A. Waldman, and S. Pestka: Human leukocyte interferon purified to homogeneity. *Science* **202** :1289, 1978.
28. Berg, K., and I. Heron: SDS-polyacrylamide gel electrophoresis of purified human leukocyte interferon and the antiviral and anticellular activities of the different interferon species. *J. Gen. Virol.* **50**:441, 1980.
29. Berg, K., and I. Heron: Antibody affinity chromatography of human leukocyte interferon. *Meth. Enzymol.* **78**:487, 1981.
30. Rubinstein, M., S. Rubinstein, P.C. Familetti, R.S. Miller, A.A. Waldman, and S. Pestka: Human leukocyte interferon: Production, purification to homogeneity, and initial characterization. *Proc. Natl. Acad. Sci. USA* **76**:640, 1979.
31. Rubinstein, M., W.P. Levy, J.A. Mochera, C.-Y. Lai, R.D. Hershberg, R.T. Bartlett, and S. Pestka: Human leukocyte interferon: Isolation and characterization of several molecular forms. *Arch. Biochem. Biophys.* **210**:307, 1981.
32. Allen, G., and K.H. Fantes: A family of structural genes for human lymphoblastoid (leukocyte-type) interferon. *Nature (London)* **287**:408, 1980.
33. Staehelin, T., D.S. Hobbs, H.-F. Kung, C.-Y. Lai, and S. Pestka: Purification and characterization of recombinant human leukocyte interferon (IFLrA) with monoclonal antibodies. *J. Biol. Chem.* **256**:9750, 1981.
34. Levy, W.P., M. Rubinstein, J. Shively, U. Del Valle, C.-Y. Lai, J. Moschera, L. Brink, L. Gerber, S. Stein, and S. Pestka: Amino acid sequences of a human leukocyte interferon. *Proc. Natl. Acad. Sci. USA* **78**:6186, 1981.
35. Zoon, K.C., M.E. Smith, P.J. Bridgen, C.B. Anfinsen, M.W. Hunkapiller, and L.E. Hood: Amino terminal sequence of the major commponent of human lymphoblastoid interferon. *Science* **207**:527, 1980.
36. Goeddel, D.V., D.W. Leung, T.J. Dull, M. Gross, R.M. Lawn, R. McCandliss, P.H. Seeburg, A. Ullrich, E. Yelverton, and P.W. Gray: The structure of eight distinct cloned human leukocyte interferon cDNAs. *Nature (London)* **290**:20, 1981.
37. Lawn, R.M., M. Cross, C.M. Houck, A.E. Franke, P.W. Gray, and D.V. Goeddel: DNA sequence of major human leukocyte interferon gene. *Proc. Natl. Acad. Sci. USA* **78**:5435, 1981.
38. Maeda, S., R. McCandliss, M. Gross, A. Sloma, P.C. Familletti, J.M. Tabor, M. Evinger, W.P. Levy, and S. Pestka: Construction and identification of bacterial plasmids containing nucleotide sequence for human leukocyte interferon. *Proc. Natl. Acad. Sci. USA* **77**:7010, 1981.
39. Maeda, S., R. MacCandliss, T.-R. Chiang, L. Costello, W.P. Levy, N.T. Chang, and S. Pestka: Sequences of a human fibroblast interferon gene and two linked human leukocyte interferon genes. In: *Developmental Biology Using Purified Genes*, D. Brown and C.F. Fox, eds., Academic Press, New York, pp. 85, 1981.
40. Mantei, N., M. Schwarzstein, M. Streuli, S. Panem, S. Nagata, and C. Weissmann: The nucleotide sequence of a cloned human leukocyte interferon cDNA. *Gene* **10**:1, 1980.

41. Streuli, M., S. Nagata, and C. Weissmann: At least three human type α interferons: Structure of α2. *Science* **209**:1343, 1980.
42. Bowden, D.W., J. Mao, T. Gill, K. Hsiao, J.S. Lilquist, D. Testa, and G.F. Vovis: Cloning of eukaryotic genes in single-stranded phage vectors: The human interferon genes. *Gene* **27**:87, 1984.
43. Torczynski, R.M., M. Fuke, and A.P. Bollon: Human genomic library screened with 17-base oligonucleotide probes yields a novel interferon gene. *Proc. Natl. Acad. Sci. USA* **81**:6451, 1984.
44. Sloma, A.: European patent application 83102893.1 (1983).
45. Innis, M.A.: International patent application PCT/US83/00032 (1983).
46. Daugherty, B., D. Martin-Zanca, B. Kelder, K. Collier, T.C. Seamans, and S. Pestka: Isolation and bacterial expression of a murine alpha leukocyte interferon gene. *J. Interferon Res.* **4**:635, 1984.
47. Shaw, G.D., W. Boll, H. Taira, N. Mantei, P. Lengyel, and C. Weissmann: Structure and expression of cloned murine IFN-α genes. *Nucleic Acids Res.* **11**:555, 1983.
48. Dijkema, R., P. Pouwels, A. DeReus, and H. Schellekens: Structure and expression in *Escherichia coli* of a cloned rat inteferon-α gene. *Nucleic Acids Res.* **12**:1227, 1984.
49. Gold, P., and S. Pestka, (manuscript in preparation).
50. Taira, H., R.J. Braeze, B.M. Jayaram, P. Lengyel, M.W. Hunkapiller, and L.E. Hood: Mouse interferons: Amino terminal amino acid sequence of various species. *Science* **207**:528, 1980.
51. Feinstein, S.I., Y. Mary, Y. Chernajovsky, L. Maroteaux, U. Nir, V. Lavie, and M. Revel: Family of human α-interferon-like sequences. *Mol. Cell Biol.* **5**:510, 1985.
52. Hauptmann, R., and P. Swetly: A novel class of type I interferons. *Nucleic Acids Res.* **13**:4739, 1985.
53. Capon, D.J., H.M. Shepard, and D.V. Goeddel: Two distinct families of human and bovine interferon-α genes are coordinately expressed and encode functional polypeptides. *Mol. Cell Biol.* **5**:768, 1985.
54. Velan, B., S. Cohen, H. Grosfeld, and A. Shafferman: Isolation of bovine interferon-α genes and their expression in bacteria. *Meth. Enzymol.* **119**:464, 1986.
55. Velan, B., S. Cohen, H. Grosfeld, M. Leitner, and A. Shafferman: Bovine interferon α genes. *J. Biol. Chem.* **260**:5498, 1985.
56. Bewley, T.A., H.L. Levine, and R. Wetzel: Structural features of human leukocyte interferon A as determined by circular dichroism spectroscopy. *Int. J. Peptide Protein Res.* **20**:93, 1982.
57. Manavalan, W., C. Johnson Jr., and P.D. Johnston: Prediction structure type for human leukocyte interferon subtype A from circular dichroism. *FEBS Lett.* **175**:227, 1984.
58. Hayes, T.G.: Chou-Fasman analysis of the secondary structure of fibroblast and leukocyte interferons. *Biochem. Biophys. Res. Commun.* **95**:872, 1980.
59. Wetzel, R.: Assignment of the disulfide bonds of leukocyte interferon. *Nature (London)* **289**:606, 1981.
60. Morehead, H., P.D. Johnston, and R. Wetzel: Roles of the 29-138 disulfide bond of subtype A of human α interferon in its antiviral activity and conformational stability. *Biochem.* **23**, 2500, 1984.

61. Labdon, J.G., K.D. Gibson, R. Sun, and S. Pestka: Some species of human leukocyte interferon are glycosylated. *Arch. Biochem. Biophys.* **232**:422, 1984.
62. Berthold, W., C. Tan, and Y.H. Tan: Purification and *in vitro* labeling of interferon from human fibroblast cell line. *J. Biol. Chem.* **253**:2506, 1978.
63. Heine, K.J.W., and A. Billian: Purification of human fibroblast interferon by adsorption to controlled pore-glass and zinc-chelate chromatography. *Meth. Enzymol.* **78**:448, 1981.
64. Okamura, H., W. Berthold, L. Hood, M. Hunkapiller, M. Inoue, H. Smith-Johannsen, and Y.H. Tan: Human fibroblast interferon: Immunosorbent column chromatography and N-terminal amino acid sequence. *Biochem.* **19**:3831, 1980.
65. Friesen, H.-J., S. Stein, M. Evinger, P.C. Familletti, J.A. Moschera, J. Meienhofer, J. Shively, and S. Pestka: Purification and molecular characterization of human fibroblast interferon. *Arch. Biochem. Biophys.* **206**:432, 1981.
66. Kenny, C., J.A. Mochera, and S. Stein: Purification of human fibroblast interferon produced in the absence of serum by Cibacron Blue F3GA-agarose and high performance liquid chromatography. *Meth. Enzymol.* **78**:435, 1981.
67. Smith-Johannsen, H., and Y.H. Tan: Isolation of Hu-IFN-β by immunosorbent and high-pressure liquid chromatography. *J. Interferon Res.* **3**:473, 1983.
68. Stein, S., C. Kenny, H.-J. Friesen, J. Shively, U. Del Valle, and S. Pestka: NH_2-terminal amino acid sequence of human fibroblast interferon. *Proc. Natl. Acad. Sci. USA* **77**:5716, 1980.
69. Knight, E.,Jr., and D. Fahey: Human fibroblast interferon: An improved purification. *J. Biol. Chem.* **256**:3609, 1981.
70. Havell, E.A., Y.K. Yip, and J. Vilcek: Correlation of physiochemical and antigenic properties of human leukocyte interferon subtypes. *Arch. Virol.* **55**:121, 1977.
71. Taniguchi, T., N. Montei, M. Schwarzstein, S. Nagata, M. Muramutsu, and C. Weissmann: Human leukocyte and fibroblast interferons are structurally related. *Nature (London)* **285**:547, 1980.
72. Branca, A.A., and C. Baglioni: Evidence that types I and II interferons have different receptors. *Nature (London)* **294**:768, 1981.
73. Merlin, G., E. Falcoff, and M. Aguet: ^{125}I-labelled human interferons alpha, beta and gamma: comparative receptor-binding data. *J. Gen. Virol.* **66**:1149, 1985.
74. DeLey, M., J. VanDamme, A. Billiau, and P. DeSomes: Properties of antibodies directed against human immune interferon. *J. Virol. Methods* **3**:149, 1981. 75. Cavalieri, R.L., E.A. Havell, J. Vilcek, and S. Pestka: Synthesis of human interferon by *Xenopus laevis* oocytes: Two structural genes for interferons in human cells. *Proc. Natl. Acad. Sci. USA* **74**:3287, 1977.
76. De Maeyer-Guignard, J., M.G. Tovey, I. Greeser, and E. De Maeyer: Purification of mouse interferon by sequential affinity chromatography on poly (U)-and antibody-agarose columns. *Nature (London)* **271**:622, 1978.
77. Iwakura, Y., S. Yonehara, and Y. Kawade: Purification of mouse L-cell interferon. *J. Biol. Chem.* **253**:5074, 1978.

78. Kawakita, M., B. Cabrer, H. Taira, M. Rebello, E. Slattery, H. Weidoli, and P. Lengyel: Purification of interferon from mouse Ehrlich ascites tumor cell. *J. Biol. Chem.* **253**:598, 1978.
79. Cabrer, B., H. Taira, R.J. Broeze, T.D. Kempe, K. Williams, E. Slattery, W.H. Konigsberg, and P. Lengyel: Structural characteristics of interferons from mouse Ehrlich ascites tumor cells. *J. Biol. Chem.* **254**:3681, 1979.
80. Vonk, W.P., and J. Trapman: Large scale one-step purification of murine interferon-beta using a monoclonal antibody. *J. Interferon Res.* **3**:169, 1983.
81. Jayaram, B.A., H. Schmidt, O. Yoshie, and P. Lengyel: Simple procedure for the isolation of mouse interferon-beta. *J. Interferon Res.* **3**:177, 1983.
82. Taniguchi, T., S. Ohno, Y. Fujii-Kuriyama, and M. Muramatsu: The nucleotide sequence of human fibroblast interferon cDNA. *Gene* **10**:11, 1980.
83. Goeddel, D.V., H.M. Shepard, E. Yelverton, D. Leung, R. Crea, A. Sloma, and S. Pestka: Synthesis of human fibroblast interferon by *E. coli*. *Nucleic Acids Res.* **8**:4057, 1980.
84. Houghton, M., M.A.W. Eaton, A.G. Stewart, J.C. Smith, S.M. Doel, G.H. Catlin, H.M. Lewis, T.P. Patel, J.S. Emtager, N.H. Carey, and A.G. Porter: The complete amino acid sequence of human fibroblast interferon as deduced using synthetic oligodeoxyribonucleotide primers of reverse transcriptases. *Nucleic Acids Res.* **8**:2885, 1980.
85. Derynck, R., J. Content, E. DeClerq, G. Volckaert, J. Tavernier, R. Devos, and W. Fiers: Isolation and structure of a human fibroblast interferon gene. *Nature (London)* **285**:542, 1980.
86. Higashi, Y., Y. Sokawa, Y. Watanabe, Y. Kawade, S. Ohno, C. Takaoka, and T. Taniguchi: Structure and expression of a cloned cDNA for mouse interferon-β. *J. Biol. Chem.* **258**:9522, 1983.
87. Houghton, M., I.J. Jackson, A.G. Porter, S.M. Doel, G.H. Catlin, and N.H. Carey: The absence of introns within fibroblast interferon gene. *Nucleic Acids Res.* **9**:247, 1981.
88. Mark, D.F., S.D. Lu, A.A. Creasey, R. Yamamoto, and L.S. Lin: Site specific mutagenesis of the human fibroblast interferon gene. *Proc. Natl. Acad. Sci. USA* **81**:5662, 1984.
89. Shepard, H.D., D.W. Leung, N. Stebbing, and D.V. Goeddel: A single amino acid change in IFN-β1 abolishes its antiviral activity. *Nature (London)* **294**:563, 1981.
90. Wheelock, E.F.: Interferon-like virus inhibitor induced in human leukocytes by phytohemegglutinin. *Science* **149**:310,1965.
91. Yip, Y.K., R.H.L. Pang, C. Urban, and J. Vilcek: Partial purification and characterization of human γ (immune) interferon. *Proc. Natl. Acad. Sci. USA* **78**:1601, 1981.
92. Hsu, Y.-R., and T. Arakawa: Structural studies on acid unfolding and refolding of recombinant human interferon γ. *Biochem.* **24**:7959, 1985.
93. Epstein, L.B.: The special significance of interferon-gamma, In: *Interferon and the immune system*, J. Vilcek and E. De Maeyer, eds. Elsevier Science Publisher, B.V., pp. 185, 1984.
94. Schultz, R.M., and W.J. Kleinshcmidt: Functional identity between murine γ interferon and macrophage activating factor. *Nature (London)* **305**:239, 1983.

95. Yip, Y.K., B.S. Barrowclough, C. Urban, and J. Vilcek: Purification of two subspecies of human γ (immune) interferon. *Proc. Natl. Acad. Sci. USA* **79**:1820, 1982.
96. Braude, I.A.: Purification of human γ interferon to essential homogeneity and its biochemical characterization. *Biochem.* **23**:5603, 1984.
97. Friedlander, J., D.G. Fischer, and M. Rubinstein: Isolation of two discrete human interferon-γ (immune) subtypes by high-performance liquid chromatography. *Anal. Biochem.* **137**:115, 1984.
98. Rinderknecht, E., B.H. O'Conner, and H. Rodriguez: Natural human interferon-γ. *J. Biol. Chem.* **259**:6790, 1984.
99. Yip, Y.K., B.S. Barrowclough, C. Urban, and J. Vilcek: Molecular weight of human gamma interferon is similar to that of other human interferons. *Science* **215**:411, 1982.
100. Kelker, H.C., J. Le, B.-Y. Rubin, Y.K. Yip, C. Nagler, and J. Vilcek: Three molecular weight forms of natural human interferon-γ revealed by immunoprecipitation with monoclonal antibody. *J. Biol. Chem.* **259**:4301, 1984.
101. Pestka, S., B. Kelder, P.C. Familletti, J.A. Moschera, R. Crowl, and E.S. Kempner. Molecular weight of the functional unit of human leukocyte, fibroblast and immune interferons. *J. Biol. Chem.* **258**:9706, 1983.
102. Osborne, L.C., J.A. Georgiades, and H.M. Johnson: Large-scale production and partial purification of mouse immune interferon. *Infect. Immun.* **23**:80, 1979.
103. Georgiades, J.A., and H.M. Johnson: Partial purification and characterization of mouse immune interferon. *Meth. Enzymol.* **78**:545, 1981.
104. Gribaudo, G., F. Cofano, A. Negro-Ponzi, and S. Landolfo: Mouse gamma interferon produced by a cloned T-cell lymphoma. I. Purification and physiochemical characterization. *J. Interferon Res.* **4**:91, 1984.
105. Gribaudo, G., F. Cofano, M. Prat, C. Baiocchi, G. Cavallo, and S. Landolfo: Natural murine interferon-γ. *J. Biol. Chem.* **260**:9936, 1985.
106. Gray, P.W., and D.V. Goeddel: Structure of the human immune interferon gene. *Nature (London)* **298**:859, 1982.
107. Gray, P.W., D.W. Leung, D. Pennica, E. Yelverton, R. Najarian, C.C. Simonsen, R. Derynck, P.J. Sherwood, D.M. Wallace, S.L. Berger, A.D. Levinson, and D.V. Goeddel: Expression of human immune interferon cDNA in *E. coli* and monkey cells. *Nature (London)* **295**:503, 1982.
108. Devos, R. H. Cheroutre, Y. Taya, W. Degrave, H. Van Heuverswyn, and W.Fiers: Molecular cloning of human immune inerferon cDNA and its expression in eukaytic cells. *Nucleic Acids Res.* **10**:2487, 1982.
109. DeGrado, W.F., Z.R. Wasserman, and V. Chowdhry: Sequence, and structural homologies among type I and type II interferons. *Nature (London)* **300**:379, 1982.
110. Gray, P.W., and D.V. Goeddel: Cloning and expression of murine immune interferon cDNA. *Proc. Natl. Acad. Sci. USA* **80**:5842, 1983.
111. Derynck, R.: More about interferon cloning. In: *Interferon Vol. 5*, I. Gresser, ed., Academic Press, New York, pp. 181, 1983.
112. Cerretti, D.P., K. McKereghan, A. Larsen, D. Cosman, S. Gillis, and P.E. Baker: Cloning, sequence, and expresion of bovine interferon-γ. *J. Immunol.* **136**:4561, 1986.

113. Dijkema, R., P.H. Van der Meide, P.H. Pouwels, M. Caspers, M. Dubbeld, and H. Schellekens: Cloning and expression of the chromosomal immune interferon gene of the rat. *EMBO J.* **4**:761, 1985.
114. Robert-Galliot, B., M.J. Commoy-Chevalier, P. Georges, and C. Chany: Phosphorylation of recombinant interferon-gamma by kinases released from various cells. *J. Gen. Virol.* **66**:1439, 1985.
115. Kung, H.-F., and E. Bekesi: Phosphorylation of human immuen interferon (IFN-γ). *Meth. Enzymol.* **119**:296, 1986.
116. Langer, J.A., A. Rashidbaigi, and S. Pestka: Preparation of ^{32}P-labeled murine immune interferon and its binding to the mouse immune interferon receptor. *J. Biol. Chem.*, in press.
117. Rashidbaigi, A., H.-F. Kung, and S. Pestka: Characterization of receptors for immune interferon in U937 cells with ^{32}P-labeled human recombinant immune interferon. *J. Biol. Chem.*: **260**:8514, 1985.
118. Arakawa, T., C.G. Parker, and P.-H. Lai: Sites of phosphorylation in recombinant human interferon-γ: *Biochem. Biophys. Res. Commun.* **136**:679, 1986.
119. Miller, D.L., H.-F. Kung, and S. Pestka: Crystallization of recombinant human leukocyte interferon A. *Science* **215**:689, 1982.

TABLE I. Classification and General Properties of Interferons

Class	IFN-α	IFN-β	IFN-γ
Nomenclature	Leukocyte	Fibroblast	Immune
Type (a)	I	I	II
Primary natural source	Leukocytes	Fibroblasts	T-Cells
pH 2 Stability (b)	+	+	-
Number of Species	>15	1 (c)	1
N-Linked Glycosylation	Some Species	+	+
Presence of Introns in the Genes	-	-	+
Chromosomal Location (d)	9 Short Arm	9 Short Arm	12 Long Arm
Chromosomal Location of Binding Sites (e)	21	21	6 Long Arm

(a) The type designation represents an old classification.

(b) pH 2 stability is a generalization not always valid. There are reports of acid sensitive IFN-α (11,12).

(c) Some additional species related to IFN-β have been reported, but these may be completely different interferon types (13).

(d) The interferon genes were localized to the specified human chromosomes (14-16).

(e) Functional assay (17,18) or more direct receptor binding studies have been used to localize the genes for human interferon receptors (19,20).

Figure 1.

AMINO ACID SEQUENCES OF HUMAN IFN-α SPECIES

```
                     S1       S10          S20  S23  1        10          20          30          40          50          60          70
IFN-α consensus      MALSFSLLMA  VLVLSYKSIC  SLG  CDLPQTHSLG  NRRALILLAQ  MGRISPFSCL  KDRHDFGFPQ  EEFDGNQFQK  AQAISVLHEM  IQQTFNLFST
IFN-αK (α6)          ...P.A....  LV...C..S.  ..D  ..........  H..TMM....  .R...L....  ......R...  ..........  .E.......V  ..........
IFN-α5 (αG)          ...P.V....  LV..NC....  ...  .........S  ...T.MIM..  ..........  ..........  ..........  ..........  ..........
IFN-αA (α2)          ...T.A..V.  L....C..S.  .V.  ..........  S..T.M....  .RK..L....  ..........  ...-......  .ET.P.....  ...I......
IFN-αD (α1)          ..SP.A...V  LV...C..S.  ...  ....E....D  ...T.M....  .S....S...  M.........  ..........  .P.......L  ...I....T.
IFN-αH1 (αH2)        ...P...M..  LV...C..S.  ...  .N.S.....N  ...T.M.M..  .R........  ......E...  ..........  ..........  M.........
IFN-αB2 (α8)         ...T.Y..V.  LV......FS  ...  ..........  ..........  .R........  ......E...  ....DK....  ..........  ..........
IFN-αB               ...T.Y.MV.  LV......FS  ...  ..........  ..........  .R........  ......E...  ....DK....  ..........  ..........
IFN-α4b              ..........  ..........  ...  ..........  ..........  .....H....  .........E  .....H....  T.........  ..........
IFN-αC               ..........  ..........  ...  ..........  ........G.  ..........  ......RI..  ..........  ..........  ..........
IFN-αL (Ψα10)        ..........  .........*  ...  .......T.R  ........G.  ..........  ......RI..  ..........  ..........  ..........
IFN-αJ1 (α7)         ..R......V  ..........  ...  .........R  ..........  ..........  ....E.R..E  .....H....  T.........  ..........
IFN-αJ2              ..R......V  ..........  ...  .........R  ..........  ..........  ....E.R..E  .....H....  T.........  ..........
IFN-αI               ..........  ..........  ...  ..........  ..........  ..........  ...P...L..  ..........  T.........  ..........
IFN-αF               ..........  ..........  ...  ..........  ..........  ..........  ..........  ..........  ..........  ..........
IFN-αWA              ..........  ..........  ...  ..........  ..........  .....H....  ...Y......  .V........  .....AF...  ..........
IFN-αGx-1            ...P...M..  LV...C..S.  ...  .N.S.....N  ...T.MIM..  ..........  ..........  ..........  ..........  ..........
IFN-α76              ..........  ..........  ...  ..........  ..........  .....H....  .........E  .....H....  ..........  ..........
IFN-α88                              ......  ...  ..........  ..........  ..........  .......L..  ..........  T.........  ..........


                             80          90         100         110         120         130         140         150         160    166
IFN-α consensus      KDSSAAWDES  LLEKFSTELY  QQLNDLEACV  IQEVGVEETP  LMNEDSILAV  RKYFQRITLY  LTEKKYSPCA  WEVVRAEIMR  SFSFSTNLQK  RLRRKD
IFN-αK (α6)          ....V....R  ..D.LY....  ..........  M...W.GG..  ..........  ..........  ..........  ..........  ...S.R...E  .....E
IFN-αG (α5)          .....T...T  ..D..Y....  .........M  M......D..  ...V....T.  ..........  ..........  ..........  ...L.A...E  .....E
IFN-αA (α2)          .........T  ..D..Y....  ..........  ..G...T...  ..K.......  ..........  .K........  ..........  ...L.....E  S..S.E
IFN-αD (α1)          .........D  ..D..C....  ..........  M..ER.G...  ...V......  K...R.....  ..........  ..........  .L.L.....E  .....E
IFN-αH1 (αH2)        .N.......T  .....YI..F  ..M.......  ..........  ..........  K.........  .M........  ..........  ..........  ......
IFN-αB2 (α8)         .......L.T  ..DE.YI..D  .......S..  M.....I.S.  ..Y.......  ..........  .......S..  ..........  ...L.I....  ..KS.E
IFN-αB               .......L.T  ..DE.YI..D  .......VLC  D.....I.S.  ..Y.......  ..........  .......S..  ..........  ...L.I....  ..KS.E
IFN-α4b              E......EQ.  ..........  ..........  ..........  ...V......  ..........  ..........  ..........  .L........  ......
IFN-αC               E......EQ.  ..........  ..........  ..........  ..........  ..........  .I.R......  ..........  .L........  ......
IFN-αL (Ψα10)        E......EQ.  ........I.  ..........  ..........  ..........  ..........  .I.R......  ..........  .L........  ......
IFN-αJ1 (α7)         E......EQ.  ..........  ..........  ..........  .....F....  ..........  .M........  ..........  ........K.  G.....
IFN-αJ2              E......EQ.  ..........  ..........  ..........  .....F....  ..........  .M........  ..........  ..........  ......
IFN-αI               E......EQ.  ..........  ....N.....  .....M....  ..........  ..........  ..........  ..........  .L........  I.....
IFN-αF               .....T.EQ.  .........N  .....M....  ..........  ...V......  K.........  ..........  ..........  ...L.KIF.E  .....E
IFN-αWA              .........T  ..D..YI..F  ..........  T.......IA  ..........  ..........  .MG.......  ..........  ..........  G.....
IFN-αGx-1            .....T...T  ..D..Y....  .........M  M......D..  ...V....T.  ..........  ..........  ..........  ...L.A...E  .....E
IFN-α76              E......EQ.  ..........  ..........  ..........  ..........  ..........  ..........  ..........  .L........  ......
IFN-α88              E......EQ   ..........  ....N.....  .....M....  ..........  ..........  ..........  ..........  .L........  ......
```

Figure 2.

AMINO ACID SEQUENCES OF IFN-α SPECIES

	S1 S10	S20	S24	1 10	20	30	40	50	60	70
Mu-IFN-α consensus	MARLCAFLMV	LAVMSY-WST	CSLG	CDLPQTHNLR	NKRALTLLVQ	MRRLSPLSCL	KDRKDFGFPQ	EKVDAQQIQK	AQAIPVLSEL	TQQILNIFTS
Mu-IFN-αA	.........T	.L....-...	....	....	....	....	......R...	.........N	.......Q..	...V......
Mu-IFN-α1	....	......-.P.	....	....	....	....	....	........K.	....	....
Mu-IFN-α2	........VM	.I....-..I	....	....H.Y...	.....KV.A.	....PF....	...Q.....L	....N.....	.......RD.	...T..L...
Mu-IFN-α4	I	.VM...Y..A	....	....H.Y..G	.......V.EE	....P.....	L	....N.....	....L..RD.	......L...
Mu-IFN-α5	....	.P.L..-.P.	....	....	.........K	....	....	...G.....E	....	...V......
Mu-IFN-α6	....	......-...	....	.......K..	........I.	....	....	....TLK...	EK.......V	....
Mu-IFN-α6k	....	...L..-.P.	....	....	...L.....K	....	....	...G.....E	.......T..	.....TL...
Ra-IFN-α1	.........S	.V.V..-..A	.C..	....H.....	...VF...A.	......V...	....Y....L	....G.....	.......H..	.....SL...
Mo-IFN-αD	..LPF.L..A	.V.L.C-K.G	....	....E..S.D	.R.TMM..K.	.S.I..S...	M..H......	QEF.GN.F..	.P..S..H..	I..TF.L..T
Hu-IFN-α consensus	MALSFSLLMA	VLVLSY-KSI	CSLG	CDLPQTHSLG	NRRALILLAQ	MGRISPFSCL	KDRHDFGFPQ	EEFDGNQFQK	AQAISVLHEM	IQQTFNLFST

	80	90	100	110	120	130	140	150	160	167 169
Mu-IFN-α consensus	KDSSAAWNAT	LLDSFCNDLH	QQLNDLQACL	MQEVGVQEPP	LTQEDSLLAV	RKYFHRITVY	LREKKHSPCA	WEVVRAEVWR	ALSSSANLLA	RLSEEKE
Mu-IFN-αA	.......D.S	....	......K..V	....	.....Y....	.T........	....	....	.M....K...	......E
Mu-IFN-α1	....	....	.......G..	..Q.....F.	.....A....	....	....	....	........V.G	..R...
Mu-IFN-α2	.A........	....	.......T..	..Q.......	.....A....	....	....	....	.....V...P	......E
Mu-IFN-α4	..L..T....	....	......K..V	..-----...	....	.T........	..K....L..	...I......	.....T....	....
Mu-IFN-α5	....	.......EV.	......K..V	........S.	....	....	.......L..	....	.....V....	...K.E.
Mu-IFN-α6	.......D..	...T.....Y	....	V...RL....	....V.....	....	....	....	........V.G	..R...
Mu-IFN-α6k	....	.........H	.L.....G..	..Q.EI.AL.	....	.T.......F	....	....	......K...	..N.DE
Ra-IFN-α1	.E..T..D..	.........Q	...SG.....	..Q.....S.	....	.E........	...N......	....K.....	.........MG	..R..RNES
Mo-IFN-αD	.......DED	...K..TE.Y	......E..V	..QER.G.T.	.MNA..T...	K...R...L.	.T...Y....	.......IM.	SF.L.T..QE	..RRKE
Hu-IFN-α consenus	KDSSAAWDES	LLEKFSTELY	QQLNDLEACV	IQEVGVEETP	LMNEDSILAV	RKYFQRITLY	LTEKKYSPCA	WEVVRAEIMR	SFSFSTNLQK	RLRRKD

Figure 3.

AMINO ACID SEQUENCES OF IFN-α-LIKE SPECIES

```
                     S1        S10             S20  S23  1         10         20         30         40         50         60         70
Bo-IFN-αD             ..PAWS....  L.L...NA..  ...       .H..HS...A K..V.T..R.  LR.V..S...  Q..N..A...  .ALG.S.L..  .........V T.H.......
Bo-IFN-α*D            ..FVL.....  LVLV..GPGG  ...       ...SPN.V.V G.QN.R..G.  .R.L..RF..  Q..K..A...  .MVEVS...E  ..........  L..S....HK
Hu-IFN-α*D            ...L.P..A.  LVMT..SPVG  ...       .....N.G.L S.NT.V..H.  .R.....L..  ...R..R...  .MVK.S.L..  .HVM......  L..I.S..H.
Hu-IFN-α consensus    MALSFSLLMA  VLVLSYKSIC  SLG       CDLPQTHSLG NRRALILLAQ  MGRISPFSCL  KDRHDFGFPQ  EEFDGNQFQK  AQAISVLHEM  IQQTFNLFST

                               80          90         100        110        120        130        140        150        160        170
Bo-IFN-αD             EG.A.V....  ..D.LR.A..  ...T..Q..L R..EG.LPA.  .LK...S...  ......L...  .Q..RH....  ......QV..  A..S.....E  .F....
Bo-IFN-α*D            ER....T.TT  ...QLL.G.H  ...D..D..L GLLT.GGDSA  .GRTGPT..M  KR.P.G.HV.  .Q..G..D..  ..I..LE...  .L.S..S..E  ...MM.GDLK  SP
Hu-IFN-α*D            ER.....NMT  ..DQLH....  ...QH..T.L L.V..EG.SA  GAISSPA.TL  .R...G.RV.  .K.....D..  .....M...K  .LFL...M.E  ...S..RDLG  SS
Hu-IFN-α consensus    KDSSAAWDES  LLEKFSTELY  QQLNDLEACV IQEVGVEETP  LMNEDSILAV  RKYFQRITLY  LTEKKYSPCA  WEVVRAEIMR  SFSFSTNLQK  RLRRKD
```

Figure 4.

AMINO ACID SEQUENCES OF IFN-β SPECIES

```
                                     S10                  S20 S21
IFN-β consensus    M T x R C L L Q x A   L L L C F S T T A L   S
Hu-IFN-β           . . N K . . . . I .   . . . . . . . . . .   .
Mo-IFN-β           . . N K . . . . I .   . . . . . . . . . .   .
Bo-IFN-β1          . . Y . . . . . M V   . . . . . . . . . .   .
Bo-IFN-β2          . . H . . . . . M V   . . . . . . . . . .   .
Bo-IFN-β3          . . Y . . . . P M V   . . . . . . . . . .   .
Mu-IFN-β           . N N . W I . H A .   F . . . . . . . . .   .

                                      10                   20                   30
IFN-β consensus    x S Y x L L x F Q Q   R x S x x x C Q K L   L x Q L x x x x x x
Hu-IFN-β           M . . N . . G . L .   . S . N F Q . . . .   . W . . N G R L E Y
Mo-IFN-β           M . . N . . G . L .   . S . S F Q . . . .   . W . . N G S L E Y
Bo-IFN-β1          R . . S . . R . . .   . Q . L K E . . . .   . G . . P S T S Q H
Bo-IFN-β2          R . . S . . R . . .   . R . L A L . . . .   . R . . P S T P Q H
Bo-IFN-β3          R . . S . . R . . .   . R . A E V . . . .   . G . . H S T P Q H
Mu-IFN-β           I N . K Q . Q L . E   . T N I R K . . E .   . E . . N G K I - -

                                      40                   50                   60
IFN-β consensus    C L x x R M D F x x   P E E M K Q x Q Q F   Q K E D A A L x I Y
Hu-IFN-β           . . K D . . N . D I   . . . I . . L . . .   . . . . . . . T . .
Mo-IFN-β           . . K D . . N . D I   . . . I . . P . . .   . . . . . . . T . .
Bo-IFN-β1          . . E A . . . . Q M   . . . . . . E . . .   . . . . . . I . V M .
Bo-IFN-β2          . . E A . . . . Q M   . . . . . . A . . .   . . . . . . I . V . .
Bo-IFN-β3          . . E A K . . . Q V   . . . . N . A . . .   R . . . . I . V . .
Mu-IFN-β           N . T Y . A . . K I   . . . . T E - K M -   . . S Y T . F A . Q

                                      70                   80                   90
IFN-β consensus    E M L Q N I F x I F   R x D F S S T G W N   E T I V E x L L x E
Hu-IFN-β           . . . . . . . A . .   . Q . S . . . . . .   . . . . . N . . A N
Mo-IFN-β           . . . . . . . A . .   . Q . L . . . . . .   . . . . . K . . A N
Bo-IFN-β1          . V . . H . . G . L   T R . . . . . . . S   . . . I . D . . K .
Bo-IFN-β2          . . . . Q . . N . L   T R . . . . . . . S   . . . I . D . . E .
Bo-IFN-β3          . . . . Q . . N . L   T R . . . . . . . S   . . . I . D . . V .
Mu-IFN-β           . . . . . V . L V .   . N N . . . . . . .   . . . . V R . . D .

                                     100                  110                      120
IFN-β consensus    L Y x Q x N x L K T   V L E E K x E K E N   x T x G x x M S S - - L
Hu-IFN-β           V . H . I . H . . .   . . . . . L . . . D   F . R . K L . . . - - .
Mo-IFN-β           V . H . I D H . . .   I . . . . L . . . D   F . R . K F . . . - - .
Bo-IFN-β1          . . W . M . R . Q P   I Q K . I M Q . Q .   S . T E D T I V - - - P
Bo-IFN-β2          . . E . M . H . E P   I Q K . I M Q . Q .   S . M . D T T V - - - .
Bo-IFN-β3          . . G . M . R . Q P   I Q K . I M Q E Q .   F . M . D T T V - - - .
Mu-IFN-β           . H Q . T V F . . .   . . . . . Q . - . R   L . W E - - . . . T A .

                                     130                  140                 150
IFN-β consensus    H L K x Y Y x R x x   x Y L K x K E Y x x   C A W T V V R V E I
Hu-IFN-β           . . . R . . G . I L   H . . . A . . . S H   . . . . I . . . . .
Mo-IFN-β           . . . R . . G . I L   H . . . A . . . S H   . . . . I . . . . .
Bo-IFN-β1          . . G K . . F N L M   Q . . E S . . . D R   . . . . . . Q . Q .
Bo-IFN-β2          . . R K . . F N L V   Q . . . S . . . N R   . . . . . . . . Q .
Bo-IFN-β3          . . . K . . F N L V   Q . . E S . . . N R   . . . . . . . . Q .
Mu-IFN-β           . . . S . . W . V Q   R . . . L M K . N S   Y . . M . . . A . .

                                     160          166
IFN-β consensus    L R N F x F I x R L   T G Y L R N
Hu-IFN-β           . . . . Y . . N . .   . . . . . .
Mo-IFN-β           . . . . F . . N K .   . . . . . .
Bo-IFN-β1          . T . V S . L M . .   . . . V . D
Bo-IFN-β2          . . . . S . L T . .   . . . . . E
Bo-IFN-β3          . T . . S . L M . .   . A S . . D
Mu-IFN-β           F . . . L I . R . .   . R N F Q .
```

Figure 5.

AMINO ACID SEQUENCES OF IFN-γ SPECIES

```
                      S1              S10                  S20   S23
Hu-IFN-γ              M K Y T S Y I L A F  Q L C I V L G S L G  C Y C
Bo-IFN-γ              . . . . . . F . . L  L . . G L . . F S .  S . G
Mu-IFN-γ              . N A . H C . . . L  . . F L M A V . - .  . . .
Ra-IFN-γ              . S A . R R V . V L  . . . L M A L . - .  . . .

                      1                10                   20                   30
Hu-IFN-γ              Q D P Y V K E A E N  L K K Y F N A G H S  D V A D N G T L F L
Hu-IFN-γ (protein)    e . . . . . . . . .  . . . . . . . . . .  . . . . . . . . . .
Bo-IFN-γ              . G Q F F R . I . .  . . E . . . . S S P  . . . K G . P . . S
Mu-IFN-γ              H G T V I E S L . S  . N N . . . S S G I  . . - E E K S . . .
Ra-IFN-γ              . G T L I E S L . S  . . N . . . S S S M  . A M E G K S . L .

                                       40                   50                   60
Hu-IFN-γ              G I L K N W K E E S  D R K I M Q S Q I V  S F Y F K L F K N F
Hu-IFN-γ (protein)    . . . . . . . . . .  . . . . . . . . . .  . . . . . . . . . .
Bo-IFN-γ              D . . . . . . D . .  . K . . I . . . . .  . . . . . . . E . L
Mu-IFN-γ              D . W R . . Q K D G  . M . . L . . . . I  . . . L R . . E V L
Ra-IFN-γ              D . W R . . Q K D G  N T . . L E . . . I  . . . L R . . E V L

                                       70                   80                   90
Hu-IFN-γ              K D D Q S I Q K S V  E T I K E D M N V K  F F N S N K K K R D
Hu-IFN-γ (protein)    . . . . . . . . . .  . . . . . . . . . .  . . . . . . . . . .
Bo-IFN-γ              . . N . V . . R . M  D I . . Q . . F Q .  . L . G S S E . L E
Mu-IFN-γ              . . N . A . S N N I  S V . E S H L I T T  . . S N S . A . K .
Ra-IFN-γ              . . N . A . S N N I  S V . E S H L I T N  . . S N S . A . K .

                                      100                  110                  120
Hu-IFN-γ              D F E K L T N Y S V  T D L N V Q R K A I  H E L I Q V M A E L
Hu-IFN-γ (protein)    . . . . . . . . . .  . . . . . . . . . .  . . . . . . . . . .
Bo-IFN-γ              . . K . . I Q I P .  D . . Q I . . . . .  N . . . K . . N D .
Mu-IFN-γ              A . M S I A K F E .  N N P Q . . . Q . F  N . . . R . V H Q .
Ra-IFN-α1             A . M S I A K F E .  N N P Q I . H . . V  N . . . R . I H Q .

                                      130                  140   143
Hu-IFN-γ              S P A A K T G K R K  R S Q M L F R G R R  A S Q
Hu-IFN-γ (protein)    . . . . . . † † † †  † † † †
Bo-IFN-γ              . . K S N L R . . .  . . . N . . . . . .  . . M
Mu-IFN-γ              L . E S S L R . . .  . . R C*
Ra-IFN-γ              . . E S S L R . . .  . . R C*
```

FIGURE LEGENDS

Figure 1. The amino acid sequences of Hu-IFN-α's derived from cDNA or genomic DNA sequences. These sequences include the signal peptide (S_1–S_{23}). Residues which are different from consensus sequences are shown. Residues which are common to all listed sequences are underlined in the consensus sequence. Alphabetic nomenclature (7,8,36-39) or numeric designations (6,40,41) are from different investigators. Closely related sequences are listed together (10). Sequences are listed as two classes (6). Class I are αK, α5, αA, and αD. Class II are α4b, αC, αL, αJ1, αJ2, αI and αF with an intermediate class composed of αH_1, αB_2 and αB. The order of arrangement within each class is based on the increasing differences from the consensus sequence. The α5 sequence is complete, whereas the αG sequence begins at residue 34, since only a partial length clone was isolated. Identity of αG and α5 is proposed based on the available sequences. Sequence αL (Ψα10) has a termination codon within the signal sequence and may be a pseudogene. This is indicated by an asterisk. Since the coding region for the mature protein is normal, it is possible that *in vivo* suppression of termination might lead to production of the protein. The protein sequence recently derived from another cDNA library is identical to αB_2 (α8) (42). The genomic clone IFN-αWA is from Torczynski *et al.* (43). The IFN-αGX-1 (44) and IFN-α76 (45) appear to be recombinants between, respectively, IFN-αH_1 (1-16) and IFN-αG (17-166), on the one hand and between IFN-α4b (1-50), IFN-αC (51-131) and IFN-α4b (132-166) on the other. A gap was introduced at position 44 in IFN-αA (dashed line) to provide maximum alignment with the other species.

Figure 2. The amino acid sequences of various IFN-α species. The amino acid sequences are derived from cloned DNA sequences (46-49), and from a partial sequence of natural Mu-IFN-α (50). These sequences are compared to the Hu- and Mu-IFN-α consensus sequences. Amino acids which are found in all murine, rat and monkey IFN-α sequences and in all Hu-IFN-α sequences are underlined in the murine consensus sequences. The underlined residues in the Hu-IFN-α consensus sequence represent the common amino acids in all human sequences. Gaps (dashed line) are introduced in human and murine species to provide maximum alignment.

Figure 3. Amino acid sequences of human and bovine IFN-α-like species. The amino acid sequences are derived from cloned DNA sequences (52,53) and are compared to the consensus sequence of Hu-IFN-α. The amino acid sequence of Bo-IFN-αD (53-55) is also included for comparison. The IFN-α*D species is related to Hu-IFN-αD and was originally designated as IFN-α_{II}1 (53). A closely related sequence, Hu-IFN-αω, was described by Hauptmann and Swetly (52). The nucleotide sequence of a number of pseudogenes related to the IFN-α* family have been reported (22). Amino acids which are common to all Hu-IFN-α consensus sequences are underlined. We have arbitrarily designated these species IFN-α* until a nomenclature is established.

Figure 4. The amino acid sequences of various IFN-β species. The amino acid sequences are derived from cloned DNA sequences (24,38,39,49,82-86). Numbering is according to the human sequence. Common amino acids to all the sequences are underlined. Positions where no consensus is evident are denoted as "x". Several gaps (indicated by hyphens) were introduced into the murine sequences in order to maximize alignment.

Figure 5. The amino acid sequences of various IFN-γ species. The amino acid sequences, predicted from DNA sequences (106-108, 110-113), have been aligned. The structure derived from direct amino acid sequencing of natural Hu-IFN-γ (98) is denoted as "Hu-IFN-γ (protein)". The first amino acid residue of the protein is pyroglutamate designated as "e". Various deletions which were found at the COOH-terminus of the natural protein are indicated as "t". Gaps (indicated by hyphens) were introduced in the mouse sequence to allow maximum alignment. Asterisks are shown to designate the end of the rat and mouse sequences.

IV. Cellular and Physiologic Mechanisms of Action

16. The Interferon System in the Mouse

Yoshimi Kawade

Institute for Virus Research, Kyoto University, Kyoto 606, Japan

INTRODUCTION

In the previous interferon (IFN) volume of the Texas Reports, the review on murine IFN (MuIFN) (13) centered on the evidence for the existence of the α, β and γ types in mouse IFN, and emphasized basic similarities of the mouse IFN system to the human counterpart. Since then, great progress was made in that mouse genes or cDNA for α, β and γ IFNs were cloned, and their amino acid sequences deduced. The results are briefly reviewed here. I shall also discuss some findings relevant to the functional aspects of the IFN system in the animal body.

AN OVERVIEW OF MOUSE INTERFERON GENES AND PROTEINS

Like the human IFN (HuIFN) system, the mouse IFN system comprises not less than 10 non-allelic IFN-α genes, and a single gene each of IFN-β and γ. Some of their basic properties are summarized in Table 1, in comparison with the human counterparts. More information, including the nucleotide and amino acid sequences, can be found in (36).

IFN-α. Several MuIFN-α genes (or cDNA) have been cloned, and seven were completely sequenced (Table 2). Unfortunately, the same designations of the subtypes α5 and α6 were each given by Trapman's (37) and Pitha's (15) groups to different molecular species; they are distinguished here by adding suffixes T and P, respectively. Four of the seven complete sequences (α1, α5(P), α6(T), and α6(P)) consist of 166 amino acids, and the other three (α2, α4 and αA) have an additional residue at the C-terminus. α4 is exceptional, having 5 amino acid deletions corresponding to the 103 to 107 residues, and was reported to have a low antiviral activity (16); strictly speaking, however, this conclusion must await complete purification of the protein and determination of the actual specific activity. All these MuIFN-α subtypes are homologous to the HuIFN-α_I class (36); no mouse counterparts of HuIFN-α_{II} have been reported.

Most of the known human IFN-α subspecies are non-glycosylated. In contrast, the majority of the mouse IFN-α subtypes so far sequenced have one potential N-glycosylation site, in agreement with the previous observations on natural MuIFN-α (14). Although the sugar moiety is dispensable for the biological activity, it may affect the cross-species activity in some cases (35).

IFN-α from natural sources is a mixture of various subspecies (19), but their composition in terms of the genes is not clear. In the case of virus- or double-stranded (ds) RNA-induced L cell, mRNA for IFN-α4 is predominant (together with β mRNA) (17,37), but it is not known whether the α4 protein is the dominant species in the secreted product. α1 and α2 seem to be minor components, because they are neutralized by a monoclonal antibody which hardly affects the activity of L cell IFN-α (35).

IFN-β The result of cDNA cloning (11) revealed that the polypeptide is 5 amino acids shorter than the human counterpart, but that there are 3 N-glycosylation sites in contrast to one in HuIFN-β; this accounts for the larger molecular sizes of natural MuIFN-β than that of HuIFN-β. Also, the molecular size heterogeneity sometimes observed in natural MuIFN-β preparations (13) may be attributed to variations in the sugar moiety. MuIFN-β contains only one Cys residue, and therefore no disulfide bridge. This is in sharp contrast to HuIFN-β (3 Cys), whose Cys^{31}-Cys^{141} bridge seems to be essential for the antiviral activity.

As is well known, human "type I" IFNs induced with virus or dsRNA contain either the α or the β type as the sole or predominant component. In contrast, various mouse cells almost always produce IFN-α and β concomitantly (14). The molecular mechanisms that cause the difference between human and mouse cells are not yet clarified (17).

IFN-γ. The number of amino acids deduced from the cDNA nucleotide sequence is 133, 10 amino acids shorter than the human counterpart. The C-terminal portion of natural HuIFN-γ was shown to be proteolytically split off to various lengths (30); corresponding information on natural mouse IFN-γ is yet to come, but similar splitting appears likely (9). The MuIFN-γ molecules produced in E. coli were shown to lack the last four amino acids (24). There are two potential N-glycosylation sites like the human counterpart, but their positions are different.

The overall homology in amino acid sequence between human and mouse IFNs is greatest for α and smallest for γ (Table 1); this is in accord with their degrees of cross-species antiviral activities. Also, antigenic cross-reactions were found between the α types of the two species using conventional antisera (13), but not between the β and between the γ types. For the purpose of structure-activity studies, individual IFN-α subtypes, as well as IFN-β and γ, in both glycosylated and non-glycosylated forms, can now be utilized, but so far not much information has been obtained. Also, monoclonal antibodies to MuIFN-α (35), β (4,23,35) and γ (28,31,33) have been obtained, which will be useful for the anatomy of IFN molecules. For instance, it was reported that monoclonal antibodies that react with the C-terminal part of MuIFN-γ neutralize its macrophage-activating activity, while those that react with the N-terminal part activate it, although all these antibodies neutralize the antiviral activity (31). Molecular explanation of this intriguing finding is not clear. It seems we need elucidation of the three-dimensional structure of IFN molecules for a breakthrough in the functional anatomy of the molecules.

The availability of the IFN gene base sequences in several animal species allows one to analyze the evolution of IFN genes (22,36). IFN-α and β genes are no doubt derived from a common ancestral gene by duplication; IFN-γ gene is so different in structure that at present its relationship to IFN-α/β genes is totally obscure. The divergence time of IFN-α and β genes was recently estimated to be 200-300 million years ago (or more). This roughly corresponds to the time of divergence of mammals and birds/reptiles. That is, all mammals are likely to have separate IFN-α and β genes, but this is not certain in birds and reptiles. Chicken might have only a single type of IFN, since chick IFNs of different sources are neutralized similarly by the same monoclonal antibodies (18); complete purification of chick IFN and gene cloning will be most rewarding for considering the evolution of IFN genes.

FUNCTIONING OF THE IFN SYSTEM IN VIVO

During the past two decades, much work accumulated concerning pleiotropic effects of IFN, in addition to the antiviral effects. Since various purified and recombinant IFNs recently became available, the uncertainties arising from the use of impure IFN preparations have largely disappeared. However, not much is known about the physiological (and pathological) roles of endogenous IFN in the body. For instance, exogenous IFN administered to mice was shown to affect some immune responses, but little direct evidence has been available to indicate whether, or to what extent, endogenous IFN is involved in the processes of normal immune responses (6). Neither do we know whether endogenous IFN has any role to play during normal ontogenetic development, although a possible role was suggested in activating the major histocompatibility genes in early embryos (26). Here, I shall pick up a few topics on *in vivo* IFN.

Physiological IFN

It seems possible, or even likely, that small amounts of IFN are produced by various cells on various occasions in the normal functioning of the body; the IFN will perhaps act locally in a para- or autocrine mode, and generally be below detectable levels in body fluids extracted for assay. The concept of such "physiological IFN" has been advanced by several investigators, notably Bocci (this volume). Appearance of IFN in the body without apparent inducing stimuli has been reported, e. g., in placenta (Chany, this volume), in normal mouse sera (7), in the sera of autoimmune patients (6); the significance of these IFNs is not clear.

Macrophages are usually poorly permissive for virus growth. Put in culture, they were often shown to produce low levels of IFN spontaneously (6). According to Belardelli et al. (1), peritoneal (resident) macrophages appear to be exposed to IFN *in vivo*, because administration of anti-IFN-(α,β) antibodies to mice before harvesting the macrophages made them permissive for viruses. Also, mouse peritoneal macrophages can confer antiviral resistance to fibroblasts cultured together; this seems to be caused by IFN spontaneously produced by the peritoneal cells (to undetectable levels), since the effect is abolished by added anti-IFN-(α,β) antibody (29).

IFN-γ and -α/β have been shown to act synergistically in various systems. However, a case of antagonism was also recorded. An important function of IFN-γ is the induction of Ia antigens on macrophages and other cells. IFN-α and β not only fail to induce Ia but also block this action of IFN-γ (12,20). These differential effects of IFN-γ and α/β may well be important in the regulation of immune responses. Interestingly, macrophages (thioglycollate-stimulated) from newborn mice did not respond to IFN-γ, failing to express Ia antigen. This was attributed to spontaneous production of IFN-β by the newborn macrophages, since addition of anti-β monoclonal antibody made them responsive to IFN-γ (12).

Bacteria and IFN induction

Various bacteria and their products act as IFN inducers in mice and in leukocyte cultures (Weigent, this volume), and sensitize mice (or spleen cells) for enhanced IFN induction by other inducers (10). T cell mitogens, which are good inducers of IFN-γ in cultured leukocytes, fail to induce IFN-γ when given to mice; we found that when the mice were treated with *Mycobacterium bovis* BCG or *Corynebacterium parvum* and several days later were challenged with T cell mitogens, high levels of IFN-γ appeared in the circulation (25,34). Interestingly, lipopolysaccharide (LPS), a B cell mitogen believed to be an inducer of IFN-α/β, was found to induce in bacteria-presensitized mice high levels of IFN-γ following early IFN-α/β. Induction of IFN-γ by LPS was recently reported also in cultured leukocytes (2). These results thus revealed a potentially important interplay of bacteria, IFN, and the immune and reticuloendothelial systems. These bacteria are notable for immunomodulating and anti-tumor activities. They will induce production of various effectors other than IFN; for instance, BCG-LPS is a typical regimen for inducing tumor necrosis factor in mice. These effectors will most likely be involved in the observed IFN-γ induction, as well as in the modulation of immune functions in cooperation with IFN.

Future problems

It now seems a rule, rather than an exception, that the action of a biological effector, such as IFN, interleukins and hormones, is pleiotropic. Furthermore, different effectors often interact with each other in action, either positively or negatively, or in time sequence (Vilcek, this volume). Thus, analyses of the role of IFN must take such a network into view(3).

One possible approach toward understanding the role of IFN *in vivo* is administration of anti-IFN antibodies to mice, as has been done using conventional antisera (8,21,27); such should be extended to various problems using monoclonal antibodies with high neutralizing activity. Another would be to produce transgenic mice, harboring extra mouse IFN gene with artificially inducible construction (this is already underway in this and other laboratories); or those harboring anti-sense gene that would specifically inactivate IFN mRNA. With IFN genes and proteins at hand, we seem to be facing fruitful years toward clarifying the physiological significance of IFN.

REFERENCES

1. Belardelli, F., F. Vignaux, E. Proietti, and I. Gresser: Injection of mice with antibody to interferon renders peritoneal macrophages permissive for vesicular stomatitis virus and encephalomyocarditis virus. Proc. Natl. Acad. Sci. USA 81:602, 1984.
2. Blanchard, D.K., J.Y. Djeu, T.W. Klein, H. Friedman, and W.E. Stewart II: Interferon-γ induction by lipopolysaccharide: Dependence on interleukin 2 and macrophages. J. Immunol. 136:963, 1986.
3. Borecky, L.: Interferon: The lesson learned from endocrine and immunotherapy. In: Physiology and Pathology of Interferon System, L. Borecky, and V. Lackovic, eds. Springer. Contr. Oncol. 20:318, 1984.
4. Bosveld, I.J., W.P. Vonk, R.A.C.P. Hekman, P.W. van Vliet, P. de Jonge, W. van Ewijk, and J. Trapman: Prparation and properties of monoclonal antibodies against murine interferon-β. Virology 120:235, 1982.
5. Daugherty, B., D. Marin-Zanca, B. Kelder, K. Collier, T.C. Seamans, K. Hotta, and S. Pestka: Isolation and bacterial expression of a murine alpha leukocyte interferon gene. J. Interferon Res. 4:635, 1984.
6. De Maeyer-Guignard, J., and E. De Maeyer: Immunomodulation by interferons: Recent developments. In: Interferon 6, I. Gresser, ed. Academic Press, pp. 69-91, 1985.
7. Galabru, J., N. Robert, C. Buffet-Janvresse, Y. Riviere, and A.G. Hovanessian: Continuous production of interferon in normal mice: Effect of anti-interferon globulin, sex, age, strain and environment on the levels of 2-5A synthetase and p67K kinase. J. gen Virol. 66:711, 1985.
8. Gresser, I., F. Belardelli, C. Maury, M.-T. Maunoury, and M.G. Tovey: Injection of mice with antibody to interferon enhances the growth of transplantable murine tumors. J. Exp. Med. 158:2095, 1983.
9. Gribaudo, G., F. Cofano, M. Prat, C. Baiocchi, G. Cavallo, and S. Landolfo: Natural murine interferon-γ. J. Biol. Chem. 260:9936, 1985.
10. Havell, E.A., G.L. Spitalny, and P.J. Patel: Enhanced production of murine interferon γ by T cells generated in response to bacterial infection. J. Exp. Med. 156:112, 1982.
11. Higashi, Y., Y. Sokawa, Y. Watanabe, Y. Kawade, S. Ohno, C. Takaoka, and T. Taniguchi: Structure and expression of a cloned cDNA for mouse interferon-β. J. Biol. Chem. 258:9522, 1983.
12. Inaba, K., M. Kitaura, T. Kato, Y. Watanabe, Y. Kawade, and S. Muramatsu: The contrasting effect of alpha/beta- and gamma-interferons on the expression of macrophage Ia antigens. J. Exp. Med. 163:1030, 1986.
13. Kawade, Y.: Purification and properties of murine interferon. Texas Rept. Biol. Med. 41:219, 1981-82.
14. Kawade, Y.: Characterization of mouse interferon molecules. In: Humoral Factors in Host Defense, Y. Yamamura, et al., eds. Academic Press, pp.175-189, 1983.
15. Kelley, K.A., and P.M. Pitha: Characterization of a mouse interferon gene locus. I. Isolation of a cluster of four α interferon genes. Nucleic Acids Res. 13:805, 1985.

16. Kelley, K.A., and P.M. Pitha: Characterization of a mouse interferon gene locus. II. Differential expression of α-interferon genes. Nucleic Acids Res. 13:825, 1985.
17. Kelley, K.A., and P.M. Pitha: Differential effect of poly rI·rC and Newcastle disease virus on the expression of interferon and cellular genes in mouse cells. Virology 147:382, 1985.
18. Kohase, M., H. Moriya, T.A. Sato, S. Kohno, and S. Yamazaki: Purification and characterization of chick interferon induced by viruses. J. gen. Virol. 67:215, 1986.
19. Lemson, P.J., W.P. Vonk, J.A.G.M. van der Korput, and J. Trapman: Isolation and characterization of subspecies of murine interferon alpha. J. gen. Virol. 65:1365, 1984.
20. Ling, D.P., M.K. Warren, and S.N. Vogel: Antagonistic effect of interferon-β on the interferon-γ-induced expression of Ia antigens in murine macrophages. J. Immunol. 135:1857, 1985.
21. Marcovistz, R., J. Galabru, H. Tsiang, and A.G. Hovanessian: Neutralization of interferon produced early during rabies virus infection in mice. J. gen. Virol 67:387, 1986.
22. Miyata, T., H. Hayashida, R. Kikuno, H. Toh, and Y. Kawade: Evolution of interferon genes. In: Interferon 6, I. Gresser, ed. Academic Press, pp. 1-30, 1985.
23. Murasko, D.M., and M. Rusckowski: Production, screening and characterization of a monoclonal antibody to murine interferon-β. J. gen. Virol. 64:727, 1983.
24. Nagata, K., N. Kikuchi, O. Ohara, H. Teraoka, N. Yoshida, Y. Watanabe, and Y. Kawade: Purification and characterization of recombinant murine immune interferon. Submitted for publication.
25. Okamura, H., K. Kawaguchi, K. Shoji, and Y. Kawade: High-level induction of gamma interferon with various mitogens in mice pretreated with Propionibacterium acnes. Infect. Immun. 38:440, 1982.
26. Ozato, K., Y.-J. Wan, and B.M. Orrison: Mouse major histocompatibility class I gene expression begins at midsomite stage and is inducible in earlier-stage embryos by interferon. Proc. Natl. Acad. Sci. USA 82:2427, 1985.
27. Pfau, C.J., I. Gresser, and K.D. Hunt: Lethal role of interferon in lymphocytic choriomeningitis virus-induced encephalitis. J. gen. Virol. 64:1827, 1983.
28. Prat, M., G. Gribaudo, P.M. Comoglio, G. Cavallo, and S. Landolfo: Monoclonal antibodies against murine γ interferon. Proc. Natl. Acad. Sci. USA 81:4515, 1984.
29. Proietti, E., S. Gessani, F. Belardelli, and I. Gresser: Mouse perioneal cells confer an antiviral state on mouse cell monolayers: Role of interferon. J. Virol. 57:456, 1986.
30. Rinderknecht, E., B.H. O'Connor, and H. Rodriguez: Natural human interferon-γ. J. Biol. Chem. 259:6790, 1984.
31. Schreiber, R.D., L.J. Hicks, A. Celada, N.A.Buchmeier, and P.W. Gray: Monoclonal antibodies to murine γ-interferon which differentially modulate macrophage activation and antiviral activity. J. Immunol. 134:1609, 1985.
32. Shaw, G.D., W. Boll, H. Taira, N. Mantei, P. Lengyel, and C. Weissmann: Structure and expression of cloned murine IFN-α genes. Nucleic Acids Res. 11:555, 1983.
33. Spitalny, G.L., and E.A. Havell: Monoclonal antibody to murine gamma interferon inhibits lymphokine-induced antiviral and macrophage

tumoricidal activities. J. Exp. Med. 159:1560, 1984.
34. Wada, M., H. Okamura, K. Nagata, T. Shimoyama, and Y. Kawade: Cellular mechanisms in in vivo production of gamma interferon induced by lipopolysaccharide in mice infected with Mycobacterium bovis BCG. J. Interferon Res. 5:431, 1985.
35. Watanabe, Y., and Y. Kawade: To be published.
36. Weissmann, C., and H. Weber; The interferon genes. Progr. Nucleic Acid Res. Mol. Biol. in press, 1986.
37. Zwarthoff, E.C., A.T.A. Mooren, and J. Trapman: Organization, structure and expression of murine interferon alpha genes. Nucleic Acids Res. 13:791, 1985.

TABLE 1. Characteristics of Mouse IFN Genes and Proteins in Comparison with the Human Counterparts[a)].

	IFN-α	IFN-β	IFN-γ
Number of non-allelic genes	>10(>14)	1(1)	1(1)
Chromosome location	4(9)	4(9)	10(12)
Number of introns	0(0)	0(0)	3(3)
Number of amino acids in mature protein	166(166)[b)]	161(166)	133(143)[c)]
Number of Cys	5(4,5)	1(3)	1[d)](0)
Number of N-glycans	0,1(0)	3(1)	2(2)
Homology to HuIFN			
Nucleotide	ca. 70-75%	68%	64%
Amino acid	ca. 60%	48%	40%

a) Figures in parentheses refer to human IFN.
b) See Table 2 for details of MuIFN-α; HuIFN-α2 has 165, and HuIFN-$\alpha_{II}1$ has 172.
c) The C-terminus of both Mu- and HuIFN-γ may be split off to yield shorter polypeptides in the final products (9,24,30).
d) The Cys is at the C-terminus and may be lost in the mature protein.

TABEL 2. Mouse IFN-α Subtypes that Have Been Cloned

Subtype	No. of AA[a)]	No. of glyc.[b)]	Ref.
Mα1	166	1	32,37,15
Mα2	167	1	32,37
Mα3	-[c)]	-	32
Mα4	162	1	37,15
Mα5(T)	-[d)]	(1)	37
Mα5(P)	166	1	15
Mα6(T)	166	0	37
Mα6(P)	166	1	15
MαA	167	0	5
MαB	-	-	36

a) Number of amino acid residues in the mature protein.
b) Number of N-glycosylation site. It is at Asn^{78} in each case.
c) Partially sequenced, but the result not reported.
d) One-third of N-terminal not sequenced; the remainder is identical to Mα5(P), except one residue, therefore, Mα5(P) & Mα5(T) genes may be allelic.

17. The Physiological Interferon Response

Velio Bocci

Instituto di Fisiologia Generale, Università di Siena, 53100 Siena, Italy

THE PURSUING OF AN IDEA

The idea of an interferon (IFN) response in physiological conditions was borne out by a number of observations and reflections during the late 70s (1). There were many important anatomical, physiological, microbiological and immunological observations (reviewed in 2) indicating the continuous interaction between the gut-associated lymphoid tissue (GALT) and the luminal content potentially rich with IFN inducers. On the other hand, the absence of IFN in body fluids and tissues in healthy animals was favouring the generally accepted idea (3) that IFN would be produced only during viral infections. This idea however could be misleading and, like in a puzzle, if the apparently unrelated pieces were accommodated together they would give a coherent picture: I reasoned that firstly, owing to an array of exogenous and endogenous stimuli, IFN could be produced in minimal amounts only in restricted areas; secondly, IFN could be mostly used locally according to the concept of the paracrine secretion; thirdly, that even if it was going to spill-over into the plasma pool both the dilution and a very efficient catabolic system (4) would prevent its detection. In this way animals and plants, as they live in a contaminated environment, would have the benefit of IFN effects without having either circulating IFN, or toxic effects.

Thus two types of responses were envisaged: one was the classical response to an emergency condition such as a viral infection or induction by polynucleotides with massive production of IFN and consequently more or less transient IFN plasma levels accompanied by a flu-like syndrome (5), and another called the "physiological IFN response" (2) characterized by a kind of miniature IFN production almost continuous throughout life. The latter type of response, although practically invisible, is certainly not less important than the former for survival.

A FEW BASIC ASSUMPTIONS AND THE SITES OF PRODUCTION

I will summarize a few assumptions indispensable to imagine how IFN could be produced at a continuous low, physiological level in a particular site throughout life.
The first is that exogenous and endogenous inducers act as "physiological" stimuli in the lymphoid tissue associated with the following sites: the gut (GALT), the bronchi (BALT), the skin (SALT), the spleen, bone marrow and thymus (internal-associated lymphoid tissue: IALT) and the placenta and its annexes (6).
A second assumption concerns the modality and type of production. It is necessary to emphasize that in spite of the wealth of exogenous and endogenous IFN inducers (2) only a few molecules at a time can reach the targets in the lymphoid micro-environment. Moreover depending upon the cell reactivity, the threshold level and an all or none type of response, only a few cells may be switched on to produce IFN that, in line with the prediction (2) appear to be α (acid-labile) and γ. Only in the case of the placenta has IFN β been detected (7). A short digression is needed here because I consider the expressions "preformed", "constitutive", "spontaneous" or "endogenous" IFN production not clear. It appears that normal cells do NOT produce IFN and therefore if we were to live in an uncontaminated environment, absolutely free of inducers, the physiological IFN response would be practically nonexistent. As I have discussed at length previously (2) this conclusion is supported by the substantially diminished response in germ-free animals. However, even if these animals are fed with a synthetic diet they are still undergoing endogenous stimuli. These are less readily detectable than exogenous stimuli and could be represented by hormones, interleukins, glycoproteins (acting as lectins) shed by cellular membranes and/or glycosidases and proteases released by neutrophils and macrophages in the lymph nodes, spleen and bone marrow microenvironments (2) where the protease inhibitors present in plasma may have a reduced concentration. Moreover, IFN production could occur as the result of a transient depression of IFN genes during an early step of cell differentiation (hormonal influence?), or during a phase of the cell cycle.
The response is thus envisaged as a basic and strictly localized production of IFN as well as of many other lymphokines and monokines: an IFN concentration gradient will be formed around the producer cell as IFN is released in the interstitial fluid and diffuses outwards (Figure 1). Experimental evidence supporting this view has been given by Dianzani et al. (9) and obviously in the case of a viral infection the response was massive whereas, in physiological conditions, the re-

sponse is limited to only a few cells probably far away from one another. From this it seems obvious that a state of generalized refractoriness is most unlikely to occur and, at any given time, there always will be some responsive cells. Moreover, because of the migratory characteristics of lymphocytes and monocytes, it appears probable that cells in traffic around the producer cell will bind IFN molecules to their receptors, thus transferring IFN biological effects to far distant sites.

These possibilities are linked to a third assumption which tries to explain why IFN levels are physiologically undetectable in the circulation: most of the IFN present in the pericellular environment will be used (cell binding) and catabolized locally with little spill-over into the blood stream through venous capillary absorption and lymphatics.

As I mentioned before, learning that IFN had a very rapid turnover (4) was crucial to understand that even if trace amounts of IFN continuously reached the circulation they would not become detectable. The absence of circulating IFN is an important point because it implies that normally IFN has no deleterious effects, whereas during viral diseases or IFN therapy a number of side-effects (5) have been correlated to a progressively higher IFN plasma level. On the assumption that IFN exerts mainly short-range effects at the pericellular site, one can say that the physiological response is characterized by the paracrine-type of secretion (10). This is probably common to other lymphokines and in contrast, during the acute phase response, a real endocrine-type effect becomes evident (i.e. IFN or Il 1 can reach the thermoregulatory centre or the liver to elicit fever and synthesis of acute phase proteins). Clearly the advantage of the paracrine secretion is that in normal conditions cells passing through the sites of IFN production can pick up the message and generalize defensive functions without any need of circulating IFN.

EXPERIMENTAL EVIDENCE IN FAVOUR OF THE RESPONSE

Several pieces of information have become available in the last few years:

a) Traces of m-RNA for IFN α have been isolated from several organs of normal mice (11). Although there seems to be an "apparent absence of induction", the trace of IFN m-RNA could be due to the miniature induction typical of the physiological IFN response. In my opinion there is no need to evoke intrinsic (i.e., independent from exogenous and/or endogenous stimuli) mechanisms controlling transcription of IFN genes in vivo.

b) Release of IFN α and γ by normal human blood mononuclear (B.M.) cells, rabbit tissues, peritoneal macrophages from animals reared in conventional conditions and which have probably undergone minimal induction in vivo, has been shown by several investigators (12-17). Belardelli et al. (18) did not detect any IFN but they found mouse peritoneal macrophages in antiviral state (A.S.), which may imply a previous contact with IFN in vivo. Accordingly, anti-IFN antibodies injected previously in vivo did not allow the establishment of the A.S. Furthermore Proietti et al. (19) found that freshly harvested peritoneal macrophages could transfer an A.S. to target homologous cells only and that the transfer was inhibited by specific anti-IFN α/β antibodies. Similarly injection of antibodies to IFN α/β enhanced the tumorigenicity of xenogeneic (20) and syngeneic (21) tumors in mice.

c) That IFN may have been effectively present in some microenvironments (lung and intestines) and was bound to passenger lymphoid cells is also supported by Hovanessian et al's findings (22,23), who measured definite levels of (2'-5') oligo A synthetase and protein kinase in cells and plasma samples of healthy men and mice. Interestingly enzymes levels, which are taken as markers of IFN activation (6), were very low in germ-free, pathogen-free, antibiotic-treated and anti-IFN immunoglobulin treated mice. The whole of these results could not agree better with the predictions I made in 1981 and they support the concept that the physiological IFN response is modulated mostly by exogenous and endogenous stimuli.

d) Mice during the weaning period or when under pathogen-free conditions have extremely low NK activity that rapidly increases once they feed on a normal diet (24). While at first intake of IgA and viral inhibitors present in milk (25) may inhibit IFN production, the subsequent development of the gut microflora and usual feeding (26,27) would enhance production of IFN and Il 2 (28) with consequent activation of NK cells.

e) As it was foreseen (2), bone marrow of normal subjects produces small amounts of IFN α that cannot be detected in the circulation (29). IFN α seems to have a role (inhibition, stimulation, differentiation?) in the regulation of normal hematopoiesis: this is a good example of how positive and negative factors act simultaneously or at different levels of maturation on hematopoietic cells. It would be interesting to define the endogenous inducers that activate the local production of IFN at basic rate.

f) We have mostly used physiological approaches in vivo trying to explore in rabbits, rats and mice whether IFN levels are higher in lymph and venous blood draining from a strategic area such as the GALT, in comparison to arterial blood. On the whole the results indicate that some spill-over of IFN from the GALT may indeed occur: acid labile IFN α and γ levels are consistently higher in intestinal lymph and venous blood than arterial blood (30-32).

g) Activation of intestinal lymph production and inflow which occurs during intestinal absorption can temporarily increase IFN plasma le-

vels in man (33). We noted a small and transient IFN elevation because obviously, the lymph inflow is small in relation to the size of the plasma and interstitial fluid pools and concomitant rapid IFN turnover.
h) Similarly, vigorous physical exercise caused in man a transient increase of IFN levels (34). Also in this case one or more factors such as reduced renal blood flow and/or increased lymph flow may be responsible for the increase.
i) As IFN was detected in murine placentas (35) and in human amniotic fluid (36), we investigated whether the human isolated normal placenta at term released any antiviral activity in the perfusate. All placentas so far examined released detectable activity which was attributable mostly to IFN β and some to IFN α (7).
j) Circadian variations of IFN plasma levels have been detected in rats undergoing a monophasic feeding pattern (37).
All of these results fit well within the proposed theoretical framework and represent good circumstantial evidence in favour of the existence of the physiological IFN response. However, in spite of the suggestion (1) that radioactive or fluorescein-labelled anti-IFN antibodies should be crucial in providing direct evidence of the response, so far mostly for technical reasons, we have been unable to offer clear-cut data. Probably rapid diffusion, cell-binding and degradation of IFN around the producer cells make the localization of the antigen difficult. However it is hoped that more skillfull workers than us will be able to prove experimentally what I have provisionally drawn in Figure 1.

POSSIBLE SIGNIFICANCE OF THE PHYSIOLOGICAL IFN RESPONSE? HOW TO EXPLOIT IT?

The expression "physiological IFN response" was coined mostly to focus attention upon an overlooked phenomenon, but since 1980 (1) more or less direct evidence has been presented to suggest that many other lymphokines and monokines can be produced with the same mechanisms and that the immune system operates through the interplay of several factors. Thus, although the expression can be retained today as a paradigmatic example, its meaning certainly encompasses the release of many factors essential for a correct display of immunological functions.
The response may procure a multitude of important physiological effects and briefly the host defense system could be maintained in a continuous state of alertness against viruses, tumor cells and parasites by primed lymphocytes, virus-resistant cells and stimulated NK cells, macrophages and neutrophils. Moreover enhancement of the expression of membrane antigens may favor recognition and elimination of altered cells by cytotoxic T lymphocytes. Similarly, enhancement of the immune response and possibly of antibody-dependent cell-mediated

cytotoxicity may be another facet of the response. In the bone marrow, trace levels of IFNs may exert either differentiation effects and/or chalone-like activities to balance colony-stimulating factors (29). Even though all of these effects are difficult to quantify, there is little doubt that without IFN and the consequent activation of several cellular mechanisms, life of vertebrate animals would have a very short span indeed.

It is an ongoing endeavour of this laboratory to validate the relevance of the response and its possible variations in relation to factors such as genetic background (14), sex, pregnancy, nutritional status, types of diet, environmental conditions, daily and seasonal cycles, stress, immune reactivity and ageing. There would be a great advantage if the response could be tested in vivo and if this could be achieved, one could then correlate its intensity and quality with the parameters formally indicated. This, in turn, could help in optimizing the response in abnormal responders and hopefully reduce the incidence of viral diseases and tumors.

If one accepts the concept of the physiological IFN response and of the paracrine-type of action of lymphokines, one is led to wonder why we administer IFNs and Il 2 as if they were antibiotics or cytostatic drugs. In fact administration of IFN by conventional routes may be meaningful when it is necessary to achieve a high and/or a long-lasting IFN plasma level during acute viral diseases or if IFN is meant to act as an antiproliferative drug. On the other hand, when IFN should act as an immunomodulator, these conventional routes of administration appear unsuitable because they yield high IFN plasma levels, hence toxicity, favor IFN wastage through the kidneys and achieve little interaction between IFN and effector cells. A practical way to overcome these problems would be to change the strategy of administration trying to shift most of the IFN into the lymphatic pool (10). This can be done by spreading administration of IFN through the subcutis all over the body with a high concentration of human albumin that, owing to its colloid osmotic properties, acts as an interstitial fluid expander. Multi-site SC administration of IFN-albumin leads to high lymph-plasma IFN concentration ratio, low IFN plasma levels and probably increased immunostimulatory activity. In animal models, we are trying to show that pharmacokinetic parameters obtained by using what I have called the "lymphatic route" are superior to conventional SC route. If oncologists will be willing to try it in humans and if the therapeutic index should improve, the facilitated lymphatic absorption of IFN could become an elective route for a rational administration of biological response modifiers. The many "ifs" mean that hard work is ahead of us but nonetheless I feel it important to pursue this line of research, the outcome of which could be very beneficial to the immunodepressed and tumor-bearing patients.

ACKNOWLEDGMENTS

I am very grateful to my collaborators and to many colleagues for their experimental contributions supporting the existence of the physiological IFN response. This work was financed by Progetti finalizzati: "Controllo delle malattie da infezione" e "Oncologia". C.N.R., Roma.

REFERENCES

1. Bocci, V.: Is interferon produced in physiologic conditions? Med Hypotheses 6:735, 1980.
2. Bocci, V.: Production and role of interferon in physiological conditions. Biol Rev 56:49, 1981.
3. Bocci, V.: The physiological interferon response. Immunol Today 6:1, 1985.
4. Bocci, V.: Distribution, catabolism and pharmacokinetics of interferons. In: Interferon, vol. 4: In Vivo and Clinical Studies, N.B. Finter, and R.K. Oldham, eds. Elsevier Science Publishers, pp. 47-72, 1985.
5. Scott, G.M.: Interferon: pharmacokinetics and toxicity. Phil Trans R Soc Lond B 299:91, 1982.
6. Bocci, V.: The physiological interferon response: the sites and the meaning. In: Human Lymphokines, A. Khan, and N.O. Hill, eds. Academic Press, pp. 241-255, 1982.
7. Bocci, V., L. Paulesu, and M.G. Ricci: The physiological interferon response: IV. Production of interferon by the perfused human placenta at term. Proc Soc Exp Biol Med 180:137, 1985.
8. Owen, R.L.: Sequential uptake of horseradish peroxidase by lymphoid follicle epithelium of Peyer's patches in the normal unobstructed mouse intestine: an ultrastructural study. Gastroenterol 72:440, 1977.
9. Dianzani, F., P. Gullino, and S. Baron: Rapid activation of the interferon system in vivo. Infect Immun 20:55, 1978.
10. Bocci, V.: Immunomodulators as local hormones: new insights regarding their clinical utilization. J Biol Resp Modif 4:340, 1985.
11. Tovey, M.G., and I. Gresser: Detection of interferon messenger RNA in the organs of normal mice. In: The Interferon System, F. Dianzani, and G.B. Rossi, eds. Serono Symposia 24:109-113, Raven Press, 1985.
12. Smith, T.J., and R.R. Wagner: Rabbit macrophage interferons. I. Conditions for biosynthesis by virus-infected and uninfected cells. J Exp Med 125:559, 1967.
13. Black-Olszewska, Z., and M. Cembrzynska-Novak: Synthesis of spontaneous interferon by mouse peritoneal cells in vitro. I. Attempts to elucidate the origin of spontaneous interferon. Acta Biol Med Germ

38:765, 1979.
14. Haller, O., H. Arnheiter, I. Gresser, and J. Lindenmann: Genetically determined, interferon-dependent resistance to influenza virus in mice. J Exp Med 149:601, 1979.
15. Fischer, D.G., and M. Rubinstein: Spontaneous production of interferon-γ and acid-labile interferon-α by subpopulations of human mononuclear cells. Cell Immunol 81:426, 1983.
16. Bocci, V., L. Paulesu, M. Muscettola, M.G. Ricci, and G. Grasso: The physiological interferon response. III. Preliminary experimental data support its existence. Contr Oncol 20:36, 1984.
17. Martinez-Maza, O., U. Andersson, J. Andersson, S. Britton, and M. De Ley:Spontaneous production of interferon-γ in adult and newborn humans. J Immunol 132:251, 1984.
18. Belardelli, F., F. Vignaux, E. Proietti, and I. Gresser: Injection of mice with antibody to interferon renders peritoneal macrophages permissive for vesicular stomatitis virus and encephalomyocarditis virus. Proc Natl Acad Sci USA 81:602, 1984.
19. Proietti, E., S. Gessani, F. Belardelli, and I. Gresser: Mouse peritoneal cells confer an antiviral state on mouse cell monolayers: role of interferon. J Virol 57:456, 1986.
20. Reid, L.M., N. Minato, I. Gresser, J. Holland, A. Kadish, and B.R. Bloom: Influence of anti-mouse interferon serum on the growth and metastasis of tumor cells persistently infected with virus and of human prostatic tumors in athymic nude mice. Proc Natl Acad Sci USA 78:1171, 1981.
21. Gresser, I., F. Belardelli, C. Maury, M.T. Maunoury, and M.G. Tovey: Injection of mice with antibody to interferon enhances the growth of transplantable murine tumors. J Exp Med 158:2095, 1983.
22. Hovanessian, A.G., P. Rollin, Y. Rivière, P. Pouillart, P. Sureau, and L. Montagnier: Protein kinase in human plasma analogous to that present in control and interferon-treated HeLa cells. Biochem Biophys Res Commun 103:1371, 1981.
23. Galabru, J., N. Robert, C. Buffet-Janvresse, Y. Rivière, and A.G. Hovanessian: Continuous production of interferon in normal mice: effect of anti-interferon globulin, sex, age, strain and environment on the levels of 2-5A synthetase and p67K kinase. J Gen Virol 66:711, 1985.
24. Wigzell, H.: Regulation of cytotoxic cells by interferon. In: Miami Winter Symposia, Vol. 18, L.W. Mozes, J. Schultz, W.A. Scott, and R. Werner, eds. Academic Press, pp. 403-412, 1981.
25. Matthews, T.H.J., C.D.G. Nair, M.K. Lawrence, and D.A.J. Tyrrell: Antiviral activity in milk of possible clinical importance. Lancet 1387, 1976.
26. Tagliabue, A., W. Luini, D. Soldateschi, and D. Boraschi: Natural killer activity of gut mucosal lymphoid cells in mice. Eur J Immunol 11:919, 1981.

27. Bartizal, K.F., C. Salkowski, and E. Balish: The influence of a gastrointestinal microflora on natural killer cell activity. J Reticuloend Soc 33:381, 1983.
28. Spitz, M., A. Gearing, M. Callus, L. Spitz, and R. Thorpe: Interleukin-2 in vivo: production of and response to interleukin-2 in lymphoid organs undergoing a primary immune response to heterologous erythrocytes. Immunol 54:527, 1985.
29. Zoumbos, N.C., P. Gascon, J.Y. Djeu, and N.S. Young: Interferon is a mediator of hematopoietic suppression in aplastic anemia in vitro and possibly in vivo. Proc Natl Acad Sci USA 82:188, 1985.
30. Bocci, V., M. Muscettola, L. Paulesu, and G. Grasso: The physiological interferon response. II. Interferon is present in lymph but not in plasma of healthy rabbits. J Gen Virol 65:101, 1984.
31. Bocci, V., M. Muscettola, L. Paulesu, and G. Grasso: The physiological interferon response. V. Antiviral activity present in rat lymph is neutralized by anti-mouse interferon-γ antibodies. Microbiologica 8:405, 1985.
32. Bocci, V., L. Paulesu, M. Muscettola, and L. Vanni: Presence of interferon in venous blood draining from gut-associated lymphoid tissue. Immunol Lett 12:25, 1986.
33. Bocci, V., L. Paulesu, M. Muscettola, and A. Viti: The physiologic interferon response. VI. Interferon activity in human plasma after a meal and drinking. Lymphokine Res 4:151, 1985.
34. Viti, A., M. Muscettola, L. Paulesu, V. Bocci, and A. Almi: Effect of exercise on plasma interferon levels. J Appl Physiol 59:426, 1985.
35. Fowler, A.K., C.D. Reed, and D.J. Giron: Identification of an interferon in murine placentas. Nature 286:266, 1980.
36. Lebon, P., S. Girard, F. Thepot, and C. Chany: The presence of α-interferon in human amniotic fluid. J Gen Virol 59:393, 1982.
37. Paulesu, L., M. Muscettola, V. Bocci, and A. Viti: Daily variations of plasma interferon levels in the rat. IRCS Med Sci 13:993, 1985.

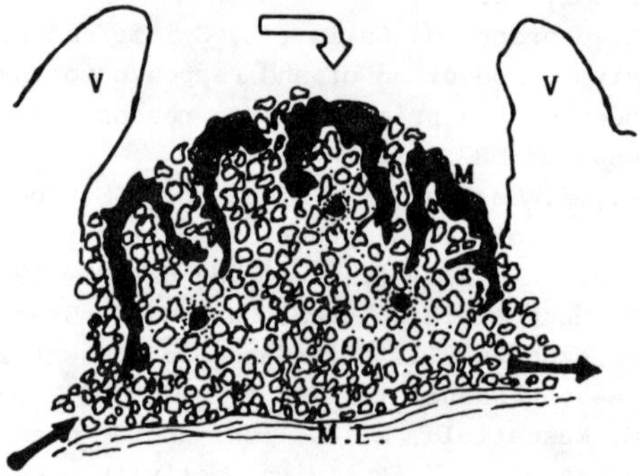

Figure 1. A provisional schematic view of the physiological IFN response in the gut-associated lymphoid tissue. Compounds acting as IFN inducers can enter the lymphoid follicle via membranous (M) epithelial cells (8) and stimulate IFN (as well as other lymphokines) production in a few responsive cells (●). The released IFN will diffuse into the interstitial fluid and activate neighbouring cells. Some IFN may be broken-down locally or leak into the lymphatic and venous capillaries. IFN-activated leukocytes will migrate and transfer IFN biological effects all over the body. Endogenous inducers are thought to act in similar way in the internal-associated lymphoid tissue. Villi (V) and muscularis layer (M.L.). The arrows indicate the inflow and outflow of leukocytes.

18. A Possible Role for IFNs α and β in the Development of IFN-γ's Antiviral State in Mouse and Human Cells

Thomas K. Hughes and Samuel Baron

Department of Microbiology, University of Texas Medical Branch, Galveston, TX 77550

INTRODUCTION

Lymphokine regulation of biological responses in some cases may be a multicomponent process. For example, evidence has indicated that in lymphoid cells, IFN-γ can induce the production of tumor necrosis factor (TNF), interleukin-1 (IL-1), and lymphotoxin (1,2,3). In addition, TNF or IL-2 can induce IFN-γ (1,4) and in fibroblasts, TNF can induce IFN-β (5). Such a cascade tends to indicate that a highly complex mechanism of events is occurring during cell activation. Thus, one may question whether an effect attributed to a particular lymphokine is actually caused by it or by another substance that it induces.

The antiviral potential of interferons α, β, and γ (IFNs α, β, and γ) have been well documented (6,7). IFNs α and β have relatively similar mechanisms of inducing the antiviral state by binding to a common receptor site on the cell (8) and exhibiting similar kinetics of sensitivity to metabolic inhibitors (9,10). In addition, the genes for IFNs α and β may be located, in close proximity, on the same chromosome (8). In contrast to IFNs α and β, however, IFN-γ demonstrates different kinetics of sensitivity to metabolic inhibitors (10), appears to bind to a different receptor on the cell and is coded for by a gene on a different chromosome (8).

IFNs α and β both appear to initiate antiviral activity in the cell through a single round of protein synthesis. IFN-γ, however, appears to require two rounds of protein synthesis, the second round of which appears to result in the antiviral state (10). The possibility therefore exists that in the first round of protein synthesis, IFN-γ may be inducing the production of a substance which in turn induces the antiviral state. If this is the case, IFN-γ itself may not be directly antiviral which others have speculated in the past (11). To test this hypothesis, we examined the possibility that IFN-γ was inducing one or both of the other IFNs, α and/or β, which in turn induced the antiviral state. Here we present evidence showing that under certain conditions a large portion of IFN-γ's antiviral activity is mediated mainly by its induction of IFN-α in mouse cells and IFN-β mainly in human cells.

RESULTS

Effects of Cell Concentration and Antibodies to IFNs α and/or β on IFN-γ's Antiviral Activity.

To determine whether IFN-γ mediated its antiviral activity by inducing another IFN, we employed the following strategy. Mouse L-929 or human embryonic lung (HEL) cells were plated at low cell densities in the presence of various concentrations of natural or recombinant IFN-γ (rIFN-γ) and high concentrations of antibody to IFN α and/or β. If IFN-γ induced another IFN(s) which subsequently caused the antiviral state, the high levels of antibody to the other IFNs would neutralize their effects. The low cell density was used to preclude IFN mechanisms that could circumvent the antibody to IFNs. Such circumventing mechanisms might include high concentrations of IFN at the interfaces of producing cells that might be inaccessible to the antibody (12) or even non-detectable (13) and transfer of the antiviral state between cells in direct contact which might occur via gap junction (14,15). Following treatment with IFN-γ and the antibodies to IFNs α and/or β, the supernatant fluids were decanted and the L-929 or HEL cells were challenged with vesicular stomatitis virus (VSV) or Sindbis virus (SbV) in the presence of the same concentrations of antibodies to IFNs α and/or β. As shown in Figures 1 and 2, L-929 or HEL cells, at low cell densities, treated with IFN-γ in the continuous presence of high concentrations of antibody to the other IFNs failed to develop an antiviral state to VSV or SbV. Specifically, the antiviral activity of mouse IFN-γ was blocked by anti-IFN-α/β antibody, while the antiviral activity of human IFN-γ was blocked by anti-IFN-β. Further characterization in the mouse system with monoclonal antibodies to IFN-α or β revealed that most of the activity was blocked by monoclonal anti-IFN-α (Figure 3). These data suggest that a large component of the antiviral activity of mouse and human IFN-γ may be due mainly to their induction of IFNs α and β, respectively. In these experiments, the antibodies were reapplied following IFN-γ removal to prevent the effect of late IFN-α and/or β production after IFN-γ treatment (discussed in the following section). It is important to note that although the antibody to IFN-α and/or β was most effective if continuously present, it was also highly effective at inhibiting the development of the antiviral state if only present during IFN-γ treatment (data not shown). This argues against the possibility that the antibody acted mainly against virus-induced IFN.

Demonstration of IFN-α/β in the Supernatant Fluids of IFN-γ Treated Cells.

We also have demonstrated the presence of IFN-α in the supernatant fluids of IFN-γ treated mouse cells. Mouse L-929 cells were treated with 50 u/ml of IFN-γ for 24 hours, washed extensively, refed with an equal volume of medium, and the supernatant fluids checked 24 hours later for the presence of IFN-α/β. Table I shows that L-929 cells produce an antiviral-like activity following treatment with natural or recombinant IFN-γ that has the characteristics of IFN-α/β, i.e., insensitivity to pH 2 and neutralized by anti-IFN α/β but not anti-IFN-γ. There was no detectable activity present in the supernatant fluids obtained from control cells. It is important to note that in a few cases, the levels of IFN-α/β produced are very low or non-detectable by direct assay (13). In addition, we have also shown that mouse spleen, bone marrow and peritoneal exudate cells produce IFNs-α and/or β following treatment with IFN-γ (Table II). These findings contrast the above demonstration of mouse L-929 cell production of apparently only IFN-α (Figure 4).

The direct detection of IFN-β in the supernatant fluids of IFN-γ-treated HEL cells has yet to be demonstrated. Previous evidence in the mouse system, though, has shown that an antiviral state can be seen in cells treated with conventional IFN inducers well before the detection of IFN in the cell supernatant fluids (13). Studies are currently underway to directly detect IFN-β in the supernatant fluids of IFN-γ treated cells in the human system.

DISCUSSION

Taken together, our findings indicate that, 1) the antiviral activity in IFN-γ treated cells could be reduced by anti-IFN-α and β in mouse and human cells, respectively, some times to the level of the virus control at low cell densities, 2) IFNs α and/or β can be demonstrated in the supernatant fluids of IFN-γ treated mouse L-929 and lymphoid cells, and 3) rIFN-γ can be used indicating that an IFN-α or β inducer other than IFN-γ is not responsible. In addition, the possibility that mycoplasma contamination of the cell cultures contributes to the induction of IFN-α or β may be addressed by the fact that the HEL cells used in these studies have been shown to be mycoplasma-free (Dr. T. Albrecht, personal communication).

An obvious question raised by these results is that, since typing of IFN preparations by neutralization with anti-IFN is a rather common procedure, why have the present findings not been seen in the past? Possible explanations include, 1) the routine use of confluent cells in contact with each other to perform plaque or cytopathic effect reduction assays might allow high concentrations of IFN-α in narrow intercellular spaces and transfer of antiviral activity between contacted cells, and 2) the use of levels of antibody that cannot overcome induction of resistance by high concentrations of locally produced IFN-α or β.

It is interesting to note that in the mouse L-929 cells, IFN-γ appears to selectively induce IFN-α. Past reports indicate that most IFN inducers generally stimulate mouse L-929 cells to coordinately produce IFN-α and β (IFN-α/β) (16). The reason for this selective induction of IFNα by IFN-γ is unknown.

The implications of these findings are numerous. For example, is IFN-γ solely an inducer of IFN or does it also directly function as an IFN? If IFN-γ directly induces a portion of the antiviral state, then it would be important to compare that antiviral state with the antiviral states induced by IFNs α and β. Are the immunomodulatory, antiproliferative or cytolytic activities attributed to IFN-γ the result of IFN-γ or another substance induced by it? Our results tend to raise serious questions about the accepted mechanisms of action of IFN-γ and its related paradigms. Important ramifications, therefore, result for research dealing with virology, immunology, cellular control mechanisms and IFN-γ and its potential applications since clinical trials are currently underway for its use as a biological response modifier (17).

ACKNOWLEDGEMENTS

We wish to thank Charlotte S. Larned for expert technical assistance.

This work was supported in part by a grant from the Elsa U. Pardee Foundation, Midland, Michigan.

REFERENCES

1. Philip, R. and L.B. Epstein: Tumor necrosis factor as immunomodulator and mediator of monocyte cytotoxicity induced by itself, γ-interferon and interleukin-1. Nature 323:86, 1986.
2. Wong, G.W.H. and D.V. Goeddel: Interferon induces the expression of tumor necrosis factor/lymphotoxin and vice versa: TNO-ISIR Meeting on the Interferon System, Clearwater Beach, FL, USA, 1985.
3. Robbins, C.H.: Immunoregulation by lymphokines: immune interferon and lymphotoxin induction of lymphokine activity in human peripheral blood leukocyte cultures. Adv. Exp. Med. Biol. 166:37, 1983.
4. Weigent, D.A., G.J. Stanton and H.M. Johnson: Interleukin-2 enhances natural killer activity through induction of γ interferon. Infect. Immun. 41(3):992, 1983.
5. Kohase, M., D. Henriksen-DeStefano, L.T. May, J. Vilcek and P. Seghal: Induction of B_2-Interferon by tumor necrosis factor: A homeostatic mechanism in the control of cell proliferation. Cell 45:659, 1986.
6. Finter, N.B. ed. Interferon and interferon inducers. North Holland, Amsterdam. 1983.
7. Baron S., F. Dianzani and G.J. Stanton, eds.: The Interferon System: A Review to 1982. In: Texas Reports on Biology and Medicine, Vol. 35. 1982.
8. Smith-Johannsen, H., Y-T. Hou, X-Y. Liu and Y.H. Tan: Regulatory control of interferon synthesis and action. In: Interferons and their applications. P.E. Cane and W.A. Carter eds. Handbook of Experimental Pharmacology 71:101, 1984.
9. Dianzani, F., C.E. Buckler and S. Baron: Effect of cyclohexamide on the antiviral action of interferon. Proc. Soc. Exp. Biol. Med. 130:519, 1969.
10. Dianzani, F., M. Rucca, A. Scupham and J.A. Georgiades: Immune and virus induced interferons may activate the cell by different derepressional mechanisms. Nature 183:400, 1980.

11. Georgiades, J., S. Baron, W.R. Fleischmann, M. Langford, D.A. Weigent and G.J. Stanton: Immune interferon. In: Interferons and their applications. P.E. Cane and W.A. Carter eds. Handbook of Experimental Pharmacology 71:305, 1984.
12. Dianzani, F. and S. Baron: Unexpectedly rapid action of human interferon in physiological conditions. Nature 257:682, 1975.
13. Buckler, C.E., K.T. Wong and S. Baron: Induction of the interferon system by various inducers. Proc. Soc. Exp. Biol. Med. 127:1258, 1968.
14. Blalock, J.E. and S. Baron: Interferon induced transfer of viral resistance between animal cells. Nature 268:422, 1977.
15. Blalock, J.E.: A small fraction of cells communicates the maximal sensitivity to a population. Proc. Soc. Exp. Biol. Med. 162:80, 1979.
16. Iwakura, U., S. Yokehara and Y. Kawade: Purification of mouse L cell interferon. Essentially pure preparation with associated cell growth inhibitory activity. J. Biol. Chem. 253:507, 1978.
17. Vadhan-Raj, S., C.F. Nathan, S.A. Sherwin, H.F. Oettgen and S.E. Krown: Phase 1 trial of recombinant interferon γ by 1 hour i.v. infusion. Cancer Treat. Rep. 70(5):609, 1986.
18. Campbell, J.B., J. Greenberger, M.A. Kochman and S.L. White: A microplaque reduction assay for human and mouse interferon. Canad. J. Microbiol. 21:1247, 1975.

TABLE I. Natural and recombinant mouse IFN-γ induce IFN-α/β in mouse L-929 cells.

	Residual activity (u/ml) after treatment:		
IFN-γ (u/ml)	pH 2	Anti-γ	Anti-α/β
0	0	0	0
Natural (100)	20	20	0
Natural (30)	8	8	0
Recombinant (50)	ND	8	0

Legend to Table I: Mouse L-929 cells ($5x10^6$/flask 20 ml in EMEM 10%) were grown in 75 cm^2 tissue culture flasks (Costar, Cambridge, MA) and incubated 24 hours at 37°C in 4% CO_2. Following incubation, the indicated concentrations of IFN-γ or media alone were placed on the cells. Twenty-four hours later, the cells were washed 3x with EMEM 2%, and refed with 5 ml EMEM 2%. After another 24 hours, the supernatant fluids were harvested. Following treatment with acid (pH 2) anti-mouse IFN-γ antiserum (200u/ml), or anti-mouse IFN-α/β antiserum (100u/ml), the fluids were assayed for IFN activity in a microplaque reduction assay.

Table II: Mouse spleen, bone marrow and peritoneal exudate cells produce IFNs α and/or β in response to IFN-γ

Antiviral Cell	IFN-γ	pH2	Treatment Anti-α	Anti-β	Residual Activity (U/ml)
MoSpl	−	−	−	−	<3
"	+	+	−	−	35
"	+	+	+	−	<3
"	+	+	−	+	25
"	+	+	+	+	<3
BM	−	−	−	−	<3
"	+	+	−	−	10
"	+	+	+	−	3
"	+	+	−	+	<3
"		+	+	+	<3
PEC	−	−	−	−	<3
"	+	+	−	−	100
"	+	+	+	−	100
"	+	+	−	+	100
	+	+	+	+	5

Legend to Table II: Mouse spleen (MoSpl), bone marrow (BM) or peritoneal exudate cells were harvested from non-sensitized C3H/HeJ mice as described elsewhere (37). One to $5x10^6$ cells/well were placed in 24 well tissue culture plates (Costar, Cambridge, MA) in Eagle's minimal essential medium supplemented with 2% fetal bovine serum and penicillin/streptomycin (100 μ/100 μg/ml), with or without 50 μ/ml natural IFN-γ. Following 24 hours of incubation at 37°C, 4% CO_2, the supernatant fluids were harvested. The supernatant fluids were then acid treated at pH 2 for 24 hours to inactivate residual IFN-γ. Samples were then normalized to pH 7.4 and the antiviral activities were determined on mouse L-929 cells, after treatment with media or 125 units of anti-mouse IFN-α or anti-mouse IFN-β (Yamas Shoyu Co., Ltd., Japan).

Figure 1. A large component of IFN-γ's antiviral activity is blocked by antibody to IFN α/β in sparsely populated cell cultures.

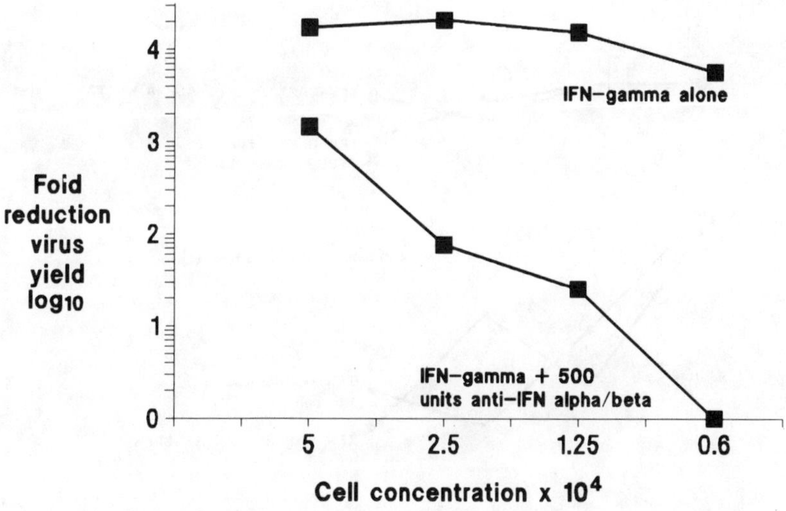

Legend to Figure 1. Mouse L-929 cells were placed in 96 well tissue culture plates (Costar Cambridge, MA) at the indicated cell concentrations in 0.1 ml Eagles Minimal Essential Medium with 10% fetal bovine serum, penicillin/streptomycin (100 units/100 μg/ml) and gentamycin (50 mg/ml) (EMEM 10%). Twenty-four hours later medium or natural IFNγ (22) was added at a concentration of 50 u/ml in the presence or absence of 500 neutralizing units of rabbit anti-mouse IFN α/β (kindly provided by Dr. Doug Weigent). Following 24 hours incubation, the supernatant fluids were decanted and the cells infected with vesicular stomatitis virus (VSV) at a multiplicity of infection (MOI) of .05. Virus was harvested 48 hours later and the yields were quantified on mouse L-929 cells using a slightly modified microplaque assay (18).

Figure 2. A large component of the antiviral activity of human rIFN-γ appears to be mediated by its induction of IFN-β in HEL cells.

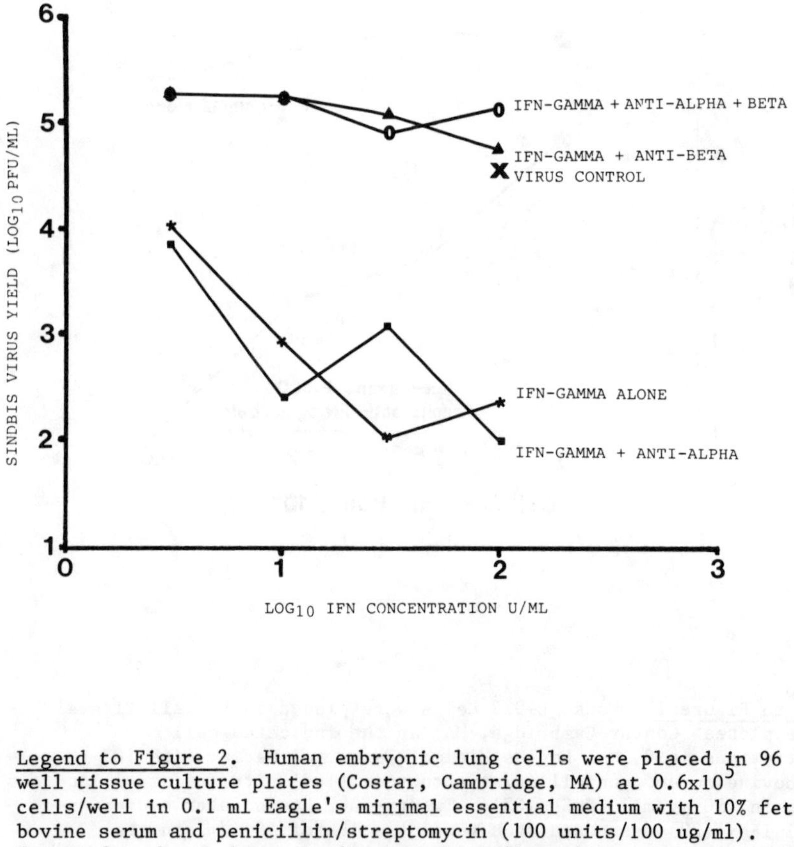

Legend to Figure 2. Human embryonic lung cells were placed in 96 well tissue culture plates (Costar, Cambridge, MA) at $0.6x10^5$ cells/well in 0.1 ml Eagle's minimal essential medium with 10% fetal bovine serum and penicillin/streptomycin (100 units/100 ug/ml). Twenty-four hours later, medium or the indicated concentrations of recombinant human interferon-γ (Biogen, Inc.) was added in the absence or presence of 125 units of rabbit anti-human IFN-α and/or β (NIH, Bethesda, MD). Following 24 hours of incubation, the supernatant fluids were decanted and the cells were infected with Sindbis virus at an MOI of 0.5. Virus was harvested 24 hours later and the yields were quantified on mouse L-929 cells using a slightly modified microplaque assay (18).

Figure 3. Recombinant IFN-γ's antiviral activity is inhibited by monoclonal antibody to mouse IFN-α.

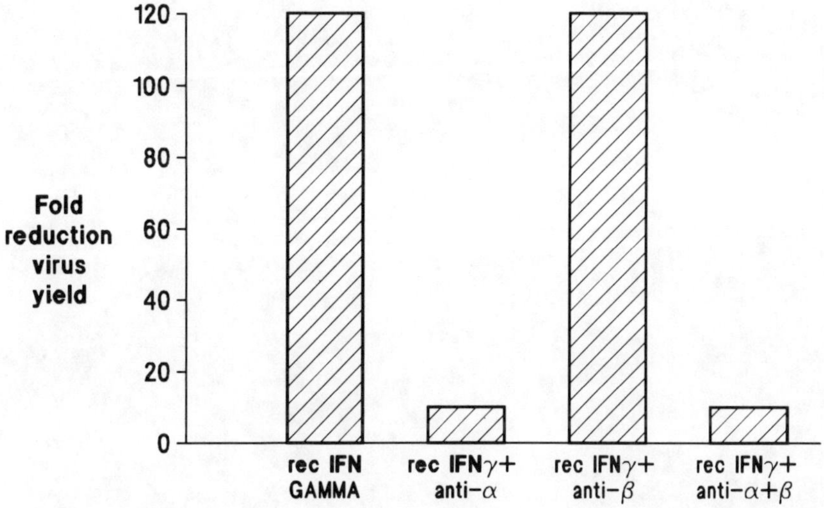

Legend to Figure 3. Mouse L-cells were plated at a concentration of 0.6×10^4 cells/well in microtiter plates. Twenty-four hours later 10u/ml recombinant mouse IFN-γ was placed in the well with monoclonal anti-mouse IFN-α (250 neutralizing units), monoclonal anti-mouse IFN-β (250 neutralizing units), a combination of the two (250 neutralizing units final), or media alone. Twenty-four hours later, the cells were washed 3 times and infected with VSV (MOI=.05). Virus yields were quantified as before.

19. Interleukin-1 and Tumor Necrosis Factor as Inducers of Interferon

A. Billiau, J. Van Damme, and G. Opdenakker

Rega Institute for Medical Research, University of Leuven, B-3000 Leuven, Belgium

INTRODUCTION

IL-1 : What's in a Name

The term interleukin-1 stands for a family of protein molecules which constitute the active principle in a number of factors produced mainly by mononuclear phagocytes, and previously identified descriptively by biological activity in various assay systems (for review see ref. 6, 15). These biological activities relate to the specific immune response as well as to aspecific or natural host resistance.

Investigators concerned with the antigen-specific immune response originally described IL-1 as LAF (lymphocyte activating factor). LAF-activity can best be described as the ability to make T-cells responsive to antigen-presentation, thereby inducing production of IL-2, the T-cell growth factor.

In aspecific host resistance the actions of IL-1 are multiple and defined at different levels of organization. At the level of the single cell IL-1 can be considered as the active principle of :

1) FAF (fibroblast activating factor) which causes proliferation of certain fibroblasts in certain conditions.

2) MCF (monocytic cell factor) which induces production of collagenase and prostaglandin (PG) release by synovial cells.

3) "22K" antiviral factor which exerts an interferon-like antiviral effect on certain fibroblasts.

As defined at the organ level, IL-1 is the active principle of :

1) EP (endogenous pyrogen) which upon injection in animals causes fever, probably by inducing PG-synthesis in the anterior hypothalamus.

2) LEM (leukocytic endogenous mediator) which, upon injection in animals, causes the so-called acute phase response, i.e. a response seen in various infections and traumatic situations and characterized by a

biphasic neutropenia/neutrophilia reaction, hyposideremia and -zincemia, hypercupremia and higher serum levels of so-called acute phase reactants (e.g. serum amymoid A, C-reactive protein, ...). While the neutropenia and subsequent neutrophilia are due to effects of IL-1 on endothelial cell adhesive properties and on bone marrow function, the other components of the acute phase response are mediated by effects of IL-1 on protein synthesis in hepatocytes.

3) Catabolin which is defined as a factor causing breakdown of muscle protein, cartilage and bone. Some of the effects are mediated by prostaglandin synthesis. Cartilage breakdown seems to be due to induction of proteoglycanase in chondrocytes; bone resorption can be referred to activation of osteoclasts.

IL-Molecules

Already before recombinant DNA technology was there to help resolve the molecular nature of IL-1, it had become usual to distinguish two types of IL-1, both having a MW of 17,000 but differing in isoionic point (pI) : the pI-5 and pI-7 forms. Molecular cloning of human IL-1 has revealed the existence of at least two peptides with a quite different amino acid sequence, currently designated as IL-1(α) and IL-1(β) (1,4,9,11,13,14). Both are synthesized as precursor proteins of about 30,000. Cleavage generates one or possibly several biologically active peptides, the most prominent of which is a peptide of 17,000 constituting the carboxyterminal half of the precursor. The significance of the exceptionally long prepeptide is at present unclear.

The Producing Cell(s)

Not only blood monocytes but mononuclear phagocytes from every existing source (peritoneum, lung, liver, spleen, synovia, bone marrow) as well as certain macrophage cell lines have been shown to produce IL-1. Besides, certain other cells, some of which may play a role in antigen presentation or in aspecific host resistance, are also shown to be good IL-1 producers: corneal epithelium, epidermal keratinocytes (ETAF = epidermal thymocyte activating factor), Langerhans' cells, astrocytes and other glial cells, renal mesangial cells, dendritic cells. Contrary to older literature data on the cell source of EP, neutrophils are poor producers of IL-1, if producers at all.

Stimuli for Production

The list of exogenous substances or agents that may activate macrophages to produce IL-1 is inordinately long. Bacteria (e.g. Staphylococci), bacterial products (e.g. lipopolysaccharide) or plant lectins (e.g. ConA) are the ones that are mostly used in the laboratory. We may assume that, in vivo, a mononuclear phagocyte produces IL-1 whenever it has recognized and/or ingested a foreign agent. It is not excluded, however, that endogenous mediators produced by other cells may play a role in this process by facilitating triggering of the macrophage. Thus, lymphokines produced by T-cells have been found to trigger and/or modulate production of IL-1 by phagocytes. Candidate molecules for this function are CSF and interferon-γ. IL-1 production is associated by enhanced expression of Class II antigens (Ia or DR) on the cell membrane and there is some evidence that such expression is in fact a prerequisite for the cell to be able to react to IL-1 inducing stimuli.

THE ANTIVIRAL EFFECT OF IL-1

Early Studies : The Interferon-Like "22K"-Factor

Crude or partially purified lymphokine/monokine preparations obtained from ConA-stimulated human peripheral blood mononuclear cells (PBMC) were found to contain, besides IFN-γ, a second interferon-like antiviral factor (18,19). It was called 22K-factor because, on gel filtration columns, it migrated as a protein with Mr = 22,000 as opposed to 45,000 for IFN-γ. This interferon-like factor was serologically distinct from IFN-γ and IFN-α, but was neutralizable by highly specific polyclonal antibodies directed against HuIFN-β. Despite this apparent serological relationship, the 22K factor differed from classical HuIFN-β by a variety of criteria. Thus, in contrast to HuIFN-β, it was strictly species specific and it acted only on a very limited array of human cells. Most significantly, while HuIFN-β could be bound to affinity columns of anti-IFN-β antisera, the 22K factor failed to be bound by such columns, although they were prepared from sera that neutralized its biological activity. Also antisera raised against highly purified 22K-factor, failed to neutralize HuIFN-β although they did neutralize antiviral activity of 22K. These observations were decisive in formulating the hypothesis that the antiviral activity of 22K factor was due to its ability to induce IFN-β.

The Active Principle of 22K Factor is (an) IL-1

Identification of 22K factor as (an) IL-1 resulted from concurrent efforts to characterize the active principle biochemically, and to detect other possible biological activities (20). Increasingly pure preparations of 22K factor were found to possess various activities assigned to IL-1. The most significant of these were : pyrogenicity (EP-activity), induction of neutropenia and neutrophilia (LEM-activity), mouse thymocyte activation (LAF-activity) and induction of collagenase in synovial cells (MCF-activity).

Purification studies allowed to obtain the 22K factor in pure form and to determine its Mr value as 17,000 on SDS-PAGE analysis. Amino-acid sequence analysis yielded an N-terminal sequence that, on confrontation with that derived from molecular cloning of IL-1 cDNA revealed extensive homology and allowed to define the correct proteolytic cleavage site on the 31,000 Mr precursor protein (2,20). As a result of these studies it can now be certified that the active principle of 22K factor is IL-1(β).

A final piece of evidence demonstrating IFN-β-mediated antiviral activity of IL-1 is the observation (table 1) that recombinant-DNA derived IL-1(α) as well as IL-1(β) have in vitro antiviral activity that can be blocked by specific antisera against IFN-β.

One of the activities of 22K factor was not "classical" for IL-1, i.e. the ability of 22K-factor to induce colony formation in human bone marrow culture. However, this effect has now been demonstrated to be indirect as it is due to the ability of IL-1 to induce production of colony stimulating factor(s) in phagocytic adherent cells present in most bone marrow cultures, unless care has been taken to remove them (3,8).

Mechanism(s) of Action

The postulate that the *in vitro* antiviral effect of IL-1 is due to induction of HuIFN-β is based on 3 lines of evidence : (1) The antiviral effect is blocked by antisera that are specific for HuIFN-β, e.g. by a serum raised against *E.coli*-derived recombinant HuIFN-β (18). (2) The antiviral activity of IL-1 is preferentially seen in cells that are known to be sensitive to induction of IFN-β by classical IFN-β-inducers, such as double-stranded RNA and that are exquisitely sensitive to the antiviral effect of IFN-β (18). (3) If such cells are treated with IL-1 in association with the metabolic inhibitors actinomycin D and cycloheximide, amounts of HuIFN-β are produced that are consistently higher than in control cultures receiving only the inhibitors (21). (4) The amounts of IFN-β-specific mRNA in (IL-1 + cycloheximide)-treated cultures is significantly higher than that in cultures treated with cycloheximide only (21).

Obviously, the amounts of IFN-β induced by IL-1 are minute, and although it may be argued that in the microenvironment of the cells, they may be sufficient to explain the antiviral effect, one may ask the question whether other induced molecules may be involved. Especially relevant to this criticism is the observation that IL-1 is able, without the help of metabolic inhibitors, to induce increased levels of the mRNA for a protein called "26K" (5). According to some investigators the gene product of this mRNA has interferon-like antiviral activity (17,22). More so, although the amino-acid sequence has no homology with that of IFN-β, the antiviral activity has been found to be blocked by highly specific antisera against IFN-β, reason why 26K has been called IFN-β_2. Until these controversies are resolved, the question of the role of 26K in the antiviral effect of IL-1 should be held in abeyance.

Biological Significance

Production of IL-1 occurs in the body as part of the host response to various acute, infectious or traumatic events. There is, however, evidence that IL-1 is also produced in chronic disease states characterized by persistent or intermittent inflammation. What could be the role of IFN-β induced by this IL-1 ? Aside from their direct antiviral effect, interferons can exert many other actions : inhibition of cell growth, enhancement of cytotoxic lymphocytes, inhibition of local inflammatory responses, ... Each of these actions could be invoked as a basis for rationalizing on the "usefulness" of IL-1's ability to induce IFN-β. One could speculate that production of IL-1 simply provides the organism with an increased base level of resistance to virus infection. One could also hypothesize that the IFN-β acts to some extent as a negative feed-back on the growth promoting activity of IL-1 on fibroblasts, or as a feed-back mechanism controlling inflammation, etc...

Sofar there is no evidence to support any of these speculations.

ANTIVIRAL EFFECT OF TUMOR NECROSIS FACTOR

Tumor necrosis factor (TNF) is a monokine produced by mononuclear phagocytes under rather similar circumstances as IL-1. This factor is defined by its ability to cause cell death in certain tumor cell lines. Recently it has become increasingly clear that IL-1 has TNF-activity on certain cells (10,12). TNF, on the other hand, possesses nearly all of the biological activities that are characteristic for IL-1 (7,16). We have found that recombinant DNA-derived human TNF has antiviral activity on fibroblasts which is similar to that of IL-1(β) in that it can also be blocked by specific antisera against HuIFN-β (see Table 1). It is therefore likely that this activity of TNF is also due to induction of HuIFN-β in fibroblasts.

REFERENCES

1. Auron, PE, AC Webb, LJ Rosenwaser, SF Mucci, A Rich, SM Wolff, and CA Dinarello: Nucleotide sequence of human monocyte interleukin 1 precursor cDNA. Proc Nat Acad Sci USA 81:7907, 1984.
2. Billiau A, G Opdenakker, J Van Damme, M De Ley, G Volckaert, and J Van Beeumen: Interleukin 1: amino acid sequencing reveals microheterogeneity and relationship with an interferon-inducing monokine. Immunol Today 6:235, 1985.
3. Billiau A, J Van Damme, G Opdenakker, WE Fibbe, JHF Falkenburg, and J Content: Interleukin-1 as a cytokine inducer. Immunobiol, in press, 1986.
4. Cameron P, G Limjuco, J Rodkey, C Bennett, and JA Schmidt: Amino acid sequence analysis of human interleukin 1 (IL-1). Evidence for biochemically distinct forms of IL-1. J Exp Med 162:790, 1985.
5. Content J, L De Wit, P Poupart, G Opdenakker, J Van Damme, and A Billiau: Induction of a 26 kDa protein mRNA in human cells treated with an interleukin-1-related, leukocyte-derived factor. Eur J Biochem 152:253, 1985.
6. Dinarello CA: An update on human interleukin-1 : from molecular biology to clinical relevance. J Clin Immunol 5:287, 1985.
7. Dinarello CA, JG Cannon, SM Wolff, HA Bernheim, B Beutler, A Cerami, IS Figari, MA Palladiono Jr, and JV O'Connor: Tumor necrosis factor (Cachectin) is an endogenous pyrogen and induces production of interleukin 1. J Exp Med 163:1433, 1986.
8. Fibbe WE, J Van Damme, A Billiau, PJ Voogt, N Duinkerken, PMC Kluck, and JHF Falkenburg: Interleukin-1 (22K factor) induces release of granulocyte-macrophage colony stimulating activity from human mononuclear phagocytes. Blood, submitted, 1986.
9. Furutani Y, M Notake, M Yamayoshi, JI Yamagishi, H Nomura, M Ohue, R Furuta, T Fukui, M Yamada, and S Nakamura: Cloning and characterization of the cDNAs for human and rabbit interleukin-1 precursor. Nucleic Acids Res 13:5869, 1985.

10. Lachman LB, CA Dinarello, MD Llansa, and IJ Fidler: Natural and recombinant human interleukin 1-β is cytotoxic for human melanoma cells. J Immunol 136:3098, 1986.
11. Lomedico PT, U Gubler, CP Hellmann, M Dukovich, JG Giri, YCE Pan, K Collier, R Seminonow, AO Chua, and SB Mizel: Cloning and expression of murine interleukin-1 cDNA in Escherichia coli. Nature 312:458, 1984.
12. Lovett D, B Kozan, M Hadam, K. Resch, and D Gemsa: Macrophage cytotoxicity: interleukin-1 as a mediator of tumor cytostatis. J Immunol 136:340, 1986.
13. March CJ, B Mosley, A Larsen, DP Cerretti, G Braedt, V Price, S Gillis, CS Henney, SR Kronheim, K Grabstein, PJ Conlon, TP Hopp, and D Cosman: Cloning, sequence and expression of two distinct human interleukin-1 complementary DNAs. Nature 315:641, 1985.
14. Matsushima, K, TD Copeland, K Onozaki, and JJ Oppenheim: Purification and biochemical characteristics of two distinct human interleukin-1 from the myelomonocytic THP-1 cell line. Biochemistry, in press, 1986.
15. Oppenheim JJ, EJ Kovacs, K Matsushima, and SK. Durum: There is more than one interleukin-1. Immunol Today 7:45, 1986
16. Pober JS, MP Bevilacqua, DL Mendrick, LA Lapierre, W Fiers, and MA Gimbrone Jr: Two distinct monokines, interleukin 1 and tumor necrosis factor, each independently induce biosynthesis and transient expression of the same antigen on the surface of cultured human vascular endothelial cells. J Immunol 136:1680, 1986.
17. Revel M, R Ruggieri, and A Zilberstein: Expression of HuIFN-β_2 genes in rodent cells. In: The Biology of the Interferon System 1985, H. Schellekens, and W.E. Stewart II, eds. Elsevier, pp. 207-216, 1986.
18. Van Damme J, A Billiau, M De Ley, and P De Somer: An interferon-β-like or interferon-inducing protein released by mitogen-stimulated human leukocytes. J Gen Virol 64:1819, 1983.
19. Van Damme J, M De Ley, H Claeys, A Billiau, C Vermylen, and P De Somer: Interferon induced in human leukocytes by concanavalin A: isolation and characterization of γ- and β-type components. Eur J Immunol 11:937, 1981.
20. Van Damme J, M De Ley, G Opdenakker, A Billiau, P De Somer, and J Van Beeumen: Homogeneous interferon-inducing 22K factor is related to endogenous pyrogen and interleukin-1. Nature 314:266, 1985.
21. Van Damme J, G Opdenakker, A Billiau, P De Somer, L De Wit, P Poupart, and J Content: Stimulation of fibroblast interferon production by a 22K protein from human leukocytes. J Gen Virol 66:693, 1985.
22. Weissenbach J, Y Chernajovsky, M Zeevi, L Shulman, H Soreq, U Nir, D Wallach, M Perricandet, P Tiollais, and M Revel: Two interferon mRNAs in human fibroblasts: in vitro translation and Escherichia coli cloning studies. Proc Natl Acad Sci USA 77:7152, 1980.

Table 1. Antiviral Activity of Natural and Recombinant IL-1, and of Recombinant TNF

Cytokine preparation	Antiviral activity ($\log_{10}$ AVU/ml)[a] in the presence of :		
	no antibody	anti-IL-1β	anti-HuIFN-β
Natural IL-1β (22K factor)[b]	4.00	<1.00 (<0.1%)	<1.00 (<0.1%)
Natural IL-α[c]	4.35	4.20 (71%)	<2.50 (<1.4%)
Natural IL-1β[c]	5.35	2.60 (0.2%)	<2.50 (<0.1%)
Recombinant IL-1α[d] (pI5)	4.55	4.70 (140%)	<2.50 (<0.9%)
Recombinant IL-1β[e] (pI7)	4.80	3.25 (2.8%)	<2.50 (<0.5%)
Recombinant TNF-α[f]	4.00	3.50 (30%)	<0.50 (<0.03%)

[a] Average (n = 2) antiviral activity against VSV on MG-63 cells.

[b] Derived from human buffy coat cells induced with ConA, purified to electrophoretic homogeneity (20).

[c] Courtesy of Dr. K. Matsushima, Laboratory of Molecular Immunoregulation, NCI, Frederick, MD. The material was prepared as described in ref. 14.

[d] Courtesy of Dr. C. Dinarello, Tufts University School of Medicine, Boston, MA, U.S.A.; origin of product: Genzyme Inc., Boston, MA.

[e] Courtesy of Dr. C. Dinarello.

[f] Courtesy of Dr. C. Dinarello; origin of product: Genentech Inc., South Francisco, Cal. (see ref. 7).

20. Interactions of Interferon-Gamma with Other Lymphokines/Cytokines

Jan Vilček,[a] Rena Feinman,[a] Vito J. Palombella,[a] Hanna C. Kelker,[a] Masafumi Tsujimoto,[b] and Junming Le[a]

[a]Department of Microbiology and Kaplan Cancer Center, New York University Medical Center, New York, NY 10016; [b]Suntory Institute for Biomedical Research, Osaka 618, Japan

INTRODUCTION

The aim of this brief review article is to highlight some of the recognized interactions of interferon (IFN)-gamma with other lymphokines/cytokines. Two types of interactions will be discussed. First we shall evaluate the modulation of IFN-gamma production by two other cytokines, i.e., interleukin-1 (IL-1) and IL-2. In the second part we shall review information on how IFN-gamma and other cytokines can mutually affect each others' activities. Discussion of other cytokines will be limited to tumor necrosis factor (TNF) and lymphotoxin (LT).

The advent of recombinant DNA technology has made available purified, homogeneous preparations of an ever increasing number of cytokines. In addition to recombinant IFNs, already available for experimentation for several years, it is now possible to obtain *E. coli*-derived preparations of IL-1-alpha, IL-1-beta, IL-2, TNF and LT. Availability of these reagents has greatly advanced our understanding of the mechanisms and diversities of their actions. However, it should be remembered that in the intact organism these cytokines rarely, if ever, act separately from one another. Typically, two or more cytokines may be induced coordinately in the same microenvironment. In addition, induction of one cytokine may turn on the synthesis of another one in what has been termed the "lymphokine cascade" or "cytokine network". For this reason, the effort to understand the interactions of cytokines that can be formed in the same microenvironment is not a purely academic pursuit.

ROLE OF IL-1 AND IL-2 IN THE CONTROL OF IFN-GAMMA SYNTHESIS

The proliferative response of T lymphocytes upon their exposure to antigens or nonspecific mitogens requires the generation of IL-2 and the induction of T cell responsiveness to IL-2 controlled by the expression of an inducible IL-2 receptor. Both events require the presence of accessory cells. Accessory cells, in turn, provide two major functions. As is well known, accessory cells are needed for the HLA-restricted presentation of antigen and -- more to the point in the present context -- they are the source of IL-1.

The fact that monocytes are required for the production of IFN-gamma by T cells was demonstrated many years ago in the pioneering studies of Epstein et al. (1). In promoting IFN-gamma production both major functions of the accessory cells, i.e, antigen presentation and the generation of IL-1, can play a role. Recent studies have shown that IL-1 exerts at least two major actions in T cells: it promotes the generation of IL-2 by helper T cells (the original function associated with "lymphocyte activation factor", as IL-1 used to be called) and it induces IL-2 receptor (Tac antigen) expression on helper and suppressor T cells (2-4). Thus, although IL-1 is required for IFN-gamma production, it is possible that it promotes IFN-gamma production indirectly via its ability to induce IL-2 production and IL-2 responsiveness (4). It is interesting that a reciprocal stimulation of IL-2 production by IFN-gamma has also been demonstrated (5).

The role of IL-2 in the control of IFN-gamma production was probably first recognized by Farrar et al. (6) and more rigorously defined by Torres et al. (7). Availability of recombinant IL-2 made it possible to demonstrate unequivocally that the addition of IL-2 to cultures of mononuclear cells, in the absence of antigen or mitogen, led to an induction of IFN-gamma production (8,9). Interestingly, IL-2 failed to induce IFN-gamma in cultures of highly purified T cells, but did so readily in the presence of monocytes (4,9). IL-1 alone also failed to stimulate IFN-gamma release from purified T cells. In contrast, IL-1 and IL-2 added together to cultures of isolated T cells, in the absence of any other stimulus, induced IFN-gamma yields similar to those seen in mixed cultures of T cells and monocytes stimulated with IL-2 (4).

These results indicated that the presence of IL-1 and IL-2 is sufficient to turn on IFN-gamma synthesis in isolated T cells, but are these two mediators required for antigen- or mitogen-induced IFN-gamma synthesis under physiological conditions? Available evidence suggests strongly that IL-2 is an important regulator of IFN-gamma synthesis in cells stimulated with antigen or mitogen. Whether all IFN-gamma synthesis by antigen- or mitogen-stimulated T cells is completely dependent on the generation of IL-2 and whether IL-2 serves as the actual inducing stimulus for IFN-gamma is less certain.

A comparison of the kinetics of IFN-gamma and IL-2 mRNA synthesis in mitogen-stimulated cells showed that the two mRNAs appear at the same time (10). If IL-2 were required for IFN-gamma induction, it would be expected that the appearance of IL-2 should precede the generation of IFN-gamma. On the other hand, treatment with monoclonal antibody to the human IL-2 receptor (anti-Tac) inhibited IFN-gamma production in mitogen- or antigen-activated cultures (4,9,11). Since gamma-irradiation of the cells before mitogenic stimulation did not affect the inhibitory action of anti-Tac (9), it is clear that the effects of IL-2 and anti-Tac on IFN-gamma production are separate from their effects on cell proliferation. However, the inhibitory effect of anti-Tac was not complete, raising the possibility that at least a portion of the IFN-gamma yield was produced independently from the generation of IL-2. We found that when anti-Tac was added to PHA-stimulated mononuclear cells, IFN-gamma produced within the first 4 to 6 hours after the addition of PHA was inhibited much less strongly than the IFN-gamma yield produced by 24 or 48 hours after stimulation (unpublished data). This result suggested that the initial burst of IFN-gamma production may be IL-2-independent, while generation of the bulk of IFN-gamma requires amplification by endogenously produced IL-2. A similar conclusion was reached by Grabstein et al. (12).

COOPERATIVE ACTIONS BETWEEN IFN-GAMMA AND TUMOR NECROSIS FACTOR

IFN-gamma and TNF in Tumor Cell Cytotoxicity

TNF is a monocyte/macrophage produced protein, originally detected in the serum of animals injected with endotoxin (13). TNF is functionally and structurally related to lymphocyte-derived LT. Both TNF and LT show cytolytic or cytostatic activities on some tumor cells in culture and cause hemorrhagic necrosis of some tumors in experimental animals. Recently, TNF was shown to be identical with a protein termed cachectin, defined as a hormone inhibiting lipoprotein lipase activity and synthesis (14). Other recently identified biological activities of TNF include activation of polymorphonuclear leukocytes and a mitogenic activity in normal fibroblasts. These and other recent findings indicate that TNF is a cytokine with a broad repertoire of biological activities in addition to the cytolytic/cytostatic activity on tumor cells (reviewed in ref. 13,14).

TNF and the structurally related LT interact with IFNs at several levels. LT is known to be a product of activated lymphocytes, synthesized in response to specific antigens or mitogens. Conditions eliciting LT production are very similar to conditions leading to IFN-gamma synthesis (15). TNF is known to be mainly a product of monocytes/macrophages (13-15). Both TNF and LT are often produced in cultures of mononuclear leukocytes along with IFN-gamma (16). It has also been shown that IFNs can promote the production of TNF and LT (17,18). Several groups showed that IFN (in particular IFN-gamma) can markedly enhance the susceptibility of tumor cells to the cytotoxic action of LT or TNF (16,19). In an attempt to explain the synergism between IFN-gamma and TNF we (20) and others (21,22) have examined the effect of various IFNs on TNF binding to cell surface receptors. Incubation of several different cell lines with IFN-gamma caused a significant increase ($\sim$30-100%) in TNF binding (20). This increase was less marked and less regularly seen with IFN-alpha or IFN-beta. Increased binding of TNF in cells incubated with IFN-gamma was shown to be due to an increased expression of TNF receptors without a demonstrable change in the binding affinity. We have also shown that IFN-gamma caused a stimulation in the synthesis of the TNF receptor protein, probably resulting from a direct stimulation of transcription (23).

These studies suggested that in some cell lines there may be a causal relationship between the stimulation of TNF receptor synthesis and the synergistic enhancement of TNF cytotoxicity by IFN-gamma. For instance, IFN gamma and TNF were markedly synergistic in the HT-29 cell line, while IFN-alpha and IFN-beta showed only a slight enhancing effect on TNF cytotoxicity. At the same time, IFN-gamma was shown to cause a significant enhancement of TNF receptor expression in the HT-29 cell line, while IFN-alpha and -beta did not (20). On the other hand, no such correlation between increased TNF receptor expression and sensitivity to TNF action was found in other cell lines. In several tumor cell lines that are resistant to TNF action IFN-gamma caused an increase in TNF binding without a concomitant increase in the sensitivity to TNF cytotoxicity. In the A673 human rhabdomyosarcoma line, highly sensitive to the cytotoxic action of TNF, treatment with IFN-gamma increased TNF binding, but failed to produce a substantial increase in the sensitivity to TNF action over a wide range of TNF concentrations. Finally, in the FS-4 line of human fibroblasts, in which TNF is growth-stimulatory, IFN-gamma also increased TNF binding but at the same time exerted an inhibitory effect on the TNF-mediated mitogenic effect (24,25).

On balance, it is likely that increased TNF receptor expression after incubation of cells with IFNs is not a major mechanism of synergism between IFNs and TNF (26). The magnitude of the modulatory effects of IFNs on the level of TNF receptor expression may be too small to appreciably alter the biological response to TNF. Synergism between TNF and IFNs is probably due to the activation of separate inhibitory pathways whose combined cytotoxic actions are greater than the sum of their separate actions. Although the precise mechanism of the synergistic cytotoxic activities of IFNs and TNF on tumor cells has not been explained, attempts are being made to exploit this phenomenon in experimental cancer therapy.

Implications for Monocyte Cytotoxicity

Lysis of tumor cells by monocytes/macrophages is believed to represent one of the major mechanisms of host defense against tumors. It was shown that IFN-gamma is a potent activator of monocyte/macrophage cytotoxicity for tumor cells and that IFN-gamma is in fact the long-sought T cell product termed "macrophage-activating factor" (27,28). TNF has been considered as a possible mediator of tumor cells lysis by monocytes because (a) TNF is known to be both a monocyte product and a protein cytotoxic for some tumor cells, and (b) some agents that induce an increase in monocyte cytotoxicity (e.g., lipopolysaccharide or IFN-gamma) are also known to stimulate TNF production (13,17,18). In recent studies we obtained more direct evidence for the role of TNF as a mediator of monocyte cytotoxicity for tumor cells. First we found that the A673 human rhabdomyosarcoma cell line was unusually sensitive to the "spontaneous" cytotoxicity of human peripheral blood monocytes (29). In subsequent experiments, we showed that A673 cells also were the most sensitive to the cytotoxic action of recombinant human TNF among 10 different randomly selected human tumor cell lines (unpublished data). Along similar lines, we and others demonstrated that the sensitivity of HT-29 cells to purified TNF could be increased by their incubation with IFN-gamma (24,30), and separate experiments showed that incubation of HT-29 cells with IFN-gamma also produced a marked increase in their susceptibility to monocyte cytotoxicity (29).

In our effort to examine the function of TNF as a mediator of monocyte cytotoxicity more directly we employed two main experimental approaches (31). One, we examined the effect of a specific monoclonal antibody against TNF on monocyte-mediated cytotoxicity. Two, we developed clones of A673 cells differing in their susceptibility to the cytotoxic action of recombinant TNF and we then compared the relative sensitivities of these cloned lines to monocyte lysis. Both experimental approaches have indicated that TNF is indeed a major mediator of monocyte cytotoxicity for tumor cells.

Further support for the role of TNF in monocyte killing came from experiments employing the HT-29 cell line. Although HT-29 cells were relatively resistant to monocyte cytotoxicity as well as to the cytotoxic action of TNF, their resistance in both types of assays could be overcome by IFN-gamma (24,29,30). Increased sensitivity of HT-29 cells to monocyte cytotoxicity induced by IFN-gamma was likely due to their sensitization to the lytic action of TNF because the enhanced monocyte lysis was inhibited in the presence of neutralizing MAb to TNF (31).

In summary, IFN-gamma affects TNF-mediated monocyte cytotoxicity for tumor cells at two different levels: (a) it can enhance TNF production, and (b) it can sensitize target cells to the lytic action of monocyte-derived TNF. Both of these actions are likely to be important in the host defense against malignancies.

Other Cooperative Actions Between IFN-Gamma and TNF

Murphy et al. (32) showed that activated T cells produce factors inhibiting colony formation with granulocyte/macrophage (GM) precursor cells from human bone marrow. Physicochemical analysis revealed that inhibition was due to the combined action of IFN-gamma and LT present in the conditioned medium. Neither IFN-gamma nor LT alone were inhibitory, but a mixture of the two lymphokines inhibited colony formation by up to 70%. The authors suggested that the simultaneous production of INF-gamma and LT may represent a mechanism of suppression of hematopoiesis by activated T cells in some cases of bone marrow failure. Broxmeyer et al. (33) observed a similar synergism between TNF or LT and IFN-gamma on colony formation with various hematopoietic precursor cells.

TNF or LT may also synergize with IFN-gamma in promoting differentiation of myelomonocytic precursor cells along the monocytic pathway (34, G. Trinchieri, personal communication). Another event promoted by TNF or LT and IFN-gamma in which cooperativity may be seen is the activation of neutrophils (35-37). It is apparent that the synergism of IFN-gamma with LT and TNF is not restricted to events involving cytolysis.

ACKNOWLEDGEMENTS

We thank Dr. T. Noguchi for many helpful discussions and continuous support, and Cristy Minton for preparation of the manuscript. Work from the authors' laboratory was supported by NIH grants AI-07057, AI-12948 and by a grant from Suntory Limited.

REFERENCES

1. Epstein, L.B., M.J. Cline, and T.C. Merigan: PPD-stimulated inteferon: in vitro macrophage-lymphocyte interaction in the production of a mediator of cellular immunity. Cell Immunol 2:602, 1971.
2. Smith, K.A., L.B. Lachmann, J.J. Oppenheim, and M.F. Favata: The functional relationship of the interleukins. J Exp Med 151:1551, 1980.
3. Kaye, J., S. Gillis, S.B. Mizel, E.M. Shevach, T.R. Malek, C.A. Dinarello, L.B. Lachman, and C.A. Janeway: Growth of a cloned helper T cell line induced by a monoclonal antibody specific for the antigen receptor: Interleukin 1 is required for the expression of receptor for interleukin 2. J Immunol 133:1339, 1984.
4. Le, J., J.-X Lin, D. Henriksen-DeStefano, and J. Vilček: Bacterial lipopolysaccharide-induced interferon-gamma production: roles of interleukin 1 and interleukin 2. J Immunol 136:4525, 1986.
5. Boraschi, D., S. Censini, and A. Tagliabue: Interferon-gamma reduces macrophage-suppressive activity by inhibiting prostaglandin E_2 release and inducing interleukin 1 production. J Immunol 133:764, 1984.
6. Farrar, W.L., H.M. Johnson, and J.J. Farrar: Regulation of the production of immune interferon and cytotoxic T lymphocytes by interleukin 2. J Immunol 126:1120, 1981.
7. Torres, B.A., W.L. Farrar, and H.M. Johnson: Interleukin 2 regulates immune interferon (IFN-gamma) production by normal and suppressor cell cultures. J Immunol 128:2217, 1982.
8. Kasahara, T., J.J. Hooks, S.F. Dougherty, and J.J. Oppenheim: Interleukin 2-mediated immune interferon (IFN-gamma) production by human T cells and T cell subsets. J Immunol 130:1784, 1983.

9. Vilček, J., D. Henriksen-DeStefano, D. Siegel, A. Klion, R.J. Robb, and J. Le: Regulation of IFN-gamma induction in human peripheral blood cells by exogenous and endogenously produced interleukin 2. J Immunol 135:1851, 1985.
10. Efrat, S., S. Pilo, and R. Kaempfer: Kinetics of induction and molecular size of mRNAs encoding human interleukin-2 and gamma interferon. Nature 297:236, 1982.
11. Reem, G.H. and N.-H. Yeh: Interleukin 2 regulates expression of its receptor and synthesis of gamma interferon by human T lymphocytes. Science 225:429, 1984.
12. Grabstein, K., S. Dower, S. Gillis, D. Urdal, and A. Larsen: Expression of interleukin 2, interferon-gamma, and the IL2 receptor by human peripheral blood lymphocytes. J Immunol 136:4503, 1986.
13. Old, L.J.: Tumor necrosis factor (TNF). Science 230:630, 1985.
14. Beutler, B., and A. Cerami: Cachectin and tumour necrosis factor as two sides of the same biological coin. Nature 320:584, 1986.
15. Kelker, H.C., J.D. Oppenheim, D.S. Stone-Wolff, D. Henriksen-DeStefano, B.B. Aggarwal, H.C. Stevenson, and J. Vilček: Characterization of human tumor necrosis factor produced by peripheral blood monocytes and its separation from lymphotoxin. Int J Cancer 36:69, 1985.
16. Stone-Wolff, D.S., Y.K. Yip, H.C. Kelker, J. Le, D. Henriksen-DeStefano, B. Rubin, E. Rinderknecht, B.B. Aggarwal, and J. Vilček: Interrelationships of human interferon-gamma with lymphotoxin and monocyte cytotoxin. J Exp Med 159:828, 1984.
17. Wallach, D., D. Aderka, S. Budilovsky, and T. Hahn: Inteferon enhances the production of lymphotoxins and potentials their cytotoxic effet. In: The Biology of the Interferon System, E. DeMaeyer, and H. Schellekens, eds. Elsevier, Amsterdam, pp. 293-303, 1983.
18.Nedwin, G.E., L.P. Svedersky, T.S. Bringman, M.A. Palladino Jr., and D.V. Goeddel: Effect of interleukin 2, interferon-gamma and mitogens on the production of tumor necrosis factors alpha and beta. J Immunol 135:2492, 1985.
19. Williamson, B.D., E.A. Carswell, B.Y. Rubin, J.S. Prendergast, and L.J. Old: Human tumor necrosis factor produced by human B cell lines: Synergistic cytotoxic interaction with human interferon. Proc Natl Acad Sci 80:5397, 1983.
20. Tsujimoto, M., Y.K. Yip, and J. Vilček: IFN-gamma enhances expression of cellular receptors for tumor necrosis factor. J Immunol 136:2441, 1986.
21. Ruggiero, V., J. Tavernier, W. Fiers, and C. Baglioni: Induction of the synthesis of tumor necrosis factor receptors by interferon-gamma. J Immunol 136:2445, 1986.
22. Aggarwal, B.B., T.E. Essalu, and P.E. Hass: Characterization of receptors for human tumour necrosis factor and their regulation by gamma-interferon. Nature 318:665, 1985.
23. Tsujimoto, M., and J. Vilček: Tumor necrosis factor receptors in HeLa cells and their regulation by interferon-gamma. J Biol Chem 261:5384, 1986.
24. Vilček, J., D. Henriksen-DeStefano, V.J. Palombella, and M. Tsujimoto: Interactions between tumor necrosis factor and interferons. In: The Biology of the Interferon System 1985, W.E. Stewart and H. Schellekens, eds. Elsevier, pp. 249-256, 1986.
25. Vilček, J., Palombella, V.J., D. Henriksen-DeStefano, C. Swenson, R. Feinman, M. Hirai, and M. Tsujimoto: Fibroblast growth-enhancing activity of tumor necrosis factor and its relationship to other polypeptide growth factors. J Exp Med 163:632, 1986.
26. Tsujimoto, M., R. Feinman, and J. Vilček: Differential effects of type I IFN and IFN-gamma on the binding of tumor necrosis factor to receptors in two human cell lines. J Immunol 137, in press.
27. Roberts, W.K., and A. Vasil: Evidence for the identity of murine gamma interferon and macrophage activating factor. J Interferon Res 2:519, 1982.

28. Le, J., W. Prensky, Y.K. Yip, Z. Chang, T. Hoffman, H.C. Stevenson, I. Balazs, J.R. Sadlik, and J. Vilček: Activation of human monocyte cytotoxicity by natural and recombinant immune interferon. J Immunol 131:2821, 1983.
29. Feinman, R., D.S. Siegel, J. Le, and J. Vilček: Interferon-gamma enhances target cell sensitivity to monocyte killing. Cell Immunol 99:287, 1986.
30. Fransen, L., J. Van Der Heyden, R. Ruysschaert, and W. Fiers: Recombinant tumor necrosis factor: its effect and its synergism with interferon-gamma on a variety of normal and transformed human cell lines. Eur J Cancer Clin Oncol 22:419, 1986.
31. Feinman, R., D. Henriksen-DeStefano, M. Tsujimoto, and J. Vilček: Tumor necrosis factor is an important mediator of tumor cell killing by human monocytes. Submitted for publication.
32. Murphy,M., R. Loudon, M. Kobayashi, and G. Trinchieri: Gamma interferon and lymphotoxin, released by activated T cells, synergize to inhibit granulocyte/monocyte colony formation. J Exp Med 164:263, 1986.
33. Broxmeyer, H.E., D.E. Williams, L. Lu, S. Cooper, S.L. Anderson, G.S. Beyer, R. Hoffman, B.Y. Rubin: The suppressive influences of human tumor necrosis factors on bone marrow hematopoietic progenitor cells from normal donors and patients with leukemia: synergism of tumor necrosis factor and interferon-gamma. J Immunol 136:4487, 1986.
34. Perussia, B., E.T. Dayton, V. Fanning, P. Thiagarajan, J. Hoxie, and G. Trinchieri: Immune interferon and leukocyte-conditioned medium induce normal and leukemic myeloid cells to differentiate along the monocytic pathway. J Exp Med 158:2058, 1983.
35. Shalaby, M.R., B.B. Aggarwal, E. Rinderknecht, L.P. Svedersky, B.S. Finkle, and M.A. Palladino: Activation of human polymorphonuclear neutrophil functions by interferon-gamma and tumor necrosis factor. J Immunol 135:2069, 1985.
36. Klebanoff, S.J., J. Vadas, M. Harlam, L.H. Sparks, J.R. Gamble, J.M. Agosti, and M. Walterdorph: Stimulation of neutrophils by tumor necrosis factor. J Immunol 136:4220, 1986.
37. Tsujimoto, M., S. Yokota, J. Vilček, and G. Weissman: Tumor necrosis factor provokes superoxide anion generation from neutrophils. Bioch Bioph Res Comm Biochem Biophys Res Commun 137:1094, 1986.

21. Inhibition of Cell Growth by Interferon: An Analysis Using Quiescent Fibroblasts Stimulated by Growth Factors

D. Leavesley, J. Taylor-Papadimitriou, and E. Rozengurt

Imperial Cancer Research Fund, P.O. Box 123, Lincoln's Inn Fields, London WC2A 3PX, England

INTRODUCTION

In addition to their well described activity as antiviral agents interferons (IFN's) are known to inhibit the mitogenic effect of growth factors. The mechanisms underlying the interferon-induced inbition of cell growth are however poorly understood. Moreover, while it is clearly established in vitro that IFN can act as a growth regulating agent which inhibits growth factor-stimulated cell proliferation the role of IFN as a regulator of cell growth in vivo is not at all clear.

Quiescent fibroblasts arrested in the G_1/G_0 phase of the cell cycle can be stimulated to proliferate by the addition of serum or growth factors which act in a synergistic manner (1,2) and interferons added simultaneously with the mitogens can inhibit the stimulation of DNA synthesis and cell division (3). Quiescent mouse and human fibroblasts therefore provide a unique system for the investigation of interferon induced inhibition of cell growth because after addition of mitogens, the cells move synchronously into the cell cycle, thus allowing a kinetic analysis of molecular events. In this paper we will briefly examine the data relating to the effects of IFN on i) the early regulatory signals induced by mitogens in 3T3 cells, and ii) the later nuclear and late G1 events preceding DNA synthesis. A consideration of the data has allowed us to draw some conclusions regarding the kinetics of IFN action as an inhibitor of the mitogenic response in 3T3 cells and to demonstrate that this effect is dissociable from the antiviral action of IFN.

1. Early Signals in Mitogenesis

The first step in the interaction of polypeptide growth factors and IFN is with specific cell surface receptors. The binding to high affinity receptors by both agents is known to alter the membrane in several ways (1,4) and it is therefore possible that binding of IFN to its receptor could alter growth factor receptor binding and in this way inhibit mitogenesis. However, a direct inhibition of the binding of growth factors to their receptor by IFN has not been observed (5) and long term effects on the level of receptor expression have not been examined.

Binding of growth factors to receptors triggers cellular events within seconds and minutes which include changes in ion fluxes, in levels of cAMP, and in the activity of protein kinase C. These events have recently been discussed in detail (2) and are summerized in figure 1.

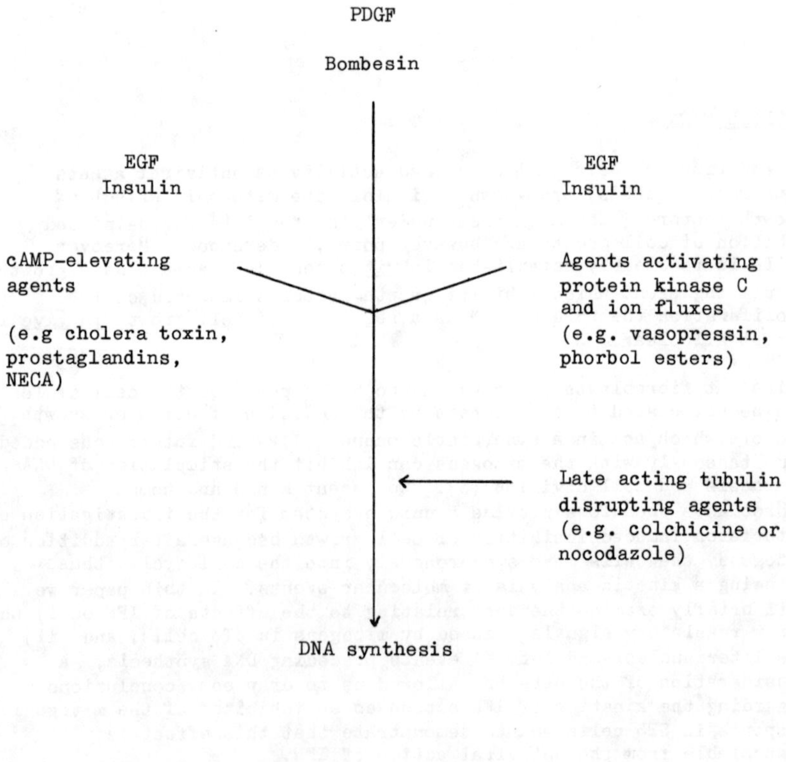

Figure 1. Early signals generated by growth factors; synergistic action of cyclic AMP-elevating agents, and agents affecting protein kinase C. EGF and insulin can synergize with agents shown on either the left or right side and with each other. Tubulin disrupting agents can enhance the DNA synthesis stimulated by any combination of growth factors, and are still effective added several hours after the other mitogens.

Several important points should be noted from this integrated signal framework. While most growth active hormones and peptides are mitogenic only when in the presence of other growth factors, PDGF, PDGF-like growth factors (e.g. FDGF) and bombesin are mitogenic alone (2,6). Agents which synergize are capable of intiating only some of these early signals and in some cases it can be shown that agents which synergize initiate complementary signals (e.g. a cAMP elevating agent and vasopressin). PDGF and Bombesin are able to induce both arms of the signal network, which appear necessary for the mitogenic stimulation of DNA synthesis.

We have examined the effect of IFN on some of the early mitogenic signals. We find that activation of the sodium potassium pump is not inhibited (3) and neither is the increase in intracellular levels of cyclic AMP (7), nor the activation of protein kinase C by phorbol esters (Rodriguez-Pena and Rozengurt, pers. commun). It has also been found that PDGF-induced Ca^{2+} mobilization in 3T3 cells is not affected by IFN treatment (Williams, B. pers. commun.). It would therefore appear that the IFN induced inhibition of mitogenesis is not mediated by an effect on the early mitogenic signals.

2. Events in Early G1

Soon after the early signals the induction of expression of certain genes is observed. The proto-oncogenes c-*fos* and c-*myc* are transiently induced within 15 minutes and 60 minutes respectively (8-10). Messenger RNA coding for β actin and ornithine decarboxylase (ODC) are also induced with similar kinetics to c-*myc* and are maximal after about 3 hours (11). Other genes identified only by the increases in the corresponding mRNA have also been studied, but their function remains unknown (12,13).

Results from several studies on the influence IFN has on these early G1 events are, with one or two exceptions, consistant. The increase in ODC induced by mitogens was shown some time ago to be strongly inhibited by IFN treatment (14) probably at the transcriptional level (15). Recently inhibition of induction of ODC mRNA has been demonstrated (16) and these investigators also find that the induction of c-*fos*, c-*myc* and β actin mRNA is inhibited by simultaneous IFN treatment in 3T3 cells. Transfection of these cells with activated c-*myc* can overcome this IFN inhibition suggesting it is acting on transcription (17). Work from Tominaga and Lengyel (18) shows on the other hand that pretreatment with IFN can enhance the transcription of c-*fos* and c-*myc* in growth arrested Balb 3T3 cells stimulated by PDGF, even though under these conditions mitogenesis is inhibited. Moreover, IFN may affect the level of c-*myc* mRNA by an indirect mechanism (19). These results as well as data from Kerr et al. using an active 2-5A analog (Watling and Kerr unpublished results) and Zullo et al (20) suggest that the inhibition of expression of the proto-oncogenes c-*myc* and c-*fos* is not necessary for the inhibition of cell growth by interferon.

Occasional reports of IFN stimulation of mitogenesis (21-23) and the recent demonstration of the mitogenic activity of dsRNA (22) and antiviral activity of PDGF (24) may indicate that elements of the IFN and mitogenic pathways, at least in part, converge. From the results outlined above the early mitogenic events are not inhibited and some may in fact be enhanced. It cannot be excluded that the early mitogenic signals and those from the IFN-receptor interaction leading to the antiviral state share common elements and thus IFN does not inhibit them. The antiproliferative activity of IFN must be manifest either in a divergent pathway or in later events.

3. Events in Late G1

We recently reported the surprising observation that pre-exposure of quiescent 3T3 cells to IFN prior to stimulation with growth factors does not inhibit DNA synthesis when the IFN is removed up to 2 hours after the mitogenic stimulus (25). Such treatment however, did lead to a sustained antiviral state and markedly inhibits ODC induction. A more detailed analysis revealed that IFN needs to be present for many hours in G1 and may be added several hours after the mitogenic stimulus and still establish an effective inhibition (see fig 2). In these experiments we used both a mixture of complementary mitogens (e.g. vasopressin and insulin) and purified PDGF. From the data it may be concluded that neither the induction of the proto-oncogenes, βactin and ODC, nor the early regulatory signals, are the prime targets for IFN antigrowth activity in the 3T3 system. The corollary is that events occuring later in G1 are implicated as the targets for IFN antigrowth activity.

In the schematic framework shown in figure 1 tubulin disrupting agents act synergistically with other growth factors even when added late in G1 (26-28). The kinetics for their action mirror the kinetics of interferons' inhibitory effect on DNA synthesis i.e. they can be added late in G1 and still stimulate DNA sythesis. By inference the suggestion can be made that IFN may be acting, at least in part, via the microtubules. This idea is supported by the observations that colchicine is able to abolish the growth inhibitory effect of IFN (29,30). Elements of the cytoskeleton have previously been implicated in the antiviral and antiproliferative activity of IFN (3), and clearly their role in these actions warrants further study.

CONCLUSIONS

Analysis of the data related to IFN activity in inhibiting cell proliferation in quiescent 3T3 cells indicates that inhibition of the early signals is not involved. Moreover, the early nuclear events, and altered expression of some proto-oncogenes do not appear to be primary targets, their inhibition being neither necessary nor sufficient for proliferation inhibition. The kinetic evidence indicates that late events in G1 are a major target of IFN action. It is not unlikely that the IFN pathway and the mitogenic pathways are distinct and independant initially but converge at some event(s) late in G1 stimulated by growth factors but inhibted by IFN. Kinetic evidence suggests a possible role for the involvement of the microtubule network in this restriction event. As the antiproliferative and antiviral states are kinetically dissociable one

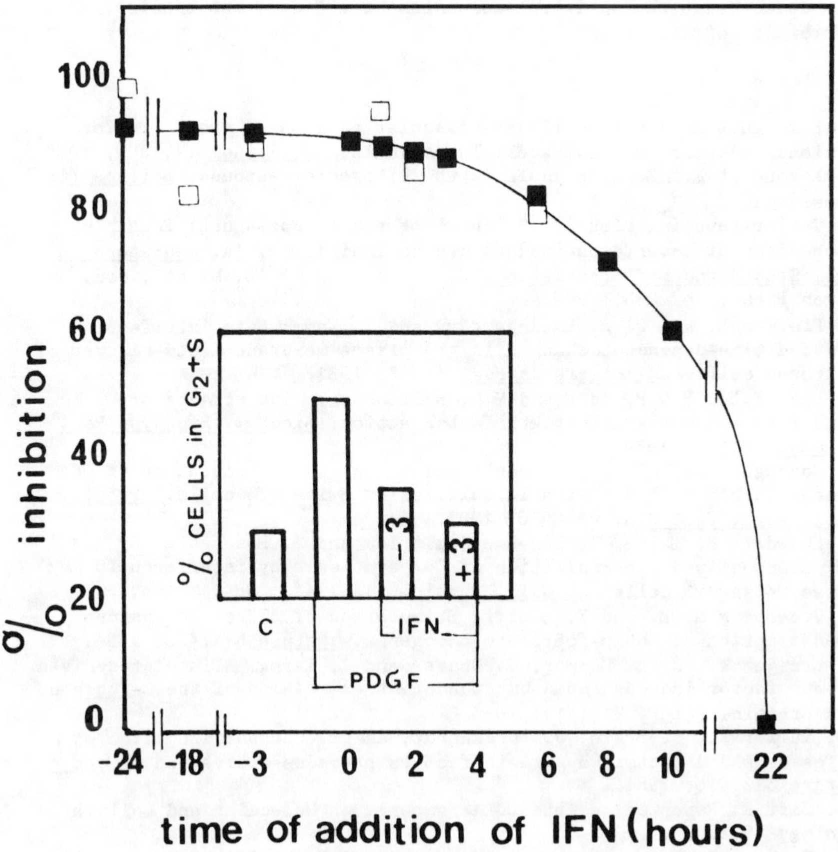

Figure 2. Time of addition of interferon and inhibition of DNA synthesis in Swiss 3T3 cells stimulated to divide by PDGF. IFN (1000 units/ml) was added at the times indicated to quiescent Swiss 3T3 cells, before and after additon of PDGF (time 0). [3H]dT was added with the PDGF (0.5 units/ml) and cells processed at 30 hours for estimation of radioactivity incorporated into TCA-precipitable material (■ average of 3 experiments) or percentage labelled cells (□). The c.p.m. or percentage of labelled cells were expressed as a percentage of the corresponding figure for cultures stimulated by PDGF in the absence of IFN to calculate the percentage inhibition of labelling. Inset: Parallel cultures stimulated with PDGF and treated with IFN 3 hours before and 3 hours after were analyzed by cytofluorometry 30 hours after addition of PDGF, and the percentage cells in $G_2 + S$ estimated. C refers to unstimulated cells.

may deduce that the antiviral mechanism of IFN does not require inhibition of this event.

REFERENCES

1. Rozengurt E. and M. Collins: Molecular aspects of growth factor action: receptors and intracellular signals. J. Pathol 141:309, 1983.
2. Rozengurt E.: Early Signals in the mitogenic response. Science (in press) 1986.
3. Taylor-Papadimitriou J., N. Ebsworth and E. Rozengurt: Possible mechanisms of interferon-induced growth inhibition. In: Mediators in Cell Growth and Differentiation, R. J. Ford and A. L. Maizel, eds. Raven Press, pp. 283, 1985.
4. Pfeffer L. M., F. R. Landsbergery and I. Tamm: Beta interferon induced time-dependant changes in the plasma membrane lipid-bilayer of cultured cells. J. Interferon Res. 1:613, 1981
5. Lin, S.L., P.O.P. Ts'o and M.D. Hollenberg: The effects of interferon on epidermal growth factor action. Biochem. Biophys. Res. Commun. 96:163, 1980.
6. Rozengurt E. and J. W. Sinnett-Smith: Bombesin stimulation of DNA synthesis and cell division in cultures of Swiss 3T3 cells. Proc. Natl. Acad. Sci. USA. 80:2936, 1983.
7. Ebsworth N. M., J. Taylor-Papadimitriou and E. Rozengurt: Cyclic AMP does not mediate inhibition of DNA synthesis by interferon in mouse Swiss 3T3 cells. J. Cell. Physiol. 120:146, 1984.
8. Greenberg M. E. and E. B.Ziff: Stimulation of 3T3 cells induces transcription of the c-fos proto-oncogenes. Nature 311:433, 1984.
9. Kruijer W., J. A. Cooper, T. Hunter and I. Verma: Platelet-derived growth factor induces rapid but transient expression of the c-fos gene and protein. Nature 312:711, 1984.
10. Muller R., R. Bravo, J. Burckhardt, and T. Curran: Induction of c-fos gene and protein by growth factors precedes activation of c-myc. Nature 312:716, 1984.
11. Ziff E: Reported to 15th UCLA Symposia on Molecular and Cellular Biology 1986.
12. Cochran B. H., J. Zullo, I. M. Verma and C. D. Stiles: Expression of the c-fos gene and of an fos-related gene is stimulated by platelet-derived growth factor. Science 226:1080, 1984.
13. Cochran B. H., A. C. Reffel and C. D. Stiles: Molecular cloning of gene sequences regulated by platelet-derived growth factor. Cell 33:939, 1983.
14. Sreevalson T., J. Taylor-Papadimitriou and E. Rozengurt: Selective Inhibition of serum-stimulated events in 3T3 cells. Biochem. Biophys. Res. Commun. 87:679, 1979.
15. Sreevalson T., E. Rozengurt, J. Taylor-Papadimitriou and J. Burchell: Differential effects of interferon on DNA Synthesis, 2-deoxyglucose uptake and ornithine decarboxylase activity in 3T3 cells stimulated by polypeptide growth factors and tumour promoters. J. Cell. Physiol. 104:1, 1980.
16. Einat M., D. Resnitzky and A. Kimchi: Inhibitory effects of interferon on the expression of genes regulated by platelet-derived growth factor. Proc. Natl. Acad. Sci. USA. 82:7608. 1985.
17. Kimchi A., M. Einat, D. Resnitzky, A. Yarden, and G. Gat: Inhibition of c-myc expression and cellular proliferation by

endogenous and exogenous interferons. J. Cell Biochem. 10C: 229, 1986.

18. Tominaga S. and P. Lengyel: βInterferon alters the pattern of proteins secreted from quiescent and platelet-derived growth factor-treated balb C 3T3 cells. J. Biol. Chem. 260:1975, 1985.

19. Dani C., N. Mechti, M. Piechaczyk, B. Lebleu, P. Jeanteur and J. M. Blanchard: Increased rate of degradation of c-myc mRNA in interferon treated Daudi cells. Proc. Natl. Acad. Sci. USA. 82:4896, 1985.

20. Zullo J. N., B. B. Cochran, A. S. Huarg and C. D. Stiles: Platelet-derived growth factor and double-stranded ribonucleic acids stimulate expression of the same genes in 3T3 cells. Cell 43:793, 1985.

21. Taylor-Papadimitriou, J. The effects of interferon on the growth and function of normal and malignant cells. Symp. Soc. Gen. Microbiol. 35:109, 1983.

22. Bradley, E. C. and F. W. Ruscett: Effect of fibroblast, lymphoid and myeloid interferons on human tumor colony formation in vitro. Cancer Res. 41:244, 1981.

23. Ludwig, C.V., B.G.M., Durie, S.E. Salmon, and T.E. Moon: Tumour-Growth stimulating in vitro by interferons. Eur. J. Cancer Clin. Oncol. 19:1625, 1983.

24. Vilcek J., M. Tsujimoto, D. Henriksen-De Stefano, V. J. Palombella, M. Hirai and M. Kohase: Growth factors as interferon inducers and interferon inducers as growth factors. J. Cell. Biochem. 10C:216, 1986.

25. Taylor-Papadimitriou J., F. Balkwill, N. Ebsworth and E. Rozengurt: Antiviral and antiproliferative effects of interferons in quiescent fibroblasts are dissociable. Virol. 147:405, 1985.

26. Wang Z.-W. and E. Rozengurt: Interplay of cAMP and microtulules in modulating the initiation of DNA synthesis in 3Y3 cells J. Cell Biol. 96:1743, 1983.

27. Ball R. C., T. Albrecht, W. C. Thompson and D. H. Carney: Microtubule involvement in initiation of cellular DNA synthesis by growth factors, tumor promoters and oncognenic DNA viruses. J. Cell Biol. 10C:110, 1986.

28. Friedkin M. and E. Rozengurt: The role of cytoplasmic microtubules in the regulation of the activity of peptide growth factors. Adv. Enzyme Regul. 19:39, 1981.

29. Bourgeade M. F. and C. Chany: Inhibition of Interferon action by cytochalasin B., colchicine and vinblastine. Proc. Soc. Exp. Biol. Med. 153:501, 1976.

30. Ebsworth N.E., Rozengurt E., and J. Taylor-Papadimitriou: Microtubule-disrupting agents reverse the inhibitory effect of interferon on mitogenesis in 3T3 cells. Exp. Cell Res. 165:255, 1986.

22. Interferon Receptors

K. C. Zoon and T. Okuno

Laboratory of Immunology, Division of Virology, Office of Biologics Research and Review, Center for Drugs and Biologics, Food and Drug Administration, Bethesda, MD 20892

Laboratory of Immunology, Division of Virology, Office of Biologics Research and Review, Center for Drugs and Biologics, Food and Drug Administration, Bethesda, Maryland 20892

INTRODUCTION

There are three classes of interferon (IFN), IFN-alpha, IFN-beta, and IFN-gamma. IFN-alpha represents a family of structurally similar polypeptides composed of 165-166 amino acid residues (1,2). Human IFN-beta consists predominantly of a single glycoprotein, IFN-beta 1 (166 amino acid residues) and is approximately 30% similar to the human IFN-alpha family (2,3). IFN-gamma is a glycoprotein, which, in humans, consists of 143 amino acid and is derived from a single gene containing three introns (4); it is structurally distinct from IFN-alphas and beta (1). While all IFNs exhibit antiviral, antiproliferative and immunoregulatory activities, IFN-alphas and beta appear to be more potent with regard to their antiviral properties, while IFN-gamma appears to have greater immunomodulatory properties (5,6).

In early studies, it was demonstrated that the binding of IFN to cells was a prerequisite for the establishment of the antiviral state (7). Recently purified radiolabeled IFN preparations have been used in receptor binding studies. These studies showed that the first step necessary to initiate the biological activities of the IFN was its interaction with a specific cell-surface receptor (8). Today, we know that there are at least two specific high-affinity types of receptors on the cell surface, one which binds IFN-alpha and -beta and the other which is specific for IFN-gamma (8-11). The binding of an IFN to its receptor has been correlated with their biological responses in a number of systems (8).

BINDING CHARACTERISTICS OF RADIOLABELED IFN TO CELLS

The characterization of the binding of radiolabeled IFNs to a variety of cells has recently been reviewed (8). In many of these studies, the binding data were analyzed by the method of Scatchard (12) which enables the calculation of both the apparent dissociation constant (Kd) and the number of binding sites per cell. The apparent Kd's and number of binding sites per cell calculated from binding data derived at 0-4°C ranged from 4X10^{-9} to 4X10^{-11}M, 650 to 35,000 receptors/cell for human IFN-alphas on human and bovine cells (9,13-20); 10^{-10} to 10^{-11}M, 1,000 to 20,000 receptors/cell for mouse IFN-alpha/beta on mouse cells (21,22); approximately 10^{-9} to 10^{-10}M, 4,000 to 6,000 receptors/cell for murine IFN-beta on mouse cells (23,24); 2.4X10^{-8} to 1X10^{-10}M, 4,000 to 10,000 receptors/cell for human IFN-beta on human cells (25,26); 5X10^{-10}M, 4,000 to 12,000 receptors/cell for murine IFN-gamma on mouse cells (27,28); and 9X10^{-9} to 1X10^{-12}M, 200 to 100,000 receptors/cell for human IFN-gamma on human cells (29-34).

In our studies, the binding of ^{125}I-labeled human IFN-gamma to the human amnion cell line, WISH at 4°C was nearly maximal by 90 min. Scatchard analysis of the binding data yielded a linear plot and an apparent Kd of 8.4X10^{-10}M and 6,800 binding sites per cell. These values differ from those reported earlier and probably reflect variations in radiolabeled IFN preparations and conditions of the cells.

The existence of multiple binding sites for IFN-alpha and -gamma, respectively, have been reported by several groups, predominantly based on data that yielded curvilinear Scatchard plots (14,16). The interpretation of these results, however, is subject to careful review, for in some cases the radiolabeled IFN exhibited low biological specific antiviral activity and/or the binding data was derived under nonequilibrium conditions, i.e. temperatures which permit ligand internalization and cellular processing. An interesting observation has recently been reported by Orchansky et al. (35) which suggests the existence of two kinds of IFN-gamma binding sites. Acid-treated IFN-gamma, which exhibits a 95% decrease in its antiviral activity on WISH cells, could effectively compete with radiolabeled IFN-gamma for binding to the receptor on WISH cells but not on human peripherial blood monocytes. Moreover, IFN-gamma was found to induce an antiviral state in WISH cells, but not in monocytes. The acid-treated IFN-gamma was shown to be almost as active as IFN-gamma itself in inducing HLA-DR in WISH cells, while it was almost completely inactive as an HLA-DR inducer in monocytes. Thus, one can propose as these authors did that the observed variations in biological activity stem from the presence of different receptors on the surface of monocytes and WISH cells, one that can only bind the IFN-gamma which has its native structure and one that can also bind acid-treated IFN-gamma.

The existence of different types of receptors has been demonstrated for IFN-alpha and IFN-gamma. In addition, it is clear, that IFN-beta and IFN-alpha can interact with the same or a similar population of binding sites (9,10). However, some ambiguity exists in the relationship between the interaction IFN-gamma with the IFN-beta binding site and IFN-beta with the IFN-gamma binding site. Several studies indicated that IFN-beta inhibited the binding of radiolabeled IFN-gamma to its receptor, although the degree of blocking was less than that of IFN-gamma (27,29). It was also demonstrated that IFN-gamma competively inhibited the binding of radiolabeled IFN-beta to its binding site (26). In contrast to these data, most results indicated that IFN-gamma binding was not blocked by IFN-beta (30-32,35). In our studies, competitive inhibition of binding of IFN-gamma by IFN-beta was not observed (Fig. 1). One possible explanation for the discrepancy in the data may result from variations in the IFN preparations used; in cases where blocking of radiolabeled IFN-gamma by IFN-beta was observed, the investigators used natural IFN-beta as the competitor, which may contain contaminating compounds which could inhibit IFN-gamma binding. Additional binding studies using radiolabeled glycosylated and nonglycosylated human IFN-gamma have shown that the carbohydrate moeity of IFN-gamma does not play a major role in binding to its receptor on Daudi cells (36).

A majority of interferon receptors appear to be found on the cell surface. Pretreatment of cells with trypsin inhibits the binding of IFN to the cells (15,22,37). In addition, a major portion of IFN bound to cells at $4^{o}C$ can be removed by treatment of cells with acid or trypsin (13,24,28,38-41). Transmission electron microscopy has allowed the visualization of IFN bound to the cell surface (24,38). Furthermore, several studies have demonstrated the binding of IFN to the plasma membrane fraction (19,24,42). Recent studies using ^{125}I-murine IFN-beta have indicated that IFN may also bind to nuclei (24). The IFN appears to bind to the nuclei with a higher affinity (Kd, $1.4X10^{-10}M$) than the plasma membrane (Kd $9.8X10^{-10}M$). Approximately, 80% of the IFN is released from the 10,000 binding sites per nucleus following trypsin treatment; thus indicating a majority of the binding sites are associated with the nuclear membrane. The biological significance of the interaction of IFN with the nucleus is currently unknown.

PURIFICATION AND CHARACTERIZATION OF IFN RECEPTORS

In order to understand the role of the IFN-receptor interaction in eliciting the biological responses of IFN, the need to characterize the receptor on the molecular level soon became apparent. Several approaches were taken to elucidate some biochemical properties of the IFN receptors; they included crosslinking the receptor with radiolabeled IFN and receptor purification.

Crosslinking studies using radiolabeled IFN preparations and a variety of cell lines have yielded some information regarding the physicochemical properties of the IFN-binding sites. A summary of the apparent molecular weights of the receptors is shown in Table 1. These values were deduced based on the assumption of a bimolecular complex of the receptor or receptor subunit and IFN. In general, one complex was observed except in the case of human IFN-beta in which case two complexes were visualized by SDS PAGE following crosslinking of Daudi cells with radiolabeled IFN-beta(ser) (26). The apparent molecular weights of the receptors ranged from 95,000 to 210,000 for HuIFN-alpha, 103,000-128,000 for HuIFN-beta, 77,000 to 205,000 for human IFN-gamma and were approximately 95,000 for MuIFN-gamma and 109,000 and MuIFN-beta. The radiolabeled IFN-receptor complexes appear to be specific in that they are not formed in the presence of their respective unlabeled IFN. Several studies indicate that some of the IFN receptors appear to be glycoproteins (15).

Partial purification of IFN receptors has been achieved using a variety of solubilization and chromatographic techniques (15,20,37,47). Affinity chromatography using the respective IFN as the ligand has proven to be a very powerful purification procedure (20,47); in combination with lectin chromatography, high degrees of purification have been obtained (47). The Kd of the solubilized IFN-alpha receptor derived from Namalwa cells is 0.2 to 0.5nM (20). Estimates of the molecular weight of the solubilized human IFN-alpha receptor range from 95,000 to approximately 210,000 (19,43) and 95,000 for the solubilized human interferon gamma receptor (47). To date, no laboratory has reported the purification of an IFN receptor to homogeneity.

FATE OF RECEPTOR-BOUND INTERFERONS

It has been shown that, after binding to receptors, a number of polypeptide hormones and growth factors are internalized and degraded via receptor-mediated endocytosis. It has been demonstrated for several IFN alphas, beta and gamma that cell-surface bound IFN is rapidly internalized at 37°C and then continuously degraded following an initial lag period (24,28,37,38,41,48-51). The initial lag period for human IFN alpha and gamma is approximately 15-30 min. (37-39,41,48-51). While murine IFN-gamma is apparently internalized and degraded more rapidly than human IFNs (24,28), murine IFN-alpha/beta does not appear to be internalized and degraded (22). The presence of inhibitors of lysosomal proteases, e.g. methylamine, chloroquine, inhibited the degradation of the radiolabeled IFN preparations; thus suggesting that IFN internalization is by the receptor-mediated endocytosis pathway (38-40,50). The specific association of IFN-alpha and beta with clatharin-coated pits and receptosomes was observed by transmission electron microscopy using IFN-colloidal gold (38) or immunoferritin conjugates (24). Morphometric quantitation of IFN-alpha 2-colloidal gold particles in receptosomes following incubation of the conjugate with the cells in the presence and absence of unconjugated IFN revealed that the number of particles was reduced by 80% in the presence of unconjugated IFN (38). These data suggested that the presence of the IFN-gold conjugates in receptosomes was specific and that at least a portion of the IFN-alpha 2 was internalized by receptor-mediated endocytosis. In the case of IFN-gamma, it was shown that approximately 50% of the receptor-bound HuIFN-gamma was rapidly internalized at 37°C (50). It was suggested that either an intracellular pool of the receptors existed or the receptors were recycled. Subsequently, others have shown that 46% of the total HuIFN-gamma receptor pool was expressed on the cell surface and that the occupied IFN-gamma receptors were internalized and degraded (37). These authors suggested based on unpublished data that the human gamma-IFN receptor may be recycled. On the otherhand, radiolabeled MuIFN-gamma degradation products were not detected during a 16 hr incubation period and that the reappearance of receptor is probably due to the synthesis of new receptors and not to recycling (28). The receptors for HuIFN-alpha do not appear to recycle based on kinetic data (49) and studies employing the use of the inhibitor of receptor recycling, monensin (8).

The interaction of IFNs with cells under physiological conditions is a complex interplay between ligand binding, receptor modulation, e.g. down-regulation, internalization and ligand and receptor degradation. The binding of HuIFN to the cell surface is reduced by approximately 30-50% when the cells have been treated with IFN, even when the incubation is for a short period of time and with subsaturating concentrations of IFN (8,28,51-54). This phenomena has been termed down-regulation and in some systems has been associated with a ligand-induced increase in receptor endocytosis (55). Analysis of the steady state binding, internalization, and degradation of HuIFN-alpha 2 suggested that in fact the down-regulation of the HuIFN-alpha 2 receptors by HuIFN-alpha 2 is different than that described for several growth factor and hormone receptors by their respective ligands in that the rate of endocytosis of the occupied receptors is not increased (49,55). It is proposed that the decrease in IFN binding may be a result of either a reduced rate of receptor synthesis, a reduction in the insertion of receptors into the plasma membrane, or a reduced or altered intracellular transport of the receptor. Regeneration of the binding of IFN to the cell surface following down-regulation was dependent on protein synthesis, which again suggests that the internalized receptors are not recycled back to the cell surface but are newly synthesized (8,28,48,52). Down-regulation of IFN receptors has also been observed in vivo. The binding of radiolabeled HuIFN-alpha to peripheral blood cells (54) and hairy cells (53) from patients treated with HuIFN-alpha 2 was reduced compared to pretreatment values. The clinical significance of this down-regulation is currently under investigation.

CORRELATION OF INTERFERON BINDING AND BIOLOGICAL RESPONSE

In many systems studied, those cells responsive to the biological effects of a particular IFN bind that IFN in a specific manner, while others not responsive to IFN do not specifically bind these molecules (8,13,15,22,35,56). For example, Ucer et al. (56) reported that the induction of HLA-DR by IFN-gamma was in proportion to the number of receptors on the cell surface, and Orchansky et al. (35) showed that IFN-gamma lost the activity of both binding to its receptors and inducing HLA-DR simultaneously when it was treated by low pH. However, exceptions have been observed as was shown in the case of a mouse embryonal carcinoma cell line which can bind IFN specifically but is not responsive to IFN in terms of its antiviral and antiproliferative activities (57). Some correlation has been made between the magnitude of the biological response and the degree of receptor occupancy in responsive cells (22,37). However, receptor occupancy need not be at saturation to yield a maximal response because many of the biological activities are a result of a cascade-like processes. In addition it very difficult to compare binding of IFN and the biological response because the kinetics of the two events are very different (59).

GENETICS

Analysis of the IFN-alpha and -beta sensitivity of various mutant human cells and rodent-human somatic cell hybrids led to the conclusion that the gene encoding the human IFN-alpha and -beta receptor is located on human chromosome 21 (59,60). Likewise, it has been presented that human IFN-gamma receptor gene was also located on chromosome 21, because trisomy 21 human fibroblasts were more sensitive to human IFN-gamma than were diploid controls (61). However, Shulman et al. (62) showed that antisera raised against a human-mouse hybrid cell line containing human chromosome 21 as its only human chromosome blocked binding of human IFN-alpha 2, but not human IFN-gamma, to the cell surface receptors. In addition, Raziuddin et al. (63) showed human IFN-gamma did not bind to human-mouse hybrid cells containing three copies of human chromosome 21. Finally, Rashidbaigi et al. (46) found the formation of the complex of human IFN-gamma and its receptor was formed in hamster-human or mouse-human hybrids which contain human chromosome 6. The presence of the chromosome 6 was necessary and sufficient for the formation of this complex, but those hybrid cells could not be protected by human IFN-gamma from Vesicular Stomatitis Virus killing. Thus, the majority of the evidence suggests that human IFN-gamma receptor gene is located on chromosome 6.

ACKNOWLEDGMENTS

We are grateful to Cathy Hobbs for the preparation of this manuscript.

REFERENCES

1. Goeddel, D.V., D.W. Leung, T.J. Dull, M. Gross, R.M. Lawn, P.H. McCandliss, A. Seeburg, E. Ullrich, E. Yelverton, and P.W. Gray: The structure of eight distinct cloned human leukocyte interferon cDNAs. Nature 290:20, 1980.
2. Zoon, K.C., and R. Wetzel: Comparative structures of mammalian interferons. In: Handbook of Experimental Pharmacology Vol. 71, Interferons and Their Applications, P.E. Came and W.A. Carter, eds. Springer Verlag, pp. 79-100, 1984.
3. Taniguchi, T., S. Ohno, Y. Fuju-Kuriyama, and Y. Muramatsu: The nucleotide sequence of human fibroblast interferon cDNA. Gene 10:11, 1980.
4. Gray, P.W., D.W. Leung, D. Pennica, E. Yelvertown, R. Najarion, C.C. Simonsen, R. Derynck, P.S. Sherwood, D.M. Wallace, S.L. Berger, A.D. Levinson, and D.V. Goeddel: Expression of human immune interferon cDNA in E. coli and monkey cells. Nature 295:503, 1982.
5. Pestka, S., and S.J. Tarnowski: Purification of the interferons. Pharmac Ther 29:299, 1985.
6. Nathan, C.F., H.M. Murray, M. Weibe, and B.Y. Rubin. Identification of interferon-gamma as the lymphokine which activates human macrophage oxidative metabolism and antimicrobial activity. J Exp Med 158:670, 1983.
7. Friedman, R.M.: Interferon binding: the first step in establishment of antiviral activity. Science 156:1760, 1967.
8. Zoon, K.C., and H. Arnheiter: Studies of the interferon receptors. Pharmac Ther 24:259, 1984.
9. Branca, A., and C. Baglioni: Binding to human cells of [^{125}I]-labeled alpha interferon produced in E. coli: evidence for different receptors for type I and II interferons. Nature 294:768, 1981.

10. Merlin, G., E. Falcoff, and M. Aguet: ^{125}I-labeled human interferons alpha, beta and gamma: comparative receptor-binding data. J Gen Virol 66:1149, 1985.
11. Zoon, K.C., and H. Arnheiter: The molecular characterization of interferon receptors. In: Interferon: Research, Clinical Application, and Regulatory Consideration, K.C. Zoon, P.D. Noguchi, and T.-Y. Liu, eds. Elsevier, New York, pp. 115-124, 1984.
12. Scatchard, G.: The attraction of protein for small molecules and ions. Ann NY Acad Sci 51:660, 1949.
13. Zoon, K., D. Zur Nedden, and H. Arnheiter: Specific binding of human-alpha interferon to a high affinity cell surface binding site on bovine kidney cells. J Biol Chem 257:4695, 1982.
14. Mogensen, K.E., M-T. Bandu, F. Vignaux, M. Aguet, and I. Gresser: Binding of ^{125}I-labeled human alpha interferon to human lymphoid cells. Int J Cancer 28:575, 1981.
15. Joshi, A.R., F.H. Sarkar, and S.L. Gupta: Interferon receptors. Crosslinking of human leukocyte interferon alpha 2 to its receptor on human cells. J Biol Chem 257:13884, 1982.
16. Yonehara, S., M. Yonehara-Takahashi, A. Ishii, and S. Nagata: Different binding of human interferon alpha 1 and alpha 2 to common receptors on human and bovine cells. J Biol Chem 258:9046, 1983.
17. Hannigan, G.E., D.H. Gewert, and B.R.G. Williams: Characterization and regulation of alpha-interferon receptor expression in interferon-sensitive and resistant human lymphoblastoid cells. J Biol Chem 259:9456, 1984.
18. Arnheiter, H., M. Ohno, M. Smith, B. Gutte, and K.C. Zoon: Orientation of a human leukocyte interferon molecule on its cell surface receptor: carboxyl terminus remains accessible to a monoclonal antibody made against a synthetic interferon fragment. Proc Natl Acad Sci USA 80:2539, 1983.
19. Faltynek, C.R., A. Branca, S. McCandless, and C. Baglioni: Characterization of an interferon receptor on human lymphoblastoid cells. Proc Natl Acad Sci USA 80:3269, 1983.
20. Traub, A., S. Feinstein, M. Gez, A. Lazar, and A. Mizrahi: Purification and properties of the alpha-interferon receptor of human lymphoblastoid (Namalwa) cells. J Biol Chem 259:13872, 1984.
21. Aguet, M.: High affinity binding of ^{125}I-labelled mouse interferon to a specific cell surface receptor. Nature 284:459, 1980.
22. Aguet, M., and B. Blanchard: High affinity binding of ^{125}I-labeled mouse interferon to a specific cell surface receptor. Virology 115:249, 1981.
23. Jayaram, B., H. Schmidt, O. Yoshie, H. Samanta, G. Floyd-Smith, and P. Lengyel: Interferon Action: (A) Interferons as inducers of mRNA and protein synthesis, (B) Cross-linking of mouse-beta interferon to cell surface receptors. In: Humoral Factors on Host Defense, Y. Mamura, ed. Academic Press, New York, pp. 157-174, 1983.
24. Kushnaryov, V.M., H.S. MacDonald, J.J. Sedmak, and S.E. Grossberg: Murine interferon-beta receptor-mediated endocytosis and nuclear membrane binding. Proc Natl Acad Sci USA 82:3281, 1985.
25. O'Rourke, E.C., R.J. Drummond, and A.A. Creasey: Binding of ^{125}I-labeled recombinant beta-interferon (IFN-beta Ser_{17}) to human cells. Molec Cell Biol 4:2745, 1984.

26. Thompson, M.R., Z.-Q. Zhang, A. Fourniers, and Y.H. Tan: Characterization of human beta interferon-binding sites in human cells. J Biol Chem 260:563, 1985.
27. Celada, A., P.W. Gray, E. Rinderknecht, and R.D. Schreiber: Evidence for a gamma-interferon receptor that regulates macrophage tumoricidal activity. J Exp Med 160:55, 1984.
28. Wietzerbin, J., C. Gaudelet, M. Aguet, and E. Falcoff: Binding and cross-linking of recombinant mouse interferon-gamma to receptors in mouse leukemic L1210 cells; interferon-gamma internalization and receptor down-regulation. J Immunol 136:2451, 1986.
29. Anderson, R., Y.K. Yip, and J. Vilcek: Specific binding of [^{125}I]human interferon-alpha to high affinity receptors on human fibroblasts. J Biol Chem 257:1130, 1982.
30. Sarkar, F.H., and S.L. Gupta: Receptors for human gamma-interferon: binding and crosslinking of ^{125}I-labeled recombinant human gamma-interferon to receptors on WISH cells. Proc Natl Acad Sci USA 81:5160, 1984.
31. Orchansky, P., D. Novick, D.G. Fischer, and M. Rubinstein: Type I and type II interferon receptors. J Interferon Res 4:275, 1984.
32. Littman, S.J., C.R. Faltynek, and C. Baglioni: Binding of human recombinant ^{125}I-interferon gamma to receptors on human cells. J Biol Chem 260:1191, 1985.
33. Rashidbaigi, A., H.-F. Kung, and S. Pestka: Characterization of receptors for immune interferon in U937 cells with ^{32}P-labeled human recombinant immune interferon. J Biol Chem 260:8514, 1985.
34. Finbloom, D.S., D.L. Hoover, and L.M. Wahl: The characteristics of binding of human recombinant interferon-gamma to its receptor on human monocytes and human monocyte-like cell lines. J Immun 135:300, 1985.
35. Orchansky, P., M. Rubinstein, and D.G. Fischer: The interferon-gamma receptor in human monocytes is different from the one in nonhematopoietic cells. J Immunol 136:169, 1986.
36. Littman, S.J., R. Devos, and C. Baglioni: Binding of unglycosylated and glycosylated human recombinant interferon-gamma to cellular receptors. J Interferon Res 5:471, 1985.
37. Celada, A., R. Allen, I. Esparza, P.W. Gray, and R.D. Schreiber: Demonstration and partial characterization of the interferon-gamma receptor on human mononuclear phagocytes. J Clin Invest 76:2196, 1985.
38. Zoon, K.C., H. Arnheiter, D. Zur Nedden, D.J.P. Fitzgerald, and M.C. Willingham: Human interferon alpha enters cells by receptor-mediated endocytosis. Virology 130:195, 1983.
39. Branca, A.A., C.R. Faltynek, S.B. D'Alessandro, and C. Baglioni: Interaction of interferon with cellular receptors: Internalization and degradation of cell-bound interferon. J Biol Chem 257:13291, 1982.
40. Anderson, P., Y.K. Yip, and J. Vilcek: Human interferon gamma is internalized and degraded by cultured fibroblasts. J Biol Chem 258:6497, 1983.
41. Evans, T., and D. Secher: Kinetics of internalization and degradation of surface-bound interferon in human lymphoblastoid cells. EMBO J 3:2975, 1984.
42. Zoon, K.C.: Unpublished results.
43. Eid, P., and K.E. Mogensen: Isolated interferon-alpha receptor complexes stabilized in vitro. Fed Eur Biochem Soc 156:157, 1983.

44. Sarkar, F.H., and S.L. Gupta: Receptors for human gamma interferon: Binding and cross-linking of ^{125}I-labeled recombinant human gamma interferon to receptors on WISH cells. Proc Natl Acad Sci USA 81:5164, 1984.
45. Anderson, P., and C. Nagler: Photoaffinity labeling of an interferon-gamma receptor on the surface of cultured fibroblasts. Biochem Biophys Res Commun 120:828, 1984.
46. Rashibaigi, A., J.A. Langer, V. Jung, C. Jones, H.G. Morse, J.A. Tischfield, J.J. Trill, H.-F. Kung, and S. Pestka: The gene for the human immune interferon receptor is located on chromosome 6. Proc Natl Acad Sci USA 83:384, 1986.
47. Novick, D., P. Orchansky, M. Revel, and M. Rubinstein: Purification and characterization of the receptor for human interferon-gamma. J Interferon Res 6:supplement 1, 23, 1986.
48. Faltynek, G.R., S. McCandless, and C. Baglioni: Single high affinity binding of interferon alpha 2 to receptors on human lymphoid cells: internalization and inactivation of receptors. J Cell Physiol 123:459, 1985.
49. Zoon, K.C., D. Zur Nedden, R. Hu, and H. Arnheiter: Analysis of the steady state binding, internalization and degradation of human interferon alpha 2. J Biol Chem 261:4993, 1986.
50. Anderson, P., Y.K. Yip, and J. Vilcek: Human interferon gamma is internalized and degraded by cultured fibroblasts. J Biol Chem 258:6497, 1983.
51. Feinstein, S., A. Traub, A. Lazar, A. Mizrahi, and Y. Teitz: Studies on cell binding and internalization of human lymphoblastoid (Namalva) interferon. J Interferon Res 5:65, 1985.
52. Branca, A.A., and C. Baglioni: Down-regulation of the interferon receptor. J Biol Chem 257:13197, 1982.
53. Billard, C., F. Sigaux, S. Castaigne, F. Valensi, G. Flandrin, L. Degos, E. Falcoff, and M. Aguet: Treatment of hairy cell leukemia with recombinant alpha interferon: II. In vitro down-regulation of alpha interferon receptors on tumor cells. Blood 67:821, 1986.
54. Maxwell, B.L., M. Talpaz, and J.U. Gutterman: Down-regulation of peripheral blood cell interferon receptors in chronic myelogenous leukemia patients undergoing human interferon therapy. Int J Cancer 36:23, 1985.
55. Wiley, H.S., and D.D. Cunningham: A steady state model for analyzing the cellular binding, internalization and degradation of polypeptide ligands. Cell 25:433, 1981.
56. Ucer, U., H. Bartsch, P. Scheurich, and K. Pfizenmaier: Biological effects of gamma-interferon on human tumor cells: quantity and affinity of cell membrane receptors for gamma-IFN in relation to growth inhibition and induction of HLA-DR expression. Int J Cancer 36:103, 1985.
57. Aguet, M., I. Gresser, A.G. Hovanessian, M.-T. Bandu, B. Blanchard, and D. Blangy: Specific high affinity binding of [^{125}I]-labeled mouse interferon to interferon resistant embryonal carcinoma cells in vitro. Virology 114:585, 1981.
58. Mogensen, K.E., and M.-T. Bandu: Kinetic evidence for an activation step following binding of human interferon alpha 2 to the membrane receptors of Daudi cells. Eur J Biochem 134:355, 1983.

59. Chany, C., M. Vignal, P. Couillin, N.V. Cong, and A. Boue: Chromosonal localization of human genes governing the interferon induced antiviral state. Proc Natl Acad Sci USA 72:3129, 1975.
60. Slate, D.L., L. Shulman, J.B. Lawrence, M. Revel, and F.H. Ruddle: Presence of human chromosome 21 alone is sufficient for hybrid cell sensitivity to human interferon. J Virol 25:319, 1978.
61. Weil, J., G. Tucker, L.B. Epstein, and C.J. Epstein: Interferon induction of (2'-5') oligoisoadenylate synthetase in diploid and trisomy 21 human fibroblasts: relation to dosage of the interferon receptor gene (IRFC). Human Genetics 65:108, 1983.
62. Shulman, L.M., M.E. Kamarck, D.L. Slate, F.H. Ruddle, A. Branca, C. Baglioni, B.L. Maxwell, J. Gutterman, P. Anderson, C. Nagler, and J. Vilcek: Antibodies to chromosome 21 coded cell surface components block binding of human alpha-interferon but not gamma-interferon to human cells. Virology 137:422, 1984.
63. Raziuddin, A., F.H. Sarker, R. Dutkowski, L. Shulman, F.H. Ruddle, and S.L. Gupta: Receptors for human alpha and beta-interferon but not for gamma-interferon are specified by human chromosome 21. Proc Natl Acad Sci USA 81:5504, 1984.

TABLE 1. Characterization of IFN Receptors

Receptor	Cell Line	Apparent Molecular Weight	Reference
HuIFN-alpha	Daudi	130,000	15,19
	Daudi[a]	95,000	19
	Daudi[a]	210,000	43
HuIFN-beta	Daudi	128,000 and 103,000	26
HuIFN-gamma	U937	67,000 to 87,000	37
	WISH	85,000	44
	GM258	205,000	45
	CHO-A431 hybrid	100,000	46
	Daudi	108,000	32
	HeLa	108,000	32
	Fibroblast[a]	95,000	47
MuIFN-beta	L1210	105,000	23
MuIFN-gamma	L1210	95,000	28

[a]Solubilized receptor.

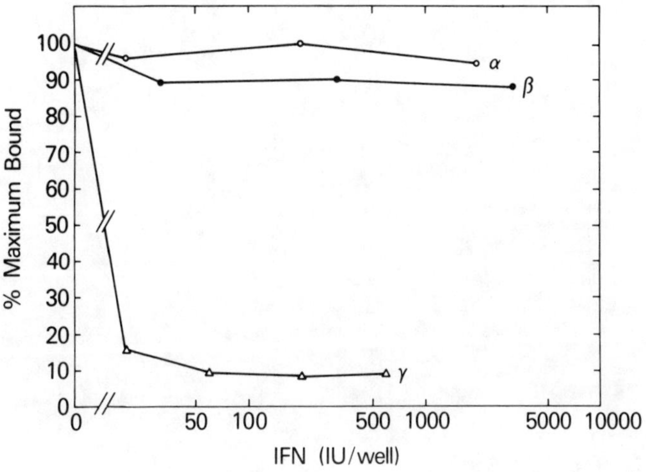

Fig. 1. Competition of ^{125}I-labeled recombinant HuIFN-gamma binding to WISH cells by unlabeled recombinant HuIFN-gamma, recombinant HuIFN-alpha 2, and natural human IFN-beta.

Confluent cultures of WISH cells in 35 mm wells were incubated with ^{125}I-labeled recombinant HuIFN-gamma (5 reference units/ml) for 2 hr at 4°C either in the absence or presence of increasing concentrations of unlabeled recombinant HuIFN-gamma, recombinant HuIFN-alpha 2, and natural human IFN-beta. The cells were washed 4 times with medium containing 10% fetal calf serum and lysed by 0.5% SDS and counted in a gamma counter.

23. Cell-to-Cell Transmission of IFN-Induced Activities

J. Edwin Blalock,[a] G. John Stanton,[b] and Douglas A. Weigent[a]

[a]Department of Physiology and Biophysics, University of Alabama at Birmingham, Birmingham, AL 35294; [b]Department of Microbiology, University of Texas Medical Branch, Galveston, TX 77550

INTRODUCTION

Many molecules which act through specific cell surface receptors frequently employ secondary messenger molecules to transmit information from the cell membrane to the nucleus (for review, see 1). The most notable of these are the polypeptide hormones which use cyclic AMP as a secondary messenger. IFN also seems to use a secondary messenger molecule(s) for information transfer both within and between cells. The first IFN-induced event transferred was viral resistance to cells of a heterologous species. Since then, we and others have shown that many IFN-induced activities, including antiproliferative and antirickettsial, suppression of antibody formation, enhancement of natural killing, and protection of target cells to killing can also be transferred between cells (2-6). This article will review our evidence for a putative IFN-induced secondary messenger, describe the activities of IFN which the putative secondary messenger transmits, and discuss the implications of IFN's inter- and intracellular information transfer.

TRANSFER OF IFN-INDUCED VIRAL RESISTANCE

While a secondary messenger molecule for IFN has not been directly shown, we designed a system for indirectly testing its existence. The rationale for this system relied on two observations: the species preference of IFN action (7), and the fact that many cells communicate via gap junctional transfer of small molecules (for review, see 8).

We reasoned that if IFN acted through a small secondary messenger molecule, this messenger might be transferred to adjacent cells and indirectly (with respect to IFN) cause them to become resistant to virus infection. This was easily testable because cells of species different from the source of the IFN are generally much less sensitive to its direct action. We found that when mouse and human cells were cocultured in the presence of mouse (Mo) IFN, both cells became resistant to virus infection (9). Under the same conditions, mouse IFN has no effect on human cells alone. The human cells in the Mo IFN treated coculture were directly shown to be resistant by challenging with poliovirus which would not grow in the mouse cell (10).

The sequence of MoIFN initiated events leading to the antiviral state were studied as possible sites for the cell-to-cell transfer of IFN-induced viral resistance in the mouse:human coculture system (11). The possibility that undetectable levels of human (Hu) IFN were produced by recipient cells was negated by the demonstration of transfer of resistance in the presence of anti-HuIFN antibody. Transfer of MoIFN sensitivity to human cells by exchange of a membrane-associated IFN receptor was unlikely since this would require the continued presence of MoIFN and resistance was transferred by MoIFN-treated cells from which the IFN was removed, prior to coculture with human cells. From kinetic data and the finding that actinomycin D blocked resistance in human cells for 3 hrs past complete transcription of mRNA for the mouse antiviral proteins, it seems unlikely that the mouse antiviral proteins or their mRNAs are the effectors of transferred resistance. If the mouse mRNA had caused the transfer, resistance should have been blocked only for the 1 hr required for transcription in the mouse cell. If mouse antiviral proteins were transferred, they should not have required de novo RNA synthesis for their action. These data further showed that a transcriptional process is required in the human cell for the development of transferred resistance. This is consistent with secondary messenger molecules which transmit the IFN signal from the membrane to the nucleus being the effectors of the transfer process. Further evidence for this idea is the requirement for cell-to-cell contact for the transfer. The cell contact requirement implies that gap junctions are involved, and they only allow passage of small molecules.

The transfer process appears to be a general phenomenon which is demonstrable with a number of cell combinations from different animal species (12). More importantly, it has been shown to operate within cells from a single species (9,13,14) and to be a major amplification system for IFN action (15). For instance, it was shown by the cloning of individual mouse L cells that there is a very marked heterogeneity among individual cells in both their sensitivity to and maximum degree of protection afforded by IFN. Further, cloned L cells of "high" IFN sensitivity can transfer their viral resistance to clones of "low" sensitivity. By studying the IFN response of individually reacting clones and a reconstituted parental population of cells, it was found that as few as 10% of these cells can determine the response of the population. This process would amplify the IFN response since sensitive, fast-responding cells would transfer resistance to less sensitive, slower-responding cells which constitute the bulk of the population. The observation that a small fraction of cells (10%) determines the response of the population shows that the transfer process plays a highly important role in the action of IFN.

The above studies were done with IFNα and β. The third major IFN type, IFNγ, was also found to cause a transfer of viral resistance (16). The transfer process was similar to that for IFNα and β, except that on a unit basis IFNγ caused the transfer more efficiently. Interestingly, although the kinetics of the response of mouse cells to MoIFNα/β and IFNγ are different, both IFNs have similar kinetics of development of transferred resistance in the human cells. This indicates that the transfer process and its expression in human cells may be similar with both IFNα/β and IFNγ whereas the initial events by which the IFNs activate mouse cells are different. Thus, IFNγ and IFNα/β probably share some common pathways to the antiviral state. Furthermore, like IFNα/β, some components of the IFNγ system are not species specific.

TRANSFER OF IFN-INDUCED VIRAL RESISTANCE BY LYMPHOCYTES

The transfer process is not limited to fibroblastoid and epithelioid cells as donors but also includes lymphocytes (17). The major difference is that the system does not require exogenous IFN for activation. This is because nonsensitized lymphocytes produce IFNα (18) when cultured with allogeneic or syngeneic tumor or virus-infected cells (19) and almost any xenogeneic cells (18). The results of other studies (20) showed that human B lymphocytes cocultivated with mouse L cells produced human leukocyte IFN (IFNα) and shortly thereafter transferred antiviral activity to the recipient cells (99% inhibition of expected virus yield). In contrast, cocultivation of T-cell populations with mouse L cells resulted in no IFN production or transfer of antiviral activity. In addition, both T and B lymphocytes pretreated with exogenous IFN or stimulated _in vitro_ by mitogens could transfer antiviral activity to human cells (4). The transfer of antiviral activity was not blocked by antibody to IFN. The data indicate that both T and B cells can be recruited by IFN to transfer antiviral activity. Thus, once cells are recruited by IFN, they can transfer antiviral activity in the absence of IFN and protect cells locally or distally from the site of infection. Additional studies (5) with T cells and, therefore, in the absence of endogenously-produced IFN showed that human T cells treated with low levels of IFN (1-10 units/ml), and washed to remove the IFN, transferred the same level of antiviral activity to recipient WISH cells as an equivalent IFN treatment alone could induce in WISH cells. Further, when T cells were pretreated with IFN (1-10 units/ml), a 2.5- to 5-fold greater level of protection developed than could be expected from the additive effect of either T cells or IFN alone. Antibody to leukocyte, fibroblast, or immune IFN blocked the antiviral effect of the respective IFN types but once initiated had no effect on the transfer of antiviral activity initiated by leukocyte, fibroblast, or immune IFN. Also, treatment of T cells with actinomycin D blocked the transfer of antiviral activity of IFN-treated T cells. Taken together, the results suggest that the increased antiviral activity is not merely an additive effect of the IFN, but represents a synergistic amplification of protection most likely due to the combination of the separate effects of IFN and IFN-induced transfer. The ability of both T and B cells to transfer antiviral activity indicates their importance in host defense against virus infections.

The lymphocyte transfer system suggests a new and efficient host immune defense against virus infection. _In vivo_, the system would be activated by IFN produced by lymphocytes in response to virus and/or virus-infected cells. Once activated, migrating lymphocytes could transfer resistance to other tissues. This transfer process also required cell contact and a transcriptional event in the recipient cells and, we assume, at least operationally, that the transferred material which caused the nuclear event is the same or similar with lymphocytes and fibroblastoid or epithelioid cells.

Most recently, we have shown that IFN caused the transfer of natural cytotoxic activity between human leukocytes in a syngeneic system (6). The design utilized two human leukocyte cell types in which the effect of IFN was transferred from IFN-treated plastic-adherent leukocytes (mostly macrophages) to E-rosette-positive cells (T cells) and the recipient cells could be separated from the donor cells prior to the assay of cytotoxic activity. This was testable because the recipient T cells lacked cytotoxic activity but could be enhanced by direct IFN treatment (21). Plastic-adherent leukocytes treated with 10-1,000 units effectively transferred cytotoxic activity at ratios as low as 40 recipient cells to one donor leukocytes. Human immune-type IFN (IFNγ) was more efficient than IFNα or IFNβ in eliciting the transfer of cytotoxic activity. The transfer occurred with IFNγ preparations of various specific activities and with recombinant IFNγ. The transferred activity had the characteristics of an IFN-induced antiviral state in that it was blocked either by actinomycin D or by prevention of cell contact. Specific antibodies to IFN had no effect on the transfer of cytotoxic activity. Protection of mouse target cells from human cytotoxic activity could also be transferred from IFN-induced human foreskin fibroblasts (HFF), which are insensitive to cytotoxic activity to the cytotoxic-sensitive mouse cells. The transfer of protection was highly efficient at ratios of one HFF cell to 16 mouse target cells. As expected, target cells alone pretreated with IFN became resistant to the action of cytotoxic cells (6,22). In additional studies, we have shown that the IFN-mediated protection of mouse L cells can also be mediated by recombinant IFNγ and blocked by treatment of the IFN with antibody to IFN. Taken together, these data support the hypothesis that the transfer of the protective effect is possible and is initiated by IFN.

TRANSFER OF OTHER IFN-INDUCED ACTIVITIES

It has recently been shown that IFN-induced activities, such as the anticellular and antirickettsial effects, are also transmissible between IFN-treated and nontreated cells. In particular, human foreskin fibroblasts, which were not sensitive to the antirickettsial activity of mouse IFNγ, acquired the ability to inhibit rickettsial growth when they were cocultured with sensitive mouse L929 cells treated with mouse IFNγ (3). Further, the transfer of IFN-induced antiproliferative activity in vitro (2) and antiviral activity in vivo has recently been demonstrated (23). IFN-treated WISH or L cells cocultured 4 hrs with xenogeneic lymphoblastoid cells were able to significantly decrease (30-50%) the cell growth rate of the lymphoblastoid cells in a dose dependent manner. The transfer of antiproliferative activity to recipient lymphoblastoid cells occurred concurrently with the transfer of antiviral activity. The decrease in the growth rate could not be attributed to the development of cellular cytotoxicity in the cell systems, or to factors released into the supernatant by the IFN-treated WISH or L cells. The mechanism of the transfer of antiproliferative activity was shown to be dependent upon stable cell contact and specifically induced by IFN, including recombinant IFNγ. Human IFN-treated human lymphocytes were also shown to transfer similar levels of antiproliferative activity to both xenogeneic mouse L cells and allogeneic human WISH cells. The transfer of antiviral activity was also demonstrated in a mouse in vivo model. Mice injected with syngeneic T lymphocytes pretreated with 10 units of IFNα/β had a 35% lower mortality rate following Semliki Forest virus challenge than did mice injected with untreated T cells ($p<0.01$). This antiviral activity could not be attributed to carryover of IFN, endogenous IFN production, or IFN-enhanced cytotoxicity present in either the inoculated cells or in host peritoneal leukocytes or spleen cells (23).

While IFN was originally described in terms of its antiviral activity (24), it is now recognized as regulating a number of cellular responses. Of particular interest is our demonstration that IFN has species specific polypeptide hormone-like activities. These included a noradrenaline-like increase in the beat frequency of cultured mouse myocardial cells (25) and corticotropin (ACTH)-like induction of melanogenesis (26) and steroidogenesis (26,27). Hormone responses such as these are known to be mediated by secondary messenger molecules and are transmissible between cells (28). Likewise, the hormonal action of IFN was transmissible. For example, human IFN did not increase the beat frequency of mouse myocardial cells. However, when human IFN was added to cocultures of mouse myocardial cells and human WISH cells, there was a dose dependent increase in the beat frequency of the myocardial cells (25). This effect was only observed when the myocardial cells were in contact with human cells. When noradrenaline was added to cocultures which had been maximally stimulated with HuIFN, there was no further increase in beat frequency, whereas noradrenaline addition to mouse myocardial cells treated with HuIFN increased their beat frequency to that of the cocultures. This indicates that IFN and noradrenaline were possibly acting through the same pathways. Both cell types in the cocultures in the presence of HuIFN also developed antiviral resistance whereas HuIFN-treated mouse myocardial cells alone did not. The observed sequence is consistent with the initiation of events in the human cell by HuIFN, and their subsequent transfer to the myocardial cell. These data showed that in conditions which can lead to transfer of IFN-induced viral resistance, transfer of the hormonal activity of IFN also occurs.

IFN also serves an important function in modulating immune responses (for review, see 29). In particular, IFN can suppress antibody production. This immunosuppression is also transferable between lymphocytes though the mechanism differs from the previously described transfer process (30). MoIFN-treated spleen cells were shown to suppress the production of antibody to sheep red blood cells (SRBC) by untreated mouse spleen cells. As expected, spleen cells not treated with IFN were not suppressive under the same conditions. Characterization of the suppressor cell activity was done by treatment of MoIFN-induced suppressor cells with antibody to MoIFN. Specific antibody did not block or reduce the suppression. However, the immunosuppressive effects of the IFN used to induce the suppressor cells was blocked by its preincubation with this antibody. Thus, the suppressor cell activity was induced by IFN, did not require the continued presence of IFN and could be attributed to either a direct or indirect action of suppressor cells. Direct evidence for such a mediator was obtained by incubating high concentrations of IFN-treated cells for 2 hr at 37°C and adding the supernatants to untreated cultures. The PFC response was suppressed over 95%, and the suppression was not affected by prior incubation of suppressor supernatants with antibody to IFN, thus providing further evidence that IFN was not directly involved in the suppression. Thus, IFN induced suppressor cells, which in turn produced a suppressor factor that was capable of suppressing the *in vitro* antibody response. The factor is devoid of antiviral activity, which suggests that IFN regulates the immune response by a mechanism(s) that is different from its antiviral property. This differentiates the cell interactions that are involved in immunosuppression by IFN from the cell-to-cell interactions that are associated with the transfer of IFN-induced viral resistance and hormonal activity.

SUMMARY

In conclusion, many of the activities of IFN are transmissible between cells and may involve more than one transfer mechanism. These mechanisms probably involve secondary messenger molecules which are shared with hormones and act at the transcriptional level. The transfer system seems to be a major amplification process for IFN action. It will be interesting in the future to determine the processes involved.

ACKNOWLEDGEMENTS

These studies were supported by U.S. Army Medical Research and Development Command contract DAMD 17-78-C-8048 to J.E.B. and by Public Health Service Grant EY01715 from the National Eye Institute to G.J.S.

REFERENCES

1. Cutrecasas, P.: Hormone-receptor interactions and the plasma membrane. In: Cell Membrane Biochemistry, Cell Biology and Pathology, G. Weissmann and R. Clairborne, eds. H.P. Publishing Co., Inc., New York, p. 177, 1975.

2. Lloyd, R.E., J.E. Blalock, and G.J. Stanton: Cell to cell transfer of IFN induced antiproliferative activity. Science 221:953, 1983.

3. Turco, J. and H.H. Winkler: Comparison of the properties of antirickettsial activity and interferon in mouse lymphokines. Infect Immun 42:27, 1983.

4. Weigent, D.A., M.P. Langford, G.J. Stanton, and J.E. Blalock: Interferon induced transfer of viral resistance by human B and T lymphocytes. Cell Immunol 87:678, 1984.
5. Weigent, D.A., R.E. Lloyd, J.E. Blalock, and G.J. Stanton: Synergism of antiviral activity in cell cultures treated with low concentrations of IFN and IFN treated lymphocytes. Proc Soc Exp Biol Med 177:257, 1984.
6. Weigent, D.A., J.E. Blalock, and G.J. Stanton: Interferon induced transfer of natural killing activity between human leukocytes. J Biol Resp Mod 4:60, 1985.
7. Lockhart, R.Z., Jr.: Criteria for acceptance of a viral inhibitor as an interferon and a general description of the biological properties of known interferons. In: Interferons and Interferon Inducers, N.B. Finter, ed. North-Holland, American Elsevier, Amsterdam and New York, 1973.
8. Lowenstein, W.R.: Cellular communication by permeable membrane junctions. In: Cell Membrane Biochemistry, Cell Biology and Pathology, G. Weissmann and R. Clairborne, eds. H.P. Publishing Co., Inc., New York, p. 105, 1975.
9. Blalock, J.E. and S. Baron: Interferon-induced transfer of viral resistance between animal cells. Nature 269:422, 1977.
10. Blalock, J.E.: Methods and procedures for experiments with mixed cell population: Transfer of the antiviral state induced by interferon. Methods in Enzymology 79:353, 1981.
11. Blalock, J.E. and S. Baron: Mechanisms of interferon induced transfer of viral resistance between animal cells. J Gen Virol 42:363, 1979.
12. Hughes, T.K., J.E. Blalock, and S. Baron: Various heterologous cells exhibit interferon induced transfer of viral resistance. Arch Virol 58:77, 1978.
13. Blalock, J.E. and G.J. Stanton: Efficient transfer of interferon induced viral resistance between human cells. J Gen Virol 41:325, 1978.
14. Blalock, J.E.: Cellular interactions determine rate and degree of interferon action. Infect Immun 23:496, 1979.
15. Blalock, J.E.: A small fraction of cells communicates the maximal interferon sensitivity to a population. Proc Soc Exp Biol Med 162:80, 1979.
16. Blalock, J.E., J. Georgiades, and H.M. Johnson: Immune-type interferon induced transfer of viral resistance. J Immunol 122:1018, 1979.
17. Blalock, J.E., D.A. Weigent, M.P. Langford, and G.J. Stanton: Transfer of interferon induced viral resistance from human leukocytes to other cell types. Infect Immun 29:356, 1980.
18. Blalock, J.E., M.P. Langford, J. Georgiades, and G.J. Stanton: Nonsensitized lymphocytes produce leukocyte interferon when cultured with foreign cells. Cell Immunol 43:197, 1979.
19. Trinchieri, G., D. Santoli, R.R. Dee, and B.B. Knowles: Antiviral activity induced by culturing lymphocytes with tumor derived or virus transformed cells. Identification of the antiviral activity as interferon and characterization of the human effector lymphocyte subpopulation. J Exp Med 147:1299, 1978.
20. Weigent, D.A., M.P. Langford, E.M. Smith, J.E. Blalock, and G.J. Stanton: Human B lymphocytes produce leukocyte interferon after

interaction with foreign cells. Infect Immun 32:508, 1981.
21. Weigent, D.A., M.P. Langford, W.R. Fleischmann, and G.J. Stanton: Enhancement of natural killing activity by different types of interferon. In: Human Lymphokines, N.O. Hill, A. Kahn, and D.C. Dumonde, eds. Academic Press, 1982.
22. Herberman, R.B., M.E. Nunn, H.T. Holden, S. Staal, and J.Y. Djeu: Augmentation of natural cytotoxic reactivity of mouse lymphoid cells against syngeneic and allogeneic target cells. Int J Cancer 19:55, 1977.
23. Lloyd, R.E.: Cell to cell transfer of interferon-induced antiproliferative activity in vitro and antiviral activity in vivo. Ph.D. Dissertation. University of Texas Medical Branch, Galveston, Texas, 1983.
24. Isaacs, A. and J. Lindenmann: Virus interference: The interferon. Proc Roy Soc Ser B 147:258, 1957.
25. Blalock, J.E. and J.D. Stanton: Common pathways of interferon and hormonal action. Nature 283:406, 1980.
26. Blalock, J.E. and C. Harp: Interferon and adrenocorticotropic hormone induction of steroidogenesis, melanogenesis and antiviral activity. Arch Virol 67:45, 1981.
27. Chany, C., D. Mathieu, and A. Gregoire: Induction of $\Delta^4{}_3$ ketosteroid synthesis by interferon in mouse adrenal tumor cell cultures. J Gen Virol 50:447, 1980.
28. Lawrence, T.S., W.H. Beers, and N.B. Gilula: Transmission of hormonal stimulation by cell to cell communication. Nature 272:501, 1978.
29. Johnson, H.M. and S. Baron: Evaluation of effects of interferon and interferon inducers on the immune response. Pharmac Ther A 1:349, 1977.
30. Johnson, H.M. and J.E. Blalock: Interferon immunosuppression: Medication by a suppressor factor. Infect Immun 29:301, 1980.

24. The Use of Combination Therapies to Enhance Interferon Action

W. Robert Fleischmann, Jr.,[a] *and Srecko Koren*[b]

[a]Department of Microbiology, University of Texas Medical Branch, Galveston, TX 77550; [b]Medical Faculty, Institute of Microbiology, Ljubljana, Yugoslavia

INTRODUCTION

Interferons are a family of induced cellular proteins which were originally named for their ability to block virus replication (1). Interferons have since been recognized to have immunoregulatory and antiproliferative activities, as well (2). Three types of interferons have been identified in murine and human systems: IFN-α, IFN-β, and IFN-γ (3).

Recently, considerable attention has focused on the possibility of using interferons as therapeutic agents in the control of viral diseases and malignancies. Other reviews in this volume detail clinical trials with interferons against a broad range of malignancies and viral diseases. These studies show that interferons have considerable promise for the control of certain diseases such as hairy cell leukemia, juvenile laryngeal papillomatosis, condylomata acuminata, and hepatitis (see other chapters of this volume). However, interferons have not been found to be highly active against most of the malignancies and viral diseases studied. Further, interferon treatment is not without side effects.

A major challenge for the future will be to employ methods in the clinic which will enhance interferon activities while moderating the side effects. This report describes three studies which seek to address this challenge: (i) treatment with IFN-γ combined with either IFN-α or IFN-β to potentiate interferon's activities; (ii) treatment with hyperthermia combined with interferon to enhance interferon's activities; and, (iii) treatment with colony stimulating factors combined with interferon to reduce interferon's bone marrow suppressive effect.

RESULTS AND DISCUSSION

Studies with Combined Interferons Treatment

Potentiation of interferon activity was originally discovered in the murine system as a greater than additive enhancement of interferon's antiviral action by combinations of MuIFN-α/β and MuIFN-γ (4). Combinations of MuIFN-α/β and MuIFN-γ were also found to potentiate the antiproliferative (5) and antitumor (6) activities of the interferons.

Next, the roles of the individual interferons were addressed. Studies demonstrated that combinations of IFN-γ and IFN-α and combinations of IFN-γ and IFN-β potentiated interferon's action (7). The level of potentiation was found to be dependent on the concentrations of each of the interacting interferons, suggesting that they had a mutually synergistic interaction (5,8). Combinations of IFN-α and IFN-β have only an additive interaction. An example of the potency and the mutual synergistic interactions of the combined interferons is shown for a cloning study with murine B-16 melanoma cells in Table 1. As can be seen, potentiation levels increased with increasing concentrations of each of the interferons. It can also be noted that the 214-fold potentiation observed with the highest concentrations of interferons employed does not appear to represent a maximum level of potentiation achievable, since there is no hint of a plateau effect.

In light of the high potency of combination interferons against the growth of cells in culture, it was important to determine whether combinations of interferons were as potent against normal cells as against malignant cells. Thus, studies employing two paired sets of nonmalignant and malignant cells of murine epidermal origin were initiated (9). As seen in Table 2, the combination interferon treatment had only a slight effect on the growth of the nonmalignant cells and was much more potent against the malignant cells. Thus, combination interferon treatment appeared to provide a highly potent effect which was able to discriminate between nonmalignant and malignant cells.

Combination interferon studies were then extended to the human system. The results of these in vitro studies with human cells paralleled those observed with the murine system (7). Potentiation was observed for each of the human interferon activities examined: antiviral activity (7), antiproliferative activity (7), and NK-cell activation (10).

Early studies on potentiation had employed crude or 200-fold partially purified IFN-γ. Thus, there was some question as to whether the potentiating factor in the IFN-γ preparation was IFN-γ or a comigrating, contaminating protein. Studies by ourselves (11,12) and others (13) with recombinant DNA-derived interferons of murine and human origin have conclusively shown that the potentiating factors in both murine and human IFN-γ preparations are the IFN-γ molecules themselves.

Most recently, experiments have sought to quantitate potentiation in vivo in the mouse (14). Panel A of Figure 1 compares the efficacies of IFN-α and IFN-γ employed separately and in combination. Treatment with 1875 units/day of IFN-α and 83 units/day of IFN-γ separately had little or no protective effect on the survival times of mice inoculated with B-16 melanoma. However, the combined treatment with these interferons had a protective effect approximately equivalent to that of 7500 units/day of IFN-α or 332 units/day of IFN-γ (X + X = 4X; therefore, 2-fold potentiation). Panel B shows the protective effects of 7500 units/day of IFN-α and 332 units/day of IFN-γ employed separately and in combination. The combination of these interferons had a protective effect approximately equivalent to that of 60,000 units/day of IFN-α (X + X = 8X; therefore, 4-fold potentiation). It can be noted that this estimate of potentiation is a conservative one, since 30% of the mice treated with the combination of 7500 units/day of IFN-α and 332 units/day of IFN-γ survived longer than 100 days, while none of the mice treated with 60,000 units/day of IFN-α survived. Nearly identical results were observed for combinations of IFN-β and IFN-γ.

Taken together, the in vitro and in vivo studies provide a basis for the suggestion that combination interferon therapy may be useful in the control of at least some viral diseases and malignancies in man.

<u>Studies with Combined Hyperthermia and Interferon Treatment</u>.

Clinical trials have shown that fever is a frequent side effect of interferon therapy. The question arose as to whether fever was an unnecessary side effect which should be controlled, or whether it was important for interferon's potency. In vitro studies in the human system with IFN-α and IFN-β suggested that hyperthermia within the range observed for fevers in clinical trials (39.5°C), could enhance interferon activities up to 5-fold (14-17). In vivo studies in the murine system also supported an important role for fever in the antitumor activity of interferon (18,19).

The relative effects of hyperthermia on the antiproliferative activities of IFN-α, IFN-β, and IFN-γ against murine B-16 melanoma cells were studied in vitro (20). As shown in Figure 2, hyperthermia had only a slight effect on the antiproliferative activities of IFN-α and IFN-β. However, hyperthermia had a highly potent effect on the antiprolifera- tive activity of IFN-γ (14-fold enhancement). The effect of hyper- thermia on IFN-γ was shown to be synergistic and the degree of that synergism was shown to increase with increasing IFN-γ concentration.

Next, the effect of hyperthermia on the already potent antiproliferative activity of combination interferon treatment was examined in the murine system. The antiproliferative activities of various combinations of IFN-α/β and IFN-γ against B-16 melanomas were determined at 37.3°C and at 39.4°C and compared (21). Table 3 illustrates the enhanced potency of combination interferon treatment at the elevated temperature. For example, the antiproliferative activity of the combination of 83 units/ml of IFN-α/β and 8.3

units/ml of IFN-γ is enhanced 153-fold by hyperthermia. It should be noted that the activities of these concentrations of interferons are only potentiated 5.7-fold by their use in combination at 37.3°C. Thus, hyperthermia appears to enhance the antiproliferative activity of combination interferon treatment.

These studies must be extended in vitro in the human system and in vivo in the murine system before their value for the clinic can be accurately assessed. However, they do raise the possibilities that fever may be an important component in the antitumor activity of interferons and that the intentional combination of controlled hyperthermia and interferon therapy may provide a high potent antitumor effect.

Studies with Combined Colony Stimulating Factor-1 and Interferon Treatment.

Interferons have been shown to cause a myelosuppressive effect in clinical trials (22-24). In vitro and in vivo mouse models for this myelosuppressive effect have been developed.

In an in vitro study, interferon has been shown to suppress the cloning of murine bone marrow cells in a bone marrow colony growth assay (25). This suppression has been shown to be reversed by the concommitant treatment of bone marrow cells with L-cell conditioned medium which contains colony stimulating factor-1 (25). A more recent study has employed partially purified CSF-1 to determine whether CSF-1 blocked all of interferon's activities or just its bone marrow suppressive activity. Each of the three types of interferons was combined with CSF-1 for antiviral and antiproliferative studies. The data show that, while CSF-1 antagonized the in vitro bone marrow suppressive effects of each of the interferons, it did not antagonize the antiviral or antiproliferative activities of the interferons (26).

In an in vivo mouse study, all three interferons were shown to cause myelosuppression in a dose dependent manner (27). MuIFN-γ was 50-fold and 100-fold more potent than MuIFN-α and MuIFN-β, respectively, based on antiviral titers. Reductions in the total WBC count of up to 40% were observed. The reductions were rapidly established, with maximum suppression occurring with as few as three days of interferon treatment. Further, the reduction in WBC counts was a general one, with similar percent reductions in the numbers of lymphocytes, polymorpho- nuclear leukocytes, and monocytes.

Using the in vivo mouse model, the ability of CSF-1 to block the interferon-mediated suppression of the WBC count was examined (27). As shown in Table 4, treatment with CSF-1 alone did not affect the total WBC count, but it did cause a shift in the relative ratios of the leukocytes, decreasing the relative percentage of lymphocytes and increasing the percentages of polymorphonuclear leukocytes and monocytes. Combined treatment with CSF-1 and the interferons blocked the myelosuppressive activity of each of the three interferons and maintained the total WBC counts at control levels. This blockade was primarily due to large increases in the percentages of polymorphonuclear leukocytes and monocytes. The numbers of lymphocytes in mice treated with CSF-1 and interferon were not significantly enhanced relative to their numbers in mice treated with interferon alone.

More work is needed before the clinical value of CSF-1 treatment for the blockade of interferon-mediated myelosuppression can be accurately assessed. However, the data do support the concept that the simultaneous administration of colony stimulating factors and interferons may be of some use in moderating the myelosuppressive effects of interferons during interferon therapy for viral disease and malignancies.

SUMMARY

Three possible means for enhancing the efficacy of interferon therapy have been studied. First, IFN-γ can be employed in combination with either IFN-α or IFN-β to synergistically enhance or potentiate the antiviral activity, the NK cell activation ability, and the antiprolif- erative activity of the interferons. Second, hyperthermia can be employed together with interferons, particularly IFN-γ alone or in combination with IFN-α or IFN-β to synergistically enhance the antiproliferative activity of the interferons. Third, colony stimulating factor-1 can be employed in combination with interferons to moderate the bone marrow suppressive effects of the interferons.

ACKNOWLEDGEMENTS

This work was supported in part by grant number CA 26475, awarded by the National Cancer Institute, United States Department of Health and Human Services and by grant number IFN-3 from the American Cancer Society. S.K. was supported by a James W. McLaughlin Postdoctoral Fellowship.

REFERENCES

1. Issacs, A. and J. Lindenmann: Virus interference. 1. The interferon. Proc Roy Soc Lond B 147:258, 1957.
2. Baron, S., F. Dianzani, G.J. Stanton, and W.R. Fleischmann, Jr.: Introduction. In: The Interferon System: A Current Review, S. Baron, F. Dianzani, G.J. Stanton, and W.R. Fleischmann, Jr., eds. The University of Texas Press, Austin, p. 1, 1986.
3. Stewart, W.E.II, J.E. Blalock, D.C. Burke, C. Chany, J.K. Dunnick, E. Falcoff, R.M. Friedman, G.J. Galasso, W.K. Joklik, J.T. Vilcek, J.S. Youngner, and K.C. Zoon: Interferon nomenclature. Nature (Lond) 125:2353, 1980.
4. Fleischmann, W.R. Jr., J.A. Georgiades, L.C. Osborne, and H.M. Johnson: Potentiation of interferon action by mixed preparations of fibroblast and immune interferon. Infect Immun 26:248, 1979.
5. Fleischmann, W.R. Jr.: Potentiation of the direct anticellular activity of mouse interferons: Mutual synergism and interferon concentration dependence. Cancer Res 42:869, 1982.

6. Fleischmann, W.R. Jr., K. Kleyn, and S. Baron: Potentiation of antitumor effect of virus-induced interferon by mouse immune interferon preparations. JNCI 65:963, 1980.
7. Fleischmann, W.R. Jr., L.A. Schwarz, and C.M. Fleischmann: Requirement for IFN-gamma in potentiation of interferon's antiviral and anticellular activities: Identity of mouse and human systems. J Interferon Res 4:265, 1984.
8. Schwarz, L.A., C.M. Fleischmann, and W.R. Fleischmann, Jr.: Potentiation of interferon's antiviral activity by the mutually synergistic interaction of MuIFN-α/β and MuIFN-γ. J Biol Response Mod 3:608, 1984.
9. Fleischmann, W.R. Jr., R.C. Newton, C.M. Fleischmann, N.H. Colburn, and M.M. Brysk: Discrimination between nonmalignant and malignant cells by combinations of IFN-gamma plus IFN-alpha/beta. J Biol Response Mod 3:397, 1984.
10. Weigent, D.A., M.P. Langford, W.R. Fleischmann, Jr., and G.J. Stanton: Potentiation of lymphocyte natural killing by mixtures of alpha or beta with recombinant gamma interferon. Infect Immun 40:35-38, 1983.
11. Fleischmann, W.R. Jr., and C.M. Fleischmann: Potentiating effect of murine interferon-gamma-containing lymphokine preparations on the antiviral and antiproliferative effects of murine interferon-alpha/beta: Identification of the potentiation factor as murine interferon-gamma itself. Antiviral Res 4:221, 1984.
12. Fleischmann, W.R. Jr., C.M. Fleischmann, and W. Fiers: Potentiation of interferon action by mixtures of recombinant DNA-derived human interferons. Antiviral Res 4:357, 1984.
13. Czarniecki, C.W., C.W. Fennie, D.B. Powers, and D.A. Estell: Synergistic antiviral and antiproliferative activities of Escherichia coli-derived human alpha, beta, and gamma interferons. J Virol 49:490, 1984.
14. Koren, S. and W.R. Fleischmann, Jr.: Quantitation of in vivo potentiation resulting from combined interferon therapy: Antitumor effect against B-16 melanoma cells in mice. J Interferon Res, in press.
15. Heron, I. and K. Berg: The actions of interferon are potentiation at elevated temperatures. Nature 274:508, 1978.
16. Hirai, N., N.O. Hill, and K. Osther: Temperature influences on different human alpha interferon activities. J Interferon Res 4:507, 1984.
17. Groveman, D.S., E.C. Borden, J.A. Merritt, H.I. Robins, R. Steeves, and G.T. Bryan: Augmented antiproliferative effects of interferons at elevated temperature against human bladder carcinoma cell lines. Cancer Res 44:5517, 1984.
18. Yerushalmi, A., M.G. Tovey, and I. Gresser: Antitumor effect of combined interferon and hyperthermia in mice. Proc Soc Exp Biol Med 169:413, 1982.
19. Robins, H.I.: Role of whole-body hyperthermia in the treatment of neoplastic disease: Its current status and future prospects. Cancer Res (Suppl) 44:4878s, 1984.
20. Fleischmann, W.R. Jr., C.M. Fleischmann, and T.D. Gindhart: Effect of hyperthermia on the antiproliferative activities of murine α-, β-, and γ-interferon: Differential enhancement of murine γ-interferon. Cancer Res 46:8, 1986.

21. Fleischmann, W.R. Jr., C.M. Fleischmann, and T.D. Gindhart: Effect of hyperthermia on combination interferon treatment: Enhancement of the antiproliferative activity against murine B-16 melanoma. Cancer Res 46:1722, 1986.
22. Louie, A.C., J.C. Gallager, K. Sikora, R. Levy, S.A. Rosenberg, and T.C. Merigan: Follow-up observations on the effect of human leukocyte interferon on non-Hodgkin's lymphoma. Blood 58:712, 1981.
23. Sherwin, S.A., J.A. Knost, S. Fein, P.G. Abrams, K.A. Foon, J.J. Ochs, C. Schoenberger, A.E. Maluish, and R.K. Oldham: A multiple phase I trial of recombinant leukocyte A interferon in cancer patients. JAMA 248:2461, 1982.
24. Billiau, A.: The pharmokinetics and toxicology of interferon. In: Interferons: From molecular biology to clinical application, D.C. Burke and A.G. Morris, eds. Cambridge University Press, Cambridge, p. 255, 1983.
25. Klimpel, G.R., W.R. Fleischmann, Jr., K.D. Klimpel: Gamma interferon (IFN-γ) and IFN-α/β suppress murine myeloid colony formation (CFU-C): Magnitude of suppression is dependent upon the level of colony stimulating factor (CSF). J Immunol 129:76, 1982.
26. Koren, S., G.R. Klimpel, and W.R. Fleischmann, Jr.: Macrophage colony stimulating factor (CSF-1) blocks the myeloid suppressive but not the antiviral or antiproliferative activities of murine alpha, beta, and gamma interferons in vitro. J Biol Response Mod, in press.
27. Koren, S., G.R. Klimpel, and W.R. Fleischmann, Jr.: Treatment of mice with macrophage colony stimulating factor (CSF-1) prevents the in vivo myelosuppression induced by murine alpha, beta, and gamma interferons. J Biol Response Mod, in press.

TABLE 1. Fold Potentiation of the Antiproliferative Activity of Interferons Observed for Various Concentrations of Interferons.

IFN-γ Concentration	IFN-α/β Concentration 29 U/ml	88 U/ml	260 U/ml
0.7 U/ml	5.5	5.7	3.6
2.1 U/ml	5.0	5.5	7.5
6.2 U/ml	4.9	10	67
19 U/ml	3.8	25	214

[Adapted and reproduced with permission from Fleischmann, Cancer Res. 42:869 (1982)]

TABLE 2. Antiproliferative activity of combination interferon treatments against nonmalignant and malignant cells.[a]

Cell Pair Treated	IFN Treatment IFN-α/β (500 U/ml)	IFN-γ (50 U/ml)	Fold Inhibition Nonmalignant Cells	Malignant Cells
D-1/D-11a	–	+	0.9	1.4
	+	–	1.1	2.2
	+	+	1.9	6.0
JB-1/JB-8	–	+	1.0	1.6
	+	–	1.8	2.4
	+	+	2.4	18

[a][Adapted and reproduced with permission from FLEISCHMANN et al., J. Biol. Response Mod. 3:397 (1984)].

Table 3. Synergistic enhancement of interferon's antiproliferative effect by combination interferon treatment at hyperthermic temperature

IFN-γ concentration (units/ml)	Parameter	IFN-α/β concentration 28 units/ml	83 units/ml	250 units/ml
0.31	Observed % of clones at 39.4°C	27.5	18.5	7.3
	Expected % of clones at 37.3°C	72.4	63.8	41.1
	Fold potentiation and enhancement	2.6	3.4	5.6
0.93	Observed % of clones at 39.4°C	14.0	7.3	1.5
	Expected % of clones at 37.3°C	67.5	59.5	38.3
	Fold potentiation and enhancement	4.8	8.2	26
2.8	Observed % of clones at 39.4°C	3.5	1.5	0.75
	Expected % of clones at 37.3°C	65.4	57.6	37.1
	Fold potentiation and enhancement	19	38	50
8.3	Observed % of clones at 39.4°C	1.5	0.25	0
	Expected % of clones at 37.3°C	43.5	38.3	24.7
	Fold potentiation and enhancement	29	153	IND[a]

[a] IND, indeterminant.

[Reproduced with permission from Fleischmann, et al., Cancer Res. 46:1722 (1986).]

TABLE 4. Effect of Mu Interferon and CSF-1 Treatment on the WBC Differential Count

		Absolute Number of Cells[1]			Relative Number of Cells (%)	
		Control	CSF-1	Statistical Significance	Control	CSF-1
Lymphocytes	Control	10,222± 930[2]	7,725±1,764	$p<0.025$[3]	88.0±3.0	76.5±3.2
	MuIFN-α	7,222±1,022	8,068± 809	NS	87.6±1.8	68.5±3.7
	MuIFN-β	6,882±1,078	7,659±1,050	NS	86.8±2.8	71.3±6.3
	MuIFN-γ	6,004±1,325	7,391±1,210	NS	86.2±3.1	72.4±5.4
Segmented Polymorphonuclear Leukocytes	Control	1,015± 346	1,817± 461	$p<0.025$	8.8±3.1	18.0±2.9
	MuIFN-α	803± 164	3,071± 693	$p<0.001$	9.8±1.8	26.0±4.9
	MuIFN-β	813± 322	2,421± 814	$p<0.005$	10.0±2.8	22.5±6.6
	MuIFN-γ	732± 255	2,096± 342	$p<0.001$	10.6±1.9	20.8±4.0
Monocytes	Control	298± 56	595± 174	$p<0.01$	2.6±0.5	5.8±0.4
	MuIFN-α	213± 54	681± 82	$p<0.001$	2.6±0.5	5.8±1.0
	MuIFN-β	274± 82	750± 197	$p<0.005$	3.4±0.5	6.0±1.4
	MuIFN-γ	216± 97	703± 152	$p<0.001$	3.0±0.8	7.0±1.9

[1]Total number of each type of white blood cells/mm^3 on day 4. These values were obtained by multiplying the differential percentage of each type of cell for each mouse by the total WBC count for each mouse. The averages and standard deviations were then determined.

[2]Mean ± standard deviation.

[3]Probabilities comparing CSF-1 treatment with control treatment were determined by Student's t-test.

[Reproduced with permission from Koren, Klimpel, and Fleischmann, J. Biol. Response Mod., in press (1986)].

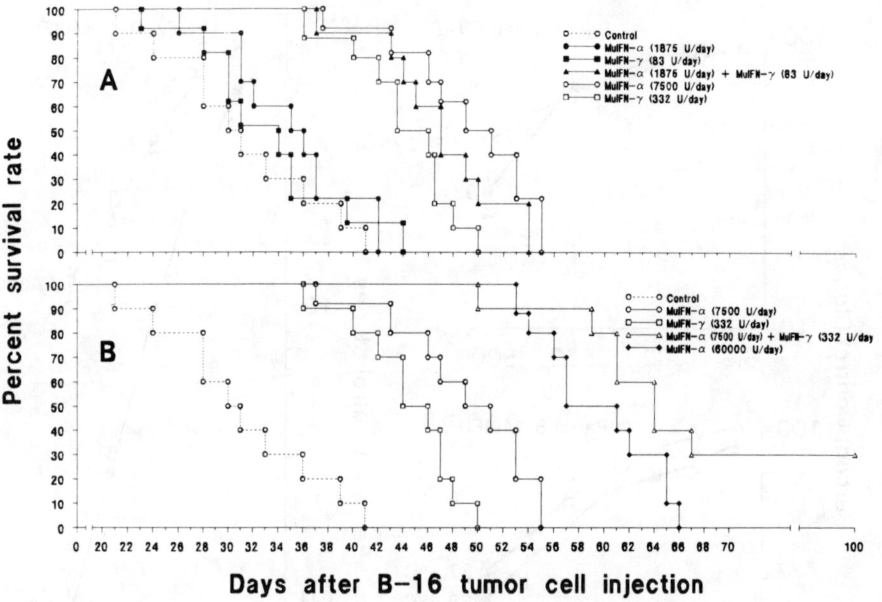

Figure 1. The effect of various concentrations of MuIFN-α and MuIFN-γ, used alone and in combination, on mortality of mice inoculated with B-16 melanoma cells. Each mouse was injected subcutaneously with 10^6 B-16 melanoma cells. Beginning 24 h later, mice were injected with 13 daily injections of mock interferon, MuIFN-α alone, MuIFN-γ alone, or different combinations of both interferon types. The survival rate was recorded until 100 days after the inoculation of tumor cells. The data were plotted as the percent survival rate for each treatment group.

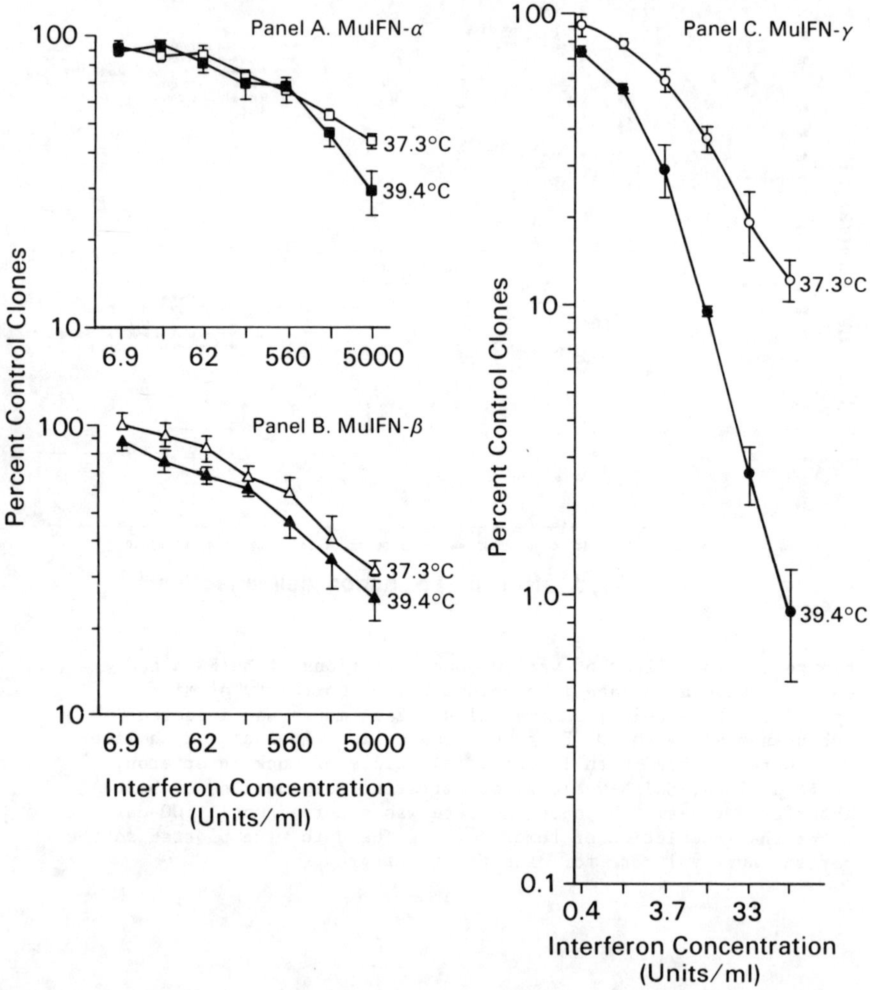

Figure 2. Effect of hyperthermia on various interferon concentrations. Log phase murine B-16 melanoma cells were plated at 300 cells/35 mm Petri dish into growth medium or serial dilutions of MuIFN-α (Panel A), MuIFN-β (Panel B), or MuIFN-γ (Panel C). Replicate sets of Petri dishes were incubated for 6 days at 37.3°C or 39.4°C in Napco Model 5300 incubators. Experiments were performed in triplicate or quadruplicate. Points: mean of three experiments; bars: standard error of the mean. [Reproduced with permission from Fleischmann, et al., Cancer Res. 46, 8 (1986)].

25. Interactions of the Interferon and Endocrine Systems

Eric M. Smith[a] and J. Edwin Blalock[b]

[a]Psychiatry and Behavioral Sciences and Microbiology, University of Texas Medical Branch, Galveston, TX 77550; [b]Physiology and Biophysics, University of Alabama at Birmingham, Birmingham, AL 35294

INTRODUCTION

A polypeptide hormone-like mode of action for interferon (IFN) is supported by its high specific activity, indirect mode of inducing antiviral activity, plus the evidence that IFN does not need to be internalized but acts through cell surface receptors (1,2,3). In the previous edition of this series, we discussed the ability of the IFN's to induce hormone-like activities in endocrine cells by activating intracellular pathways or by binding to specific hormone receptors (4). Since this was published, insight into the hormonal actions of IFN has continued. In particular, the administration of large doses of IFN and other lymphokines or biological response modifiers in clinical trials has allowed the hormone-like activities to be observed *in vivo*.

Mechanisms of IFNs Hormonal Activity

An idea that hormones and IFN might act through similar mechanisms developed when it was shown that the activity of both IFN (5) and hormones (6) could be transferred to receptor-less cells through cellular connections. The most direct way to test for a common mechanism of action was to see if IFN on hormone sensitive cells from the appropriate species would induce a hormone-like response. Mouse IFN α/β when applied to cultures of mouse myocardial cells caused a dose dependent noradrenaline-like increase in their beat frequency (7). This stimulation was species specific as HuIFN-β failed to cause an increased beat frequency. Conversely, noradrenaline (10^{-8}M or greater) induced a dose dependent IFN-like antiviral state in the mouse myocardial cells. The hormonal induction was tissue specific because noradrenaline induced antiviral activity in myocardial cells which bear α/β adrenergic receptors but not in human amnion (WISH) cells or mouse L cells which lack the receptor. Under co-culture conditions suitable for IFN induced transfer of viral resistance (7), exposure of co-cultures of mouse myocardial and human WISH cells to either HuIFN-β or noradrenaline caused an increased beat frequency in the myocardial cells and development of antiviral activity in the WISH cells, respectively. Taken together, these results strongly suggest that the effects of noradrenaline and IFN on the beat frequency and antiviral activity of mouse myocardial cells occur through a common transmissible mechanism. In contrast to many hormones, virtually all nucleated cells within a species are sensitive to that species' IFNs and presumably have IFN receptors. The ubiquitous nature of IFN receptors coupled with a common pathway(s) of IFN and hormone action predicts that IFN should have many hormonal activities (4). In fact, we expect that IFN may have as many actions as there are specialized cells on which the actions are measured. As a means to examine the generality of IFN induced hormonal responses, in vitro systems for the induction of steroidogenesis and melanogenesis were tested for induction by IFN (8). ACTH (corticotropin) and MoIFN α/β, but not HuIFN-β, induced steroid production, cell rounding, and antiviral activity in mouse adrenal tumor (Y-1) cells (8-10). ACTH and HuIFN-β, but not MoIFN α/β, induced melanin as well as an antiviral state in human melanoma (Foss) cells. Since these original studies other activities of IFN on endocrine cells have been found. IFN-α will inhibit human chorionic gonadotropin stimulation of testosterone production by porcine Leydig cells (11). Also, IFN has been found to have apparently conflicting effects on insulin production, both inhibiting (12) and inducing (13) it's production. Thus, the hormonal action of IFN and the antiviral activity of hormones appear to be a general phenomenon.

Superficially, cyclic AMP seems a candidate for the common component of the IFN and hormone systems since cyclic AMP will increase myocardial cell beat frequency (6,14,15), steroidogenesis (16), and melanogenesis (17). Although IFN can in certain conditions elevate cyclic AMP levels (18,19), cyclic AMP alone cannot account for the antiviral effects as it is not antiviral (20) and IFN does not stimulate cyclic AMP in all cells (18,19). A more likely situation is that cyclic AMP and/or other small molecules are responsible (7).

Another mode of action for IFN seems to be through activation of hormone receptors. Previously IFN has been shown to have its binding to the receptor blocked by cholera toxin and thyrotropin. Unfortunately, no biological response could be induced by these inhibitors (21-23). We had found that HuIFN-α's antiviral activity could be neutralized by an antiserum to γ-endorphin, an endogenous opiate (24) and examined the ability of IFN to bind and activate opiate receptors. This was initially determined in vitro by measuring the ability of IFN-α to compete with ^{3}H-dihydromorphine in binding to opiate receptors on the particulate fraction of mouse brain lysate (25-27). 500 antiviral units of crude HuIFN-α ($1x10^4$ U/mg) would block 50% of the specific binding of $4x10^{-9}$M ^{3}H-dihydromorphine and this inhibition was dose dependent. Neither human IFN-β or IFN-γ at similar doses bound significantly to opiate receptors.

IFN was also able to bind opiate receptors in vivo (26,27). Intracerebral injection of as little as 500 U of IFN-α induced an endorphin-like analgesia and catatonia in mice. The fact that both physical binding and biological effects were immediately reversible and preventable by the opiate antagonist, naloxone, suggests the effect was mediated through opiate receptors. Naloxone has no antiviral activity by itself and has no effect on IFN-α's antiviral activity which suggests that opiate and the IFN-α receptors are not related. Interestingly, as the IFN was purified there was a corresponding reduction in opiate receptor binding activity both *in vitro* and *in vivo* by approximately a factor of 10. Essentially homogenous IFN-α still retained opiate receptor binding activity, however, which suggested that the IFN-α preparation might contain multiple species of endorphin-related molecules. Analysis of the preparation by SDS-polyacrylamide gel electrophoresis showed the endorphin-like activity associated principally in two regions of the gel. One region was associated with IFN antiviral activity at a molecular weight range of 18,000 to 24,000 daltons (d). The majority of the endorphin-like material had no antiviral activity, and being less than 10,000 d in size seemed to correspond to β-endorphin (3623 d) or the even smaller gamma and alpha endorphins (approx. 1700 d). Recombinant HuIFN-α was also able to bind opiate receptors *in vitro* and *in vivo*. The recombinant IFN-α was similar to the purified natural IFN-α in that 4 times more antiviral units than with crude IFN-α were required to inhibit equal dihydromorphine binding. The ability of recombinant IFN-α to bind opiate receptors shows that this activity is inate to the IFN-α molecule and not just contaminants that associated with natural IFN-α. Thus, it seems that endorphin-like activity from Newcastle disease virus (NDV)-infected lymphocytes can be associated with at least 2 species of molecules, IFN and a low molecular weight endorphin-like peptide(s) both of which bind opiate receptors *in vivo* and *in vitro*. Presumably the low molecular weight endorphin-like moiety is synthesized along with a corticotropin-like molecule concommitantly with IFN (25).

Interactions Between IFN and the Neuroendocrine System

Besides analgesia and catatonia, IFN has been shown to have other opiate-like effects *in vivo*. Dafney (28) has found that IFN will prevent tolerance and dependence to morphine and natural brain opioids. HuIFN-α but not HuIFN-γ injections to morphine dependent rats significantly modifies the naloxone-induced abstinence syndrome. This response occurs in a characteristic dose-dependent manner. It is interesting to note that the dipeptide Z-Pro-D-Leu will suppress the abstinence syndrome in morphine dependent rats (29) and this peptide is part of the sequence of human IFN (30).

Gresser showed IFN could enhance the excitability of cultured neurons (31). Extending this finding, Dafney's group has shown IFN can alter single brain cell activity (32). Microiontophoretic application of HuIFN-α but not IFN-γ had an effect on cells of the sematosensory cortex, dorsal hippocampus, ventromedial hypothalmus (VMH) and the parafasciculus thalmus. Except for the VMH, IFN-α caused an increase in both the percentage of excited cells and the intensity of the firing in these structures. In the VMH, a decrease in the firing rate could be seen in the majority of the cells and an increase in the remaining 30% or so of all cells responding to the IFN-α. In another paper, comparisons of 2 IFN-α preparations and one of IFN-γ showed Cantell's HuIFN-α and Hoffman-LaRoche recombinant IFN-α were the most potent at altering brain cell firing rates (33). This was also found to be true for these two and a third preparation of IFN-α for altering naloxone-induced abstinence in morphine addicted rats (34). Thus, these and the previously described studies show IFN can directly modulate nervous system activity. This provides a possible mechanism to explain the neurological and behavioral side effects seen with application of large doses of IFN (35).

Activation of the Hypothalamic-Pituitary-Adrenal Axis by IFN and Other Biological Response Modifiers

It is well known that during infections there is a rise in circulating corticosteroid hormones (36). This rise can be initiated by injection of lymphokines containing lymphocyte culture supernatant fluids (37), which suggests it is a lymphocyte product indirectly mediating the effect. Several mechanisms seem possible. One might involve activation of the central nervous system, resulting in hypothalamic releasing hormones being produced and stimulating the pituitary-adrenal circuit. Another possibility is through lymphocyte production of a corticotropin (ACTH)-like molecule (25). We showed that NDV infection of hypophysectomized mice induced ACTH production by spleen cells (38). Presumably, this exogenous source of ACTH caused the rise in serum corticosterone, in the absence of pituitary ACTH. However, another mechanism which may have played a role in this last paradigm is IFN. IFN was probably induced by the NDV challenge and at least two laboratories have shown IFN acts directly on adrenal cells to induce steroidogenesis (8,9). Furthermore, IFN has been reported not to induce primary cultured pituitary cells to produce ACTH (N.R. Hall, personal communication). Thus, with the rise in IFN-α during a virus infection the increased corticosteroids could be a result of IFN acting on adrenal cortex cells. Injection with purified IFN in clinical trials, directly tests this hypothesis of IFN's ability to induce cortisol *in vivo*. Roosth *et al*. (39) found the serum cortisol levels of cancer patients receiving IFN to be significantly raised. The study consisted of 7 patients with solid tumors, all treated with doses of 0 to $1.2 \times 10^{(8)}$ units of recombinant IFN-α2 over a 7 week period. In comparison with a placebo injection, all patients had a significant increase in cortisol levels with $10 \times 10^{(6)}$ units or more of IFN-α2. Fifty percent of the subjects showed an increase with only 1×10^6 units of IFN.

It is interesting to compare these results with studies in which other lymphokines or biological response modifiers have been administered in clinical trials. Highly purified interleukin 2 (IL-2) when administered intravenously caused a rise in both ACTH and cortisol levels in cancer and AIDS patients (40). A thymic hormone, thymosin, will induce pituitary ACTH release and subsequent corticosteroid production *in vitro*, and *in vivo* in monkeys (41). We have found that two monokines associated with endotoxic shock and the acute phase response, IL-1 and hepatocyte stimulating factor (HSF), induce cultured pituitary cells to produce ACTH (42). HSF was over three times more potent on a molar basis than CRF, the classic inducer. Presumably, *in vivo* this would result in increased circulating cortisol levels. No specific lymphokine receptors have been identified yet on pituitary or adrenal cells but persumably they are present. Certainly in the case of IFN, most nucleated cells have surface receptors. Thus, it appears that many leukocyte products as well as IFN are capable of "signalling" or activating the neuroendocrine system.

Glucocorticoids are not the only "stress" hormones that are involved with the IFN system. ACTH, which induces glucocorticoids, will inhibit mitogen induction of IFN-γ (43) while vasopressin, a pituitary hormone and a CRF, replaces the IL-2 requirement for IFN-γ production (44). Thus, induction of the hypothalamic-pituitary-adrenal axis by IFN-γ may result in a negative feedback loop and interference with the lymphokines production. Another interaction between IFN and the neuroendocrine systems has been reported by Koff and Dunegan (44,46). ACTH completely blocked the capacity of mouse recombinant IFN-γ to activate murine peritoneal macrophages to a tumoricidal state (45). The neurotransmitters norepinephrine, vasoactive intestinal peptide, and neurotensin also modulated IFN-γ activation of macrophages. In contrast, norepinephrine and epinephrine, but not ACTH, suppress IFN-γ activation of macrophages to lyse herpes simplex virus infected cells (46). Thus, not only is IFN capable of activating the hypothalamic-pituitary-adrenal axis but it's induction and activities are sensitive to feedback from the neuroendocrine signals.

IMPLICATIONS

The hormonal activities of the IFN molecule itself, as well as the production of both IFN-α associated and non-associated hormone-like substances by IFN inducers imply that along with any antiviral, anticellular or immunomodulatory activities, the IFN system may affect the host response on a more general scale at the organ, system, or entire organism level. Contrarywise, the ability of hormones to induce antiviral activity in specialized tissues suggests that in addition to their known functions, they may protect tissues against viruses and maintain differentiation. The molecules that are classically known as hormones show intimate associations in their production and actions. Likewise, it now appears that IFN and known hormones impinge on each other's production and action. An understanding of these interactions or "side effects" may allow more effective, natural, and safer application of the IFNs.

ACKNOWLEDGEMENTS

We thank Joy Cleveland for expert technical assistance on the more recent studies and Gloria Collins for typing the manuscript. These studies were supported in part by the Office of Naval Research (#N00014-84-K-0486) and a grant from the National Institutes of Health (#AM 33839-01A1).

REFERENCES

1. Ankel, H., C. Chany, B. Galliot, M.J. Chevalier and M. Robert: Antiviral effect of interferon covalently bound to sepharose. Proc Natl Acad Sci USA 70:2360, 1973.

2. Baron, S: The biological significance of the interferon system. In: Interferon, M.B. Finter, ed. North Holland, Amsterdam, p 292-292, 1966.
3. Chany, C., H. Ankel, B. Galliot, M.J. Chevalier, and A. Gregoire: Mechanism of action and biological properties of insoluble interferon. Proc Soc Exp Biol Med 147:293, 1974.
4. Smith, E.M. and J.E. Blalock: The hormonal nature of the interferon system. Tex Rpts Biol Med 41:350, 1982.
5. Blalock, J.E. and S. Baron: Interferon-induced transfer of viral resistance. Nature 269:422, 1977.
6. Lawrence, T.S., W.H. Beers, and N.B. Gilula: Transmission of hormonal stimulation by cell-to-cell communication. Nature 272:501, 1978.
7. Blalock, J.E. and J.D. Stanton: Common pathways of interferon and hormonal action. Nature 283:406, 1980.
8. Blalock, J.E. and C. Harp: Interferon and adrenocorticotropic hormone induction of steroidogenesis, melanogenesis and antiviral activity. Arch Virol 67:45, 1981.
9. Chany, C., S. Rousset, M.F. Bourgeade, D. Mathieu and A. Gregoire: Roles of receptors and the cytoskeleton in reverse transformation and steroidogenesis induced by interferon. Ann N Y Acad Sci 350:254, 1980.
10. Campbell, J.B., J. Grunberger, M.A. Kochman, and S.L. White: A microplaque reduction assay for human and mouse interferon. Can J Microbiol 21:1247, 1975.
11. Orava, M., K. Cantell, and R. Vihko: Human leukocyte interferon inhibits human chorionic gonadotropin stimulated testosterone production by porcine Leydig cells in culture. Biochem Biophys Res Comm 127:809, 1985.
12. Shimuzu, F., M. Shimizu and K. Kamiyama: Inhibitory effect of interferon on the production of insulin. Endocrinol 117:2081, 1985.
13. Rhodes, C.J. and K.W. Taylor: Effect of human lymphoblastoid interferon on insulin synthesis and secretion in isolated human pancreatic islets. Diabetelogia 27:601, 1984.
14. Krause, E.G., W. Halle, E. Kallabis and A. Wollenberger: Positive chronotropic response of cultured isolated rat heart cells to N , 2'-O-Dibutyryl-3',5'-adenosine monophosphate. J Molec Cell Cardiol 1:1, 1970.
15. Goshina, K: Antagonistic influence of dibutyryl cyclic AMP and dibutyryl cyclic GMP on beating rate of cultured mouse myocardial cells. J Molec Cell Cardiol 8:713, 1976.
16. Schimmer, B.P: Adenylate-cyclase activity in adrenocorticotropic hormone sensitive and mutant adrenocortical tumor cell lines. J Biol Chem 247:3134, 1972.
17. Kreiner, P.W., C.J. Gold, J.J. Keirms, W.A. Brock and M.W. Bitensky: MSH-sensitive adenyl cyclase in the Cloudman melanoma. Yale J Biol med 46:583, 1973.
18. Grollman, E.F., G. Lee, S. Ramos, P.S. Lazo, H.R. Kaback, R.M. Friedman and L.D. Kohn: Relationships of structure and function of the interferon receptor to hormone receptors and establishment of the antiviral state. Can Res 38:4172, 1978.
19. Meldolesi, M.F., R.M. Friedman and L.D. Kohn: An interferon-induced increase in cyclic AMP levels precedes the establishment of the antiviral state. Biochem Biophys Res Comm 79:239, 1977.

20. Friedman, R.M. and I. Pastan: Interferon and cyclic-3',5'-adenosine monophosphate: Potentiation of antiviral activity. Biochem Biophys Res Comm 36:735, 1969.
21. Friedman, R.M. and L.D. Kohn: Cholera toxin inhibits interferon action. Biochem Biophys Res Comm 70:1078, 1976.
22. Kohn, L.D., R.M. Friedman, J.M. Holmes and G. Lee: Use of thyrotropin and cholera toxin to probe the mechanism by which interferon initiates its antiviral activity. Proc Nat Acad Sci USA 73:3695, 1976.
23. Besancon, F. and H. Ankel: Inhibition of interferon action by glycoprotein hormones. C R Acad Sci D 283:1807, 1976.
24. Blalock, J.E. and E.M. Smith: Human leukocyte interferon. Structural and biological relatedness to adrenocorticotropic hormone and endorphins. Proc Natl Acad Sci USA 77:5972, 1981.
25. Smith, E.M. and J.E. Blalock: Human lymphocyte production of corticotropin and endorphin-like substances: Association with leukocyte interferon. Proc Natl Acad Sci USA 78:7530, 1981.
26. Blalock, J.E. and E.M. Smith: Human leukocyte interferon (HuIFN-alpha): Potent endorphin-like opioid activity. Biochem Biophys Res Comm 101:472, 1981.
27. Smith, E.M., L.D. Dion and J.E. Blalock: Opiate receptor mediated effects of IFN-alpha and lymphocyte derived endorphin-like peptides. In Endocoids, H. Lal, F. LaBella and J. Lane, eds. Alan R. Liss, Inc., pp. 259-264, 1985.
28. Dafny, N: Interferon: A candidate as the endogenous substance preventing tolerance and dependence to brain opioids. Prog Neuro Psychopharmacol Biol Psychiat 8:351, 1984.
29. Walter, R., R.F. Ritzmann, H.N. Bhargava, T.C. Rainbow, L.B. Flexner and W.A. Krivoy: Induction 2-Pro-D-Leu of development of tolerance to and physical dependence on morphine in mice. Proc Natl Acad Sci USA 75:4573, 1978.
30. Wetzel, R., L.J. Perry, D.A. Estell, N. Lin, H.L. Levine, B. Shinker, F. Fields, M.J. Ross and J. Shively. Properties of human alpha-interferon purified from E. coli extracts. J Interferon Res 1:381, 1981.
31. Cavet, M.C., I. Gresser: Interferon enhances the excitability of cultured neurons. Nature 278:559, 1979.
32. Reyes-Vasquez, C., B. Prieto-Gomez, J.A. Georgiades and N. Dafny: Alpha and gamma interferons' effects on cortical and hippocampal neurons: microiontophoretic application and single cell recording. Intern J Neuroscience 25:113, 1984.
33. Dafny, N., B. Prieto-Gomez and C. Reyes-Vasquez: Does the immune system communicate with the central nervous system? J Neuroimmunol 9:1, 1985.
34. Dafny, N. and C. Reyes-Vasquez: Three different types of alpha-interferons alter naloxone-induced abstinence in morphine-addicted rats. Immuno Pharmacol 9:13, 1985.
35. Blalock, J.E. and E.M. Smith: Structure and function relationship of interferon (IFN) and neuroendocrine hormones. In: The Biology of the Interferon System, E. DeMayer, G. Galasso and H. Schellekens, eds. Elsevier/North Holland Biomedical Press, 1981.
36. Munck, A., P.M. Guyre and N.J. Holbrook: Physiological functions of glucocorticoids in stress and their relation to pharmacological actions. Endocrine Reviews 5:25, 1984.

37. Besedovsky, H.O., A. del Rey, and E. Sorkin: Lymphokine-containing supernatants from Con-A stimulated cells increase corticosterone blood levels. J Immunol 126:385, 1981.
38. Smith, E.M., W.J. Meyer and J.E. Blalock: Virus-induced corticosterone in hypophysectomized mice: A possible lymphoid adrenal axis. Science 218:1311, 1982.
39. Roosth, J., R.B. Pollard, S.L. Brown and W.J. Meyer: cortisol stimulation by recombinant interferon alpha 2. J Neuroimmunol in press, 1986.
40. Lotze, M.T., L.W. Frana, S.O. Sharrow, R.J. Robb and S.A. Rosenberg: In vivo administration of purified human interleukin 2. J Immunol 134:157, 1985.
41. Healy, D.L., G.D. Hodgen, H.M. Schulte, G.P. Chrousos, D.L. Loriaux, N.R. Hall and A.L. Goldstein: The thymus-adrenal connection: Thymosin has corticotropin-releasing activity in primates. Science 222:1353, 1983.
42. Woloski, B.M.R.N.J., E.M. Smith, W.J. Meyer, F.M. Fuller and J.E. Blalock: Corticotropin-releasing activity of monokines. Science 230:1035, 1985.
43. Johnson, H.M., B.A. Torres, E.M. Smith, L.D. Dion, and J.E. Blalock: Regulation of lymphokine (γ-interferon) production by corticotropin. J Immunol 132:246, 1984.
44. Johnson, H.M., W.L. Farrar, and B.A. Torres: Vasopressin replacement of interleukin 2 requirement in gamma interferon production: Lymphokine acitivity of a neuroendocrine hormone. J Immunol 129:983, 1982.
45. Koff, W.C. and M.A. Dunegan: Modulation of macrophage-mediated tumoricidal activity by neuropeptides and neurohormones. J Immunol 135:350, 1985.
46. Koff, W.C. and M.A. Dunegan: Neuroendocrine hormones suppress macrophage-mediated lysis of herpes simplex virus-infected cells. J Immunol 136:705, 1986.

26. Interferon as a Regulator of Hematopoiesis

Gary R. Klimpel and Victor E. Reyes

Department of Microbiology, University of Texas Medical Branch, Galveston, TX 77550

INTRODUCTION

The mechanism(s) underlying the regulation of normal hematopoiesis and hematologic disorders, such as aplastic anemia, have been studied intensely during the past several years. The development of *in vitro* and *in vivo* assay systems for measuring different aspects of hematopoiesis has led to the discovery of a number of different lymphokines, monokines, and cytokines which are believed to play important roles in regulating the survival, proliferation, and terminal differentiation of different hematopoietic progenitor cells (1,2). The type of mature cells which develop in the presence of these factors determines the nomenclature of these glycoproteins. In the murine system, colony stimulating factors (CSF) which stimulate the growth of progenitor cells of neutrophil-granulocyte (G-CSF), of macrophages (M-CSF or CSF-1), of macrophages and granulocytes (GM-CSF), and of mixed colonies containing erythrocytes, granulocytes, macrophages, and megakaryocytes (interleukin 3, IL3) have been purified to homogeneity, their genes sequenced, and their receptors characterized (1,2). Although much has been learned about the *in vitro* growth and differentiation of different progenitor cells, the regulation of these differentiation processes by lymphocytes and/or lymphokines is still not completely understood. Recently, different interferons (IFN) have been identified as potentially important molecules for regulating different aspects of hematopoiesis. These observations, made by many different laboratories (3-6), are discussed in regards to the important questions of: a) What regulates hematopoietic cell differentiation and gene expression? and b) What goes wrong with the normal control mechanisms in hematologic malignancy?

Suppressive Effects of IFNs on Hematopoiesis

It is now well established that IFNα, IFNβ, and/or IFNγ can inhibit different aspects of hematopoiesis both *in vitro* (3-6) and *in vivo* (7-10). IFNγ and/or IFNα/β have been shown to inhibit murine myeloid progenitor cells (6,11). This inhibition was believed to be mediated by the well established antiproliferative effect of the different IFNs. Murine pluripotent hematopoietic stem cells have also been shown to be inhibited by IFNα/β (12). *In vivo* administration of IFNs also has been shown to be myelosuppressive (7-10). Koren et al. (8) have shown that significant myelosuppression occurs *in vivo* after mice were given MuIFNα, MuIFNβ, or MuIFNγ. *In vivo* administration of IFN to irradiated mice was also shown to completely inhibit the proliferation of injected syngeneic bone marrow cells (7). Recently, we have shown that mice undergoing graft versus host disease have high levels of IFNα/β in their sera and have proposed that this IFN may contribute to bone marrow failure which is associated with GVHD (13).

Human recombinant IFNα, IFNβ, and IFNγ have been shown to be potent suppressors of myeloid colony formation. *In vitro* colony formation of human bone marrow granulocyte-macrophage (CFU-GM), erythroid (BFU-E), and multipotential (CFU-GEMM) progenitor cells is inhibited by these IFNs (3-5). In fact, patients who receive IFNα or IFNγ for therapeutic purposes commonly develop some degree of granulocytopenia and thrombocytopenia (9,10).

The magnitude of hematopoietic suppression observed in both human and murine systems appears to be dependent upon the concentration of other growth factors present in the assay. In both human and murine assays for myeloid differentiation, the suppressive action of IFN can be antagonized by increasing the concentration of CSF (3,6). *In vitro* suppression by IFN was most dramatic when suboptimal concentrations of CSF were used in these assays. Recently, CSF has also been shown to antagonize the myelosuppressive effects of murine IFNs *in vivo* (8).

Although the above studies document recombinant IFN as acting directly upon a hematopoietic cell, IFN may also effect hematopoiesis by an indirect effect through activation of different suppressor cell circuits (15,16) and/or natural killer (NK) cells (17). Thus, in severe hematopoietic suppression both IFN and a suppressor cell may be required.

IFN and Aplastic Anemia

Both clinical and laboratory observations have implicated IFN as a mediator of hematopoietic suppression in aplastic anemia (2). Circulating IFN has been found in 40-50% of patients with aplastic anemia (20). More importantly, high levels of IFNγ were found in bone marrow sera from these patients (20). Myeloid and erythroid colony formation by aplastic bone marrow was improved when antisera to IFNγ was included in the *in vitro* cultures (2,19). Suppressor T lymphocytes (HLA-DR$^+$, OKT8$^+$, Tac$^+$) present in the bone marrow of aplastic anemia patients have been shown to spontaneously produce IFNγ and to mediate suppression of myeloid and erythroid progenitor colony formation (18). Peripheral blood T lymphocytes obtained from these patients or mitogen-stimulated T lymphocytes from normal individuals have also been shown to inhibit colony formation by bone marrow myeloid and erythroid progenitor cells. Suppression mediated by these T cells was shown to be mediated by IFNγ and possibly by IFNα (18). The possibility that IFN acts on suppressor cells, that other factors are acting in concert with IFN, and/or that synergistic interactions are occurring between different IFNs or between IFNs and other factors have not been clearly addressed with regards to aplastic anemia patients.

Synergistic Effects of Different IFNs on Suppressing Hematopoiesis

Immune IFN (IFNγ) has been shown to be a more potent mediator of antitumor and antiproliferative activities than IFNα or IFNβ (21- 23). Further, combinations of IFNγ with either IFNα or IFNβ interact synergistically to enhance the antiviral and antitumor activities of IFN (21-23). IFNγ is also more potent than IFNα or IFNβ at suppressing human and murine in vitro CFU-GM (5,6). Additionally, murine IFNγ is significantly more potent than IFNα or IFNβ at inducing in vivo myelosuppression (8). Mixtures containing IFNγ and IFNα or IFNβ have synergistic effects on the suppression of both human (4) and murine (6) in vitro CFU-GM. Recently, IFNγ was shown to act synergistically with a factor from NK cells at inhibiting in vitro CFU-GM (17). In addition, IFNγ and lymphotoxin (LT) or tumor necrosis factor (TNF) act synergistically in suppressing tumor cell growth (24). Synergistic interactions between different IFNs or between IFNγ and other factors which suppress hematopoietic cells may have important implications in normal hematopoietic regulation, in certain disease processes, and in clinical trials in which IFNs are used to treat patients with certain malignancies.

IFN as a Mediator of Hematopoietic Differentiation.

IFNγ has been shown to be highly immunosuppressive for both humoral and cell-mediated immune responses (25,26). IFNγ, however, also appears to be necessary for many cell-mediated immune responses. For example, IFNγ production is necessary for the in vitro (27) and in vivo (28) generation of alloantigen induced cytotoxic effector T cells. Although IFNs have been shown to suppress different aspects of hematopoiesis, low levels of IFN may play an important role in normal hematopoiesis. The presence of IFN in normal bone marrow sera and in the supernatant of long-term cultures of bone marrow cells supports this possibility (20). In this regard, Moore et al. (28) have shown that CSF induces low levels of IFNα/β production in mouse bone marrow cells and that this IFNα/β is important in the initial differentiation of newly propagated mononuclear phagocytes. Additionally, IFN-pretreated bone marrow cells have an enhanced responsiveness to CSF (29). Thus, regulated production of low levels of IFN may be a necessary prerequisite for differentiation of different hematopoietic progenitor cells. In this regard, IFN could act as a regulator of hematopoiesis by activating genes which encode for growth factors or their receptors.

IFN Production by Bone Marrow Cells Stimulated with IL2

We have previously shown that alloantigen stimulation of mouse bone marrow cells results in high levels of IFNα/β production (30). Optimal production of IFNα/β by alloantigen stimulated bone marrow cells was dependent upon T cells resident in the bone marrow (31). We postulated that this IFNα/β production by bone marrow cells may play an important role in graft versus host disease (GVHD) and/or in regulation of hematopoiesis.

Recently, we have shown that IL2 is necessary for alloantigen-induced IFNα/β production and that mouse IL2 or recombinant human IL2 can induce high levels of IFNα/β production in mouse bone marrow cells in the absence of alloantigen (32). T cell-depleted bone marrow cells or bone marrow cells from nude mice were also shown to produce high levels of IFNα/β when cultured with IL2 (Table 1). This response was completely inhibited when cultures contained antisera to IL2 or to the mouse IL2 receptor (Table 2). Thus, non-T cells resident in the bone marrow appear to have receptors for IL2 and are involved in IFN synthesis upon IL2 stimulation. These results suggest that IL2 production in the bone marrow by activated T cells may contribute to hemopoietic suppression by inducing IFNα/β production.

In summary, IFN and/or lymphokines which induce IFN production play a more important role in the regulation of hematopoiesis than previously suspected.

REFERENCES

1. Whetton, A.D. and T.M. Dexter: Haemopoietic growth factors. Trends in Biochem 11:207, 1986.
2. Zoumbos, N., E. Raefsky, and N. Young: Lymphokine regulation of hemopoiesis. Prog Hematology XIV:201, 1986.
3. Raefsky, E.L., L.C. Platanias, N. Zoumbos, and N.S. Young: Studies of interferon as a regulator of hematopoietic cell proliferation. J Immunol 135:2507, 1985.
4. Broxmeyer, H.E., S. Cooper, B.Y. Rubin, and M.W. Taylor: The synergistic influence of human interferon γ and interferon α on suppression of hematopoietic progenitor cells is additive with the enhanced senstitivty of these cells to inhibition by interferons at low oxygen tension *in vitro*. J Immunol 135:2502, 1985.
5. Rigby, W.F.L., E.D. Ball, P.M. Geyre, and M.W. Fanger: The effects of recombinant DNA-derived interferons on the growth of myeloid progenitor cells. Blood 65:858, 1985.
6. Klimpel, G.R., W.R. Fleischmann, K.D. Klimpel: Gamma interferon (IFNγ) and IFNα/β suppress murine myeloid colony formation (CFU-C): Magnitude of suppression is dependent upon the level of colony-stimulating factor (CSF). J Immunol 129:76, 1982.
7. Cerottini, J.C., K.T. Brunner, P. Lindahl, and I. Gresser: Inhibitory effect of interferon preparations and inducers in the multiplication of transplanted allogeneic spleen cells and syngeneic bone marrow cells. Nature 242:152, 1973.
8. Koren, S., G.R. Klimpel, and W.R. Fleischmann, Jr.: Treatment of mice with macrophage colony stimulating factor (CSF-1) prevents the *in vivo* myelosuppression induced by murine alpha, beta, and gamma interferons. J Biol Resp Mod, in press.
9. Gutterman, J.U., S. Fine, J. Quesada, et al.: Recombinant leukocyte A interferon: Pharmacokinetics, single dose tolerance, and biological effects in cancer patients. Ann Int Med 96:549, 1982.

10. Gutterman, J.U., M.G. Rosenblum, A. Rios, H.A. Fritsche, and J.R. Quesada: Pharmacokinetic study of partially pure γ-interferon in cancer. Cancer Res 44:4164, 1984.
11. Dandoy, F., E. DeMaeyer, and J. DeMaeyer-Guignard: Antiproliferative action of interferon on murine bone marrow-derived macrophages is influenced by genotype of the marrow donor. J Interferon Res 1:263, 1981.
12. Gidali, J., I. Feher, and M. Talas: Proliferation inhibition of murine pluripotent haemopoietic stem cells by interferon or poly I:C. Cell Tissue Kinet 14:1, 1981.
13. Reyes, V.E. and G.R. Klimpel: Interferon (IFN) α/β synthesis during acute graft vs. host disease. Transplantation, in press.
14. Verma, P.S., G. Spitzer, A.R. Zander, J.U. Gutterman, K.B. McCredie, K.A. Dicki, and D.A. Johnson: Human leukocyte interferon preparations mediated block of granulopoietic differentiation in vitro. Exp Hematol 9:63, 1981.
15. Schnaper, H.W., T. Aune, and C.W. Pierce: Suppressor T cell activation by human leukocyte interferon. J Immunol 131:2301, 1983.
16. Aune, T.M. and C.W. Pierce: Activation of a suppressor T cell pathway by interferon. Proc Natl Acad Sci USA 79:3808, 1982.
17. Deoliantoni, G., M. Murphy, M. Kobayashi, M.K. Francis, B. Perussia, and G. Trinchieri: Natural killer (NK) cell-derived hematopoietic colony-inhibiting activity and NK cytotoxic factor. J Exp Med 162:1512, 1985.
18. Zoumbos, N.C., J.Y. Djeu, and N.S. Young: Interferon is the suppressor of hematopoiesis generated by stimulated lymphocytes in vitro. J Immunol 133:769, 1984.
19. Zoumbos, N.C., P. Gascon, J.Y. Djeu, S.R. Trost, and N.S. Young: Circulating activated suppressor T lymphocytes in aplastic anemia. New Engl J Med 312:257, 1985.
20. Zoumbos, N.C., P. Gascon, J.Y. Djeu, and N.S. Young: Interferon is a mediator of hematopoietic suppression in aplastic anemia in vitro and possibly in vivo. Proc Natl Acad Sci USA 82:188, 1985.
21. Blalock, J.E., J.A. Georgiades, M.P. Langford, and H.M. Johnson: Purified human immune interferon has more potent anticellular activity than fibroblast or leukocyte interferon. Cell Immunol 49:390, 1980.
22. Fleischmann, W.R., Jr., K.M. Kleyn, and S. Baron: Potentiation of antitumor effect of virus-induced interferon by mouse immune interferon preparations. J Natl Cancer Inst 65:963, 1981.
23. Fleischmann, W.R. Jr., J.A. Georgiades, K.C. Oborne, and H.M. Johnson: Potentiation of interferon activity by mixed preparations of fibroblast and immune interferon. Infect Immun 26:248, 1979.
24. Vilcek, J., D. Henriksen-DeStefano, V.J. Palombella, and M. Tsujimoto: Interactions between tumor necrosis factor and interferons. In: The Biology of the Interferon System, 1985.
25. Baron, S. and F. Dianzani: General considerations of the interferon system. In: The Interferon System, S. Baron and F. Dianzani, eds. Texas Reports and Biol Med 35:1, 1977.
26. Gisler, R.H., P. Lindahl, and I. Gresser: Effect of interferon on antibody synthesis in vitro. J Immunol 113:438, 1974.
27. Farrar, W.L., H.M. Johnson, and J.J. Farrar: Regulation of the production of immune interferon and cytotoxic T lymphocytes by interleukin-2. J Immunol 126:1120, 1981.

28. Landolfo, S., F. Cofano, M. Grovarelli, M. Prat, G. Cavallo, and G. Forni: Inhibition of interferon gamma may suppress allograft reactivity by T lymphocytes in vitro and in vivo. Science 229:176, 1985.
28. Moore, R.N., F.J. Pitruzzello, R.M. Robinson, and B.T. Rouse: Interferon produced endogenously in response to CSF-1 augments the functional differentiation of progeny macrophages. J Leukocyte Biol 37:659, 1985.
29. Moore, R.N., and B.T. Rouse: Enhanced Responsiveness of committed macrophage precursors to macrophage-type colony-stimulating factor (CSF-1) induced in vitro by interferons α + β. J Immunol 131:2374, 1983.
30. Klimpel, G.R., W.R. Fleischmann Jr., S. Baron, and K.D. Klimpel: Mouse bone marrow cells produce a different interferon (IFN) than do spleen cells in response to alloantigens. J. Immunol 129:946, 1982.
31. Reyes, V.E., K.D. Klimpel, and G.R. Klimpel: Interferon α/β production by alloantigen-stimulated mouse bone marrow cells is T cell dependent. J Immunol 134:3137, 1985.
32. Reyes, V.E., Z.K. Ballas, K.D. Klimpel, and G.R. Klimpel: Interleukin 2 induces interferon α/β production in murine bone marrow cells. Fed Proced 43:1437, Abs. #122, 1984.
33. Ballas, Z.K.: The use of 5-azacytidine to establish constitutive interleukin 2 producing clones of the EL4 thymoma. J Immunol 133:2165, 1984.
34. Ortega, G., R.J. Robb, E.M. Sevach, and T.R. Malek: The murine IL2 receptor. I. Monoclonal antibodies that define distinct functional epitopes on activated T cells and react with activated B cells. J Immunol 133:1970, 1984.

TABLE 1. Recombinant IL2 Induces IFNα/β Synthesis in Murine Bone Marrow Cells

Responder Cells	Inducer	IFN (units/ml)
B10 bone marrow		
Plus:	Medium	<10
	MuIL2	140
	Recombinant HuIL2	40
Nu/Nu B10 Bone Marrow		
Plus:	Medium	<10
	MuIL2	1010
	Recombinant HuIL2	280
C57Bl/6 Bone Marrow - T cell depleted		
Plus:	Medium	<10
	MuIL2	153

Legend Table 1: Bone marrow ($6x10^6$) cells were cultured in Linbro wells in a total volume of 2 mls. The bone marrow cells were cultured in the presence of either a) medium alone or b) IL2. MuIL2 was obtained from a thymoma cell line which constitutively produces IL2 (33). This IL2 (IFN-free) was partially purified and used at a concentration of 0.2 u/ml. Recombinant human IL2 was obtained from Genzyme, Inc., Boston, MA. This IL2 preparation was used at a final concentration of 5 u/ml. T cells were depleted from bone marrow cells using a cocktail which contained antisera to Thy 1.2 and Lyt 1.2 plus complement. The cultures were incubated for 5 days. At the end of 5 days of culture, the supernatants were harvested and assayed for IFN.

TABLE 2. Antisera to IL2 or to the IL2 Receptor Inhibits IFN Production by IL2-Stimulated Bone Marrow Cells

Culture Conditions		IFN (Units/ml)
C57Bl/6 bone marrow cells plus:		
	Medium	<10
	IL2	227
	IL2 plus anti-IL2 sera	<10
	IL2 plus anti-IL2 receptor sera	<10

Legend Table 2: Bone marrow ($5x10^5$) cells were cultured in 96 well microtiter plates in a total volume of 200 microliters per well. The cells were cultured in either of the following conditions: a) medium alone, b) IL2 (0.2 u/ml), c) IL2 plus anti-IL2 sera (Genzyme, Boston, MA; 1/4 final dilutions), or d) IL2 plus anti-IL2 receptor monoclonal antibody designated as 3C7 (34). The various cultures were incubated for 5 days. At the end of 5 days of culture, the supernatants were harvested and assayed for IFN.

27. Effects of Interferon on Phenotypic Expression by Cells

A. Dolei[a] *and F. Ameglio*[b]

[a]Instituto di Microbiologia e Virologia, University of Sassari, Viale San Pietro 43B, 07100 Sassari, Italy; [b]Instituto Regina Elena, Viale Regina Elena, and Laboratorio di Biologia Cellulare del CNR, Via Romagnosi 18A, 00100 Rome, Italy

INTRODUCTION

The interaction of interferons (IFN) with sensitive cells causes the induction of new effector molecules leading to a multifaceted series of biochemical events which results, in addition to the block of virus replication and/or spreading, in the regulation of cell growth and differentiation, and, lastly, modulation of several functions of the immune system (1).

IFNs have been shown to enhance excitability of neurons, macrophage phagocytosis, major histocompatibility complex (MHC) expression, and iodine uptake by thyroid cells; furthermore they may induce morphological differentiation of neuroblastoma cells. On the other hand, IFNs inhibit myotube formation, adipose conversion, spontaneous and hormone-stimulated melanogenesis, macrophage maturation, and several hormone-induced enzymatic activities; both inhibitory and stimulatory effect could be observed on erythroid differentiation, on antibody production and on the beating rate of myocardial cells, according to timing and doses of IFN treatment (for a review see 2). Moreover, IFN was shown to affect tumor-associated antigen expression (3) and to worsen some autoimmune disorders (4).

Purpose of this short review is to give a brief presentation of some of these research areas, with special emphasis to the IFN effects on MHC antigens and on some differentiation-related antigens.

IFN EFFECTS ON MHC PRODUCTS

In the last ten years many reports have appeared on the influence of IFNs on MHC products, in view of the possibility that IFN immunoregulatory properties could be due, at least in part, to the modulation of expression of the various components of Class I and Class II MHC genes. The formers are present on virtually all somatic cells, whereas the latters are normally expressed by B cells, activated T cells, macrophages and other accessory cells. Three families of Class II genes have been described: DP, DQ and DR (5).

Enhanced expression of MHC Class I and $beta_2$-microglobulin by all three IFNs has been shown both in normal and in neoplastic cells of various origin (6-11). In all instances IFN gamma was shown to be the most effective one, being required 200-600 fold lower concentrations of it to obtain the same extent of effect (12-13). In addition, higher levels of increase were obtained with IFN gamma as compared to alpha and beta IFNs. Figure 1 shows representative data obtained in human M14 melanoma and Namalva lymphoblastoid cells after a 48 h treatment with either IFN.

As for Class II expression and IFN gamma, all the published data account for an increase (reviewed in 9 and 11). When a separate analysis of the Class II subsets was provided, it was shown that the expression of DQ was increased more than that of DR (see Figure 2 and refs. 14-15).

Since 1981 it was observed in human systems that pure native IFN beta was as effective on Class II as on Class I in increasing both expression and shedding, whereas no effect of IFN alpha was found (7). The effect of IFN beta was confirmed (15). Other reports indicated an increasing action by IFN alpha on Class II expression (16-17). These contradictory results may reflect the type and stage of differentiation of the cells exposed to IFN, or the detection method used. When radioimmunoassay (RIA) is used,instead of radiobinding or immunofluorescence, both cytoplasmic and membrane antigens are detected; by this method also soluble, shed MHC molecules were determined and found increased accordingly after IFN (11).

The increased synthesis and shedding of specific MHC proteins is due to an IFN effect on specific mRNAs (18-23). Moreover, in some cases the IFN effect on MHC transcription occurred without increasing membrane expression, indicating that regulatory mechanisms operating at the translational and post-translational level were involved (24).

A biologically distinct effect of IFN is the more recently described phenomenon of the induction by IFN gamma of Class I (25) and Class II antigens. The latter was seen in a wide variety of Class II-negative cells, including hemopoietic, lymphoid, epithelial, fibroblastic and neuronal cells (reviewed in 11). An example of Class II induction on fibroblasts is shown on Table 1: treatment of cells with 200 IU/ml of recombinant IFN gamma induced levels of Class II antigens comparable, on a per cell basis, to those expressed by normal B lymphocytes. Some cell lines (reviewed in 11) could not be induced by IFN gamma to express Class II antigens, notably Class II-negative T lines, and choriocarcinoma, teratocarcinoma and neuroblastoma cells, even though the latters were induced to express Class I molecules. Collins et al.(26) studied the induction of DP, DQ and DR separately, and found levels of DQ comparable to those of the other subsets. Gonwa and Stobo (27) reported that normal monocytes became DR- and DQ-negative when kept in culture: Class II expression could be reinduced

by subsequent treatment of the cells with IFN gamma.
Thus IFNs seem to exert a rather selective effect on MHC antigens. The fact that under influence of IFN gamma a variety of Class II-negative cells are converted to positivity could be interpreted on one side as an involvement of more cell types in immune functions (such as antigen presentation)(28-31); on the other side this fact could be the initiating cause of an autoimmune phenomenon, with the possibility for a cell of presenting a self-molecule as an auto-antigen (32). The antigen presenting ability of mouse fibroblasts transfected with human Class II genes has been demonstrated (33). The Class II enhancing property of IFN, which in turn is produced during response to infections, could facilitate the induction of autoimmunity. This is in keeping with the high levels of IFN observed in autoimmune diseases (34). Finally, one must remind the potential involvement of Class I molecules: a raised cell surface concentration of such molecules, as observed after exposure to either IFN, could facilitate the activity of Class I-restricted, auto-reactive, cytotoxic T cells (35).

IFN AND DIFFERENTIATION

This topic is covered in more detail in the contribution by Rossi *et al*., elsewherein this book. Herein we outline briefly the role of IFN on the phenotypic expression by B cells.
Strong evidence supported a role for IFN in the regulation of hemopoietic cell differentiation, particularly for the monocyte/macrophage lineage (36-37, and reviewed in 9). A series of markers of the T cell lineage was instead found unchanged after treatment with IFN alpha (9).
As for B lymphocyte development, it was shown that IFN gamma is one of the differentiation factors for B cells, that together with interleukin 2 was required for the final maturation of B cells into Ig-secreting cells (38-39) and that enhances the *in vitro* antibody response (9, 40).
Interestingly, a pre-plasmacell neoplasia (41), the hairy cell (HC) leukemia, is one of the human malignancies that respond successfully to IFN therapy (1). To explain the dramatic reduction of circulating HC, followed by a similar, though often not complete, disappearance of the neoplastic clone from the bone marrow, several mechanisms have been proposed, among which direct or cell-mediated antitumor activity and a differentiating capability of IFN.
Very recently an *in vitro* study was undertaken by Fattorossi and coworkers (42), in which peripheral blood mononuclear cells from HC leukemia patients with varying HC counts were incubated with human IFN alpha 2. In these experiments the same numbers of seeded HC were recovered at the end of treatment, indicating that IFN alpha did not exert direct or indirect cytotoxicity against HC. IFN-treated cells retained their typical cytoplasmic projections; however they exhibited markedly reduced acid phosphatase and tartrate-resistant acid phosphatase activity, or became com-

pletely negative upon IFN treatment; moreover, IFN alpha was responsible for a dramatic reduction in surface Ig and FcR expression, as reported on Table 2. The latter effect came unexpected, as B cell markers were reported to be unmodified by IFN alpha (9), and IFN is known to enhance, rather than decrease FcR expression (9). These contrasting pieces of evidence may be explained by the notion that HC represent a differentiation blockade of a B cell at the pre-plasmacell level (41), and that B lymphocytes starting active Ig synthesis diminish their surface membrane Ig and FcR (43). Therefore it seems likely to infer that IFN may promote a progression of HC toward a more differentiated phenotype. Baldini et al. (44) recently reported that IFN alpha increased Class II antigens on splenic HC, while surface Ig remained unaffected. It has been proposed that HC may originate in the white pulp of the spleen (45), where their putative normal counterpart reside. In this view, circulating HC may represent a subset or evolving step of splenic HC and therefore can display a different sensitivity to IFN alpha.

Although in vitro phenomena do not necessarily reflect the in vivo situation, one may assume that IFN alpha administration in vivo may cause HC to differentiate towards the final step of the normal B cell pathway and thus halt the proliferative process.

ACKNOWLEDGEMENTS

Work supported in part by grants from CNR, Progetti Finalizzati Oncologia e Controllo Malattie da Infezione, and Gruppo Virologia, Contracts 1986.

REFERENCES

1. Dianzani, F., and G.B. Rossi, eds.: The interferon system. Raven Press, 1985.

2. Dolei, A., L. Cioè, M.R. Capobianchi, P.Palladino, L. Diamond, G.B. Rossi, F. Belardelli, E. Affabris, F. Ameglio, R.Tosi, and G.Rita: Effects of interferon on cell differentiation. Drugs Exptl Clin Res 8: 667, 1982.

3. Greiner, J., J. Schlom, S. Petska, P. Giacomini, S. Ferrone, and P. Fisher: Modulation of tumor associated antigen expression and shedding by recombinant human leukocyte and fibroblast interferons. Pharmacol Therapeutics, in the press.

4. Hooks, J.J., N.M. Moutsopoulos, S.A. Geis, N.I. Stahl, J.L. Decker, and A. L. Notkins: Immune interferon in the circulation of patients with autoimmune disease. New Engl J Med 5:301, 1979.

5. Ferrone, S., G. Solheim, and E. Moller, eds.: Human Class II histocompatibility antigens. Theoretical and practical aspects; clinical relevance. Springer Verlag, 1986.

6. Lindhal, P., P. Leary, and I. Gresser: Enhancement by interferon of the expression of surface antigens on murine L_{1210} cells. Proc Natl Acad Sci USA 70: 2785, 1973.

7. Dolei, A., F. Ameglio, M.R. Capobianchi, and R. Tosi: Human beta type interferon enhances the expression and shedding of Ia-like antigens. Comparison to HLA-A,B,C and β_2-microglobulin. Antiviral Res 1: 367, 1981.
8. Liao, S.K., P.C. Kwong, M. Khosravi, and P.B. Dent: Enhanced expression of melanoma associated antigens and beta$_2$-microglobulin on cultured human melanoma cells by interferon. J Natl Cancer Inst 68: 19, 1982.
9. Hokland, M.E.: Immunomodulatory effects of interferons on human mononuclear cells with special reference to the expression of cell surface antigens. Acta Pathol Microbiol Immunol Scand 93: 1, 1985.
10. Capobianchi, M.R., F. Ameglio, R. Tosi, and Dolei A.: Differences in the expression and release of DR, BR and DQ molecules in human cells treated with recombinant interferon gamma. Comparison to other interferons. Human Immunol 13: 1, 1985.
11. Ameglio, F., R. Tosi, N. Tanigaki, and A. Dolei: Modulation of Class II antigens by interferons. In: Human Class II histocompatibility antigens. Theoretical and practical aspects; clinical relevance, S. Ferrone, G. Solheim, and E. Moller, eds. Springer Verlag, pp. 359-373, 1986.
12. Sonnenfeld, G., D. Meruelo, H.O. McDevitt, and T.C. Merigan: Effect of type I and type II interferons on murine thymocytes surface antigens expression: induction or selection? Cell Immunol 57: 427, 1981.
13. Dolei A., M.R. Capobianchi, and F. Ameglio: Human interferon gamma enhances the expression and shedding of Class I and Class II MHC products in neoplastic cells better than interferon alpha and interferon beta. Infect Immun 40: 172, 1983.
14. Ameglio, F., M.R. Capobianchi, A. Dolei, and R. Tosi: Differential effects of gamma interferon on expression of HLA Class II molecules controlled by the DR and DC loci. Infect Immun 42: 122, 1983.
15. Giacomini, P., A. Aguzzi, S. Petska, P.B. Fisher, and S. Ferrone : Modulation by recombinant DNA leukocyte (alpha) and fibroblast (beta) interferons of the expression and shedding of HLA and tumor associated antigens by melanoma cells. J Immunol 133: 1649, 1984.
16. Basham, T.Y., W. Smith, L. Lanier, V. Morhenn, and T.C. Merigan: Regulation of expression of Class II MHC antigens on human peripheral blood monocytes and Langerhans cells by interferon. Human Immunol 10: 83, 1984.
17. Sztein, M.B., P.S. Steeg, H.M. Johnson, and J.J. Oppenheim: Regulation of human peripheral blood monocyte DR antigen expression in vitro by lymphokines and recombinant interferons. J Clin Invest 73: 56, 1984.
18. Basham, T.Y., and T.C. Merigan: Recombinant interferon gamma increases HLA-DR synthesis and expression. J Immunol 130: 1492, 1983.
19. Chen, E., R.W. Karr, J.P. Frost, T.A. Gonwa, and G.D. Ginder: Gamma interferon and 5-azacytidine cause transcriptional elevation of Class II MHC gene expression in K562 leukemia cells in the absence of differentiation. Mol Cell Biol 6: 1698, 1986.
20. Nakamura, M., T. Manser, G.D.N. Pearson, M.J. Daley, and M.L.Gefter: Effect of interferon gamma on the immune response in vivo and on gene expression in vitro. Nature 307: 381, 1984.

21. Peterlin, B.M., T.A. Gonwa, and J.D. Stobo: Expression of HLA-DR by a human monocyte cell line is under transcriptional control. J Mol Cell Immunol 1: 191, 1984.
22. Taniguchi, M., J.P-Y. Ting, S.C. Buessow, C. Boyer, Y. Gillespie,and J.A. Frelinger: Response of glioma cells to interferon gamma: increase in Class II RNA, protein and mixed lymphocyte reaction-stimulating ability. Eur J Immunol 15: 809, 1985.
23. Rahmsdorf, H.J., N. Harth, A.M. Eades, M. Litfin, M. Steinmetz, L. Forni, and P. Herrlich: Interferon gamma, mytomycin C and cycloheximide as regulatory agents of MHC Class II-associated invariant chain expression. J Immunol 136: 2293, 1986.
24. Rosa, F., D. Hatat, A. Abadie, D. Wallach, M. Revel, and M. Fellous: Differential regulation of HLA-DR mRNAs and cell surface antigens by interferon. EMBO J 9: 1585, 1983.
25. Hunt, J.S., and G.W. Wood: Interferon gamma induces Class I HLA and $beta_2$- microglobulin expression by human amnion cells. J Immunol 136:364, 1986.
26. Collins, T., A.S. Korman, C.T. Wake, J.M. Boss, D.J. Kappes,W.Fiers, K.A. Ault, M.A. Gimbrone, J.L. Strominger, and J.S. Pober: Immune interferon activates multiple Class II histocompatibility complex gene and the associated invariant chain gene in human endothelial cells and dermal fibroblasts. Proc Natl Acad Sci USA 81: 4917, 1984.
27. Gonwa, T.A., and J.D. Stobo: Differential expression of Ia molecules by human monocytes. J Clin Invest 74: 859, 1984.
28. Londei, M., J.R. Lamb, G.F. Bottazzo, and M. Feldmann: Epithelial cells expressing aberrant Class II determinants can present antigen to cloned human T cells. Nature 312: 639, 1984.
29. Basham, T.Y., B.J. Nickoloff, T.C. Merigan, and V.B. Morhenn: Recombinant gamma interferon differentially regulates Class II antigen expression and biosynthesis on cultured normal human keratinocytes. J Interferon Res 5: 23, 1985.
30. Berrih, S., F. Arenzana-Seisdedos, S. Cohen, R. Devos, D.Charron and J-L. Virelizier: Interferon modulates HLA Class II antigen expression on cultured human thymic epithelial cells. J Immunol 135: 1165, 1985.
31. Morel, P.A., S.C. Manolagas, D.M. Provvedini, D.R. Wegmann, and J.M. Chiller: Interferon gamma-induced Ia expression in Wehi-3 cells is enhanced by the presence of 1,25-dihidroxyvitamin D_3. J Immunol 136:2181,1986.
32. Tiku, M.L., S. Liu, C.W. Weaver, M. Teodorescu, and J.L.Skosey: Class II histocompatibility antigen-mediated immunologic function of normal articular chondrocytes. J Immunol 135: 2923, 1985.
33. Norcross, M.A., D.M. Bentley, D.H. Margulies, and R.N. Germain: Membrane Ia expression and antigen-presenting accessory cell function of L cells transfected with Class II MHC genes. J Exp Med 160: 1316, 1984.
34. Yttemberg, S.R., and T.J. Schnitzer: Serum interferon levels in patients with lupus erythematosus. Arthritis Rheum 25: 401, 1982.
35. Bevan, M.J.: High determinant density may explain the phenomenon of

alloreactivity. Immunol Today 5: 128, 1984.
36. Warren, M.K., S.N. Vogel: Bone marrow-derived macrophages: Development and regulation of differentiation markers by colony-stimulating factor and interferons. J Immunol 134: 982, 1985.
37. Takei, M., K. Takeda, and K. Konno: The role of interferon gamma in induction of differentiation of human myeloid leukemia cell lines ML1 and HL60. Biochem Biophys Res Comm 124: 100, 1981.
38. Nakagawa, T., T. Hirano, N. Nakagawa, K. Yoshizaki, and T. Kishimoto: Effect of recombinant IL-2 and IFN gamma on proliferation and differentiation of human B cells. J Immunol 134: 959, 1985.
39. Sidman, C.L., J.D. Marshall, L.D. Shultz, P.W. Gray, and H. Johnson: Gamma interferon is one of several direct B-cell-maturing lymphokines. Nature 309: 801, 1984.
40. Leibson, J.H., M. Gefter, A. Zlotnik, P.Marrack, and J.W. Kappler : Role of gamma-interferon in antibody producing responses. Nature 309:799, 1984.
41. Anderson, K.C., A.W. Boyd, D.C. Fisher, D. Leslie, S.F. Schlossmann, and L.M. Nadler: Hairy cell leukemia: a tumor of pre-plasma cells. Blood 65: 620, 1985.
42. Fattorossi, A., A. Dolei, J.G. Pizzolo, A. Cafolla, F. Mandelli, and F. Dianzani: Recombinant leukocyte interferon modulates hairy cell phenotype in vitro. Submitted for publication.
43. Katz, D.H.: The immune system. In Basic and Clinical Immunology, Lange Medical Publication, pp. 13-20, 1984.
44. Baldini, L., A. Cortelezzi, N. Polli, A. Neri, L. Nobili, A. Maiolo, G. Lambertenghi-Delliers, and E.E. Polli: Human recombinant interferon alpha-2C enhances the expression of Class II HLA antigens on hairy cells. Blood 67: 458, 1986.
45. Van der Oord, J.J., C. de Wolf-Peeter,and V.J. Desmet: Hairy cell leukemia: a B-lymphocytic disorder derived from splenic marginal zone lymphocytes. Blut 50: 191, 1985.

TABLE 1. Induction of Class II molecules in normal diploid fibroblasts treated with IFNs.

Treatment	RIA inhibition units$_{50}$/10^6 cells		
	48 h	72 h	96 h
None	<0.3	<0.3	<0.3
IFN alpha	<0.3	<0.3	<0.3
IFN beta	<0.3	<0.3	<0.3
IFN gamma	9.2	22.3	36.4

IFN alpha and beta: 5000 IU/ml; IFN gamma: 500 IU/ml. From Ameglio et al. (10), modified.

TABLE 2. Summary of modifications in the phenotypic profile induced by IFN alpha (1000 IU/ml) in mononuclear cells from HC leukemia patients.

Patient	% Positive Cells Control culture			IFN alpha culture		
	sIg	FcR	TRAP	sIg	FcR	TRAP
FP	36$\gamma\lambda$ (48)	45 (75)	40 (++++)	30$\gamma\lambda$ (30)	40 (27)	20 (++)
IM	80$\delta\lambda$ (52) 63$\mu\lambda$ (57)	84 (83)	85 (++++)	87$\delta\lambda$ (32) 60$\mu\lambda$ (45)	80 (69)	81 (++)
AC	81$\gamma\kappa$ (59)	77 (82)	78 (++++)	75$\gamma\kappa$ (27)	80 (31)	69 (++)
RM	20$\gamma\kappa$ (67)	20 (86)	ND	15$\gamma\kappa$ (34)	22 (51)	ND
MDC	22$\delta\kappa$ (50)	26 (73)	28 (+++)	20$\delta\kappa$ (38)	26 (20)	20 (+)

sIg: surface immunoglobulins; FcR: Fc gamma receptor; TRAP: tartrate-resistant acid phosphatase; ND: not done.
Numbers in parentheses represent the median channel of fluorescence in FACS; (+) is the intensity of the enzymatic stain. Values reported for sIg and FcR cannot be compared with each other as they were measured using different FACS settings to account for the marked dissimilarity in fluorescence intensity. From Fattorossi, Dolei, Pizzolo, Cafolla, Mandelli and Dianzani, submitted for publication (42).

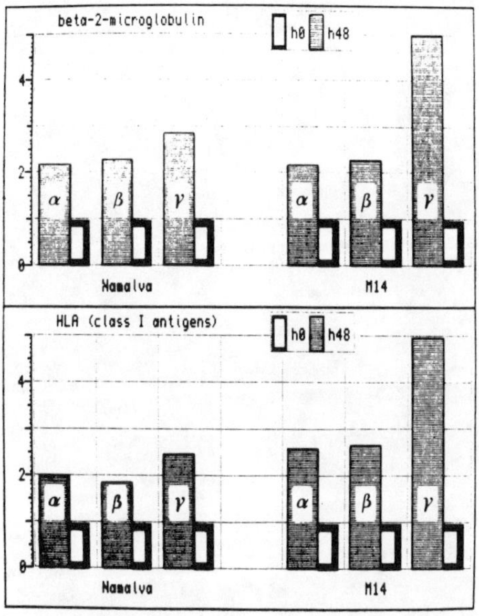

Figure 1. Expression of Class I and beta$_2$-microglobulin in Namalva and M14 human cells treated with IFNs. IFN alpha and beta: 5000 IU/ml; IFN gamma: 500 IU/ml. Data are expressed as ratio of treated/untreated values. Base means were (RIA $IU_{50}/10^6$ cells) : Namalva : Class I = 12; beta$_2$-microglobulin = 11. M14: Class I = 13 ; beta$_2$-microglobulin = 98. Cells were treated with IFN for 48h.

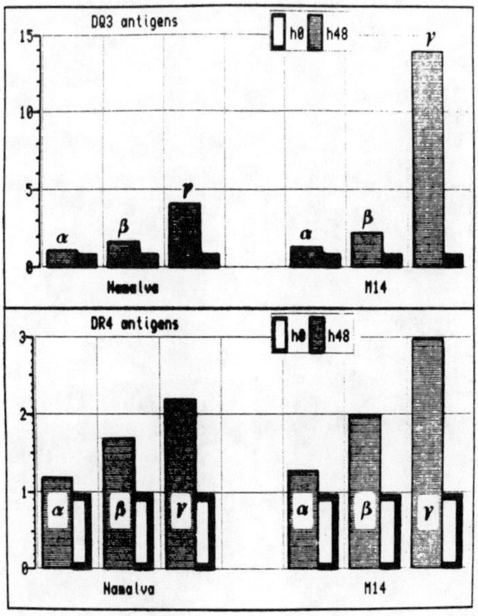

Figure 2. Expression of Class II antigens in Namalva and M14 human cells treated with IFNs. Cells were treated as in Fig. 1. Base means (RIA $IU_{50}/10^6$ cells) were: Namalva : DQ3 = 20 ; DR4 = 150. M14: DQ3 = 6; DR4 = 92. Results comparable to those obtained in Namalva cells were found in peripheral blood mononuclear cells from normal donors with different allospecificities (10).

Figure 1. Expression of Class I and Class II histocompatibility antigens in Namalva and M14 human cells treated with IFNs. IFN alpha and beta: 5000 U/ml; IFN gamma: 500 U/ml. Data are expressed as percentage [illegible] [illegible] [illegible] were [illegible] 10^6 cells [illegible] Class II [illegible] [illegible] Class I [illegible] [illegible] cells were treated with IFN for 48h [illegible]

Figure 2. Expression of Class II antigens in Namalva and M14 human cells treated with IFN. Cells were treated as in Fig. 1. [illegible] [illegible] 10^6 cells [illegible] were [illegible] Namalva: DQ3 [illegible] DR4 [illegible] M14: DQ3 [illegible] DR5 [illegible] Results comparable to those obtained in Namalva cells were found in peripheral blood mononuclear cells from normal donors with different allospecificities (10).

28. Augmentation of Surface Antigens on Human Carcinoma Cells by Recombinant Leukocyte Interferon

J. W. Greiner,[a] S. Petka,[b] P. Fisher,[c] and J. Schlom[a]

[a]Laboratory of Tumor Immunology and Biology, National Cancer Institute, NIH, Bethesda, MD 20892; [b]Roche Institute of Molecular Biology, Nutley, NJ 07110; [c]Department of Microbiology, Comprehensive Cancer Center/ Institute of Cancer Research, Columbia University, College of Physicians and Surgeons, New York, NY 10032

INTRODUCTION

Through the use of established hybridoma technology several monoclonal antibodies (MAbs) have been generated that react with specific antigenic determinants found on primary and metastatic human breast and/ or colon carcinomas (1-4). The antibodies have been tested and successfully used in immunohistochemical diagnosis as well as the isolation and characterization of the tumor antigens they recognize (3-5). One common characteristic of both human breast and colon carcinoma cell populations has been the heterogeneity in the expression of the different tumor antigens. With the MAbs as immunological probes, antigenic heterogeneity of these tumor cell populations has been defined in terms of: 1) percentage of cells expressing the antigen, 2) amount of tumor antigen expressed per cell, and 3) cellular localization of the antigen (6,7). Antigenic heterogeneity is an important consideration when designing protocols to use MAbs for the localization and treatment of human tumors. The cells within the carcinoma population which are antigen negative or low expressers of the tumor antigen will fail to bind sufficient MAb and thus escape detection and/or therapy. We have been interested in developing approaches to overcome antigenic heterogeneity through the exogenous administration of agents capable of modulating antigen expression on the surface of human tumor cells. Preliminary studies showed that retinoids, organic solvents, such as DMSO, and DNA-intercalating agents were, for the most part, ineffective in modulating tumor antigen expression. The human interferons have emerged as the most potent inducers of surface antigens on human tumor cell populations. We present here a summary of results showing modulation of class I major histocompability antigens as well as MAb-defined tumor antigens on the surface of human carcinoma cells by recombinant human leukocyte interferon. These findings suggest that the administration of such a biological response modifier could augment the overall effectiveness of a MAb for the detection and treatment of human carcinoma lesions.

RESULTS

Heterogeneity of Tumor Antigen Expression

Extensive studies to determine the range of reactivities for each of the MAbs listed in Table 1 have been published (1,2,4,8). With the use of appropriate MAbs in radioimmunoassays and cytofluorometry, the extent of heterogeneity for the expression of each tumor antigen was studied. The anti-CEA and anti-TAG-72 MAbs B1.1 and B72.3 best illustrate the antigenic heterogeneity found on the surface of human breast and colon carcinoma cells. Of more than 50 human tumor cell lines tested only the MCF-7 and LS174T cells express the B72.3 reactive TAG-72 antigen. Furthermore, within those two cell populations 5-10% of the carcinoma cells are TAG-72 positive. Both human breast and colon carcinoma cell lines express quantitatively different amounts of the cell surface B1.1-reactive CEA. Between two different human breast tumor lines, MCF-7 and MDA-MB-231, there is a seven-fold difference in the constitutive level of B1.1 binding (Table 1). Those same two breast carcinoma cell lines have qualitative differences in the expression of the 90 Kd-B6.2 antigen. Normal cell surface antigenic determinants, particularly class I and II histocompability antigens, are more homogenously expressed by human cells. As shown, the W6/32 MAb constitutively reacts with both normal and carcinoma human cells. An anti-HLA-DR MAb, which fails to react with most human carcinoma cells, interestingly shows some constitutive binding to the human breast MDA-MB-231 cell line.

Enhancement of Antigen Expression by IFN-αA

Interferon has been shown to alter the expression of normal cell surface antigenic determinants, particularly HLA (9-12). Indeed, as shown for the breast and colon carcinoma cells, treatment with the recombinant human leukocyte interferon, Hu-IFN-αA, can increase cell surface HLA expression (Table 1). Previous investigators have shown that the DR locus of HLA is highly sensitive to interferon gamma usually resulting in initiation of expression of this antigen. In agreement with other findings, IFN-αA failed to initiate human breast and colon carcinoma cells to express HLA-DR. The breast carcinoma cell line MDA-MB-231 expresses a constitutive level of HLA-DR, however, the level of expression of this antigen remained unchanged after Hu-IFN-αA treatment.

Previously, we reported that Hu-IFN-αA treatment of the human breast carcinoma cell line, MCF-7, and the colon carcinoma cell line, WiDr, resulted in a dose-dependent increase in the expression of both CEA and the 90 Kd-reactive B6.2 antigens on the surface of these cells (11,13). The increased level of binding of MAb B1.1 and B6.2 to their respective antigens could be demonstrated at antiviral levels (<50 units) which did not inhibit the growth of either cell types. In addition to the MCF-7 cells, we now report a second human breast carcinoma cell line, the MDA-MB-231, when treated with 1,000 antiviral units Hu-IFN-αA results in a more than a 5-fold increase in surface CEA expression. This cell line does not constitutively express either the 90 Kd-B6.2 reactive antigen or the high molecular weight TAG-72 antigen either before or after interferon treatment. In general, the human cells that do not exhibit a constitutive amount of surface antigen expression, remain antigen negative even after treatment with as much as 10,000 units of interferon. This is particularly important when considering interferon effects on tumor antigen expression on normal human cells (Table 1). It is conceivable that interferon administration could result in an enhanced signal (i.e., tumor antigen surface expression) originating from the tumor cell population while the surrounding normal tissue, if initially antigen negative (i.e., normal human fibroblasts) would remain so after treatment. The overall effect of this augmented signal from the tumor cell population would be an enhanced level of binding for a selective MAb thus allowing for better discrimination between normal and tumor tissue.

Furthermore, as shown in Table 2, the enhanced binding of a MAb to a human tumor cell population as a result of Hu-IFN-αA treatment seems to be a result of at least two different phenomena. Cytoflourometry and radioimmunoassay data revealed that the interferon-induced enhancement of B1.1 and B6.2 binding to the WiDr cell surface was a result of: 1) more reactive antigen expressed per cell and represented as an increase in the mean fluorescence index (MFI), and 2) a "recruitment" of previously antigen-negative or weakly antigen positive cells to become more antigen positive. In the case of both B6.2 and B1.1 binding, the WiDr cell population has become more homogeneous with >90% of the cells expressing the 90 Kd-B6.2 reactive antigen and CEA as a result of interferon treatment. These effects can be contrasted with the changes observed for HLA-A,B,C expression after interferon treatment. Constitutive W6/32 binding to the WiDr tumor cell population is homogeneous with >95% of the cells expressing the surface HLA. Interferon treatment does, however, result in an augmentation of W6/32 binding because the overall amount of antigen expressed per cell (i.e., MFI) is increased (Table 2). Thus the interferon effect on tumor antigen expression contains a component not found in the alterations of normal surface antigens. The ability of Hu-IFN- αA to convert either antigen negative or weakly antigen-positive cells to cells capable of binding significant amounts of MAb may be particularly relevant when considering that a threshold level of binding for a given MAb may be needed to effectively detect and treat carcinoma lesions.

Previously we reported (14) that clones of MCF-7 cells could be isolated that were unresponsive to the antigen-enhancing effects, yet their growth could be inhibited by Hu-IFN-αA. As shown in Table 1, both tumor associated as well as normal surface antigens on the well differentiated human colon carcinoma cell line, LS174T, were unchanged with interferon treatment. Similar to the MCF-7 clones, analysis of the LS-174T cells demonstrated an Hu-IFN-αA-mediated growth inhibition of the cells (data not shown). These results suggested that the lack of induced changes in surface antigen expression cannot be explained by the absence of an intact, functional surface interferon receptor. These results present additional evidence of biochemical pathways distal to the interferon receptor that functionally separate growth inhibition and antigen augmentation by Hu-IFN-αA.

One of the important considerations in using labeled MAbs for radiolocalization and immunotherapy of human carcinoma lesions is the amount of antibody administered to a patient. The ability to reduce the amount of administered MAb should increase the "signal:noise" ratios by reducing circulating radioactivity and thus making the detection of small lesions more efficient. We have approached this question experimentally by comparing the amount of ^{125}I-B72.3 required to maintain a reference level of binding to the MCF-7 cell surface before and after treatment with increasing titers of Hu-IFN-αA. Approximately 94 ng of the ^{125}I-labeled B72.3 was needed to evoke a signal of 1000 cpm/5x10^4 untreated MCF-7 cells. A single treatment of the breast carcinoma cells with 50 units of Hu-IFN-αA reduced the amount of B72.3 needed to maintain that same level of radioactivity to 54 ng. The reduction in the amount of ^{125}I-B72.3 input to localize 10^3 cpm was dose-dependent until only 4 ng were required after treatment with 1000 units of Hu-IFN-αA. Therefore,

Hu-IFN- A treatment of the MCF-7 cells can result in a 24-fold reduction in the amount of MAb needed to maintain the same signal at the cell surface as was initially measured on the untreated breast carcinoma cells. Thus, the ability to lower MAb input as a result of interferon treatment may be significant for the optimal use of a MAb for tumor detection and therapy.

REFERENCES

1. Colcher, D., P. Horan Hand, M. Nuti, and J. Schlom: A spectrum of monoclonal antibodies reactive with human mammary tumor cells. Proc. Natl. Acad. Sci. (USA) 78: 3199, 1981.
2. Schlom, J., J.W. Greiner, P. Horan Hand, D. Colcher, G. Inghirami, M. Weeks, S. Pestka, P.B. Fisher, P. Noguchi, and D. Kufe: Monoclonal antibodies to breast cancer-associated antigens as potential reagents in the management of breast cancer. Cancer 54: 2777, 1984.
3. Colcher, D., P. Horan Hand, M. Nuti, and J. Schlom: Differential binding to human mammary and nonmammary tumors of monoclonal antibodies reactive with carcinoembryonic antigen. Cancer Invest. 1: 127, 1983.
4. Thor, A., N. Ohuchi, C.A. Szpak, W.W. Johnston and J. Schlom: The distribution of oncofetal antigen TAG-72 defined by monoclonal antibody B72.3. Cancer Res. (in press), 1986.
5. Stramignoni, D., R. Bowen, B.F. Atkinson and J. Schlom: Differential reactivity of monoclonal antibodies with human colon adenocarcinomas and adenomas. Int. J. Cancer 31: 543, 1983.
6. Horan Hand, P., M. Nuti, D. Colcher, and J. Schlom: Definition of antigen heterogeneity and modulation among human mammray carcinoma cell populations using monoclonal antibodies to tumor-associated antigens. Cancer Res. 43: 728, 1983.
7. Greiner, J.W., J. Schlom, S. Pestka, J.A. Langer, P. Giacomini, M. Kusama, S. Ferrone and P.B. Fisher: Modulation of tumor-associated antigen expression and shedding by recombinant human leukocyte and fibroblast interferons. Pharmac. Ther. (in press), 1986.
8. Kufe, D., G. Inghirami, M. Abe, D. Hayes, H. Justi-Wheeler and J. Schlom: Differential reactivity of a novel monoclonal antibody (DF3) with human malignant versus benign breast tumors. Hybridoma 3: 223, 1984.
9. Basham, T.Y., M.F. Bourgeade, A.A. Creasey, and T.C. Merigan: Interferon increases HLA synthesis in melanoma cell: Interferon-resistant and sensitive cell lines. Proc. Natl. Acad. Sci. (USA) 79: 3265, 1982.
10. Heron, L., M. Hokland, and K. Berg: Enhanced expression of B_2-microglobulin and HLA antigen on human lymphoid cells by interferon. Proc. Natl. Acad. Sci. (USA) 75: 6215, 1978.
11. Greiner, J.W., P. Horan Hand, P. Noguchi, P.B. Fisher, S. Pestka, and J. Schlom: Enhanced expression of surface tumor-associated antigens on human breast and colon tumor cells after recombinant human leukocyte α-interferon treatment. Cancer Res. 44: 3208, 1984.
12. Giacomini, P., A. Aguzzi, S. Pestka, P.B. Fisher, and S. Ferrone: Modulation by recombinant DNA leukocyte (α) and fibroblast (β) interferons of the expression and shedding of HLA and tumor associated antigens by human melanoma cells. J. Immunol. 133: 1649, 1984.
13. Greiner, J.W., P. Horan Hand, S. Pestka, P. Noguchi, P.B. Fisher, D.

Colcher, and J. Schlom: Detection and enhancement (by recombinant interferon) of carcinoma cell surface antigens using monoclonal antibodies. In: Cancer Cells 1/The Transformed Phenotype A.J. Levine, G.F. Vande Woude, W.C. Topp and J.D. Watson, eds. Cold Spring Harbor Press, Vol. II, pp. 265-291, 1984.

14. Greiner, J.W., M. Tobi, P.B. Fisher, J.A. Langer, and S. Pestka: Differential responsiveness of cloned mammary carcinoma cell populations to human recombinant leukocyte interferon enhancement of tumor antigen expression. Int. J. Cancer 26: 159, 1985.

Table 1. Constitutive and interferon-induced levels of reactivity of monoclonal antibodies to human cells.[1]

			Surface Binding of the MAbs (cpm/5x10^4 cells)					
			Breast CA		Colon CA		Normal	
MAb	Antigen	Interferon (+/-)	MCF-7	MDA-MB-231	WiDr	LS174T	WI-38	Flow 4000
B1.1	CEA	-	6140	840	5440	6460	NEG[2]	NEG
	(180 Kd)	+	13410(2.2)[4]	4680(5.6)	12880(2.4)	6340	NEG	NEG
B6.2	90 Kd	-	3390	NEG	5080	3270	NEG	NEG
		+	8410(2.5)	NEG	12410(2.4)	2710	NEG	NEG
B72.3	TAG-72	-	1440	NEG	NEG	2610	NEG	NEG
	(>10^{6}d)	+	3160(2.2)	NEG	NEG	2440	NEG	NEG
DF3	290 Kd	-	7890	ND[3]	NEG	NEG	NEG	NEG
		+	7410	ND	NEG	NEG	NEG	NEG
W6/32	HLA-A,B,C	-	4380	2140	3880	2140	8710	6440
	(45 Kd)	+	10860(2.5)	3260(1.5)	7640(2.0)	2410	10420	8220
α-DR	HLA-DR	-	NEG	1990	NEG	NEG	NEG	NEG
	(28-34 Kd)	+	NEG	2010	NEG	NEG	NEG	NEG

[1]Cells were treated for 24-36hr with 500-2000 units Hu-IFN-αA/ml and the binding of the MAbs were measured in a radioimmunoassay using live, intact cells (11).

[2]Neg - no significant binding (<500 cpm above background).

[3]ND - not determined.

[4]Values in parentheses represent $\frac{\text{cpm - interferon treated cells}}{\text{cpm - untreated cells}}$

Table 2. Flow Cytometric Analysis of Antigenic Changes on the Surface of Human Cells After Interferon Treatment[1]

Cell Line	MAb	Untreated		+IFN-αA	
		% Pos	MFI	% Pos	MFI
WiDr	B6.2	52.2	500	97.9	685
	B1.1	48.9	610	78.9	700
	B72.3	2.8	194	3.5	187
	W6/32	95.6	760	98.5	830
	α HLA-DR	4.1	206	5.3	196
WI-38	B6.2	2.8	184	3.1	190
	W6/32	97.6	860	98.4	940

[1]Cells were cultured for 24-36 hr in the presence of 1000 units of Hu-IFN-αA/ml, then analyzed by indirect immunofluorescence and flow cytometry for surface antigen expression (11).
[2]% Pos, percentage of cells with fluorescence greater than cells stained with a negative MAb, i.e., MOPC-21, MFI, mean flluorescence intensity on a scale of 150-1000.

Table 3. Effect of Hu-IFN-αA treatment on the binding of radiolabeled B72.3 to the MCF-7 cell surface.

Hu-IFN-αA[1] Treatment (units/ml)	^{125}I-B72.3 Bound to MCF-7 Cell Surface	
	CPM/5x10^4 cells	ng B72.3/1000 cpm[2]
control	1260	94
10	1480	83
50	2140	54
500	3280	24
1500	4410	4

[1]MCF-7 cells were treated with the indicated antiviral titers of Hu-IFN-αA for approximately 30 hr.
[2]The amount of B72.3 required to localize 10^3 CPM of ^{125}I-B72.3 to the surface of 5x10^4 MCF-7 cells was determined from an antibody dilution curve ranging from 500-0.03 ng purified B72.3. Data represent the mean of 3-4 experiments.

29. Interferon Effects on Cell Differentiation

G. B. Rossi,[a] E. Affabris,[b] G. Romeo,[a] M. Federico,[a] and E. M. Coccia[a]

[a]Laboratory of Virology, Instituto Superiore di Sanità, Viale Regina Elena 299, 00161 Rome, Italy; [b]Department of Cellular and Developmental Biology, University of Rome "La Sapienza," Rome, Italy

That many different kind of alterations in eukariotic cell physiology are caused by exposure to interferon(s) (IFNs) is by now common knowledge. Indications that IFNs play a role in differentiation processes come from observation in many differentiating and differentiated systems (see Table 1). For an extensive review updated to 1984 see (53). As early as in 1971 Grossberg and Morahan (21) suggested that IFN mechanisms of action were under a repressed state in embryonic life, at a time when growth and differentiation of cells are fundamental. This is somehow supported by the data of Burke et al. (4) that indicate that pluripotent mouse teratocarcinoma cells do not produce IFNs nor are they sensitive to their action. These cells, however, do differentiate when injected into adult hosts or into a blastocyst and when culture conditions are changed. Under these conditions differentiating teratocarcinoma cells somehow release their IFN genes from the repressed state, and will respond to NDV induction with a substantial production and release of mouse IFN. Interestingly, during the establishment of the differentiated phenotype, the teratocarcinoma cells also become sensitive to IFN action, as measured by the establishment of the antiviral state. Coveney et al. (9) investigated the DNase I sensitivity, and thus the chromatin conformation of IFN-β genes during differentiation of another teratocarcinoma clone and showed patterns of IFN production (and sensitivity to) closely similar to those studied by Burke et al. (4). In murine neuroblastoma cells IFN production was, instead, depressed in differentiated cells without any apparent changes in cell sensitivity to IFN itself (61). Studies of Zusman et al. (76) showed that treatment with 10,000 U/ml of murine IFN did not affect the developmental ability of preimplantation mouse embryos with or without the zona pellucida. Further, IFN treatment did not protect the embryos from the embryotoxic effect of exposure to encephalomyocarditis virus, indicating that they are resistant to both the antiproliferative and the antiviral action of IFN. Decreased production of IFN-γ by human neonatal lymphocytes (72) and reduced IFN-γ mRNA levels in human neonatal blood mononuclear cells or purified T cells (36) as compared to human adult cells, were also reported. Oh et al. (43) measuring enhancement of human neonatal natural killer cytotoxicity (NKC) to herpes simplex virus induced by human rIFNs, reported increase of neonatal NKC by human rIFN-α, but not by human rIFN-γ. However, research on hematopoiesis is certainly the area in which most data on the effects of IFNs on cell differentiation have been accumulated. This will be discussed in the rest of this article, leaving out the effects on immunocompetent cells (i.e. Band T lymphocytes, macrophages, etc.) that need to be reviewed per se.

IFNs effects on normal and abnormal hemopoiesis

Models of hematopoiesis in mammals (for a review, see 46) include a pool of pluripotent stem cells (colony-forming unit-spleen, CFU-S). This stem cell population feeds into compartments of lineage-committed progenitors, burst-forming unit-erythroid (BFU-E) and colony-forming unit-granulo-macrophage (CFU-GM) for the erythroid and GM line, respectively. These in turn differentiate into the respective pools of late progenitors (CFU-E and G- or M-CFU) and of morphologically recognizable precursors (e.g., proerythroblasts and myeloblasts). Since 1970, studies on the hemopoietic progenitors in vitro have been performed via liquid and semisolid cultures of marrow and spleen cells additioned with growth factors for hematopoietic cells. A block of human granulopoietic differentiation has been repeatedly described by Verma et al. (68-70) in both kinds of culture assays following treatment with human leukocyte IFN. As a result of the IFN-mediated arrest of granulocyte maturation, an accumulation of granulocyte-macrophage progenitors (CFU-GM) ensues. The effect is reversible, and, in addition, is suggestive of some kind of tissue-specificity of IFN action as human fibroblast IFN is much less effective. Inhibition of the growth in agar of normal human marrow myeloid progenitors was also described by Grant et al. (19) who could show that inhibition of growth of normal human hematopoietic cells required considerably higher concentration of rIFN-αA and -.D preparations than that of cells of the human leukemia cell lines HL-60 and KG-1. In this respect Langer J.A. and Pestka (35) have recently described that the binding of human rIFN-αA to HL-60 cells increases significantly, when the cells are induced to differentiate to a neutrophil-like state by treatment with dimethylsulfoxide (DMSO) or retinoic acid. The increased binding is the result of an increase in the number of binding sites available on these cells.

As for the erythroid pathway, inhibition of growth and differentiation of murine and human erythroid progenitors (early, BFU-E, and late, CFU-E) was reported by Smith et al. (56) and Ortega et al. (44). These experiments were performed in cultures supplemented with 30-40% fetal calf serum and exposed to very crude IFN preparations. Employing electrophoretically pure mouse IFN, but still in poorly defined culture conditions, Gallien-Lartigue et al. (17) showed that exposure to IFN resulted in a pronounced inhibition of CFU-E growth and differentiation. Interestingly, analysis of hemopoietic cells from a large number of inbred mice revealed that the effect depended upon the mouse strain employed, indicating that susceptibility and/or resistance to IFN actions may depend upon the recipients' genotype. This would be of obvious interest in planning human therapeutical trials. Rossi et al. (51, 52) have carried out similar studies in which partially purified or pure mouse α/β IFN preparations were added to methyl cellulose cultures of marrow or spleen cells supplemented with 0.4-4% fetal calf serum. Preparations of erythropoietin virtually free of endotoxin were used. The pattern of IFN effects is influenced by the use of more controlled culture conditions and/or pure IFN preparations. The growth of BFU-E is markedly inhibited in the presence of 10-500 U/ml of IFN. Studies carried out by adding pure mouse IFN at sequential days of culture suggest that the main IFN target is the BFU-E , while its inhibitory effect gradually diminishes in the course of the BFU-E-CFU-E differentiation. Inhibition of CFU-E growth is marginal, and the clonogenic potential of CFU-GM is unaffected. Concentration-dependent inhibition of both erythroid and myeloid precursors using human rIFN-γ was also demonstrated (67). A more pronounced suppressive effect was seen on the BFU-E than on the CFU-E, with CFU-GM mostly resistant. In addition, a permanent T cell line, SMAA cells, established from circulating mononuclear cells of a patient with severe aplastic anemia, were shown to inhibit proliferation of purified myeloid progenitors (neutrophil and eosinophil colonies more than monocyte colonies) and erythroid colonies. This inhibition appears mediated by the release of high quantities of IFN-γ ($3x10^3$ IU/ml of culture supernatants) (24). Conversely, human immature myeloid cells from normal bone marrow were shown to be induced into terminal monocytic differentiation by exposure to a component of phytohemagglutinin-stimulated conditioned medium (PHA-CM) identified as IFN-γ (45). Recently, Herrmann et al. (25) reported that as low as 10 U/ml of the T-cell lymphokine IFN-γ induced highly purified monocytes preparations to produce GM-CSF. The response of monocytes preparations to IFN-γ was biphasic in that concentrations greater than 250 U/ml did not induce GM-CSF activity. This was due to the production of a humoral inhibitor of G/M-progenitor cells. Grabstein et al. (18) observed that when IFN-γ activates monocytes to become tumoricidal, additional stimulation by exogenously added LPS is required. No such signal was required for monocytes activation by GM-CSF.

In conclusion, it is evident that both mouse and human IFNs affect the differentiation of hematopoietic cells more often by inhibiting their growth and maturation. Examples of differentiation induction are also available and will probably become more numerous as culture conditions will improve towards the ideal of a fully chemically-defined protocol. In this respect it is only reasonable to foresee that such a development of biotechnology will enable us to reassess some of the data available. For instance, Yamamoto-Yamaguchi et al. (73), employing almost pure murine IFN preparations consisting mostly of the α type, have shown a profound inhibitory effect on the growth of bone marrow cells supplemented with macrophage-derived colony-stimulating factor. Conversely as low as 50 IU/ml IFN stimulated macrophage production. These data indicate that IFN-α preferentially affects growth and differentiation of mouse marrow cells of the macrophage lineage.

Several lines of evidence support a role for IFNs in modulating also the differentiation potential of leukemic cells. In the myeloid lineage, human IFNα (both native and recombinant) or IFN-β induce cells of the histiocytic lymphoma line U937 to move along the monocytic pathway of differentiation (23). Under the same experimental conditions, cells of promyelocytic leukemia-derived line HL-60 were not induced. Perussia et al. (45) also showed that a component of a PHA-CM identified as IFN-γ induces cells of the perypheral blood of patiens with chronic myelogenous leukemia to differentiate to monocyte-like cells. Even myeloid cells as mature as metamyelocytes (but not mature neutrophils) can be induced by this IFN-γ preparation to undergo monocyte differentiation. This may offer new insights into the understanding of monocyte recruitment and differentiation during virus infections or immune reactions. In addition human IFN-γ alone may induce an increase in monocyte differentiation markers of HL-60 (71). Induction of differentiation exerted by other inducers (12-0-tetradecanoyl-phorbol-13 acetate (TPA), retinoic acid, etc. of cells of HL-60 line, non inducea-ble to differentiate by IFN-α or IFN-β alone, can, however, instead be stimulated by IFN-α, IFN-β or IFN-γ (63, 64, 71). It is of interest that purified r-Hu-IFN-γ (45) can induce the expression of antigens characteristic of monocytes as well as changes in morphology consistent with monocytoid differentiation. Data indicate that de novo protein synthesis was induced by IFN-γ to exert its effects. Antibodies anti-IFN-γ blocked the effect. Interestingly, human IFN-γ alone is also able to induce IL-2 receptors on human peripheral blood monocytes (26). Similarly, mouse myeloid leukemic Ml cells could not be induced to differentiate into macrophages and granulocytes by IFNs, which instead "stimulated" the differentiation induced by a number of compounds (D-factor, lipopolysaccharide, poly I:C) (62). In the same cell system Lotem and Sachs (37) developed a number of mutant clones that were used to study the effect of mouse IFN-α/β on the expression of different cell genes involved in differentiation. In the erythroid lineage the effects of mouse IFN on Friend virus-induced erythroleukemic cells (FLC) have been extensively studied by Rossi et al. (for previous reviews and detailed list of references, see 53). Friend-virus induced erythroleukemic cells are erythroid precursors blocked in their differentiation pathway at the stage of proerythroblast (late CFU-E) presumably as a consequence of the chronic infection by Friend Leukemia Virus (FLV). A large majority of cell clones available show a low (0.5-2%) but definite level of spontaneous differentiation into more advanced stages of erythropoiesis such as orthochromatic normoblasts. The addition of dimethylsulfoxide (DMSO) or of several chemically related or unrelated compounds to FLC cultures causes a stochastic and massive shift towards the normoblast stage of erythropoiesis, which is a bona fide example of terminal differentiation. At this stage, in fact, a complete cessation of cell division has occurred even though the cells are still nucleated. In keeping with data obtained in other systems the IFN-α/β dose-response in FLC are bell-shaped. Doses below 500 U/ml enhance FLC "induced" differentiation (6, 12). They also appear to "induce" FLC to differentiate even in the absence of other inducers (6, 11, 12). The magnitude of the latter observation is marginal and may vary according to the FLC clone used, even though it has been documented by assessing the steady-state levels of total and cytoplasmic globin mRNA. Doses above 10,000 Units of IFN-α/β consistently decrease the percentage of differentiated cells (48-50). These effects are seen after exposure of FLC to pure preparations of mouse IFN (51).

Natural and recombinant preparation of mouse IFN-γ are also able to modulate DMSO-induced erythroid differentiation of FLC (54). Doses above 100 U/ml inhibit erythroid differentiation, lower doses (0,1-100 U/ml) do not affect the process, indicating that no enhancing effects is induced by IFN-γ in this system.

Several FLC clones have been obtained that exhibit resistance to one or more IFNs effects (1, 2) rendering the system amenable to genetic analysis and dissociation of IFN effects. Clones were screened by the acquisition of resistance to the establishment of the antiviral state. One of them (MRI 745 3C18) has been analysed in detail (1, 2, 47, 54 and unpublished observations). It appears completely resistant to the induction of the antiviral state by treatment with IFN-α/β, but partially susceptible to IFN-γ. The clones were found also resistant to the enhancement of differentiation caused by low doses of IFN-α/β, whereas they were all as susceptible as wild type parental cells to the differentiation inhibition caused by high doses of IFN-α/β. The specificity of all IFN effects on FLC was already established by using pure IFN preparations. Hence, these data suggest that at least in this system treatment with IFN-α/β results in a) the establishment of the antiviral state and the stimulation of differentiation (low doses), and b) the inhibition of differentiation (high doses), by different mechanisms. In addition, the levels of 2-5A synthetase and 67K protein kinase enzimatic activities assayed *in vitro* superimposable in extracts of IFN-α/β treated and untreated resistant cells (2, 47, 54). It appears, therefore, that when FLC are exposed to α/β IFN, the establishment of the antiviral state and the enhancement of differentiation may be related to the induction of the 2-5A and 67K protein kinase synthetase pathways whereas the inhibition of differentiation by high doses of IFN is not mediated by their induction.

Cells of the human line K562 may be considered the closest counterpart to the murine FLC. They respond to hemin or butyric acid induction with a differential expression of the embryonal globin genes. Treatment of K562 cells with Hu-IFN-α/β and -γ (at substantially higher dosages than with FLC) results in a modulation of hemoglobin production induced by butyric acid or hemin treatment (8).

In conclusion, the evidence for the existance of significant interactions of human and mouse IFNs with some differentiation pathways in leukemic cells is overwhelming. The data from K562 and FLC systems point to a somewhat "specific" relationship of IFN with erythropoiesis in general, suggesting a possible regulatory action *in vivo*. In this respect, it is tempting to remind the reader of T. Hunt's (28) statement: "reticulocyte lysates so strongly resemble interferon-treated cell extracts in their sensitivity and response to double-stranded RNA that one wonders if the erythrocyte pathway of differentiation depends on exposure to a hormone like interferon at some stage." In fact, Hovanessian and Kerr (27) showed that the 2'-5'A synthesis in rabbit reticulocyte lysates was analogous to that observed in extracts from IFN-treated cells.

Recently, 2-5A synthetase appearance and induction in chicken embryo erythrocytes during development were studied by Sokawa and Sokawa (58). Enzyme activity first appeared in the embryos on the 15th day of incubation, a marked increase being seen 1 or 2 days after hatching. It has been postulated that the 2-5A synthetase-RNase L pathway might be activated in cells not exposed to IFN, implicating a wider significance for this enzymatic system.

In fact, it has been observed that the 2-5A synthetase is distributed widely in mammalian cells and the basal enzyme levels can vastly differ among various cell lines and tissues (60). In a given cell line (Namalva) 2-5A synthetase activity may vary depending log *vs* stationary growth phases; this regulatory mechanism is apparently not activated by IFN (33) in keeping with other observations indicating that this enzyme pathway is involved in controlling cell growth in uninfected cells (30,

31). Withdrawal from stimulation with estrogens of chick oviducts (60) results in a significant increase of 2-5A synthetase activity.

In truly differentiating systems, the basal levels of 2-5A synthetase were found to be higher in the mature and immunocompetent peripheral T splenocytes than in immature T cells obtained either from the thymus of BALB/c mice or from the spleen of athymic nude mice (31). These data, taken together with those discussed above with respect to cell growth, have been interpreted as an indication that the products of 2-5A synthetase activity may be involved in the expression of cell differentiation, leading to the following general model: differentiated and non-growing cells have higher levels of 2-5A synthetase than rapidly growing and immature cells (30, 31). The model is supported by observations in the FLC system. In fact, when DMSO-induced FLC differentiate, the levels of the enzyme are low in rapidly growing cells, but increase 8-10-fold as the cells reach the stationary phase (31). The increase in enzyme levels appears to be mediated by FLC secretion of β-like IFN (16). Also in human U937 leukemic cells differentiating towards macrophage-like cells, IFN production apparently occurs, while the levels of 2-5A synthetase activity and, incidentally, those of HLA-mRNAs also increase (32). In these conditions, the administration to the cultures of anti-IFN-β antibodies prevents the elevation of the levels of both HLA-mRNAs and 2-5A synthetase activity (particularly those of the species found in the nuclear fraction), which also takes place in differentiating U937 cells (74).

The observation that the IFN-α/β-resistant clones isolated by Affabris et al. (1) are unable to "induce" the 2-5A synthetase system to any detectable level even when exposed to 10,000 U/ml of α/β mouse IFN and yet, cells of these clones do differentiate upon induction with DMSO or hexamethylenebisacetamide (HMBA) indistinguishably of parental wild type FLC, suggest that 2-5A synthetase does not play an essential role in the differentiation of FLC. Mechti et al. (39) tested simultaneously two FLC sublines and found that in DMSO-treated cultures 2-5A synthetase activity increases in one differentiating (91% B+ cells) subline but was not modified in the other differentiating (89% B+ cells) subline. In addition, HMBA, a more potent inducer of differentiation than DMSO, did not modulate 2-5A synthetase levels in either subline in face of a quasi-total cell hemoglobinization (99% B+).

In another system, mouse myeloid leukemic M1 cells exhibit detectable 2-5A synthetase activity only when they differentiate to phagocytic cells after incubation with conditioned medium (CM) from rat embryo cells, in the absence of detectable IFN activity in the supernatants. Anti-IFN serum abolished enzyme activation by CM; yet, it did not influence M1 cell differentiation to phagocytes. IFN added exogenously per se neither induced phagocyte activity of these cells nor did it enhance the CM-induced differentiation of the cells. Moreover, dexamethasone, which induces differentiation of the same cells, did not induce the enzyme activity (57). It appears that a general role of 2-5A synthetase per se (i.e. in cells not exposed to exogenous IFN) in cell differentiation is not convincingly demonstrated by the data available sofar. It cannot be excluded, however, that a localized activation of the 2-5A system (42) in intact differentiating cells may escape detection under the available experimental conditions but still play a significant biological role. However, recent data indicate that IFN decreases the expression of genes (c-myc, c-fos, ODC, and β-actin mRNA) that are turned on by the competence growth factor PDGF (Platelet Derived Growth Factor) (13, 66). Conversely, PDGF stimulates late induction of β-fibroblast IFN and 2-5A synthetase (75). These results suggest that β-fibroblast IFN and 2-5A synthetase, induced slowly by PDGF, may function as feedback inhibitors of the growth response to PDGF and/or inhibitors of cell growth in terminal differentiation.

CONCLUSIONS

During the preceeding evaluation of experimental data the following information was purposedly omitted: all effects of IFNs on cell differentiation are reversible once IFN is removed. This is taken to mean that IFNs must be continuously present throughout the whole duration of the experiments (or for a substantial part thereof) for the effects to be detectable. Removal of IFNs promptly results in disappearance of the effects and in resumption of the normal phenotype(s) or function(s) under study, unless, of course, a stably modified phenotype has been selected as a consequence of the experimental protocol. This is at variance with the development of the antiviral state, which, once established, does not require the continuous presence of IFN throughout the considerable period of time (24 hours) during which the antiviral state is detectable. Under experimental conditions mimicking the physiological ones, establishment of the antiviral state may take a very short time interval to occur, (10). One possible explanation is that IFNs induce their effects on cell differentiation through the action of secondary molecules other than those already demonstrated with respect to the antiviral state. Were this so, one could also hypothesize that a variety of secondary molecules may be produced as a consequence of exposure to IFNs. Hence the multiple and varied biologic effects of IFNs on cell physiology would find an easy and reasonable explanation.

ACKNOWLEDGEMENTS

This work was supported in part by grants from Consiglio Nazionale delle Ricerche, Rome, Italy, Progetti Finalizzati "Oncologia" No. 85.02796.44, and "Controllo delle Malattie da Infezione" No. 85.02797.52, and from the Associazione Italiana per la Ricerca contro il Cancro, Milan, Italy. The skillful secretarial assistance of Ms. C. Buschittari and Mr. G. Caricati is gratefully acknowledged.

REFERENCES

1. Affabris, E., C. Jemma, and G.B. Rossi: Isolation of Interferon-Resistant Variants of Friend Erythroleukemia Cells: Effects of Interferon and Ouabain. Virology 120:441, 1982.

2. Affabris, E., G. Romeo, M. federico, E.M. Coccia, and G.B. Rossi: Friend leukemia cell clones resistant to murine IFNs. In: The Interferon System, F. Dianzani, G.B. Rossi, eds. Serono Symposia, Raven Press, Vol. 24, pp. 373-377, 1985.

3. Blalock, J.E., and J.D. Stanton: Common pathways of interferon and hormonal action. Nature 283:406, 1981.

4. Burke, D.C., C.F. Graham, and J.M. Lehman: Appearance of interferon inducibility and sensitivity during differentiation of murine teratocarcinoma cells in vitro. Cell 13:243, 1978.

5. Calvet, M.-Ch., and I. Gresser: Interferon enhances the excitability of cultured neurones. Nature 278:558, 1979.
6. Cioè, L., A. Dolei, G.B. Rossi, F. Belardelli, E. Affabris, E. Gambari, and A. Fantoni: Potential for Differentiation, Virus Production and Tumorigenicity in Murine Erythroleukemic Cells Treated with Interferon. In: In vitro Aspects of Erythropoiesis, M. Murphy, ed. Springer Verlag, Heidelberg, pp. 159-171, 1978.
7. Cioé, L., T.G. O'Brien, and L. Diamond: Inhibition of adipose conversion of Balb/c 3T3 cells by interferon and 12-0-tetradecanoylphorbol-13-acetate. Cell Biol Int Reports 4:255, 1980.
8. Cioè, L., P. Meo, V. Sorrentino, and G.B. Rossi: Modulation of Hemoglobin Synthesis in K-562(S) Cells Treated With Interferon. Blood 61:1146, 1983.
9. Coveney, J., G. Scott, R. King, D.C. Burke, and D. Skup: Changes in the conformation of the interferon beta gene during differentiation and induction. Bioch Biophys Res Comm 121:290, 1984.
10. Dianzani, F., and S. Baron: Unexpectedly rapid action of human interferon in physiological conditions. Nature 257:682, 1975.
11. Dolei, A., M.R. Capobianchi, L. Cioè, G. Colletta, G. Vecchio, G.B. Rossi, E. Affabris, and F. Belardelli: Effects on Interferon on the expression of Cellular and Integrated Viral Genes in Friend Erythroleukemic Cells. In: Antiviral Mechanisms in the Control of Neoplasia, P. Chandra, ed. Plenum Press, London, pp. 729-739, 1979.
12. Dolei, A., G. Colletta, M.R. Capobianchi, G.B. Rossi, and G. Vecchio: Interferon Effects on Friend Leukaemia Cells. I. Expression of Virus and Erythroid Markers in Untreated and Dimethyl Sulphoxide-treated Cells. J Gen Virol 46:227, 1980.
13. Einat, M., D. Resnitzky, and A. Kimchi: Inhibitory effects of interferon on the expression of genes regulated by platelet-derived growth factor. PNAS USA 82:7608, 1985.
14. Fisher, P.B., R.A. Mufson, and I.B. Weinstein: Interferon inhibits melanogenesis in B-16 mouse melanoma cells. Bioch Bioph Res Comm 100: 823, 1981.
15. Fisher, P.B., A.F. Miranda, L.E. Babiss, S. Pestka, and I.B. Weinstein: Opposing effects of interferon produced in bacteria and of tumor promoters on myogenesis in human myoblast cultures. Proc Natl Acad Sci USA 80:2961, 1983.
16. Friedman-Einat, M., M. Revel, and A. Kimchi: Initial characterization of a spontaneous Interferon secreted during growth and differentiation of Friend Erythroleukemia cells. Mol Cell Biol 2:1472, 1982.
17. Gallien-Lartigue, O., D. Carrez, E. De Maeyer, and J. De Maeyer-Guignard: Strain dependence of the antiproliferative action of interferon on murine erythroid precursors. Science 209:292, 1980.
18. Grabstein, K.H., D.L. Urdal, R.J. Tushinski, D.Y. Mochizuki, V.L. Price, M.A. Cantrell, S. Gillis, and P.J. Conlon: Induction of macrophage tumoricidal activity by granulocyte-macrophage colony-stimulating factor. Science 232:94, 1986.
19. Grant, S., K. Bhalla, I.B. Weinstein, S. Pestka, and P.B. Fisher: Differential effect of recombinant human leukocyte interferon on human leukemic and normal myeloid progenitor cells. Bioch Bioph Res Comm 108:1048, 1982.
20. Grossberg, S.E., and S. Keay: The effects of interferon on 3T3-L1 cell differentiation. Ann NY Acad Sci 350:294, 1980.
21. Grossberg, S.E., and P.S. Morahan: Repression of interferon ac-

tion: induced dedifferentiation of embryonic cells. Science 171:77, 1971.

22. Grossberg, S.E., and J.L. Sabran: Interferon inhibition of cellular differentiation. Tex Rep Biol Med 41:332, 1982.

23. Hattori, T., M. Pack, Ph. Bougnoux, Z.-L. Chang, and T. Hoffman: Interferon-induced differentiation of U937 cells. Comparison with other agents that promote differentiation of human myeloid or monocyte-like cell lines. J Clin Invest 72:237, 1983.

24. Herrmann, F., J.D. Griffin, S.G. Meuer, and K.H. Meyer zum B''uschenfelde: Establishment of an interleukin 2-dependent T cell line derived from a patient with severe applastic anemia, which inhibits in vitro hematopoiesis. J Immunol 136:1629, 1986.

25. Herrmann, F., S.A. Cannistra, and J.D. Griffin: T cell-monocyte interactions in the production of humoral factors regulating human granulopoiesis in vitro. J Immunol 136:2856, 1986.

26. Holter, W., R. Grunow, H. Stockinger, and W. Knapp: Recombinant interferon-γ induces interleukin 2 receptors on human peripheral blood monocytes. J Immunol 136:2171, 1986.

27. Hovanessian, A.G., and I.M. Kerr: Synthesis of an oligonucleotide inhibitor of protein synthesis in rabbit reticulocyte lysates analogous to that formed in extracts from interferon-treated cells. Eur J Biochem 84:149, 1978.

28. Hunt, T.: Interferon, dsRNA and the phenotypic effector. Nature 273:97, 1978.

29. Keay, S., and S.E. Grossberg: Interferon inhibits the conversion of 3T3-L1 mouse fibroblasts into adipocytes. Proc Natl Acad Sci USA 77:4099, 1980.

30. Kimchi, A., H. Shure, and M. Revel: Regulation of lymphocyte mitogenesis by (2'-5')oligo-isoadenylate. Nature 282:849, 1979.

31. Kimchi, A., H. Shure, and M. Revel: Anti-mitogenic function of interferon-induced (2'-5')oligo(adenylate) and growth-related varations in enzymes that synthesize and degrade this oligonucleotide. Eur J Biochem 114:5, 1981.

32. Kimchi, A., R. Bendori, M. Einat, A. Yarden, D. Resnitzky, and H. Gottlieb: Production and function of IFN during the process of cell differentiation. In: The Biology of the Interferon System 1983, E. De Maeyer, and H. Schellekens, eds. Elsevier Sci. Publ., Amsterdam., pp.83-90, 1983.

33. Krishnan, I., and C. Baglioni: Elevated levels of (2'-5')oligoadenylic acid polymerase activity in growth-arrested human lymphoblastoid Namalva cells. Mol Cel Biol 1:932, 1981.

34. Lampidis, T., and D. Brouty-Boyé: Interferon inhibits cardiac cell function in vitro. Proc Soc Exp Biol Med 166:181, 1981.

35. Langer, J.A., and S. Pestka: Changes in binding of r interferon IFN-α A to HL-60 cells during myeloid differentiation. J Interferon Res 5:637, 1985.

36. Lewis, D.B., A. Larsen, and C.B. Wilson: Reduced interferon-γ mRNA levels in human neonates. Evidence for an intrinsic T cell deficiency independent of other genes involved in T cell activation. J Exp Med 1:163, 1986.

37. Lotem, J., and L. Sachs: Genetic dissociation of different cellular effects of interferon on myeloid leukemic cells. Int J Cancer 22: 214, 1978.

38. Lough, J., S. Keay, J.L. Sabran, and S.E. Grossberg: Inhibition of

chicken myogenesis in vitro by partially purified interferon. Biochem Biophys Res Comm 109:92, 1982.
39. Mechti, N., E. Affabris, G. Romeo, B. Lebleu, and G.B. Rossi: Role of interferon and 2-5A synthetase en erythroid differentiation of Friend Leukemia Cells. J Biol Chem 259:3261, 1984.
40. Multhauf, C., and J. Lough: Interferon-mediated inhibition of differentiation in a murine myoblast cell line. J Cell Physiol 126:211, 1986.
41. Nickoloff, B.J., G. Mahrle, and V. Morhenn: Ultrastructural effects of recombinant γ-interferon on cultured human keratinocytes. Ultrastruct Pathol 10:17, 1986.
42. Nilsen, T.W., and C. Baglioni: A mechanism for discrimination between viral and host mRNA in interferon-tretaed cells. Proc Natl Acad Sci USA 76:2600, 1979.
43. Oh, S.H., B. Gonik, S.B. Greenberg, and S. Kohl: Enhancement of human neonatal natural killer cytotoxicity to herpes simplex virus with use of recombinant human interferons: lack of neonatal response to . interferon. J Infect Dis 153:791, 1986.
44. Ortega, J.A., M.A. Andrew, O.W. Schorr, P.P. Dukes, and T.C. Merigan: Suppressive effect of interferon on erythroid cell proliferation. Exp Hematol 7:145, 1979.
45. Perussia, B., E.T. Dayton, V. Fanning, P. Thiagaraja, J. Hoxie, and G. Trinchieri: Immune interferon and leukocyte-conditioned medium induce normal and leukemic myeloid cells to differentiate along the monocytie pathway. J Exp Med 158:2058, 1983.
46. Peschle, C.: Hemopoietic sten and progenitor cells: recent advances of physiopathologic relevance. In: Butterworths International Medical Reviews, Haematology-Oncology, M.L.N. Willoughby, and S.E. Siegel, eds. Butterworths, London, Vol. 1, pp.263-296, 1982.
47. Romeo, G., E. Affabris, M. Federico, N. Mechti, E.M. Coccia, C. Jemma, and G.B. Rossi: Establishement of the antiviral state in α/β interferon-resistant Friend cells treated with γ interferon: induction of 67K protein kinase activity in absence of detectable 2-5A synthetase J Biol Chem 260:3833, 1985.
48. Rossi, G.B., G.P. Matarese, C. Grappelli, F. Belardelli, and A. Benedetto: Inhibition of Erythroid differentiation of Dimethyl Sulfoxide-induced Friend Leukemia Cells by Interferon. Nature 267:50, 1977.
49. Rossi, G.B., A. Dolei, L. Cioé, A. Benedetto, G. Matarese, and F. Belardelli: Inhibition of Transcription and Translation of Globin messenger RNA in Dimethyl Sulfoxide-stimulated Friend erythroleukemic cells treated with Interferon. Proc Natl Acad Sci USA 74:1655, 1977.
50. Rossi, G.B., A. Dolei, L. Cioè, A. Benedetto, G.P. Matarese, F. Belardelli, and G. Rita: Interferon and Friend Leukemia cells in culture. Tex Rep Biol Med 35:420, 1977.
51. Rossi, G.B., A. Dolei, M.R. Capobianchi, C. Peschle, and E. Affabris: Interaction of interferon with in vitro model systems involved in haematopoietic cell differentiation. Ann NY Acad Sci 350:279, 1980.
52. Rossi, G.B., A. Dolei, L. Cioé, and C. Peschle: Effect of Interferon on Erythropoietic Differentiation. Tex Rep Biol Med 41:381, 1982.
53. Rossi, G.B.: Interferons and cell differentiation. In: Interferon 1984, I. Gresser ed. Academic Press N.Y., vol. 6, pp. 31-68, 1985.
54. Rossi, G.B., E. Affabris, G. Romeo, M. Federico, E.M. Coccia, N. Mechti, and B. Lbleu: The role of two interferon-induced enzymatic activities in erythroid differentiation of Friend cells. In: The 2-5A

System: Molecular and Clinical Aspects of the Interferon-regulated Pathway, B. Williams, and R. Silverman, eds. Plenum Press, Toronto, Canada, Vol. 202, pp. 285-296, 1985.
55. Saneto, R., and H.M. Johnson: Interferon inhibition of hexose monophosphate Shunt activity as the mechanism of blocking differentiation of preadipose cell line. Bioch Biophys Res Comm 106:373, 1982.
56. Smith, K.A., T.N. Fredrickson, L.E. Mobraaten, and E. De Maeyer: The interaction of erythropoietin with fetal liver cells. II. Inhibition of the erythropoietin effect by interferon. Exp Hematol 14:164, 1976.
57. Sokawa, Y., K. Nagata, and Y. Ichikawa: Induction and function of 2'-5'oligoadenylate synthetase in differentiation of mouse myeloid leukemia cells. Exp Cell Res 135:191, 1981.
58. Sokawa, J, and Y. Sokawa: (2'-5')oligoadenylate synthetase in chicken embryo erythrocytes and immature red blood cells. J Biochem 99: 119, 1986.
59. Stadler, R., R. Müller, and C.E. Orfanos: Effect of recombinant α A-interferon on DNA synthesis and differentiation of human keratinicytes in vitro. Br J Dermatol 114:273, 1986.
60. Stark, G.R., W.J. Dower, R.T. Schimke, R.E. Brown, and I.M. Kerr: pppA2'p5'-A2'p5'A synthetase: convenient assay, species and tissue distribution and variation upon withdrawal of oestrogen from chick oviducts. Nature 278:471, 1979.
61. Stohlman, S.A., A.Y. Sakaguchi, and A. Hiti: Interferon production and activity in mouse neuroblastoma cells. Arch Virol 57:91, 1978.
62. Tomida, M., Y. Yamamoto, and M. Hozumi: Stimulation by interferon of induction of differentiation of mouse myeloid leukemic cells. Cancer Res 40:2919, 1980.
63. Tomida, M., Y. Yamamoto, and M. Hozumi: Stimulation by interferon of induction of differentiation of human promyelocytic leukemia cells. Biochem Biophys Res Comm 104:30, 1982.
64. Tomida, M., Y. Yamamoto, M. Hozumi, T. Oku, and T. Kishida: Prolongation by interferon preparation of the survival time of mice implanted with differentiation-inducible mouse myeloid leukemia cells. Leukemia Res 7:439, 1983.
65. Tomida, Y., and S. Hasegawa: Multiple effects of interferon on myogenesis in chicken myoblast cultures. Biochem Biophys Acta 20:370, 1984.
66. Tominaga, S., and P. Lengyel: β/Interferon alters the pattern of proteins secreted from quiescent and platelet-derived growth factor-treated BALB/c-3T3 cells. J Biol Chem 260:1975, 1985.
67. Toretsky, J.A., N.T. Shahidi, and J.L. Finlay: Effects of recombinant human interferon γ on hematopoietic progenitor cell growth. Exp Hematol 14:182, 1986.
68. Verma, D.S., G. Spitzer, J.U. Gutterman, A.R. Zander, K.B. McCredie, and K.A. Dicke: Human leukocyte interferon preparation blocks granulopoietic differentiation. Blood 54:1423, 1979.
69. Verma, D.S., G. Spitzer, A.R. Zander, J.U. Gutterman, K.B. McCredie, K.A. Dicke, and D.A. Johnston: Human leukocyte interferon preparation-mediated block of granulopoietic differentiation in vitro. Int Soc Exp Hematol 9:63, 1981.
70. Verma, D.S., G. Spitzer, J.U. Gutterman, M. Beran, A.R. Zander, and K.B. McCredie: Human leukocyte interferon-mediated granulopoietic differentiation arrest and its abrogation by lithium carbonate. Am J

Hematol 12:39, 1982.
71. Weinberg, J.B., M.A. Misukonis, M.M. Hobbs, and M.J. Borowitz: Cooperative effects of γ interferon and 1-α, 25-dihydroxyvitamin D3 in inducing differentiation of human promyelocytic leukemia (HL-60) cells. Exp Hematol 14:138, 1986.
72. Wilson , C.B., J. Westall, L. Johnston, D.B. Lewis, S.K. Dower, and A.R. Alpert: Decreased production of interferon-γ by human neonatal cells. Intrinsic and regulatory deficiencies. J Clin Invest 77:860, 1986.
73. Yamamoto-Yamaguchi, Y., M. Tomida, and M. Hozumi: Effect of mouse interferon on growth and differentiation of mouse bone marrow cells stimulated by two different types of colony-stimulating factor. Blood 62:597, 1983.
74. Yarden, A., H. Shure-Gottlieb, J. Chebath, M. Revel, and A. Kimchi: Autogenous production of interferon-beta switches on HLA genes during differentiation of histiocytic lymphoma U937 cells. EMBO J 3969, 1984.
75. Zullo, J.N., B.H. Cochran, A.S. Huang, and C.D. Stiles: Platelet-derived growth factor and double-stranded ribonucleic acids stimulate expression of the same genes in 3T3 cells. Cell 43:793, 1985.
76. Zusman, I., D. Engelhard, P. Yaffe, A. Ron, A. Panet, and A. Ornoy: Effects of interferon and encephalomyocarditis virus on in vitro development of preimplantation mouse embryos with and without the zona pellucida. Teratology 29:405, 1984.

TABLE 1. Effects of IFNs on differentiating and differentiated cell systems

Type of IFN	Differentiation System	Effects
Mouse IFN	Melanogenesis	Inhibition of spontaneous and melanocyte hormone stimulated melanogenesis in cultures of murine B-16 melanoma cells (14).
Hu-r IFN-αA	Myogenesis	Acceleration of myotube formation and creatine kinase (CK) isoenzyme transition from CK-BB to CK-MM in normal human myoblast cultures derived from mature skeletal muscle (15).
IFN	Myogenesis	Inhibition of CK isoenzyme transition and myotube formation of chicken embryo myogenic cells (22, 38, 65, 40).
Mouse IFN	Adipogenesis	Inhibition of adipose conversion of Balb/C 3T3 (7) and of Swiss 3T3 (29, 20, 55) cell clones.
Hu-r IFN-αA	Keratinocytes	Decrease of the amount and synthesis of non-covalently bound keratins and increase of the disulplide cross-linked keratins (59).
r-γ IFN	Keratinocytes	Increase percentage of attached cells with a mature-type, differentiated apppearance in cultures of normal human keratinocytes (41).
Hu and rat IFN	Nerve cells	Enhancement of the excitability of cat and rat nerve cells (5).
Rat IFN	Cardiac cells	Decrease of the beating rate in fulsating rat cardiac cultures (34).
Mouse IFN	Cardiac cellS	Increase in the beating frequency of mouse myocardial cells (13).

30. The Interferon System in Coordinated Development of Tissues and Loss of Malignancy in Cancerous Cells

C. Chany

Université René Descartes, Département de Microbiologie, Hôpital St. Vincent de Paul, 74 ave. Denfert-Rochereau, 75014 Paris, France

The originally described acid-stable alpha and beta interferons are known for their potent antiviral properties and for their capacity to depress cell proliferation. Although equally antiviral, acid-labile IFN gamma is a completely different molecule, as illustrated by the structure of the gene responsible for its synthesis. It is likely that the latter is more intimately associated with immune response and/or the maturation of immunecompetent cells. Since the information presently available about the biological significance of this molecule is scarce, we will exclude IFN gamma from the present review, which does not however mean that this substance could not occasionally participate directly or indirectly in the biological processes we will analyse here.

In general, malignant cells are significantly less sensitive to the different biological effects of IFNS than their normal counterpart. This can, at least partly, be attributed either to a decrease in number or a loss in quality of the IFN-specific cell membrane receptors (or both), secondary to the malignant transformation resulting in the destruction of the cytoskeleton. In spite of this, several investigators have considered IFNs as merely cytostatic drugs during antitumor therapy. As seen from what will follow, this approach is probably an over-simplification. Firstly, the biological potential of a great number of presently known IFN-alpha molecular species are far from being explored. (Some of them could have little or no anti-viral but mainly growth-regulatory properties.) Secondly, because IFNs could be induced during as yet undefined physiological conditions (1) or pathological events. We will thus analyse three sets of observations supporting the view that perhaps the most important physiological role of the IFN system could be the control of the coordinated growth of tissues, at least during fetal development, and in parallel the maintenance of the already differentiated phenotype of cells. If this assumption can be considered valid, it is not surprising that the different biological functions of these IFN molecules are affected or even controlled by other peptide mediators, some of them characterized as growth factors (2)(3)(4)(5)(6) and others ressembling lectins (7).

Apparently constitutive synthesis of interferons during foetal life.

The synthesis of IFNs is depressed in the resting cell. Besides viruses, a long list of antigens from various origins (8) are able to induce them. Among others, this list includes allogenic spleen or tumor cells. However, at the present state of knowledge, there is only one physiological circumstance during which low but detectable levels of IFN were found continuously excreted: that is, the fetal period of pregnancy, at least in humans (9),(10),(11), mice (12) and rats (unpublished data).

Alpha IFNs are present in practically all of the human amniotic fluids tested between the 16th week of pregnancy and delivery. The amounts are so low that no variations in titer could be detected during the progress of fetal development.

The site where these IFNs are synthesized could not be clearly identified. They are however more frequently seen in blood from the placenta than from the ombilical cord, or released from isolated amniotic membranes suspended in tissue culture fluid. IFNs were found in 29 out of 35 placental blood samples tested from uneventful pregnancies between the 35th week and delivery.

In one of the apparently negative blood samples, when assayed after different purification procedures (i.e. affinity columns to alpha- or beta-IFNs, cibacron-blue, ConA-sepharose chromatography), a significant amount of IFN together with lectin-like antagonists (analysed later on) were detected. A small fraction of these IFNs was of an unusually high mw.(80 KDa) reminiscent of those previously found after induction, in the amniotic membrane (13).

Comparable studies using mouse and rat placentas (unpublished data) yielded somewhat similar results, but the IFN species involved, since presently less explored, could not be identified with the same accuracy. An important point in these studies is that IFNs are only found after the 10th day of gestation, with a peak at the 17th day. This and other data discussed later suggest that IFNs are only excreted during the fetal and not the embryonic phase of pregnancy.

Substances which antagonize IFN action : sarcolectins and growth factors.

Normal or malignant animal tissues contain substances able to accelerate the restoration of the original virus sensitivity in IFN-treated cells (14). It is possible that an IFN-induced biological status cannot be continuously maintained in the cell, perhaps because under such conditions it cannot respond to growth-regulatory or other stimuli.

One group of such antagonists has been isolated, purified then characterized. They were termed sarcolectins, because of their presence in relatively important amounts in sarcomas or normal muscles

(15) from mammalian origins, but they were also found in rib cartilage (16), brain tissue (17) or placentas (11). All presently known sarcolectins share an apparent molecular size of 65 kDa (estimated by SDS PAGE electrophoresis under reducing conditions). They are all resistent to pepsin but are destroyed by other proteases. They agglutinate normal and malignant cells and have an affinity with simple sugars (7)(15). Sarcolectins from different origins share some epitopes in their antigenic structure, at least for the human and rodent species (submitted for publication). It is important to stress that they do not compete with IFN for receptors on the cell membrane and act only on the anti-viral state when established, problably working through an indirect cellular regulatory mechanism. As a result, the effects of at least two IFN-dependent secondary proteins, the 67 K protein kinase and the 2-5 A synthetase are significantly decreased or become undetectable in the cytosol (unpublished data). The other biological roles of sarcolectins are presently unknown, but they could be involved in one way or another in promoting cell proliferation.

If the IFN system can be considered as a possible, mostly negative, regulator of coordinated tissue development during fetal life (and also later), it is not surprising that growth-promoting factors or genes involved in cell multiplication can interact with this mediator. It has been reported (4) that platelet derived growth factors (PDGF) can inhibit priming of IFN induction (by this same substance) in mouse or human fibroblasts. Furthermore, pre-treatment of such cells with PDGF for 24 hours significantly decreases the capacity of IFN to induce antiviral protection in the same cells, in the following 6 hours. Opposition between these substances also extends in vitro to their effect on cell proliferation (2)(3).

IFN-induced modulation of the cell membrane can also modify the ligand affinity of the epithelial growth factor (EGF) for its specific receptor, in spite of the complete lack of direct binding competition between these two substances. Interestingly, for the same IFN concentration, short-term (1hour) treatment leads to a roughly 30% increase in receptor numbers, which is on the contrary reduced 20 hours later by about 40%. At that time, a fourfold decrease in affinity is also detected (5).

The IFN system could appear as a feedback loop after stimulation of cells with growth factors. For example, PDGF stimulates genes involved in growth such as c-*myc* and c-*fos*. Similar genes are also induced by double stranded RNA (dsRNA) or vesicular stomatitis virus (VSV). Subsequently, IFN mRNAs are also expressed, followed by corresponding secondarily induced IFN-dependent proteins.They apparently limit the effect of growth factors (6). Along the same line of thinking, the tumor necrosis factor (TNF) which is cytotoxic for many human tumor cells, can surprisingly stimulate growth in normal human fibroblasts, in which it also induces IFN-ß. This is not the case for epithelial cells in which TNF is not mitogenic (18). More recently, IFN-ß has been found as an autocrine feedback inhibitor during terminal differentiation of hematopoietic cells (19). This is in agreement with earlier data showing that low concentrations of IFN promote Friend cell differentiation while high concentrations inhibit it (20). Thus indeed the IFN system could be part of a feedback mechanism which can, when necessary, limit over-growth of cells.

Effect of IFN on proto-oncogenes involved in cell growth.

Some of the proto-oncogenes have been shown as being regularly expressed after induction of normal cell growth. For instance after antigen or lectin induced lymhocyte proliferation, c-fos is expressed generally after the first hour and c-myc somewhat later. For both, transcription can be decreased when growth-promoted cells are treated with IFN. This was reported for highly IFN-sensitive lymphoblastoid Daudi cells in which the c-myc specific 2.4 Kb mRNA transcription can drop in three hours by as much as 60%. This could possibly be attributed to an increased rate in its degradation (21)(22)(23). Similar observations were made for c-fos. It is likely that these responses are only part of the complex genetic system involved in cell growth stimulation and the IFN sensitivity of gene expression can be different from one tissue to the other.

Reconversion of transformed cells to non malignancy.

If the IFN system plays a role in cell growth regulation, it is not surprising that this system is in equilibrium with growth factors, sarcolectins, and regulates some of the proto-oncogenes involved in cell multiplication during the early G1 phase of the cycle. Therefore, it is feasible that IFN could affect the expression of modified variants of these genes. Indeed, it has been known for about 20 years (24)(25) that mouse embryonic cells transformed in vitro by the Moloney sarcoma viruses can be stably reverted to non malignancy by prolonged IFN treatment at low concentrations. The cells recover contact inhibition, no longer yield colonies in soft agar, but retain immortality. The extra-cellular matrix consisting of collagen and fibronectin is incompletely restored, but is able to provide the cell with anchorage capacity (26). The cytoskeleton is seemingly almost completely restored (27). These new characteristics of the cells are stable and, unlike the transformed controls, they are unable to induce tumors, even in nude mice. An important point is that the integrated v-mos is located on identical sites on the DNA in IFN treated or control cells, which shows that the non malignant cell stems directly from the oncogenic one. Furthermore, the v-mos is transcribed even at a higher level in the reverted cells, but apparently no completely functional protein is synthesized and no v-mos-containing virions are released. In contrast, the helper virus is unaltered and produced even in increased numbers (26)(28)(29)(30).

Thus, at least in this model, IFN does not act as an anti-viral substance, but rather as a negative regulator of a modified cellular gene expression at a post-transcriptional level.

Similar observations were made in 3T3 cells, transformed by the Harvey RAS oncogene (h-ras). After a number of serial passages, in the presence of alpha/beta mouse IFN, a significant percentage of flat cellular mutants appeared, which were then selected. These cells underwent modifications comparable with those observed in the previous model and also became stably non malignant for nude mice (31). Interestingly, agents inducing demethylation of cellular DNA (such as 5-asacytosine) were able to revert these flat mutant cells to malignancy. In contrast with cells transformed by h-ras, cells transformed by the Kirsten sarcoma virus (k-ras) were not only insensitive to IFN action, but were seemingly even stimulated in their growth and malignancy (32) (33).

In other models such as rat cells transformed by the Rous sarcoma virus, the $pp60^{src}$ expression was, even after a short 24-hour treatment, significantly reduced, with a parallel decrease in tyrosine phosphokinase activity. The cells recovered a less malignant phenotype with partial restructuration of their actin fibres and simultaneously their growth rate was reduced (34)

Besides these genetically defined cancer cells, undefined ones, obtained by radiation or chemical processes, were comparably sensitive to the "demalignifying" effect of IFNs. This also results in the more or less complete restructuration of the filamentous elements of the cells (35).

General conclusions.

Besides anti-viral protection, our understanding of the possible physiological role of the IFN system has greatly benefited from the recent observation that IFNs are continuously excreted in the amniotic fluid and the placenta during the fetal phase of pregnancy. No such substances are found during the first period, when the embryon differentiates. Furthermore, it is common knowledge that during this phase no functional IFN receptors can be detected on the cell membranes. These arguments also support the view that IFN is not directly involved in differentiation. During the fetal phase, the constitutive mode of synthesis of this substance could be either effective or only apparent, due to a series of successive inductions of different IFN species, when needed for growth regulation in different areas. Since some of them have unusually heavy apparent molecular sizes, it is possible that such IFNs are less active in anti-viral protection, but contribute rather to the regulation of tissue growth. Unfortunately, with the methods presently available, we are unable to estimate variations in release or in the quality of these IFNs. Another point worth mentioning and explaining is the sole presence of alpha-IFN in the amniotic fluid and the parallel detection of beta-variants in the placenta. Since long-term IFN treatment can induce anticytolytic resistance in target cells, both against NK (36) (37) and T lymphocytes (38) 39), it is also possible that the IFN system can occasionally promote tolerance to protect the fetus versus the immune response of the mother. It cannnot be excluded that similar mechanisms could also take place postpartum, during acquired tolerance. Equilibrium between IFNs on one hand and sarcolectins or growth factors on the other, all simultaneously present in placental blood and probably also elsewhere, suggests that they are part of a control system of coordinated growth. This view is also supported by the observation that PDGF or TNF induce IFN, perhaps as a feedback loop to control out-of-hand cell growth, occasionally in an autocrine fashion. In the immune system Interleukin 2 and IFN-gamma could have a similar relationship (40).

In some circumstances, because of the known capacity of IFNs to protect cells from the integration of almost any foreign DNA (41), it is possible that the IFN system contributes to maintaining the integrity of the genome.

When there is a pathological expression of growth, mediated by oncogenes, either carried by viruses or transferred by other means, IFNs can still protect the cells from becoming malignant. As shown here, once the cell is transformed, the molecular lesion responsible for the oncogenic manifestation can, at least in some cases, be stably repaired. It is presently unknown how much of these observations can be extended to the different branches of oncology. It is likely, however, that these are not isolated phenomena. Indeed, in some human malignancies where IFNs seem to have a significant anti-tumor effect (such as hairy cell or chronic myelogenic leukemias), the presently described model has serious chances of being the mechanism of action. As a result, when treated cells are able to recover a differentiated status (even if IFN is not directly responsible for this process), they could rejoin their normal developmental cycle oriented towards differentiation. In most tissues, this eventually leads to cell death and epuration by the immune system before renewal. The role of IFNs in "demalignifying" cancer cells could be the starting point for new investigations in this area of human therapeutics.

Acknowledgements :

The author is indebted to Dr. F. Chany-Fournier for revising and to Mrs. L. Sergent, M.C Rufino for helping in the preparation of this manuscript.

1 . Bocci, V. The physiological interferon response. Immunology Today. 6, 1, 7-9, 1985.
2 . Inglot, A.D., Oleszak, E. and Kistelow. Antagonism in action between mouse or human interferon and platelet growth factor. Arch. Virol. 63, 291, 1980.
3 . Oleszak, E. and Inglot, A.D. Platelet derived growth factor (PDGF) inhibits antiviral and anticellular action of interferon in the synchronized mouse or human cell. J.Interferon Res. 1, 37, 1980.
4 . Chudzio, T. and Inglot, A.D. Platelet derived growth factor (PDGF) inhibits priming in the synchronous mouse or human fibroblasts producing interferon. J.Interferon Res. 1, 31, 1980.
5 . Zoon, K., Nedden, D.Z., Hu, R., Karasaki, Y., Komoriya, A. and Arnheiter, H. In Interferon System, Serono Symposia Dianzani, F. Rossi, G.B. Raven Press, Vol. 24, p.363-365, 1985.
6 . Zullo, J.N., Cochran, B.H., Huang, A.S. and Stiles, C.D. Platelet derived growth factor and double-stranded ribonucleic acids stimulate expression of the same genes in 3T3 cells. Cell, 43, 793-800, 1985.
7 . Jiang, P.H., Chany-Fournier, F., Robert-Galliot, B., Sarragne, M., Chany, C. Sarcolectin : An interferon antagonist extracted from hamster sarcomas and normal muscles. Isolation, Characterization and Purification. J.Biol.Chem, 258, 12361-12367, 1983.
8 . Svet-Moldavsky, G. J., Chernyakhovskaya, I. Yu. Interferon and the interaction of allogeneic normal and immune lymphocytes with L-cells. Nature, 215, 1299-1300, 1967.
9 . Lebon, P., Girard, S., Thepot, F., Chany, C. Presence constante d'interferon de type alpha dans les liquides amniotiques humains. C.R. Acad. SCI, (Paris), 293, 69-71, 1981.
10. Lebon, P., Girard, S., Thepot, F., Chany. C. Presence of alpha-interferon in human amniotic fluid. J.Gen.Virol., 59, 393-396, 1982.
11. Duc-Goiran, P., Robert-Galliot, B., Lopez, J. and Chany, C. Unusual apparently constitutive interferons and antagonists in human placental blood. Proc. Natl. Acad. Sci.(USA), 82, 5010-5014, 1985.
12. Fowler, A.H., Reed, C.D. and Giron, D.J. Identification of interferon in murine placentas. Nature (London) 286, 266, 1980.
13. Duc-Goiran, P., Robert-Galliot, B., Chudzio, T., Chany, C. Unusual human interferons produced by virus-infected amniotic membranes. Proc. Natl. Acad. Sci. (USA), 30, 2628-2631, 1983
14. Fournier, F., Rousset, S., Chany, C. Un facteur tissulaire antagoniste de l'action de l'interferon. C.R. Acad. Sci. (Paris), 266, 2306-2308, 1968.
15. Jiang, P.H., Chany-Fournier, F., Sarragne, M., Grégoire, A., Chany, C. Detection of an interferon antagonist, sarcolectin, in human sarcomas and muscles. Int. J. Cancer, 34, 625-632, 1984.
16. Chany-Fournier, F., Pauloin, A., Chany, C. Isolation, preliminary characterization and interferon antagonistic effect of a mammalian lectin-like substance. Proc. Nalt. Acad. Sci. (USA), 75, 2333-2337, 1978.

17. Brown, P., Sarragne, M., Chany, C., Gibbs, J., Gajdusek,D.C. In : Effects of interferon on cells, viruses and the immune system, (A.Geraldes, Ed.) Academic Press, 337-343, 1975.
18. Vilcek, J., Tsujimoto, M., Henriksen de Stephano, D., Hirai, M., and Kohase, M. Growth factors as IFN inducers and IFN inducers as growth factors. J. of Cellular Biochemistry Suppl. 10C, 216, 1986.
19. Resnitzky D., Yarden, A., Zipori D. and Kimchi, A. Autocrine ß-related interferon controls c-myc suppression and growth arrest during hematopoietic cell differentiation. Cell, 46, 31-40, 1986.
20. Rossi, G.B.,Matarese, G.P., Grapelli, C., Belardelli, F., Benedetto, A. Interferon inhibits dimethyl sulphoxide-induced erythoid differentiation of Friend leukemia cells. Nature, 267, 50-52, 1977.
21. Jonak, G.J. and Knight, F. Selective reduction of c-myc mRNA in Daudi cells by interferon. Proc. Natl. Acd. Sci. (USA), 81, 1747-1750, 1984.
22. Dani, C.H., Mechti, N., Piechaezyk, M.,Lebleu, B., Jeanteur, Ph. and Blanchard, J.M. Increased rate of degradation of myc RNA and interferon-treated Daudi cells. Proc. Natl. Acad. Sci. (USA) 82, 4896-4899, 1985.
23. Kimchi, A., Einat, M., Resnitzky, D., Yarden, A. and Gat, G. Inhibition of c-myc expression and cellular proliferation by endogenous and exogenous interferons. Ucla Symposia on Molecular & Cellular Biology, Abstract M.29, 229, Suppl. 10C, 1986.
24. Chany, C., Vignal, M. Etude du mécanisme de l'état réfractaire des cellules à la production d'interféron, après induction répétées. C.R. Acad. Sci. (Paris), 1798-1800, 1968.
25. Chany, C., Vignal, M. Effect of prolonged interferon treatment on mouse embryonic fibroblast transformed by murine sarcoma virus. J. Gen. Virol., 7, 203-210, 1970.
26. Gerfaux, J., Rousset, S., Chany-Fournier, F., Chany, C. Interferon effect on collagen and fibronectin distribution in the extracellular matrix of murine sarcoma virus-transformed cells. Cancer Res. 41, 3629-3634, 1981.
27. Bourgeade, M.F., Rousset, S. Paulin, D., Chany, C. Reorganization of the cytoskeleton by interferon in MSV-transformed cells. J. Interferon Res., 1, 323-332, 1981.
28. Chany, C., Gerfaux, J., Sergiescu, D. Persistent expression of the v.mos gene in reconverted non tumorigenic cells after long term IFN treatment. The Biology of the Interferon system, 317-325, 1985.
29. Sergiescu, D., Gerfaux, J., Joret, A.M., Chany, C. Persistent expression of v-mos oncogene in transformed cells that revert to nonmalignancy after prolonged treatment with interferon. Proc. Natl. Acad. Sci. (USA) 83, August, in press, 1986.
30. Gerfaux, J., Sergiescu, D., Vignal, M., Joret, A.M., Chany,C. Stable reversion to non malignancy by long term interferon treatment of cells expressing the v-mos oncogene. UCLA Symposia on Molecular & Cellular Biology, Abstract M.50, 236 Suppl. 10C, 1986.

31. Samid, D., Chang, E., Friedman, R. Biochemical correlation of phenotype reversion in interferon treated mouse cells transformed by a human oncogene. Biochem. and Biophys. Res.Commun. 119, 21-28, 1984.
32. Emanoil-Ravier, R. Pochart, F., Canivet, M. Garcette, M., Tobaly-Tapiero, J. and Peries, J. Interferon mediated regulation of myc and Ki-ras oncogene expression in long term treated murine viral transformed cells. J. of Interferon Res., 5, 613-619, 1985.
33. Brouty-Boye, D., Wybier Franqui, J., Calvo, C., Feunteun, J. and Gresser, I. Reversibility of the transformed and neoplastic phenotype IV effect of long term interferon treatment of $C_3H/10T1/2$ cells transformed by methylcholanthrene and SV40 virus. Int. J.Cancer, 34, 107-112,1984.
34. Lin, S. L., Garber, E.A., Wang, E., Caliguiri, L.A., Schellekens, H., Goldberg, A.R. and Tamm I. Reduced synthesis of $pp60^{src}$ and expression of the transformation-related phenotype in interferon-treated Rous sarcoma virus-transformed rat cells. Molecular and Cellular Biology, Sept., 1656-1664, 1983.
35. Brouty-Boyé, D., Cheng Yih-Shyun E. and Chen Lan Bo. Association of phenotypic reversion of transformed cells induced by interferon with morphological and biochemical changes in the cytoskeleton. Cancer Research, 41, 4174, 1981.
36. Trinchieri C., Santoli, D. Antiviral activity induced by culturing lymphocytes with tumor derived or virus transformed cells enhancement of human natural killer cell activity by interferon and antagonistic inhibition of susceptibility of target cells to lysis. J. Exp. Med. 147, 1314, 1978.
37. Moore, M., White, W.J., Potter, M.R. Modulation of target cell susceptibility to human natural killer cells by interferon. Int. J. Cancer, 25, 565, 1980.
38. Bergeret, M., Gregoire, A., Chany, C. Protective effect of interferon on target cells exposed to cellular cytotoxicity. Immunology, 40, 637, 1980.
39. Bergeret, M., Fouchard, M., Gregoire, A., Chany, C.,Zagury, D. Interferon effect on cytolytic T lymphocytes in a single cycle assay. Immunology, 48, 101, 1983.
40. Dubois, M.F., Vignal, M., Le Cunff, M., Chany, C. Interferon inhibits the transformation of mouse cells by exogenous cellular or viral genes. Nature, 303, 433-435, 1983.
41. Vilcek, J., Henriksen-Destefano, D., Robb, R.J. and Le, J. Interleukin-2 as the inducing signal for interferon-gamma in peripheral blood leukocytes stimulated with mitogen or antigen. The Biology of the Interferon System, Kirchner and Schellekens, eds., 1984.

31. Interferon Production by Leucocytes

H. Kirchner and Margarita Salas

Institute of Virus Research, German Cancer Research Center, 280 Im Neuenheimer Feld, 6900 Heidelberg, Federal Republic of Germany

INTRODUCTION

Interferons according to our belief represent a coherent system of molecules intimately involved in the defense of the organisms against infections (for a review see 1, 2). From their known effects it can be readily deduced that they serve as potent amplifier molecules. They activate a variety of potent effector cells (macrophages, NK cells) in addition to the immune-specific cells primarily recognizing the antigen. Furthermore, it has become evident that most interferons are produced in vitro by the effector cells of the immune system. From this point of view it seems to be appropriate to learn more about their producer cells within the lymphoreticular and hemopoietic system and how this production is regulated. Therefore the main emphasis of this chapter will be on interferon production by various types of leucocytes. It is, however, likely, that other cells besides leucocytes are producing interferon. This, for example, is firmly established for fibroblasts in vitro, but for very few other cell types. Thus, it is often quoted that "all nucleated cells are producing interferon", but as far as we could analyse the literature, for most cells this remains to be shown. We are aware of some data about epidermal cells producing interferon (3). However, it will be definitively of interest if differentiated cells such as hepatocytes, muscle cells, neurons etc. are indeed capable of interferon production.

Most of the work to be described has been done in vitro using various types of leucocyte cultures. Much less is known about the in vivo situation. However, new data will be expected soon using powerful molecular probes and techniques to identify the cells in tissues and organs producing interferon upon injection of an inducer. This, in particular, is expected from the technique of in situ hybridization for identifying interferon producing cells (4).

Heterogeneity of the Interferon System

It is now well established that there are many different interferons that may be grouped into three main classes. It seems quite possible that additional classes and subtypes will be identified. Alpha-Interferons (IFN-α) are the products of a multi-gene family whereas there are probably only two genes for interferon beta (IFN β) in man and only one for interferon gamma (IFN-γ). It is not surprising that this heterogeneity of the molecules is paralleled by a heterogenity of producer cells within the system of white blood cells.

Local Interferon Production

So far, it largely represents an enigma at which sites interferon is produced in vivo. In particular, it is not known where the serum interferon comes from. Yet, it is assumed by many investigators that the main role of interferon is a local one and therefore the most important sites of interferon production are in various tissues and not in the circulation. Interferons are biologically very active molecules and therefore their production is regulated (see below). The possibility that interferon will be found in the serum is restricted to certain diseases, particularly of viral nature .

Interferon production by leucocytes

Gresser was the first to show that leucocytes upon viral challenge in vitro produce interferon (5). Since then Cantell and his coworkers have developed practically important procedures to produce interferon in leucocyte cultures (6). However, our understanding which subtypes of leucocytes (lymphocytes) produce the different interferons is still incomplete.

Purity of Cells Used for Interferon Production

It is essential that close attention is paid to the methods used to prepare pure cultures of different types of leucocytes. A small percentage of contaminating cells of different cell types than those selected for may yield erroneous data. Several years ago one has predominantly used depletion techniques to address the question as to which cells produce various types of interferon (7). This has been proven unsatisfactory and now methods of positive selection are available and preferably used in such studies. It is also convenient if transformed cell lines or leukemia cells of a given phenotype are available. The latter, however, may not always yield results identical to those obtained with their normal counterparts. Some tumor cells are frozen in certain differentiation stages and may or may not express the interferon gene.

T lymphocytes

T lymphocytes clearly are producers of IFN γ. This has been found in many experiments in which enriched T lymphocytes were used. It has been also suggested from the nature of the stimulants used to induce IFN γ, since all of these represented agents known to activate T lymphocytes. They have included for example allogeneic cells, specific antigens, antibodies against T lymphocyte surface antigens (anti-OKT-3) and many of the so-called phyto-mitogens (lectins). To our knowledge, Marcucci et al. (8) were the first to use pure T cell lines to prove that murine T-cell lines were producing IFN γ. Similar data have been subsequently reported for a human T cell line (9). Since then numerous workers have reported this type of results and it is definitively proven that T lymphocytes are producers of IFN γ. So far, it cannot be excluded that other leucocytes are also producing IFN γ but there are very few data to support this possibility.

It is of great interest that the production of IFN γ may be also triggered by another lymphokine, i.e. by interleukin-2 (IL-2) (10). In view of the cascade of lymphokines, the conclusion is attractive that activators of T lymphocytes induce the production of IL-2 first which then serves as a physiological inducer of IFN γ. As it appears, not all IFN-γ production is inhibited by the addition of anti-IL-2 (11), and thus, the situation may be more complex in that there may be also some production of IFN-γ that is independent of IL-2 induction. We have been lately interested in two novel inducers of IFN-γ, namely zinc ions (12) and the mycoplasma mitogen MAS (13).

The next question is if T lymphocytes are capable of producing other interferons besides IFN γ. There have been data from a number of laboratories, indicating that human T cell leukemia cells are producing both IFN α and IFN β (14, 15). Using murine T cell lines we have found that they produced IFN β provided they were stimulated with an appropriate agent such as 10-carboxymethyl-9 acridanone (16). Alternatively, they produce IFN α when other inducers are utilized. From these data it appears that T lymphocytes are the producers of all three major classes of interferons.

It is obvious that in given T cell population only a small percentage of the cells are producing IFN γ. Quite a few studies have been directed at the question which T cell subtypes are producing the different interferons. Abb et al., ourselves and a number of other investigators have found that T cells of the helper type as well as T cells of the suppressor/cytotoxic are capable of producing IFN γ (17-19). Additional studies have suggested that it is the activated T cell (carrying I-a on the surface) which produces IFN γ (20). This seems to be an intriguing possibility, since it is one of the major biological effects of IFN γ to induce the expression of I-a on various cell types. It is attractive to speculate that there may be a loop between Ia-expression and IFN γ production.

Macrophages

Macrophages play a central role in antiviral defense in animal models and part of their effects are probably due to their interferon production (21). Typical for mouse cells in general is that the genes of IFN α and IFN β are jointly activated leading to a mixed product containing both IFN α and IFN β. Thus, it is usually found that murine macrophages are simultaneously producing both IFN α and IFN β. We were surprised to find that upon stimulation with CMA murine macrophages were producing IFN β exclusively. On the other hand, when the same cells were stimulated with NDV, both genes were expressed (22, 23).

In the human system, it has been suggested that the main producer cell of natural IFN α in a leucocyte culture is the macrophage (24). Roberts et al. have shown this for induction of interferon by influenza virus (25). Furthermore, enriched cultures of human monocytes are producing high titers of IFN α (26). It remains to be determined if this IFN α is a mixture of several subtypes or a monospecies preparation.

B Lymphocytes

Human lymphoblastoid cell lines transformed by EBV spontaneously produce small quantities of interferon and upon stimulation with viruses they produce high titers composed of various subtypes of IFN α and of some IFN β (27).

This again is an example of joint expression of the IFN α and IFN ß genes. The lymphoblastoid cell lines represent B cells albeit in a transformed state. There are very few indications that normal B lymphocytes of either human or murine origin produce interferon. However, Weigent et al. found that human leucocytes enriched for B lymphocytes produce IFN α upon interactions with foreign cells (28). Other investigators studying this type of interferon induction have reached different conclusions. Thus, three groups have concluded, that the cells producing interferon upon cocultivation with tumor cells were non-T, non-B cells i.e. Null cells (see below) (29-31). The studies of Abb et al. have also suggested that $BA\text{-}1^{+}B$ cells did not contribute to the interferon production in response to allogeneic tumor cells (32).

NK Cells

Some years ago the term "Null-cells" was used for a cell population (e.g. of human blood leucocytes) that has been thouroughly depleted of T cells, B cells and phagocytic cells. Probably, the Null cells show overlapping with NK cells and perhaps the term Null cells should be abondened. It is also obvious that the approaches based on depletion techniques are insufficient to definitively settle the question as to which cell types produce certain subtypes of interferons.

NK cells are a heterogenous group of cells the exact lineage of which within the hemopoietic system still remains unclear. Recently, monoclonal antibodies for NK cells have been developed, yet they appear to crossreach with other cells. NK cells, particularly in human blood share a characteristic morpholocial appearance in that they possess granula and therefore have been also designated as LGL (large granular lymphocytes). Several investigators have reported that LGL are producers of IFN γ (33). The situation may be confused by one problem: Certain preparations of IFN α are acid-labile and thus, some of the interferons produced by NK cells may not represent IFN γ but acid-labile IFN α. The studies of Abb, however, using the Leu 7 and Leu 11b antibodies for complement dependent mass cytolysis have not supported the notion that NK cells may be producers of IFN γ, nor of IFN-α (17, 34).

Bone Marrow Cells

Shah et al. have reported that normal human bone marrow stromal cells can be induced to produce high levels of IFN ß (35). They did not produce IFN γ, although a low level of IFN α was apparently produced. The cell cultures used in these studies were karyotypically normal and not virus-transformed. Murine bone marrow derived macrophages are a convenient system of pure and well characterized cells derived from the bone marrow, which are good producers of IFN α/ß when induced by a number of different agents (36). They appear to be unable to produce IFN γ when typical inducers of this interferon subtype are added and spontaneous interferon production is not apparent. However, it is of interest that with certain inducers (CMA) IFN ß is produced exclusively whereas with other inducers both IFN ß and IFN α is produced (22, 23). The molecular mechanisms of this differential gene activation remain to be defined.

Granulocytes

There has been an early report that bovine granulocytes produce an antiviral factor (37), but at that time it was not possible to definitively determine the nature of this antiviral factor. So far, to our knowledge, there are no reports about interferon production by granulocytes. Such experiments are in fact difficult to perform because of the short-term survival of granulocytes in culture. We have attempted to approach this problem by using HL-60, a myeloblastic cell line, with a potential to differentiate either into granulocytes or into macrophages. No interferon production was observed in granulocytes obtained by such protocols. Yet, the data were not fully convincing, since the macrophages obtained in the same protocol were also negative for interferon production. In additional experiments we have used granulocytes purified from human peripheral blood and have been unable to induce interferon production in cultures of these cells (38).

Regulation of Interferon Production by Leucocytes

It is obvious that a system as powerful as the interferon system must be carefully regulated, as is the case for hormonal systems and the immune system. There are several possibilities how this regulation might work, including genetic (immunogenetic) control and control by cellular interactions.

Immunogenetic Aspects of Interferon Production

Clearly, the production of IFN γ upon allogeneic stimulation is under immunogenetic control. For example, it has been found that differences even in minor loci alone is sufficient to cause the induction of IFN γ (39). Interferon production in response to the mitogen MAS is controlled by the I-E region of H-2 (13). It is also clear that in murine systems the production of IFN α/β in the intact animal in response to viral challenge is genetically controlled (40). So far, very little is known if similarly in man, the interferon response for example towards virus infection is under genetic control.

Helper Cell Problem

Quite a number of immunological reactions require interactions between different cellular components of the immune system and it has been suggested that this in certain instances may be also necessary for interferon production. For example, older studies have shown that the production of IFN-γ by T lymphocytes requires the help of macrophages (41). Whereas this has been confirmed by several laboratories, it is evident that T cells principally are able to produce IFN-γ without the help of other cells. This has been unequivocally shown by using cloned T cell lines (8).

Spontaneous Production of Interferon by Leucocytes

Transformed B cells produce small quantities of interferon spontaneously i.e. without addition of an inducer and the same is found for some T cell lines. In both situations the interferons produced appear to represent IFN α. Very little is known, if normal leucocytes produce interferon of any type spontaneously. However, Fischer and Rubinstein have reported that the low-density subpopulation of normal human peripheral blood mononuclear leucocytes obtained by percoll gradients produced significant levels of interferon in the absence of an inducer (42). According to this report the interferon represented a mixture of IFN-α and IFN-γ. It is a question of general interest, what the significance of such spontaneous production is. Certainly, it cannot be ruled out, that it represents the response to some inducer that is contained in the tissue culture medium. Alternatively, the cells are already activated in vivo and thus, interferon production is continued when they are placed in tissue cultures.

Percentage of Interferon Producers

In any given leucocyte population it is of importance to determine the number of interferon producing cells. There are not many data addressing this problem. However, it has been found that even in murine fibroblast cultures when they are maximally induced for interferon production, only 15-40% of the cells are actively engaged in interferon synthesis (4). In cultures of macrophages, similarly only small percentage of cells is producing interferon at any given time.

Interferon Production in vivo

At this time the question as to which types of leucocytes (or other cells) produce the different types of interferons in vivo remains unsolved. This is partucularly noteworthy in regard to IFN-γ, since attempts to induce IFN γ in vivo by simple protocols in experimental animals have been largely unsuccesful. So far, it always was necessary to have double-stimulation protocol. In contrast to the situation observed with IFN α/β, the latter yielded limited amounts of interferon only.

There used to be agreement that in healthy individuals no interferon can be detected in the serum of other body fluids. However, Bocci some years ago has postulated the existence of a "physiological interferon response" and recently, data have become available to support such a response (43). Since interferon is probably produced in the tissues it may be more relevant to look in the lymphatic vessels for "physiologic interferon" than in the blood (44).

Interferon has been detected in the serum of patients with certain autoimmune disease and chronic virus infections. In fact, it seems logical to assume that these two conditions are causing interferon production since viral infection induces the production of IFN-α, whereas conceivably autoimmunity causes the production of IFN-γ. In this context it is of interest that IFN-γ may indeed be produced in the socalled syngeneic MLC (45). It remains to be determined if more physiologic stimuli are indeed capable of induction of interferon that appears in the serum of healthy individuals. An interesting report of Bocci et al. has suggested that physical exercise causes the appearance of serum interferon in man (46).

Conclusions

1. Perhaps, many different cell types produce interferon, but for very few this has been firmly established, including fibroblasts and leucocytes.
2. From in vitro studies it is quite obvious that a number of different leucocytes produce different types of interferon. These include T cells and macrophages, both in human and murine systems. The T cells are the producers of IFN γ, whereas macrophages contribute significantly to the production of IFN-α. In murine systems the production of IFN β by macrophages has been also documented. It is not clear if B cells or granulocytes produce interferon at all. The place of the NK cells within the hemopoietic system is still uncertain

and it is also unclear if they are producers of interferon.

3. The question as to which cells produce interferon in vivo is largely unsettled, but it is hoped that by the methods of in situ hybridization and other new approaches, experimental access to this problem will be possible.

References

1. Kirchner, H.: Interferons, a group of multiple lymphokines. Springer Sem Immunopathol 7:347, 1984.

2. Kirchner, H.: The interferon system as an integral part of the defense system against infections. Antiviral Research 6:1, 1986.

3. Schuller, G. B., Roe, J. L., Fowler, A. K., and Hellmann, K. B.: Isolation and characterization of interferon-producing reticuloendothelial cells from mouse epidermis. Clin Immunol Immunopathol 31:331, 1984.

4. Zawatzky, R., De Maeyer, E., and De Maeyer-Guignard, J.: Identification of individual interferon-producing cells by in situ hybridization. Proc Natl Acad Sci USA 82:1136, 1985.

5. Gresser, I.: Production of interferon by suspensions of human leucocytes. Proc Soc Exp Biol Med 108:799, 1961.

6. Strander, H., and Cantell. K.: Production of interferon by human leucocytes in vitro. Ann Med Exp Biol Fenn 44:265, 1966.

7. Kirchner, H. and Marcucci, F.: Interferon production by leucocytes. In: Interferons and the Immune System, J. Vilcek and E. De Maeyer, eds. Elsevier Science Publishers, pp. 7-34, 1984.

8. Marcucci, F., Waller,M., Kirchner, H., and Krammer, P.: Production of immune interferon (IFN-γ) by murine T cell clones from long term cultures. Nature 291:79, 1981.

9. Nathan, I., Groopman, J. E., Quan, S. G., Bersch, N., and Golde, D. W.: Immune (γ) interferon produced by a human T-lymphoblast cell line. Nature (London) 292:842, 1981.

10. Handa, K., Suzuki, R., Matsui, H., Shimizu, Y., and Kumagai, K.: Natural killer (NK) cells as a responder to interleukin 2 (IL 2). II. IL-2 induced interferon γ production. J Immunol 130:988, 1983.

11. Salas, M., and Kirchner, H.: unpublished observation.

12. Salas, M., and Kirchner, H.: Interferon production in human leucocyte cultures stimulated by Zn^{2+}, in preparation.

13. Kirchner, H., Nicklas, W., Giebler, D., Keyssner, K., Berger, R., and Storch, E.: Induction of interferon gamma in mouse spleen cells by culture supernatants of mycoplasma arthritidis. J Interferon Res 4:389, 1984.

14. Larsson, E., Lundgren, E., Nilsson, K., and Strannegard, Ö.: A human neoplastic hematopoietic cell line producing a fibroblast type of interferon. Dev Biol Stand 42: 193, 1979.

15. Morris, A. G., Morser, J., and Meager, M.: Spontaneous production of gamma interferon and induced production of beta interferon by human T-lymphoblastoid cell lines. Infect Immun 35:533, 1982.

16. Storch, E., Kirchner, H., Brehm, G., Hüller,K., and Marcucci, F.: Production of interferon beta by murine T cell lines induced by 10-carboxymethyl-9-acridanone. Scand J Immunol 23:195, 1986.

17. Abb, J., Abb, H., and Deinhardt, F.: Characterization of human interferon-gamma-producing leukocytes with monoclonal antileukocyte antibodies. Med Microbiol Immunol 171:215, 1983.

18. Marcucci, F., Klein, B., Altevogt, P., Landolfo, S., and Kirchner, H.: Concanavalin A-induced interferon gamma production by murine spleen cells and T cell lines. Lack of correlation with Lyt 1,2 phenotype. Immunobiol 219:227,

1984.
19. Conta, B. S., Powell, M. B., and Ruddle, N. H.: Production of lymphotoxin, IFN-γ, and IFN-α by murine T cell lines and clones. J Immunol 130:2231, 1983.
20. Schober, I., Braun, R., Munk, K., Leroux, M., and Kirchner, H.: Ia-positive T lymphocytes are the producer cells of interferon gamma. Exp Cell Res 152:348, 1984.
21. Kirchner, H., Engler, H., Schröder, C.H., Zawatzky, R., and Storch, E.: Herpes Simplex Virus type 1-induced interferon production in peritoneal exudate cells of the mouse. J Gen Virol 64:437, 1983.
22. Brehm, G., Storch, E., and Kirchner, H.: Purification and characterization of interferons induced by 10-carboxymethyl-9-acridanone in murine macrophage cultures. Nat Immun Cell Growth Regulation 5:50, 1986.
23. Brehm, G., and Kirchner, H.: Analysis of the interferons induced in mice in vivo and in vitro by Newcastle disease virus and by polyinosinic-polycytidylic acid. J Interferon Res 6:21, 1986.
24. Saksela, E., Virtanen, I., Hovi, T., Secher, D. S., and Cantell, K.: Monocyte is the main producer of human alpha interferons following Sendai virus induction. Proc Med Virol 30:3, 1983.
25. Roberts, N.J., Jr., Douglas, R.G., Jr. Simons, R. M. and Diamond, M. E.: Virus-induced interferon production by human macrophages. J Immunol 123:365, 1979.
26. Opitz,I., and Kirchner, H.: unpublished data.
27. Havell, E. A., Yip, Y. K., and Vilcek, J.: Characteristics of human lymphoblastoid (Namalwa) interferon. J Gen Virol 38:51, 1977.
28. Weigent, D.A., Langford, M.P., Smith, E.M., Ballock, J. E., and Stanton, G. J.: Human B lymphocytes produce leucocyte interferon after interaction with foreign cells. Infect Immun 32: 508, 1981.
29. Kirchner, H., Peter, H.H., Hirt, M. M., Zawatzky, R., and Bradstreet, P.: Studies of the producer cell of interferon in human lymphocyte cultures. Immunobiol 156:65, 1979.
30. Timonen, T., Saksela, E., Virtanen, I., and Cantell, K.: Natural killer cells are responsible for the interferon production induced in human lymphocytes by tumor cell contact. Eur J Immunol 10:422, 1980.
31. Rönnblom, L., Ramstedt, U., and Alm, G. V.: Properties of human natural interferon-producing cells stimulated by tumor cell lines. Eur J Immunol 13:471, 1983.
32. Abb, J., Abb, H., and Deinhardt, F.: Phenotype of human α-interferon producing leucocytes identified by monoclonal antibodies. Clin exp Immunol 52:179, 1983.
33. Djeu, J. Y., Stocks, N., Zoon, K., Stanton, G. J., Timonen, T., and Herberman, R.B.: Positive self regulation of cytotoxicity in human natural killer cells by production of interferon upon exposure to influenza and herpes viruses. J Exp Med 156:1222, 1982.
34. Abb, J., Abb, H., and Deinhardt, F.: Relationship between natural killer (NK) cells and interferon (IFN) alpha-producing cells in human peripheral blood. Studies with a monoclonal antibody with specificity for human natural killer cells. Immunobiol 167:359, 1984.
35. Shah, G., Dexter, T. M., Lanotte, M.: Interferon production by human marrow stromal cells. Br J Haematol 54:365, 1983.
36. Havell, E. A., and Spitalny, G. L.: The induction and characterization of interferon from pure cultures of murine macrophages. Ann N Y Acad Sci 350:413, 1980.
37. Rouse, B. T., and Babiuk, L.A.: Mechanisms of recovery from herpesvirus infections - a review. Can J Comp Med 42:414, 1978.

38. Kapp, A., Kirchner, H., Wokalek, H., and Schopf, E.: Modulation of granulocyte oxidative response to recombinant interferon α_2 and γ. Arch. Derm. Res., in press.
39. Schirrmacher, V., Landolfo, S., Zawatzky, R., and Kirchner, H.: Immunogenetic studies of the resistance of mice against highly metastatic DBA/2 tumor cell variants. II. Influence of minor histocompatibility antigens on tumor resistance, γ interferon induction and cytotoxic response. Invasion and Metastatis 1:175, 1981.
40. De Maeyer, E., and De Maeyer-Guignard, J.: Influence of animal genotype and age on the amount of circulating interferon induced by mouse mammary tumor virus. J Gen Virol 2:445, 1968.
41. Epstein, L.B., Cline, M.J., and Merigan, T.C.: The interaction of human macrophages and lymphocytes in the phytohemagglutinin-stimulated production of interferon. J Clin Invest 50:744, 1971.
42. Fischer, D.G. and Rubinstein, M.: Spontaneous production of interferon-γ and acid-labile interferon-α by subpopulations of human mononuclear cells. Cell Immunol 81:426, 1983.
43. Bocci, V.: The physiological interferon response. Immunology Today 6:7, 1985.
44. Bocci, V., Muscettola, M., Paulesu, L., and Grasso, G.: The physiological interferon response. V. Antiviral activity present in rat lymph is neutralized by anti-mouse interferon-γ antibodies. Microbiologica 8:405, 1985.
45. Berger, R., Landolfo, S., Balzi, E., and Kirchner, H.: Syngeneic mixed lymphocyte reaction causes the production of interferon gamma. Immunobiol 165:225, 1983.
46. Viti, A., Muscettola, M., Paulesu, L., Bocci, V., and Almi, A.: Effect of exercise on plasma interferon levels. J Appl Physiol 59:426, 1985.

32. Interferon Production during Immunologically Related Diseases

John J. Hooks and Barbara Detrick

Immunology and Virology Section, Laboratory of Immunology, National Eye Institute, NIH, Bethesda, MD 20892

INTRODUCTION

It is clear that the IFNs can be produced by cells which participate in immune responses (1,2). Moreover, components of the immune system, such as IL2 and anti-T cell antibody, can induce these cells to produce IFN (3). A number of recent studies have focused on the concept that the IFNs can also act as regulatory proteins in immune reactivity. These regulating actions range from altering T cell reactivity and antibody production to enhancing the expression of MHC class II antigens (1,4,5). Based on these observations, it is not surprising that the production of the IFNs may be altered during immunologically related disorders. This brief review will highlight some of the data demonstrating this fact. We will also examine some of the possible consequences of this altered production during immunologically related diseases.

IFN PRODUCTION DURING IMMUNOLOGICALLY RELATED DISORDERS

IFN production during the course of an immune response influences the magnitude of immune reactions. This event can be envisioned as part of our biological control mechanisms. However, this process of IFN production may be augmented or depressed during the course of certain disease states and it may then either appropriately modify certain responses or contribute to some of the clinical manifestations. How this normal process of IFN production may become aberrant in selected immunologically mediated diseases will be reviewed in this section.

Alterations in the IFN system can be evaluated in three ways: by the abnormally high presence of IFN in the circulation, by the identification of IFN at a localized site, or by the aberrant production of IFN by mononuclear cells tested in vitro. Modifications in the IFN system have been associated with four human immunologically related disorders: autoimmunity, immunodeficiencies, selected lymphoid malignancies and certain infections (6).

Autoimmunity and immunodeficiency are most usually associated with the elevated presence of circulating IFN. IFNs have been described in the sera of patients with systemic lupus erythematosus (SLE), rheumatoid arthritis, scleroderma, Sjogren's syndrome, vasculitis, Behcet's syndrome and Vogt-Koyanagi-Harada's syndrome as well as the virus induced immunodeficiency, AIDS (reviewed in 1,6). IFN-alpha, both acid labile and acid stable forms, are found in SLE and AIDS patients, while IFN-gamma is found in the circulation of patients with Behcet's syndrome (7-11). These studies indicate that IFN is present in the sera of patients with collagen vascular disorders and selected immunodeficiencies but is not frequently detected in other immunologically associated disorders. The presence of an acid-labile IFN-alpha in AIDS patients may be associated with the proposed etiologic agent, HTLV III. We recently described the production of an acid-labile IFN-alpha by B cells infected with either HTLV I or EBV virus (12). Whether or not the presence of acid-labile IFN alpha in SLE patients is associated with an etiologic agent or with a virus which may be activated during the course of this immunoregulatory disorder remains to be determined. Nevertheless, the presence of this IFN may contribute to some of the immunoregulatory alterations observed in this disease (1, 6-11).

A second way to evaluate IFN production in immunologically related disorders is to indentify, by immunocytochemical analysis, the presence of IFN at a localized site. We have recently identified IFN-gamma in association with the infiltration of T lymphocytes and the activation of MHC class II antigens in the salivary glands of patients with Sjogren's syndrome and in the eyes of patients with ocular inflammation (Hooks and Detrick, unpublished data). These studies indicate that IFN-gamma induced MHC class II antigen expression may serve as a local amplification system in autoimmune and inflammatory diseases.

A third way to evaluate IFN production in immunologically related disorders is to monitor IFN-gamma production in vitro by patient mononuclear cells. Studies from a number of laboratories show that IFN-gamma plays a vital role in the lymphokine circuit (1). In fact, a defect in the production of IFN-gamma or other lymphokines can be indicative of an underlying aberration in regulatory signals. Peripheral blood leukocytes can be stimulated in vitro with T cell mitogens to produce IFN-gamma. Whether or not cells have the ability to produce appropriate amounts of IFN-gamma can be used to analyze T cell function and to monitor lymphokine production.

Alterations in the ability of mononuclear cells to produce IFN-gamma is observed in certain immunologically related disorders. A depressed production of IFN-gamma is associated with infections such as measles, simian foamy virus infections, tuberculosis and leprosy, with autoimmune disorders such as SLE; with immunodeficiencies such as AIDS and in lymphoid malignancies such as chronic lymphocytic leukemia of the B cell type (1,13). We have recently described this defect in patients with retinitis pigmentosa (14). In these patients, the subnormal production of IFN-gamma is associated with a diminished expression of MHC class II antigens (5, 15).

Conversely, the excessive production of IFN-gamma has also been identified. An elevated and spontaneous production of IFN-gamma was found in a lymphoproliferative disorder (chronic lymphocytic leukemia of the T cell type) and Behcet's syndrome (11,15).

IMPLICATIONS OF IFN PRODUCTION IN THE REGULATION OF THE IMMUNE RESPONSE

We will address two general aspects of IFN production during immunologically related disorders. First, the production of IFN, especially IFN-alpha, may be related to a causative agent. AIDS induced by HTLV III may well be an example of this. AIDS is frequently associated with the presence of circulating acid labile IFN-alpha (10). In fact, we have found that HTLV I infected B lymphocytes can produce this acid labile form of IFN-alpha (12). Alternatively, the altered immune reactivity may activate latent viruses or predispose the host to certain viruses which are the inducers of the observed IFN. Whether or not the IFN-alpha produced in SLE is associated with a causative agent or the activation of a virus is a very important unanswered question.

The second aspect addresses the consequences of IFN production. For example we have seen that the process of IFN production may be augmented or depressed during the course of certain disease states. Since the IFNs are potent immunoregulatory proteins, they may either appropriately modify some responses or contribute to some of the clinical manifestations. Recent studies on immune abnormalities in autoimmune and inflammatory diseases have focused on two areas: polyclonal B cell activation and MHC class II antigen expression. Interestingly, recent studies on immunoregulatory functions of IFNs have focused on these same two areas.

Using recombinant mouse IFN-alpha, investigators have reevaluated the effect of IFNs on B lymphocytes. These studies indicate that IFN acts directly on B cells resulting in maturation of the cell and immunoglobulin secretion. Thus IFN influences differentiation by acting as one of the helper factors in the stimulation of B lymphocyte antibody responses (17, 18). Hypergammaglobulinemia and polyclonal B cell activation are hallmarks of SLE and AIDS. Since these are the two diseases most frequently associated with the prolonged presence of IFN-alpha, it is possible that this IFN may be contributing to these abnormalities.

Studies during the past few years have shown that lymphokines, such as IFN-gamma and IL2, may play a major role in facilitating immune responses. One such activity which appears unique to the IFNs is their ability to modulate the expression of cell surface antigens (1,4,5). For example, IFN-gamma is a potent manipulator of the MHC antigens. More specifically, its ability to modulate the synthesis and expression of class II antigens, reflects IFN-gamma's major contribution as a regulatory protein. Usually, cells bearing class II antigens can present antigen to T lymphocytes resulting in the initiation and perpetuation of immune responses (5,19,20). Through these processes, it appears that lymphokines, such as IFN-gamma, may help to mediate certain immunopathologic processes and may be required to augment the host defense against certain infections and malignancies. It is thus apparent that the production of IFN-gamma in certain chronic autoimmune and inflammatory diseases may be a part of a series of inappropriate effector mechanisms resulting in target organ destruction.

A number of recent reports describe the inappropriate or deviant expression of HLA-DR antigen in conditions in which an immunologic role has been postulated. For example, class II antigens have been detected on the surface of the thyroid epithelial cell in autoimmune thyroiditis (21), on renal tubular cells in graft versus host disease (22), on bile duct epithelial cells in primary biliary cirrhosis (23), on salivary gland duct cells in Sjogren's syndrome(24), on retinal pigment epithelial (rpe) cells in autoimmune and inflammatory eye diseases (25), and more recently on these rpe cells in selective degenerative processes (15). In each of these examples the cells do not express HLA-DR antigens under normal physiologic conditions but are activated to express the antigen during the immunologically mediated diseases. In these conditions it is postulated that IFN-gamma was the inducer of class II antigen expression. In this context, we have identified T cell infiltrations, IFN-gamma production and MHC class II antigen expression in the eye during inflammatory eye diseases and in the salivary gland during Sjogren's syndrome (Hooks and Detrick, unpublished data). It is possible that lymphokine induced MHC class II antigen expression may serve as a local amplification system in these autoimmune diseases.

As a final note, it may be appropriate to briefly comment on another new and exciting aspect of this intimate relationship between IFN-gamma and class II antigens. Recent data now implicate both of these regulatory molecules in cellular differentiation. Certainly the influence of IFN-gamma on hemopoitesis and the maturation of selected lymphoid cells as well as tumor cells can be viewed as instrumental in the immunobiology of the host (4, 26, 27). This area awaits further definition with the hope that this novel role for IFN-gamma broadens our understanding not only for the immune system in particular, but also for basic biological control systems in general.

SUMMARY

Immunologically related diseases such as autoimmune diseases and immunodeficiencies represent variations in immune reactions which arise out of dysfunctions in immunoregulation. The IFNs can act as potent immunoregulatory proteins. This report summarizes how the production of IFN may occur in immunologically related diseases and how the presence of these proteins may participate in the immune reactions which are provoked. A better understanding of how lymphokines, such as IFN, can modify immune reactions may provide insight into ways to restore immune balance.

REFERENCES

1. Hooks, J., and B. Detrick-Hooks: Immunoregulatory functions of interferon. In: Biological response modifiers (BRM's). P. Torrence (ed.) Academic Press, pp 57-75, 1985.
2. Kirchner, H., F. Marcucci. In: Interferons and the Immune System, J. Vilcek and E. DeMaeyer, eds. Elsevier Science Pub., Vol. 2, pp. 7-34, 1984.
3. Kasahara, T., J. J. Hooks, S. F. Dougherty, J. J. Oppenheim: Interleukin 2-mediated immune interferon (IFN-γ) production by human T cells and T cell subsets. J Immunol 130:1784, 1983.
4. Basham, T. Y., T. C. Merigan: Recombinant interferon-γ increases HLA-DR synthesis and expression. J Immunol 130:1492, 1983.
5. Detrick, B., D. A. Newsome, C. M. Percopo, J. J. Hooks: Class II antigen expression and gamma interferon modulation of monocytes and retinal pigment epithelial cells from patients with retinitis pigmentosa. Clin Immunol Immunopathol 36:201, 1985.
6. Hooks, J. J. and B. Detrick-Hooks: Interferon in autoimmune diseases and other immunoregulatory disorders. In: Interferons and the immune system, J. Vilcek and E. DeMaeyer, eds. Elsevier Press, pp. 165-174, 1984.
7. Hooks, J. J., H. M. Moutsopoulos, S. Geis, N. Stahl, J. Decker, A. L. Notkins: Immune interferon in the circulation of patients with autoimmune disease. N Eng J Med 301:5, 1979.
8. Hooks, J. J., G. W. Jordan, T. Cupps, H. S. Moutsopoulos, A. S. Fauci, A.

L. Notkins: Multiple interferons in the circulation of patients with systemic lupus erythematosus and vasculitis. Arth and Rheum 25:396, 1982.
9. Preble, O. T., R. J. Black, R. M. Friedman: Systemic lupus erythematosus: presence in human serum of an unusual acid-labile leukocyte interferon. Science 216:429, 1982.
10. DeStefano, E., R. M. Friedman, A. E. Friedman-Kien, J. J. Goedert, D. Henriksen, O. T. Preble, J. A. Sonnabend, J. Vilcek: Acid -labile human leukocyte interferon in homosexual men with Kaposi's sarcoma and lymphadenopathy. J Infec Dis 146:451, 1982.
11. Ohno, S., F. Kato, H. Matsuda, N. Fujii, T. Minagawa: Detection of gamma interferon in the sera of patients with Behcet's disease. Infect Immun 36:202, 1982.
12. Boumpas, D.T., J. J. Hooks, M. Popovic, G. C. Tsokos, D.L. Mann: Human T-cell leukemia/lymphoma virus I and/or Epstein-Barr virus-infected B-cell lines spontaneously produce acid-labile α-interferon. J Clin Immunol 5:340, 1985.
13. Vilcek, J., A. Klion, D. Henriksen-DeStefano, A. Zemtsou, D. Davidson, M. Davidson, A. E. Friedman-Klen, J. Le: Defective gamma-interferon production in peripheral blood leukocytes of patients with acute tuberculosis. J Clin Immunol 6:146, 1986.
14. Hooks, J. J., B. Detrick-Hooks, S. Geis, D. A. Newsome: Retinitis pigmentosa associated with a defect in the production of interferon-gamma. Am J Ophthalmol 96:755, 1983.
15. Detrick, B., M. Rodrigues, C.-C. Chan, M. O. M. Tso, J. J. Hooks: Expression of HLA-DR antigen on retinal pigment epithelial cells in retinitis pigmentosa. Amer J Ophthal 101:584, 1986.
16. Hooks, J. J., B. F. Haynes, B. Detrick-Hooks, L. F. Diehl, T. Gerrand, A. S. Fauci: Gamma (immune) interferon production by leukocytes from a patient with a T_G cells proliferative disease. Blood 59:198, 1982.
17. Leibson, H. J., M. Gefter, A. Zlotnick, P. Marrack, J. W. Kappler: Role of gamma-interferon in antibody producing responses. Nature 309:799, 1984.
18. Sidman, C. L., J. D. Marshall, L. D. Shultz, P. W. Gray, H. M. Johnson: Gamma interferon is one of several direct B cell-maturing lymphokines. Nature 309:801, 1984.
19. Cowing, C., S. H. Pincus, D. H. Sachs, H. B. Dickler: A subpopulation of adherent accessory cells bearing both 1-A and I-E or C subregion antigens is required for antigen-specific murine T lymphocyte proliferation. J Immunol 121:1680, 1978.
20. Pober, J. S., M. A. Gimbrone, R. S. Cotran, C. S. Reiss, S. J. Burakoff, W. Fiers, K. A. Ault: Ia expression by vascular endothelium is inducible by activated T cells and by human γ interferon. J Exp Med 157:1339, 1983.
21. Hanafusa, T., R. Pujol-Borrell, L. Chiovato, R. C. G. Russell, D. Doniach,

and G. F. Bottazzo: Aberrant expression of HLA-DR antigen on thyrocytes in Graves' disease: relevance for autoimmunity. Lancet ii:1111, 1983.
22. Hall, B. M., G. G. Duggin, J. Philips, A. G. Bishop, J. S. Horvath, D. J. Tiller: Increased expression of HLA-DR antigens on renal tubular cells in renal transplants: relevance to the rejection response. Lancet ii:247, 1984.
23. Ballardini, G., R. Mirakian, F. B. Bianchi, E. Pisi, D. Doniach, G. F. Bottazzo: Aberrant expression of HLA-DR antigens on bileduct epithelium in primary biliary cirrhosis: relevance to pathogenesis. Lancet ii:1009, 1984.
24. Moutsopoulos, H. M., J. J. Hooks, C. C. Chan, Y. Dalavanga, B. Detrick: HLA-DR antigen expression in glandular tissue from patients with Sjogren's syndrome. Ann Rheumatic Diseases (in press), 1986.
25. Chan, C. C., B. Detrick, R. B. Nussenblatt, A. Palestine, L. S. Fujikawa, J. J. Hooks: Expression of HLA-DR antigen on retinal pigment epithelial cells from patients with uveitis. Arch Ophthal 104:725, 1986.
26. Houghton, A. N., T. M. Thomson, D. Gross, H. F. Oeltgen, L. J. Old: Surface antigens of melanoma and melanocytes. J Exp Med 160:255, 1984.
27. Perussia, B., E. T. Dayton, V. Fanning, P. Thiugarujan, J. Hoxie, G. Trinchier: Immune interferon and leukocyte-conditioned medium induce normal and leukemic myeloid cells to differentiate along the monocyte pathway. J Exp Med 158:2058, 1983.

33. Interferon Effects on Cellular and Humoral Immunity

E. De Maeyer and J. De Maeyer-Guignard

Institut Curie-Biologie, Bât. 110, Campus d'Orsay, 91405 Orsay, France

INTRODUCTION

The interest for the immunomodulating properties of interferons is still widening and in this short overview we can only deal with the most recent developments ; a more detailed and historical treatment of the subject can be found in several previous publications (1,2,3,4). The main emphasis of the past two years has been on the immunomodulating properties of IFN-gamma ; this is because IFN-gamma, as a product of activated T-cells, is an obvious component of the immune system, whereas this relationship seems more distant in the case of IFN-alpha IFN-beta. In this respect we must agree with a point recently made by J.L. Virelizier : "There is a tendency ... to neglect the regulatory functions of non-specifically induced IFN-alpha and IFN-beta. This is a dangerous drift, because the latter constitute the bulk of the early IFN production during acute infections and may well participate in the modifications of immune responsiveness caused by such infections. IFN-alpha and beta are able to increase NK activity (whereas IFN-gamma has very little, if any, effects on NK function) suppress or enhance antibody formation according to the timing used, activate macrophages for cytotoxity and monokine secretion and enhance the expression of MHC class I antigens. Neglecting such powerful effects of IFN-alpha and IFN-beta would be unwise". (5)*

---

* May we add that in several publications coming from highly respectable immunology laboratories, murine IFN preparations made by mouse fibroblasts are designated as Mu IFN-beta, wheras such preparations generally consist of about equal mixtures of IFN-alpha and IFN-beta. It is evidently not widely enough appreciated that murine fibroblasts can make both alpha and beta interferons (6,7).

EXPRESSION OF CELL SURFACE MOLECULES : ANTIGENS AND RECEPTORS

Antigens of the MHC complex

Modulation of the expression of antigens of the major histocompatibility complex (MHC) is one of the chief effects by which interferons influence the immune system, and this area has recently witnessed an intense activity. The structural genes of the MHC are on chromosome 17 in the mouse and on chromosome 6 in man. Class I antigens (H-2 in mouse, HLA A,B,C in man) are involved in the restriction of cytotoxic T cells and are expressed on most cells in the body, whereas class II antigens are principally expressed at the surface of the cells of the immune system. In the mouse, the polymorphic class I molecules are encoded by three distinct loci, H-2K,H-2D and H-2L. Each class I antigen furthermore is associated non-covalently with a second polypeptide chain, beta 2 microglobulin, encoded by a gene which is not part of the MHC, and located on a different chromosome. Class II antigens consist of the association of two polypeptide chains, encoded by genes of the I region of the MHC cluster in the mouse and of the HLA-DR locus in man. Class II antigens are of utmost importance in cell-to-cell recognition and interaction, and quantitative variation of these antigens appears to play a central role in immunoregulation (8). The expression of MHC class II antigens is constitutive on Langerhans and dendritic cells, and is inducible on monocytes, macrophages, T and B lymphocytes. Class II antigens can also be present on some cells with no known immune function, such as for example malignant melanoma cells. It was previously shown that recombinant HuIFN-gamma can increase synthesis and expression of MHC II antigens (HLA-DR) on human monocytes (9). Recent evidence indicates that recombinant Hu IFN-gamma also induces the expression of class II antigens (HLA-DR and HLA-DC) on tumor cells of various origins such as melanoma cells, glioma cells and cells from several human carcinoma lines (10,11). The inducibility of class II antigens by IFN-gamma appears to be a general characteristic of human melanoma cell lines and also of non malignant melanocytes, which do not normally express these antigens. Normal fibroblasts can also express class II antigens when induced with IFN-gamma (10). Besides expression and shedding of class II antigens, shedding of specific melanoma antigens is also significantly increased by IFN-gamma (12). Theoretically, such shedding could play a role in the host's immune response to premalignant and malignant melanocytes (13). So far, however, there is no formal evidence that shedding of HLA-DR or melanoma antigens is in fact immunostimulatory (12). Recombinant Hu IFN-gamma is able to induce expression and shedding of HLA Class II antigens on melanoma cells that have become resistant its antiproliferative effect (14) ; this shows that the antiproliferative and antigen modulating effects of IFN-gamma take place by a different mechanism. At the same time these data suggest a way by which tumor cells that are resistant to the antiproliferative effect of interferon in vitro could still be inhibited in vivo. We must emphasize, however, that there is no formal evidence so far for an immunostimulatory role, followed by tumor rejection, of the increased expression of of class II MHC antigens by interferons. However, in a system of adenovirus 12 transformed cells, it has been demonstrated that the increased expression of the MHC class I antigens by Mu IFN-alpha/beta significantly reduces tumorigenicity in immunocompetent hosts (15).

A systematic study of the induction by recombinant Mu IFN-gamma of class I (H-2K^k) and class II (I-A^k) antigens in the mouse has shown a widespread, but selective, increase of these antigens in most tissues. Of the lymphatic-hematopoietic system, the bone marrow showed the most significant increase of both class I and class II antigen. Of the nonlymphoid organs, most tissues showed increased class I antigen expression on endothelial cells and more numerous dendritic cells bearing the class II antigen. Antigen expression returned to baseline after cessation of treatment with IFN-gamma. This suggests the possibility of both rapid upward and downward regulation of antigen expression by IFN-gamma (16,17). Variable expression of class II antigens could represent a regulatory mechanism for local immune reactions; this is particularly important in the central nervous system, in which normally no class II antigens are expressed. Induction of class II antigens by IFN-gamma has been observed in human glioma cells (18) and astrocytes can be induced by IFN-gamma to express class II antigens at their surface and then become able to stimulate T cells. Thus, IFN-gamma can mediate immune-specific interactions between astrocytes and T cells, and stimulate immune responses in the brain (19) ; this is not necessarily always beneficial, and under certain circumstances such immune stimulation in the brain could conceivably cause disease. Not all cells derived from the central nervous system seem to be inducible for class II antigens by IFN-gamma, and cells from a murine neuroblastoma line could be stimulated to express class I but not class II antigens. Similarly, Hu IFN-gamma induced class I HLA and b2-microglobulin expression but not class II antigens on human amnion cells (20). This shows that IFN-gamma can regulate the levels of class I and class II antigens independently ; the differentiation state of the target cell seems to have a strong influence on this effect (21).

IFN-gamma has been shown to modulate HLA class II antigen expression on cultured thymic epithelial cells, and this finding raises the possibility that IFN-gamma participates in the mechanisms that assure the permanent expression of these antigens on thymic epithelial cells in vivo, with potentially important functional consequences in terms of education for self recognition (22). This raises the question of the natural immunoregulatory role of IFN-gamma: could one of the major functions of IFN-gamma be the stimulation of class II surface antigens with resulting interaction of cells belonging to the immune system ? Certainly, stimulation of class II antigens, as opposed to antigens belonging to class I, seems to be a specific function of IFN-gamma, since under most circumstances IFN-alpha or IFN-beta, although capable of stimulating class I antigens, do not stimulate the expression of class II antigens (9,23). In fact, in one instance Mu IFN-beta has been shown to exert an antagonistic effect on the induction of class II antigens on murine macrophages by Mu IFN-gamma (24). There are, however, examples of stimulation of class II antigens in man by Hu-IFN-alpha and in mouse by Mu IFN-alpha/beta (25,26,27). In addition, both Hu IFN-alpha and Hu IFN-gamma can increase the level of synthesis of class II HLA mRNAs in several human B lymphoid as well as melanoma cell lines ; however, this increase in mRNA levels does not always result in concomitant expression of the corresponding antigens at the cell surface, which indicates that other regulatory mechanisms, operating at the translational level, are involved (28).

IFN-gamma manifestly is the prime inducer of expression of class II antigens, and IFN-alpha and IFN-beta only play a secondary role in this respect; expression of class I antigens on the other hand is usually readily induced by all three interferon species. Some cells are more susceptible to induction than others, and high and low class I (HLA) responder lines to Hu IFN-alpha have been isolated from the human thymus leukemia cell line Molt 4 (29). In fact, some cells can be completely resistant to the induction of class I antigens by interferon, as shown by the fact that two H-2 negative variants of the murine YAC-1 lymphoma line remained H-2 negative in spite of treatment with either Mu IFN-beta or IFN-gamma ; interestingly, these two variants were as susceptible as wild-type cells to other effects of interferon such as the antiviral and cell growth inhibitory effect (30).

A natural role for Hu IFN-beta in the turning on of class I HLA antigens during cell differentiation is strongly suggested by experiments in which the appearance of class I antigens during differentiation from cells of a lymphoma line to macrophages is inhibited by treatment with anti IFN-beta serum. This observation points to interferons as natural modulators during the normal differentiation process of cells derived from the hematopietic system (31).

<u>Effects on other cell-surface molecules</u>

Enhanced expression of histocompatibility antigens is but

one manifestation of the ability of interferons to stimulate the expression of genes coding for cell-surface molecules important for immune reactions. The number of cellular receptors for tumor necrosis factor (TNF) is significicantly enhanced by treatment with IFN-gamma and also, but to a lesser extent, IFN-alpha and beta (32,33,34). Other cell surface receptor molecules influenced by IFN-gamma treatment are interleukin-2 receptors on human peripheral blood monocytes which are enhanced (35) and transferrin receptors on murine peritoneal macrophages which are down regulated by Mu IFN-gamma treatment (36,37). Fc receptors on the other hand are increased on mouse peritoneal macrophages after treatment with either Mu IFN-gamma or Mu IFN-alpha/beta (38).

INTERACTION WITH INTERLEUKIN 2 (IL 2)

T helper cells both produce and respond to IL 2, whereas the majority of cytolytic and suppressor T cells do not produce IL 2 but proliferate in response to IL 2 derived from T helper cells. IFN-gamma administered to mice three days before antigen administration significantly enhances T helper cell activity, and in addition, enhances interleukin 2 (IL 2) production (39). Conversely, treatment of con A induced human thymocytes with IL 2 or SEA induced mouse spleen cells resulted in enhanced IFN-gamma con A synthesis (40,41,42). In these studies, IL 2 by itself did not induce IFN-gamma ; however, in human peripheral blood mononuclear cells, IL 2 by itself did elicit significant levels of IFN-gamma synthesis. In the latter study, significantly higher doses of IL 2 were used, and when lower amounts were added to the cultures, the presence of PHA was required to induce IFN-gamma synthesis (43). Stimulation of NK cell activity by IL 2 however does not occur through IFN-gamma induction, but is a direct effect of IL 2 (64,44,45,46). An interesting observation is the switch from IFN-alpha/beta synthesis to IFN-gamma synthesis caused by IL-2 treatment of murine splenocyte cultures induced with LPS : IL 2 down regulates IFN-alpha/beta induction by LPS, and stimulates IFN-gamma synthesis (47).

MACROPHAGE ACTIVATION

Macrophages play a central role in immunoregulation, since, in addition to being antigen-presenting cells in conjunction with class II MHC antigens, they are able to destroy tumor cells, and kill pathogens after phagocytosis with release of free radicals such as hydrogen peroxide (48). To become optimally effective, macrophages have to be activated, and interferons, and more especially IFN-gamma, are very effective activators of macrophage function (4). There is, however, evidence that macrophage activating factors, other than interferons, could also play a role (49). Recombinant IFN-gamma stimulates the peroxide-releasing capacity of human macrophages about twentyfold, and thereby enhances their ability to kill toxoplasmas (50). Administration of recombinant Hu IFN-gamma to cancer patients similarly enhances the secretion of hydrogen peroxide by their monocytes (51). Endogenous IFN-gamma production in Listeria monocytogenes infected mice activates the macrophages of these animals with enhanced clearance of the bacteria, resulting in resolution of the infection (52,53). After activation by IFN-gamma, macrophages can destroy herpes simplex virus infected cells without harming uninfected cells. This activation, however, can be inhibited by norepinephrine and epinephrine, which suggests a mechanism by which stress-related hormones can decrease resistance to some viral infections (54). A comparison of recombinant MuIFN-gamma with natural murine IFN-alpha/beta showed IFN-gamma to be a remarkably potent activator of tumoricidal macrophages, 100 to 1000 fold more efficient than IFN-alpha/beta in terms of antiviral units (55). A comparison of several in vitro immunomodulating activities of recombinant IFN-alpha/beta and gamma has shown that for some activities (for example inhibition of the proliferative response of T cells to PHA) IFN-alpha and beta are more efficient, whereas for others, (for example stimulation of immunoglobulin synthesis), IFN-gamma is a more efficient modulator (56).

EFFECTS ON B CELLS

Although the effect of interferon on antibody formation is one of the first immunomodulating activities described, the action of interferons on B cells have recently received relatively little attention. Studies on the effects of interferons on antibody formation have frequently given apparently contradictory results of either suppression or enhancement (56,57). Various natural and recombinant Hu IFN-alpha species stimulated IgG and IgM synthesis by human B cells in vitro ; the effect was most pronounced in the presence of helper T cells (58). In vitro, Ig synthesis can be induced in B cell cultures with a variety of stimuli, provided that T cells or cytokines are present ; two of these mediators are IL 2 and IFN-gamma (59,60,61). Recombinant Hu IFN-gamma in conjunction with IL 2 induces IgM and IgG secretion in a portion of Staphylococcus aureus stimulated B cells, which raises the possibility that IFN-gamma is one of the differentiation factors for B cells (62). In contrast to these results is the inhibition of IgE and IgG1 synthesis observed when IFN-gamma is added to cultures of LPS stimulated, T depleted mouse spleen cells that have been enhaced with supernatant from con-A stimulated supernatants of a helper T-cell clone (63). Stimulation as well as inhibition of immune functions, depending on the experimental conditions, has often been observed with all three species of interferon.

CONCLUSIONS

In view of the limited space available for this overview, it has not been possible to do justice to all the aspects of current research on immunomodulation by interferons, and we have therefore put the emphasis on some of the most recent publications (1984,1985, and 1986) on this subject. The interest for this subject of is still expanding, which attests to its importance.

REFERENCES

1. De Maeyer-Guignard, J., and E. De Maeyer. In: Interferon 6, , I. Gresser, ed. Academic Press, London, pp. 69-91, 1985.
2. De Maeyer, E. and J. De Maeyer-Guignard. Phil. Trans. R. Soc. Lond. B299:77, 1982.
3. Epstein, L.B. In: Interferon 3, I. Gresser, ed. Academic Press, London, pp. 13-44, 1981.
4. Lucas, D.O. and L.B. Epstein. In: The Reticuloendothelial System, S.M. Reichard, J.P. Filkins eds. Plenum Publishing Corporation, pp.143-168, 1985.
5. De Maeyer, E. Ann. Inst. Pasteur/Immunol. 136D:67, 1985 (8th Forum of Immunology).
6. De Maeyer-Guignard, J., M.G. Tovey, I. Gresser, and E. De Maeyer. Nature 271:622, 1978.
7. De Maeyer-Guignard, J., A. Cachard, and E. De Maeyer. Virology 120:472, 1982.
8. Janeway, C.A. Jr., K. Bottomly, J. Babich, P. Conrad, S. Conzen, B. Jones, J. Kaye, M. Katz, L. McVay, D.B. Murphy and J. Tite. Immunology Today 5:99, 1984.
9. Basham, T., and T.C. Merigan. J. Immunol. 130:1492, 1983.
10. Houghton, A.N., T.M. Thomson, D. Gross, H.F. Oettgen, and L.J. Old. J. Exp. Med. 160:255, 1984.
11. Piguet, V., S. Carrel, A.C. Diserens, J.P. Mach, and N. De Tribolet. J. Natl. Cancer Inst. 76:223, 1986.
12. Gershon, H.E., Yan-De Kuang, G. Scala, and J.J. Oppenheim. J. Leukocyte Biol. 38:279, 1985.
13. Herlyn, M., D. Guerry, and H. Koprowski. J. Immunol. 134:4226, 1985.
14. Ziai, M.R., L. Imberti, A. Tongson, and S. Ferrone. Cancer Res. 45:5877, 1985.
15. Hayashi, H., K. Tanaka, F. Jay, G. Khoury, and G. Jay. Cell 43:263, 1985.
16. Skoskiewicz, M.J., R.B. Colvin, E.E. Schneeberger, and P.S. Russell. J. Exp. Med. 162:1645, 1985.
17. Momburg, F., N. Koch, P. Möller, G. Moldenhauer, G.W. Butcher, and G.J. Hammerling. J. Immunol. 136:940, 1986.
18. Takiguchi, M., J.P.-Y. Ting, S.C. Buesson, C. Boyer, Y. Gillespie, and J.A. Frelinger. Eur. J. Immunol. 15:809, 1985.
19. Fierz, W., B. Endler, K. Reske, H. Wekerle, and A. Fontana. J. Immunol. 134:3785, 1985.

20. Hunt, J.S., and Wood, G.W. J. Immunol. 136:364, 1986.
21. Wong, G.H.W., I. Clark-Lewis, A.W. Harris, and J.W. Schrader. Eur. J. Immunol. 14:52, 1984.
22. Berrih, S., F. Arenzana-Seisdedos, S. Cohen, R. Devos, D. Charron, and J.L. Virelizier. J. Immunol. 135:1165, 1985
23. Kelley, V.E., W. Fiers, and T.B. Strom. J. Immunol. 132:240, 1984.
24. Ling, P.D., M.K. Warren, and S.N. Vogen. J. Immunol. 135:1857, 1985.
25. Sztein, M.B., P.S. Steeg, H.M. Johnson, and J.J. Oppenheim. J. Clin. Invest. 73:556, 1984.
26. Kim, K.J., G. Chaouat, W.M. Leiserson, J. King, and E. De Maeyer. Cell. Immunol. 76:253, 1983.
27. Dolei, A., M.R. Capobianchi, and F. Ameglio. Infection & Immunity 40:172, 1983.
28. Rosa, F., D. Hatat, A. Abadie, D. Wallach, M. Revel, and M. Fellous. EMBO J. 2:1585, 1983.
29. Burrone, O.R., R.F. Kefford, D. Gilmore, and C. Milstein. EMBO J. 4:2855, 1985.
30. Piontek, G.E., K. Taniguchi, H.G. Ljungren, A. Grönberg, R. Kiessling, G. Klein, and K. Kärre. J. Immunol. 135:4281, 1985.
31. Yarden, A., H. Shure-Gottlieb, J. Chebath, M. Revel, and A. Kimchi. EMBO J. 3:969, 1984.
32. Aggarwal, B.B., T.E. Eessalu, and P.E. Hass. Nature 318:665, 1985.
33. Ruggiero, V., J. Tavernier, W. Fiers, and C. Baglioni. J. Immunol. 136:2445, 1986.
34. Tsujimoto, M., Y.K. Yip, and J. Vilcek. J. Immunol. 136:2441, 1986.
35. Holter, W., R. Grunow, H. Stockinger, and W. Knapp. J. Immunol. 136:2171, 1986.
36. Hamilton, T.A., P.W. Gray, and D.O. Adams. Cell. Immunol. 89:478, 1984.
37. Weiel, J.E., D.O. Adams, and T.A. Hamilton. J. Immunol. 134:293, 1985.
38. Vogel, S.N., D.S. Finbloom, K.E. English, D.L. Rosenstreich, and S.G. Langreth. J. Immunol. 130:1210, 1983.
39. Frasca, D., L. Adorini, S. Landolfo, and G. Doria. J. Immunol. 134:3907, 1985.
40. Reem, G.H. and N.H. Yeh. J. Immunol. 134:953, 1985.
41. Johnson, H.M., T. Vassallo, and B.. Torres. J. Immunol. 134:967, 1985.
42. Vilcek, J., D. Henriksen-Destefano, D. Siegel, A. Klion, R.J. Robb, and J. Le. J. Immunol. 135:1851, 1985.
43. Svedersky, L.P., G.E. Nedwin, D.V. Goeddel, and M.A. Palladino, Jr. J. Immunol. 134:1604, 1985.
44. Brunda, M.J., D. Tarnowski, and V. Davatelis. Int. J. Cancer 37:787, 1986.
45. van de Griend, R.J., C.P.M. Ronteltap, C. Gravekamp, D. Monnikendam, and R.L.H. Bolhuis. J. Immunol. 136:1700, 1986.
46. Rook, A.H., J.J. Hooks, G.V. Quinnan, H.C. Lane, J.F. Manischewitz, A.M. Macher, H. Masur, A.S. Fauci, and J.Y. Djeu. J. Immunol. 134:1503, 1985.

47. Blanchard, D.K., J.Y. Djeu, T.W. Klein, H. Friedman, and W.E. Stewart II. J. Immunol. 136:963, 1986.
48. Virelizier, J.L., and F. Arenzana-Seisdedos. Med. Biol. 63:149, 1985.
49. Kleinerman, E.S., R. Zicht, P.S. Sarin, R.C. Gallo, and I.J. Fidler. Cancer Res. 44: 4470, 1984.
50. Nathan, C.F., H.W. Murray, M.E. Wiebe, and B.Y. Rubin. J. Exp. Med. 158:670, 1983.
51. Nathan, C.F., C.R. Horowitz, J. de la Harpe, S. Vadhan-Raj, S.A. Sherwin, H.F. Oettgen, and S.E. Krown. Proc. Natl Acad. Sci USA 82:8686, 1985.
52. Havell, E.A., G.L. Spitalny, and P.J. Patel. J. Exp. Med. 156:112, 1982.
53. Buchmeier, N.A., and R.D. Schreiber. Proc. Natl. Acad. Sci. USA 82:7404, 1985.
54. Koff, W.C., and M.A. Dunegan. J. Immunol. 136:705, 1986.
55. Varesio, L., E. Blasi, G.B. Thurman, J.E. Talmadge, R.H. Wiltrout, and R.B. Herberman. Cancer Res. 44:4465, 1984.
56. Shalaby, M.R., P.K. Weck, E. Rinderknecht, R.N. Harkins, J.W. Frane, and M.J. Ross. Cell. Immunol. 84:380, 1984.
57. Johnson, H.M., B.G. Smith, and S. Baron. J. Immunol. 114:403, 1975.
58. Neubauer, R.H., L. Goldstein, H. Rabin, and N. Stebbing. J. Immunol. 134:299, 1985.
59. Brunswick, M. and P. Lake. J. Exp. Med. 161:953, 1985.
60. Romagnani, S., M.G. Giudizi, R. Biagiotti, F. Almerigogna, C. Mingari, E. Maggi, C-M. Liang, and L. Moretta. J. Immunol. 136:3513, 1986.
61. Lê thi Bich-Thuy, C. Queen, and A.S. Fauci. Eur. J. Immunol. 16:547, 1986.
62. Nakagawa, T., T. Hirano, N. Nakagawa, K. Yoshizaki, and T. Kishimoto. J. Immunol. 134:959, 1985.
63. Coffman, R.L., and J. Carty. J. Immunol. 136:949, 1986.
64. Sayers, T.J., A.T. Mason, and J.R. Ortaldo. J. Immunol. 136:2176, 1986.

47. Blanchard, D.K., [illegible] Djeu, J.Y., Klein, T.W., Friedman, H., and W.E. Stewart II. J. Immunol. 136:963, 1986.
48. Vitetta, E.S., [illegible] and [illegible] African [illegible], Med. Biol. 53:146, 1975.
49. [illegible] Goldstein, [illegible], B. [illegible] Sachs, [illegible] and T.J. Fidler. Cancer Res. 44:5470, 1984.
50. Kasahara, K., [illegible] Murray, M.E. [illegible] and J.Y. [illegible] Immunol. [illegible]:176, 1983.
51. [illegible], C.D., D.E. Hosevitz, [illegible], S. [illegible] A. [illegible], J. [illegible], and S.C. [illegible] Proc. Natl. Acad. Sci. [illegible] 1984.
52. [illegible] J. [illegible] 1984.
53. [illegible] Proc. Natl. Acad. Sci. 82:7400, 1985.
54. [illegible] and [illegible] Johnson. J. Immunol. 136:[illegible], 1986.
55. Varesio, [illegible], [illegible], M.E. [illegible], [illegible], Ralph, [illegible] and [illegible] Cancer Res. 44:[illegible], 1984.
56. Chantry, [illegible], P.R. [illegible] Kindleysides, [illegible], [illegible], and [illegible] Cell. Immunol. [illegible]:[illegible], 1984.
57. Johnson, H.M., B.G. [illegible] and [illegible] Baron. J. Immunol. 116:[illegible], 1976.
58. [illegible], [illegible] Goldstein, [illegible] and [illegible] J. Immunol. [illegible], 1985.
59. [illegible], [illegible] and [illegible] J. Exp. Med. 152:[illegible], 1984.
60. [illegible], [illegible] Robertson, [illegible], [illegible] Kenney, J. Immunol. [illegible]:[illegible], 1986.
61. [illegible], [illegible] and A. [illegible] J. Immunol. [illegible], [illegible].
62. Nakagawa, [illegible], [illegible] Hirano, [illegible] Yoshizaki, and [illegible] Kishimoto. J. Immunol. [illegible]:[illegible], 1985.
63. [illegible] and [illegible] Carey. J. Immunol. [illegible]:[illegible], 1984.
64. [illegible], [illegible], and [illegible]. J. Immunol. 116:216, 1986.

34. Antitumor Mechanisms of Interferons

S. Tyring[ab] *and S. Baron*[b]

[a]University of Alabama at Birmingham, Birmingham, AL 35294; [b]Department of Microbiology, University of Texas Medical Branch, Galveston, TX 77550

Introduction

Interferons (IFN) have been demonstrated to exert antitumor action against a wide range of neoplasms. This has been shown both in vitro, in experimental animals and in the clinical situation. Although IFN was originally described as an antiviral protein, it has been demonstrated to exert antitumor action on many cells transformed by chemical carcinogens, radiation, etc., as well as by oncogenic viruses. Interferon can kill tumor cells directly or indirectly via a number of effector cells. In addition, IFNs may act indirectly via their hormonal effects, inhibition of tumor viruses, inhibition of oncogene expression, immunomodulation and modulation of cell membrane macromolecules. This chapter will discuss various mechanisms by which IFNs may act to inhibit or eradicate tumor targets.

A. DIRECT ANTITUMOR EFFECTS OF INTERFERONS

Although all IFNs have antiproliferative activity against a wide range of normal and tumor cells, IFN gamma is considered more potent than IFN alpha or IFN beta per antiviral unit. In addition, IFNs have been shown to be cytolytic for certain tumor cell lines (18). Combinations of IFN gamma and IFN alpha have been shown to be synergistic in their antiproliferative actions in vitro and in a mouse model (5). The direct cytolytic activities of human IFN preparations have also been demonstrated to synergise (18). IFN gamma has been shown to be the molecule responsible for synergy in partially purified preparations of IFN gamma by use of recombinant IFN gamma as well as lack of synergy by IFN gamma preparations treated with an antibody to the IFN gamma molecule. (5, 18). The mechanism by which IFNs directly kill tumor cells has not been elucidated but the process does appear to require protein synthesis.

Results of clinical trials of IFN gamma combined with IFN alpha or IFN beta have thus far not been reported. This combination, however, may have greater efficacy with less toxicity than high concentrations of individual IFNs. This is based on the observation that such combinations have greater anticellular effects on malignant cells than nonmalignant cells in paired sets (8).

B. INDIRECT ANTITUMOR EFFECTS OF INTERFERONS

1. Activation of Effector Cells

In addition to their direct effects, IFNs act on tumor cells indirectly through their activation of the host's cell-mediated immune system. IFN activates and enhances the antitumor activity of NK (natural killer) cells, macrophages, sensitized T cells and ADCC (antibody-dependent cellular cytotoxicity). IFN gamma is significantly more efficient than other IFNs in enhancement of NK activity (23) and in macrophage activation (11). Interferon, however, may also protect some tumor cells from the cytolytic action of these cells with IFN gamma being more potent than other IFNs (13, 19). Observations are being made to determine whether high doses of IFN gamma will reverse the protective effects due to the presence in the preparation of an inhibitor of IFN action (7). The net antitumor effect of IFN, therefore, is the sum not only of its direct and indirect actions, but also of its positive and negative effects on tumor growth. In the vast majority of tumors treated with IFNs in the clinical situation as well as those tumor cell lines examined _in vitro_, the net effect has been partial or total destruction of the tumor cells. As can be seen in Table 1, IFNs have activity against a wide range of tumors, but the degree of eradication depends on the type of IFN employed as well as the presence of effector cells. IFN gamma can be seen to be the most potent IFN per antiviral unit both in its direct and in its cell-mediated actions. The use of unseparated PBMCs (peripheral blood mononuclear cells) allows evaluation of effector cells which act early in the immune response to tumor (e.g. NK cells) as well as those which act later (e.g. macrophages).

The kinetics of direct- and effector-cell-mediated tumor target killing can be seen in Figure 1. Synergy between IFN alpha and IFN gamma has been reported to potentiate NK activity (20) and may partially explain enhanced cytolysis of melanoma targets in Figure 1. Since complete eradication of these targets was not observed until 48 - 72 hours, other effector cells may also be synergistically activated by these combined IFNs. Although IFNs are known to activate macrophages, the majority of late killing was probably not due to this effector since removal of adherent cells by 3 to 24 hours cultivation in plastic culture vessels did not significantly decrease the cytolytic action of IFN-activated PBMC. One candidate effector for this late killing, however, is the IFN gamma activated T cell (GAT) (21).

Such in vitro assays of the antitumor action of IFNs have only occasionally proven to be of value in predicting the clinical efficacy of IFNs. As illustrated in Table 2, however, we have found a good correlation between the results of an in vitro cytotoxic assay for IFNs and the response of epithelioma-bearing animals to these IFNs. Especially notable is the observation that combined IFNs plus effector cells were able to completely eradicate these tumor cells both in vitro and in vivo.

2. Other Indirect Antitumor Actions of Interferons

Treatment of cancer patients with IFN alpha has been shown to augment expression of Fc receptors on monocytes. IFN gamma, however, augments Fc receptor expression on a number of tumor cell lines and normal cells in vitro to a greater degree than does IFN alpha (12). The Class II major histocompatibility antigen, HLA-DR, is required by macrophages to present antigen to helper T cells. IFN gamma is a more efficient inducer of HLA-DR expression on a number of normal and tumor cells, but IFN alpha is a stronger inducer of Class I MHC antigens (HCA-A, B, C) (17). Other receptors also are modulated (2) but their significance is still being investigated.

Interferons induce activities of at least two enzymes, a protein kinase and a 2′, 5′-oligoadenylate synthetase. These enzymes have been suggested to be responsible for some of the anticellular (and antiviral) effects of IFN, but no simple correlation exists between these enzymatic activities and the establishment of the anticellular (or antiviral) effects of IFN.

Another potential mechanism of the anticellular action of IFNs that is under active investigation is oncogene suppression. IFN has been demonstrated to inhibit the expression of such proto-oncogenes as C-myc and c-Ha-ras in certain human target cells (4). The relationship between this activity, however, and the anticellular action of IFN remains unclear. It has also been demonstrated that IFN treatment of virally-transformed as well as x-ray-transformed cells can lead to a reversion of the transformed phenotype (3). Removal of IFN from such cells, however, resulted in a partial reversion to the transformed phenotype.

Interferons can have a positive or negative effect on antibody synthesis depending on when IFN is added to antibody-producing cells (9). IFN gamma is many times more potent than other IFNs. Studies suggest that the IFN gamma enhancing effect on the antibody response is mediated by helper T cells, whereas its suppressive effect on antibody responses is a direct effect on the B cell. The effect of IFNs on production of antibody to tumor associated antigens, however, remains poorly understood.

Interferons are known to have many hormonal effects (14) some of which are thought to play a role in their antitumor actions. Most notable is the effect of IFNs on synthesis of and response to various prostaglandins which, in turn, are known to significantly influence the growth of tumor cells (16).

C. SYNERGY OF INTERFERONS WITH OTHER ANTITUMOR AGENTS

As previously discussed, IFN gamma can act synergistically with IFN alpha or IFN beta in both direct and cell-mediated mechanisms. In addition, IFNs can act synergistically with a number of other cancer therapies. For example, IFN treatment of a cancer patient could be synergistic with surgery by serving to eliminate metastases. This would be useful in killing pre-existing metastases as well as eliminating metastatic cells generated by surgery thereby offsetting the immunosuppressive effects of the surgery.

Interferons block progression of cells through the G_1 phase. Therefore, simultaneous administration of IFN and chemotherapeutic agents which have their most potent effect when cells are in the S-phase might be synergistic. This has been proven to be the case in vitro with IFN and mitomycin-C or 5-fluorouracil (10).

In vitro gamma or x-irradiation has been observed to synergise with IFN beta against human cervical carcinoma cells, and with IFN alpha or IFN gamma against synchronous human hypernephroma cells (1). In these cases IFN is thought to act as a radiosensitizer in addition to its direct effects on tumor cells. In addition, IFN may also function in a clinical situation to reverse radiation associated reductions of NK activity as well as reductions in NK activity associated with the malignancy itself.

Both the antiviral and anticellular actions of IFNs are known to be potentiated at elevated temperatures. This not only indicates that fever found during viral infections and some neoplastic diseases would potentiate host defense mechanisms, but also suggests that treatment of tumors with hyperthermia combined with IFN might be synergistic. Recent studies using the mouse melanoma B-16 demonstrated that elevated temperatures (i.e. 39-40°C) had a more dramatic enhancing effect on the antiproliferative activity of IFN gamma than of either IFN alpha or IFN beta. Furthermore, it was observed that the direct synergistic antiproliferative activity of combined IFNs can be further enhanced by hyperthermia (6).

The anticellular actions of IFNs have been shown to be enhanced when added to tumor cells in combination with a number of other lymphokines. These include interleukin-2, lymphotoxin, and tumor necrosis factors (15, 22).

CONCLUSION

Interferons have been demonstrated to exert their antitumor effects through a number of direct and indirect mechanisms. In almost every case IFN gamma has proved more potent than other IFNs. While IFN alpha has been clinically tested against a wide range of tumors with very promising results in some cases (e.g. hairy cell leukemia and condyloma acuminatum), clinical trials with IFN gamma are in their early stages. It therefore remains to be seen whether the exciting laboratory findings with IFN gamma will be reflected in the clinic. Also pending are reports of clinical studies with combination IFN treatment as well as IFNs combined with various other modes of cancer therapy. Many questions remain to be answered relating to dosage, toxicity to the host, duration of treatment, sequencing of treatments and which cancers are best treated with IFNs. Therefore many basic and clinical studies remain until the full antitumor potential of IFNs is realized.

REFERENCES

1. Chang, A.Y.C. and P.C. Keng: Effects of gamma interferon and radiation on synchronized human hypernephroma cells. Pro Am Assoc Cancer Res 26:281, 1985.
2. Chany, C., S. Rousset, and F. Chany-Fournier: Role of membrane receptors in the biological effects of interferon. Tex Rep Biol Med 41:307, 1982.
3. Chany, C. and M. Vignal: Effect of prolonged interferon treatment on mouse embryonic fibroblasts transformed by murine sarcoma virus. J Gen Virol 7:203, 1970.
4. Clemens, M.: Interferons and oncogenes. Nature 313:531, 1985.
5. Fleischmann Jr., W.R. and C.M. Fleischmann: Potentiating effect of murine-gamma-containing lymphokine preparation on the antiviral and antiproliferative effects of murine interferon alpha/beta: Identification of the potentiation factor as murine interferon gamma itself. Antiviral Res 4:221, 1984.
6. Fleischmann Jr., W.R., C.M. Fleischmann, and T.D. Gindhart: Effect of hyperthermia on combination interferon treatment: Enchancement of the antiproliferative activity against murine B-16 melanoma. Cancer Res 46:1722, 1986.
7. Fleischmann Jr., W.R., J.A. Georgiades, L.C. Osborne, F. Dianzani, and H.M. Johnson: Induction of an inhibitor of interferon action in a mouse lymphokine preparation. Infect Immun 26:949, 1979.
8. Fleischmann Jr., W.R., R.C. Newton, C.M. Fleischmann, W.M. Colburn, and M.M. Brysk: Discrimination between nonmalignant and malignant cells by combinations of IFN gamma plus IFN alpha/beta. J Biol Response Modifiers 3:397, 1984.
9. Johnson, H.M. and S. Baron: The nature of the suppressive effect of interferon and interferon inducers on the in vitro

immune response. Cell Immunol 25:106, 1976.
10. Le, J., Y.K. Yip, and J. Vilcek: Cytolytic activity of interferon gamma and its synergism with 5-fluorouracil. Int J Cancer 34:495, 1984.
11. Pace, J., S.W. Russell, and P.A. LeBlanc: Comparative effects of various classes of mouse interferons on macrophage activation for tumor cell killing. J Immunol 134:977, 1985.
12. Perussia, B., E.T. Dayton, R. Lazarus, et al.: Immune interferon induces the receptor for monomeric IgG_1 on human monocytic and myeloid cells. J Exp Med 158:1092, 1983.
13. Sarzotti, M., S. Baron, S.K. Tyring, and G.R. Klimpel: Interferon-mediated protection of B-16 melanoma cells from cytotoxicity by activated macrophages. Cell Immunol (in press, 1986).
14. Smith, E.B. and J.E. Blalock: The hormonal nature of the interferon system. Tex Rep Biol Med 41:350, 1982.
15. Soehnlen, B., R. Liu, and S.E. Salmon: Recombinant tumor necrosis factors exhibit antitumor activity against clonagenic tumor cells and synergism with gamma interferon. Proc of AACR 26:303, 1985.
16. Stringfellow, D.A.: Interferon induction: hyporesponsiveness and prostaglandins. Tex Rep Biol Med 41:116, 1982.
17. Sztein, M.B., P.S. Steeg, H.M. Johnson, and J.J. Oppenheim: Regulation of human peripheral blood monocyte DR antigen expression in vitro by lymphokines and recombinant interferons. J Clinical Invest 73:556, 1984.
18. Tyring, S., G. Klimpel, M. Brysk, V. Gupta, G.J. Stanton, W.R. Fleischmann, Jr., and S. Baron: Eradication of cultured human melanoma cells by immune interferon and leukocytes. JNCI 73:1067, 1984.
19. Wallach, D.: Interferon-induced resistance to the killing by NK cells: A preferential effect of IFN gamma. Cell Immunol 75:390, 1983.
20. Weigent, D.A., M.P. Langford, W.R. Fleischmann, Jr., and G.J. Stanton: Potentiation of lymphocyte natural killing by mixtures of alpha or beta interferon with recombinant gamma interferon. Infect Immun 40:35, 1983.
21. Weigent, D.A., M.P. Langford, W.R. Fleischmann, Jr., and G.J. Stanton: Enhancement of natural killing activity by different types of interferon. In: Human Lymphokines, N.O. Hill, A. Kohn, and D.C. Dumonole, eds. Academic Press, 1982.
22. Williams, T.W. and J.A. Bellant: In Vitro synergism between interferons and human lymphotoxin: enhancement of lymphotoxin-induced target cell killing. J Immunol 130:518, 1983.
23. Zarling, J.M., J. Sosman, L. Eskra, E.C. Borden, J.S. Horoszewica, and W.A. Carter: Enhancement of T cell cytotoxic responses by purified human fibroblast interferon. J Immunol 121:2002, 1978.

TABLE 1

Cytolysis of Human Tumor and Normal Cells by Interferons and Peripheral Blood Mononuclear Cells

Tumor Cells	% Surviving Cells[a]						
	IFN alpha[b]		IFN beta		IFN gamma		No IFN
	No PBMC	PBMC[c]	No PBMC	PBMC	No PBMC	PBMC	PBMC
Melanoma (6)[d]	86	38	83	40	65	<1	113
Adenocarcinoma (4)	72	28	65	21	34	10	47
Astrocytoma (1)	93	35	84	34	95	15	97
Large cell carcinoma (2)	88	37	78	24	40	12	56
Squamous cell carcinoma (4)	60	15	52	13	38	4	32
Renal cell carcinoma (1)	100	29	89	30	89	13	82
Normal cells (3)	74	47	79	45	65	13	78

a - Percentage surviving cells after 72 hours incubation with PBMC and/or IFN (relative to controls without PBMC or IFN). Viability was determined via trypan blue exclusion. Two-fold differences are significant at $P < 0.05$.

b - Concentration of each IFN = 200 u/ml.

c - Effector:target cell ratio = 100:1. The number of PBMC in actual contact with each target cell was estimated to be 3 - 6.

d - Number of different lines tested. Each line was studied on average of three times.

TABLE II

Comparison of Anticellular Effects of IFNs on Mouse JB-8 Epithelioma Cells *in vitro* and *in vivo*

Treatment	In Vitro: % of cells viable after 72 h (mean of 5 exp ± S.E.)	Average tumor volume as % of control	In Vivo[a]: Number of sites with tumors as % of control
Medium + spleen cells (S.C.)[b]	63 ± 11[c]	96	85
IFN alpha/beta 10^4 U/ml	51 ± 8	86	70
IFN alpha/beta 10^4 U/ml + S.C.	27 ± 5	77	65
IFN gamma 10^2 U/ml	37 ± 6	64	65
IFN gamma 10^2 U/ml + S.C.	14 ± 4	46	50
IFNs alpha/beta + gamma	4 ± 2	13	15
IFNs alpha/beta + gamma + S.C.	0 ± 0	0	0

a - Values were determined nine weeks after bilateral subcutaneous injection of 10^5 JB-8 cells followed by seven daily intralesional injections of IFN alpha/beta and/or IFN gamma with or without spleen cells. Each *in vivo* value is the average of two experiments with ten mice per experimental group.

b - Spleen cells:target cell ratio = 100:1

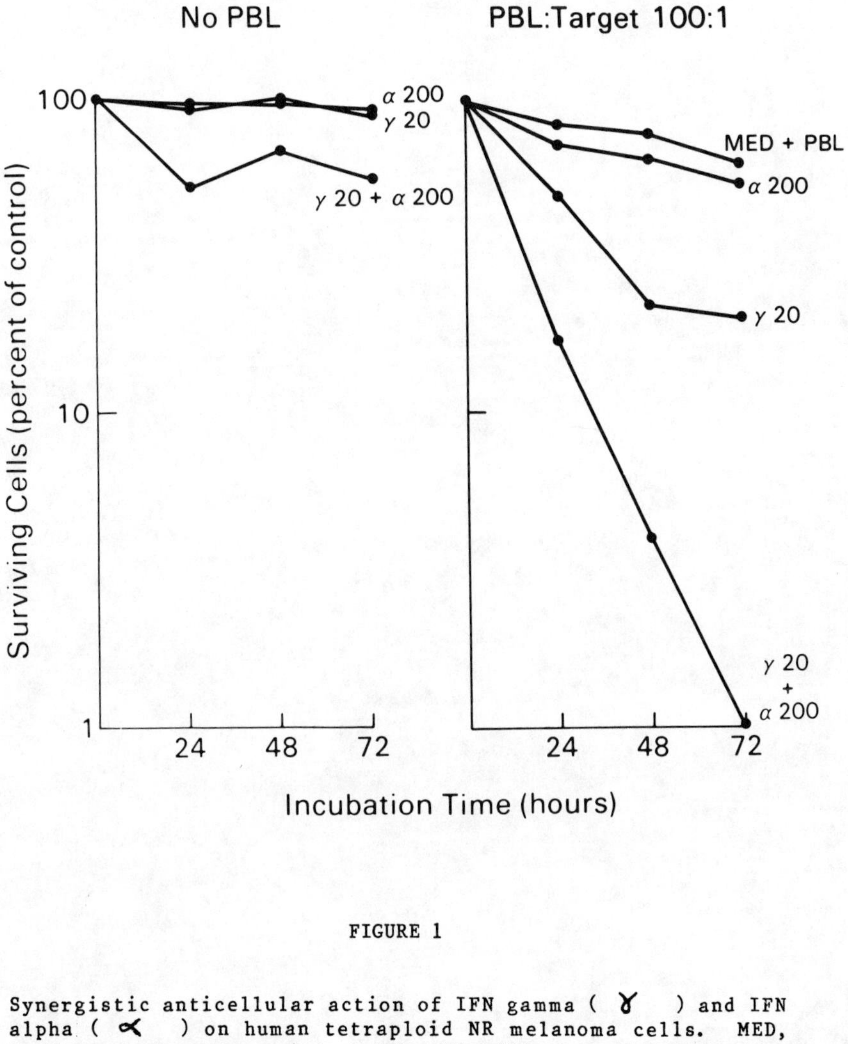

FIGURE 1

Synergistic anticellular action of IFN gamma (γ) and IFN alpha (α) on human tetraploid NR melanoma cells. MED, medium; numbers are units of IFN. Viability was determined at each time period via trypan blue exclusion.

35. Interferons and Bacterial Infections

M. Degrè, H. Rollag, and G. Bukholm

Department of Virology, National Institute of Public Health, and Institute of Bacteriology, National Hospital of Norway, University of Oslo, Oslo, Norway

INTRODUCTION

The possibility that interferons (IFN) have a role in the pathogenesis of bacterial infections has been raised by several authors previously. To date only few experimental studies have been published showing that pretreatment of mice with exogenous IFN can give protection against infection with several different bacterial species, e.g. Diplococcus pneumoniae, Hemophilus influenzae, or Salmonella typhimurium (1,2,3,4). Inoculation of mice with bacteria or bacterial products with capacity to induce IFN may also give protection against a subsequent bacterial infection (Baron, personal communication). There is obviously a need to confirm and extend these studies. However, there is av wide range of studies, that indirectly support the idea that IFN might play a role in the complex host defense not only against virus but also against bacterial infections. Firstly, IFNs are frequently present in the organism during bacterial infections, and secondly IFNs influence several physiological cell functions involved in the antibacterial defense.

PRODUCTION OF INTERFERONS DURING BACTERIAL INFECTIONS

IFN can be present in vivo during bacterial infections. Baron and coworkers (5) demonstrated IFN activity in middle ear fluids obtained from patients with bacterial acute otitis media. The bacteria included both Gram + cocci as Streptococcus pneumonia, Str. pyogenes and Staphylococcus aureus, and Gram negative rods as H. influenzae. The IFN was characterized as leukocyte (α) interferon. IFN was also present in the serum or in the cerebrospinal fluid during bacterial meningitis (6,7,8).

A wide range of bacteria, including those mentioned above, can induce IFN production in experimental animals. Either viable bacteria (9,10) or formaldehyde or phenol inactivated bacteria (9-16), inoculated intraperitoneally into mice induced circulating IFN activity up to 10^3 U/ml. The IFN was mostly of type I, predominantly of leukocyte (α) type, but under certain circumstances also IFN-γ was produced. Structural parts or extracts of bacteria have IFN inducing properties (10, 15-21). IFN is also induced by bacteria in spleen cell (9,22,23) or leukocyte cultures (9, Kishida, personal communication).

Bacterial infections, especially in the respiratory tract frequently occur in the wake of preceding viral infections. High titers of IFN, induced by the virus, may be present in the lungs at the time of bacterial invasion. Bacterial infection can, in fact, augment IFN levels induced by other agents as endotoxin or poly I:C (24). Also IFN-γ can be produced in sensitised host in response to bacterial infections, i.e. Mycobacterium bovis or Listeria monocytogenes (25,26) or bacterial products as M protein from S. pyogenes, or by tetanus or diphteria toxoid (27,28).

MECHANISM OF INTERFERON EFFECT ON BACTERIAL INFECTIONS.

The protective effect of IFNs against bacterial infections is not completely understood. There is no direct activity of IFNs on extracellular bacteria, although one early report stated that extracellular multiplication of Shigella flexneri is inhibited by IFN containing preparations (29). A possible effect on intracellular multiplication of some bacteria is most likely mediated by the host cell. Modifying effect of physiological cell functions, including those participating in the hosts antimicrobial defense, is thought to be the major factor.

Immune defense

The complex effect of IFNs on the immune defense is well established and it is reviewed elsewhere in this volume. However, it should be mentioned in the present context, that modifications of the humoral immune response, stimulation of B-cell maturation, enhanced or reduced antibody production, and effects on various paramethers of cell mediated immunity, as lymphocyte response to repeated antigenic stimulation, antibody dependent and antibody independent cytolysis of cells, NK- cell activity might have a relevanse to the antibacterial defense, especially against intracellular bacteria. Thus, IFN-α enhanced the natural cytotoxicity of peripheral blood mononuclear cells against Shigella infected cells (30).

Phagocytic activity

Phagocytic activity of polymorphonuclear leukocytes and macrophages is a major defense factor against bacterial infections. There is a general concensus that treatment of phagocytic cells with moderate concentrations of IFN-α/β enhances the ingestion of particles mediated by Fc, C3b and non-specific receptors (31-36). Although, the mechanism of this effect is not clear, it is most likely due to enhanced expression of surface receptors (36,38-40) and alteration of cytoskeletal structure of the phagocytizing cells (40). Intracellular levels of cAMP are stimulated by IFN treatment, but this phenomenon does not seem to be a mediator for the increased phagocytosis (41). IFN-γ effect is quantitatively different, but generally also stimulatory to macrophage functions, including phagocytosis (Rollag, H. and Degrè, M.: To be published), although in some experiments IFN-γ depressed ingestion of bacteria mediated by the non-specific receptors.

TABLE 1. Phagocytosis of non-opsonized and IgG-opsonized E.coli by human monocytes cultivated for 7 days without IFN and then treated for 24 h with an IFN-α, IFN-β, or IFN-γ preparation

Interferons	Non-opsonized E.coli	IgG-opsonized E.coli
IFN-α 10^2 U/ml	102	145
IFN-α 10^3 U/ml	104	152
IFN-β 10^2 U/ml	99	143
IFN-β 10^3 U/ml	98	124
IFN-γ 10^1 U/ml	76	141
IFN-γ 10^2 U/ml	84	137

Phagocytosis was assessed using ^{32}P-labelled E.coli

Adherence and penetration of bacteria

For several bacterial species there is a high degreee of correlation between cell invasive properties of bacteria *in vitro* and their ability to produce disease in man. This process can be modified by treatment of cells with IFNs. The first step of this process, adherence of bacteria to the cell membrane, does not seem to be influenced by IFN treatment(42) at least in our experimental system. However, penetration of several *Salmonella* and *Shigella* species into epithelial cells is inhibited by physiological concentrations of natural or recombinant IFNs (4,42-45). It is interesting that *Shigella* enterotoxin abolishes IFN effect on invasiveness (Bukholm et al. to be published) and invasiveness of *Shigella* into cells that lack receptor for the toxin is reduced by IFN treatment, but not in cells which have receptors for the toxin. The inhibitory effect of IFN seems to be dependent on active protein synthesis in the host cell, because low temperature and the ribosomal 60S subunit inactivators, cycloheximide and Shigella toxin abolished the effect.

TABLE 2. Effect of cycloheximide and S. flexneri toxin on the invasiveness of S. typhimurium in Hep-2 cell cultures treated with human leukocyte IFN (500 U/ml)

Treatment of cells	% infected cells	No of bacteria per infected cell	No of bacteria per 100 cells
IFN	6	2.3	14
IFN + shigella toxin	49	3.0	146
IFN + cyclohex. 1ug/ml	39	3.6	141
IFN + cyclohex.100ug/ml	28	3.9	108

The fate of intracellular bacteria

The ingested bacteria are normally inactivated and degraded by the cells. This process might be influenced by IFN treatment of the cells. Only very limited data are available and the results are different in various systems. Some authors found an inhibition of intracellular growth of the ingested bacteria in IFN treated cells (46,47, Whitaker-Dowling,P. personal communication), while others found an enhanced intracellular multiplication or no effect (48-50). Also the effect on intracellular lysosomalenzymes might be stimulatory or inhibitory (49,50).

TABLE 3. Effect of human leukocyte IFN on invasiveness of *S. flexneri* in A 549 cells

IFN titre	% infected cells	No of bacteria per infected cell	No of bacteria per 100 cells
0	43	5.9	251
100	30	3.9	120
500	9	5.8	50
1000	8	4.1	31

SUMMARY

IFN modifies several physiological cell functions that are part of the host defense against bacterial infection. These modifications probably influence the total defense of the organism but much remains to be clarified.

REFERENCES

1. Giron,. D.J., J.P. Schmidt, R.J. Ball, and F.F. Pindak: Effect of interferon inducers and interferon on bacterial infections. *Antimicrob Agents Chemother*, 1:80, 1972.
2. Degrẽ, M. and H. Rollag Jr: Pathogenesis of Sendai virus infection in mice. *Acta path microbiol scand*, Sect. B. 88:177, 1980.
3. Izadkhah, Z., A.D. Mandel, and G. Sonnenfeld: Effect of treatment of mice with sera containing gamma interferon on the course of infection with Salmonella typhimurium strain LT-2. *J Interferon Res*, 1:137, 1980.
4. Bukholm, G., B.P. Berdal, C. Haug, and M. Degrẽ: Mouse fibroblast interferon modifies Salmonella typhimurium infection in infant mice. *Infect Immun*, 45:62, 1984.
5. Howie, V., R.B. Pollard, K. Kleyn, B. Lawrence, T. Peskuric, K. Paucker, and S. Baron: Presence of interferon during bacterial ototis media. *J Infect Dis*,145:811, 1982.
6. Gresser, I. and K. Naficy: Recovery of an interferon-like substance from the cerebrospinal fluid. *Proc Soc Exp Biol Med*, 117:285, 1964.
7. Haahr, S: The occurence of interferon in the cerebrospinal fluid in patients with bacterial meningitis. *Acta Path Microbiol Scand*, 73:264, 1968.
8. Michaels, R.H., M.M. Wienberger, and M. Ho: Circulating interferon-like viral inhibitor in patients with meningitis due to Haemophilus influenzae. *N Engl J Med* 272:1148, 1965.
9. Baron, S., V. Howie, M. Langford, E.M. Macdonald, G.J. Stanton, J. Reitmeier, and D.A. Weigent: Induction of interferon by bacteria, protoza and viruses: defensive role. *Tex Rep Biol Med*, 41:150, 1982.

10. Nakane, A., T. Minigawa, and I. Yasuda: Induction of alpha/beta interferon and gamma interferon in mice infected with Listeria monocytogenes during pregnancy. *Infect Immun*, 50:877, 1985.

11. Degrê, M., and H. Dahl: Production of an interferon-like agent following inoculation with bacterial vaccine. Proc Soc Exp Biol Med 137: 233 1971.
12. Degrê, M., and H. Dahl: Interferon production and prevention of viral infections in mice by components of a mixed bacterial vaccine. Acta path Microbiol Scand, Sect. B, 82:904, 1974.
13. Singer, S.H., and M.C. Hardegree: Induction of interferon by bacterial vaccines and allergenic extracts. J Allergy 47:332, 1971.
14. Kandefer-Szerszen, M: Typhoid-paratyphoid (TAB) vaccine as interferon inducer in mice. Acta Microbiol Pol 22:156,1973.
15. Stinebring, W.R., and J.S. Youngner: Patterns of interferon appearance in mice injected with bacteria or bacterial endotoxin. Nature, 204:713, 1964.
16. Youngner, J.S., and W.R. Stinebring: Interferon appearance stimulated by endotoxin, bacteria, or viruses in mice pre-treated with Escherichia coli endotoxin or infected with Mycobacterium tuberculosis. Nature, 208:456, 1965.
17. DeClercq, E., and T.C. Merigan: An active interferon inducer obtained from Hemophilus influenzae type B. J Immunol, 103:899, 1969.
18. Grossberg, S.E., G. Burleson, P. Morahan, and P. Jameson: A bacterial protein inducing antiviral resistance and high titers of interferon. Progr immunobiol Standard, 5:274, 1972.
19. Kato, N., I.Nakashima, and M. Ohta: Interferon production in mice by the capsular polysaccaride of Klebsiella pneumoniae. Infect Immun, 12:1, 1975.
20. Barot-Ciorbaru, R., J. Wietzerbin, J-F. Petit, J. Chedid, E. Falcoff and E. Lederer: Induction of interferon synthesis in mice by fractions from Nocardia. Infect Immun, 19:353: 1978.
21. Cavaillon, J-M., Y. Riviere, J. Svab, L. Montagnier, and J.E. Alouf: Induction of interferon by Streptococcus pyogenes extracellular products. Immunol Letters, 5:323, 1982.
22. Blanchard, D.K., T.W. Klein, H.Friedman, and W.E. Stewart II: Kinetics and characterization of interferon production by murine spleen cells stimulated with Legionella pneumophila antigens. Infect Immun, 49:719, 1985.
23. Heremans, H., M. De Ley, A. Billiau, and P. De Somer: Interferon induced in mouse spleen cells by Staphylococcus aureus. Cellular Immunol, 71:353, 1982.
24. Havell, E.A.: Augmented capacity for alpha and beta interferon production during bacterial infection. Ann Rep Trudeau Inst 1982/83, 38.
25. Salvin, S.B., J.S. Youngner, and W.H. Lederer: MIgration inhibitory factor and interferon in the circulation of mice with delayed hypersensitivity. Infect Immun 7:68, 1973.
26. Havell, E.A., G.L. Spitalny, and P.J. Patel: Enhanced production of murine interferon by T cells generated in response to bacterial infection. J Exp Med, 156:112, 1982.
27. Green, J.A., S.R. Cooperband, and S. Kibirck: Immune-specific induction of interferon production in cultures of human blood lymphocytes. Science, 164:1415, 1969.
28. Weigent, D.A., E.H. Beachey, T.Huff, J.W. Peterson, G.J. Stanton, and S. Baron: Induction of human gamma interferon by structurally defined

polypeptide fragments of group A streptococcal protein. Infect Immun, 43:122, 1984.

29. Green, J.A.: Inhibition of Shigella flexneri by lysates of cells treated with interferon-containing preparations. Infect Immun, 7:1006, 1973.

30. Klimpel, G.R., D.W. Niesel, and K.D. Klimpel. J Immunol, In press, 1986.

31. Huang, K.Y., R.M. Donahoe, F.B. Gordon, and H.R. Dressler: Enhancement of phagocytosis by interferon containing preparations. Infect Immun, 4:581, 1971.

32. Imanishi, J., Y. Yokota, T.J. Kishida, T. Mukainaka, and A. Matuso: Phagocytosis enhancing effect of human leukocyte interferon preparation on human peripheral monocytes in vitro. Acta Virol, 19:52, 1975.

33. Hamburg, S.I., H.B. Fleit, H.C. Unkeless, and M. Rabinovitch: Mononuclear phagocytes: Responders to and producers of interferon. Ann NY Acad Sci, 350:72, 1980.

34. Degrê, M., and Rollag, H: Influence of interferon on the in vivo phagocytic activity of reticuloendothelial system cells. J Reticuloendothel Soc, 25:489, 1979.

35. Rollag, H., and M. Degrè: Effect of interferon preparations on the uptake of non-opsonized Escherichia coli by mouse peritoneal macrophages. Acta path microbiol scand, Sect B, 89:153, 1981.

36. Rollag H., M. Degrê, and G. Sonnenfeld: Effects of interferon α/β and interferon-γ preparations on phagocytosis by mouse peritoneal macrophages. Scand J Immunol, 20:149, 1984.

37. Melby, K., T. Midtvedt, M. Degrè: Effect of leukocyte interferon on phagocytic activity of polymorphonuclear leukocytes. Acta path microbiol scand, Sect. B. 90:181, 1982.

38. Vogel, S.N., D.S. Finebloom, K. English, D.L. Rosenstreich, and S.G. Langreth: Interferon-induced enhancement of macrophage Fc-receptor expression: β-interferon treatment of C3H/HeJ macrophages results in increased numbers and density of Fc receptors. J Immunol 130:1210, 1983.

39. Guyre, P.M., P.M. Morganelli, and R. Miller: Recombinant immune interferon increases immunoglobulin G Fc-receptors on cultures human mononuclear phagocytes. J Clin Invest, 72,393, 1983.

40. Wang, E., J. Michl, L.M. Pfeffer, S.C. Silverstein, and I. Tamm: Interferon suppresses pinocytosis but stimulates phagocytosis in mouse peritoneal macrophages: Related changes in cytoskeletal organization. J Cell Biol, 98:1328, 1984.

41. Degrê, M. and H. Rollag: Effect of murine beta-interferon preparation on phagocytosis and cyclic AMP levels in mouse peritoneal macrophages. J Interferon Res, 2:151, 1982.

Bukholm, G., K. MOdalsli, and M. Degrè: Effect of measles virus infection and interferon treatment on invasivenes of Shigella flexneri in HEp-2 cell cultures. J Med Microbiol, In press, 1986.

43. Bukholm, G. and M. Degrè: Effect of human leukocyte interferon on invasiveness of Salmonella species in HEp-2 cell cultures. Infect Immun, 42:1198, 1983.

44. Bukholm, G. and M. Degrè: Effect of human gamma interferon on invasiveness of Salmonella typhimurium in HEp-2 cell cultures. J Interferon Res, 5:45, 1985.

45. Niesel, D.W., C.B. Hess, Y.C. Cho, K.D. Klimpel, and G.R. Klimpel: Natural and recombinant interferons inhibit epithelial cell invasion by Shigella species. Infect Immun, In press, 1986.
46. Gober, L.L., A.E. Friedman-Kien, E.A. Havel, and J. Vilcek: Suppression of the intracellular growth of Shigella flexneri in cell cultures by interferon preparations and polyinosinic-polycytidylic acid. Infect Immun, 5:370, 1972.
47. Turco, J. and H.H. Winkler: Cloned mouse interferon-γ inhibits the growth of Rickettsia prowazekii in cultured mouse fibroblasts. J Exp Med, 158:2159, 1983.
48. Douvas, G.S., D.L. Looker, A.E. Vatter, and A.J.Crowle: Gamma interferon activates macrophages to become tumoricidal and Leishmanicidal but enhances replication of macrophage-associated Mycobacteria. Infect Immun, 50:1, 1985.
49. Rollag, H., B. Mørland, and M. Degrě: Effect of homologous beta-interferon preparation on degradation if Escherichia coli and on lysosomal enzyme activities in mouse peritoneal macrophages. Acta path microbiol immunol scand, Sect. B, 90:113, 1982.
50. Degrě, M., G. Sonnenfeld, H. Rollag, and B. Mørland: Effect of gamma interferon preparations on in vitro phagocytosis and degradation of Escherichia coli by mouse peritoneal macrophages. J Interferon Res, 1:505, 1981.

[illegible] Kessel, D.W. [illegible] R. [illegible] K.D. Kl[illegible] [illegible] Altered [illegible] and [illegible] of [illegible] by [illegible] [illegible] 1958.

46. [illegible] A.E. [illegible] and [illegible] [illegible] of the [illegible] of [illegible] [illegible] by [illegible] [illegible] the [illegible]-[illegible] [illegible] 1972.

47. [illegible] and [illegible] [illegible] [illegible] 1958.

48. [illegible] [illegible] and [illegible] [illegible] [illegible] [illegible]

49. [illegible] R. [illegible] and [illegible] [illegible] of [illegible] [illegible] [illegible] on [illegible] [illegible] [illegible] [illegible] 90-91 [illegible]

50. [illegible] [illegible] and [illegible] [illegible] the [illegible] [illegible] [illegible] of [illegible] [illegible] [illegible]

36. Interferons and Protozoal Infections

Gerald Sonnenfeld, Felipe Kierszenbaum, Cheryl L. Gould, Antonie L. W. DeGee, and John M. Mansfield

Department of Microbiology and Immunology, School of Medicine, University of Louisville, Louisville, KY 40292; Department of Microbiology and Public Health, Michigan State University, East Lansing, MI 48824; Department of Veterinary Science, University of Wisconsin, Madison, WI 53706

There have been many reports in the literature over almost a twenty year period indicating that interferon production is induced after exposure of animals to protozoan parasites (1-8). The nature of the protozoa that induce interferon runs the gamut from plasmodia to trypanosomes, and interferon production has been reported in cases of experimental animal infection or natural human infection (6,7). When first reported, these reports were difficult to reconcile with the biological role of interferons, as interferons were originally described as antiviral agents (9).

In recent years, knowledge of the biological activities of interferons has been greatly expanded (10). It has become clear that interferons have many activities in addition to their antiviral activities (10). These include regulation of immune responses (11) and regulation of normal and tumor cell growth and differentiation (10). These findings encouraged the consideration of a role for interferon in resistance to parasite infections. Such a role could include either a direct effect of interferons on parasites, or regulation by interferons of the host's immune defenses against parasites. In addition, interferon produced during the course of a protozoan parasite infection could help the host ward off secondary viral infections.

The focus of this review is on recent developments in the interactions of protozoan parasites with the interferon system, with particular attention paid to the possible immunoregulatory activities of interferon. The interactions of the interferon system with African and South American trypanosomes, the major area of interest in our laboratories, will be the area of greatest concentration.

TRYPANOSOMA CRUZI

Trypansoma cruzi is the South American trypanosome causing Chagas' disease (12). Infection with this intracellular parasite leads to damage in heart muscle, the central nervous system, and gastrointestinal tissue. Successful vaccination or chemotherapeutic treatment of the disease have been difficult to achieve (13). Early reports of Rytel and Marsden and others (4,8) had suggested that an interferon-like antiviral agent was produced in the sera of mice that had been infected with *T. cruzi*.

In our laboratories, mice were infected with different strains of *T. cruzi*. The Tulahuén and Y strains infect reticuloendothelial cells and myocardial cells, but are not entirely alike (14). Mice infected with either strain of *T. cruzi* produced an antiviral substance in their sera during the acute phase of infection. Mice infected with the Tulahuén strain produced peak levels of the antiviral substance within 24 hrs of infection, while mice infected with the Y strain required 72 hrs of infection to reach peak production (14). The earlier production of antiviral activity in mice infected with the Tulahuén strain could have been due to earlier arrival of the parasite at reticuendothelial cells responsible for interferon production.

The early antiviral activity produced after *T. cruzi* infection has been characterized as interferon-α/β (15). There was no interferon-γ produced early in the course of infection, but others have noted that interferon-γ was produced during the chronic stages of *T. cruzi*-infection of some strains of mice (J. Wietzerbin, personal communication). When mice infected with the Tulahuén strain of *T. cruzi* were treated with five daily doses of exogenous interferon-α/β beginning on the day of infection, the course of the parasitemia was altered (15). Enhanced resistance was evidenced by a transient decrease in parasitemia in interferon-α/β-treated mice as compared to mock interferon-treated mice (15). Similar results have been found when *T. cruzi*-infected mice were treated with interferon inducers (16). Others have shown that treatment mice with an antibody directed against interferon-α/β did not alter the course of infection of those mice with *T. cruzi* (17). However, those studies were preliminary in nature, and the antibody may not have eliminated all interferon-α/β from local sites of infection. The antibody also had no effect on interferon-γ, which also may play a role in resistance. In total, the above data suggest that interferons may play a role in mediating resistance of mice to infection with *T. cruzi*.

As preliminary evidence accrued to suggest a possible role for interferon in resistance to murine Chagas' disease, studies were begun to determine the mechanisms of interferon-induced resistance. Initial studies were carried out with interferon-α/β. When murine cell cultures were treated with interferon-α/β, no alterations in parasite uptake were seen when the cultures were subsequently infected with *T. cruzi* (18). This suggested that the interferon-α/β had no direct effect on the murine target cell. However, when the trypanosomes were pretreated with interferon-α/β, a decreased uptake of parasites by the cells was observed (18). This suggested a direct interaction between the interferon-α/β and the trypanosomes, and raises the intruiging possibility that there may be a receptor on the trypanosomes for interferon-α/β. Subsequent studies with purified interferons indicated that interferon-β was responsible for the effects that were observed with the earlier more crude preparations.

With regard to interferon-γ, it appears that the effect of the interferon is increased uptake and oxidative killing of T. cruzi by phagocytic cells (19,20). This mechanism for protection would be in accordance with the role of interferon-γ as a major macrophage activator for resistance to infectious diseases (21).

It is possible, therefore, to envision a two-step defense mechanism for enchanced resistance of mice to T. cruzi infection. First, in the early acute phase of infection, interferon-beta is produced by non-specific stimulation of cells by the trypanosome. This interferon-β may minimize uptake of parasites and thereby decrease the ability of the parasites to replicate. Once the infection becomes established and the interferon-β defense is overwhelmed, interferon-γ is produced as part of the cell-mediated immune response to the trypanosome. The interferon-γ then maximizes uptake of trypanosomes into phagocytic cells and increases the efficiency of killing of the trypanosomes by those cells. The validation of this hypothesis requires further experimentation. In addition, the interaction of the interferon system with other immune defenses against T. cruzi, including natural killer cell activity (22), requires further study to determine if these defense systems can be manipulated to provide greater protection against Chagas' disease.

TRYPANOSOMA BRUCEI

African trypanosomes, including subspecies Trypanosoma brucei, are the causative agents of African sleeping sickness (23). Trypanosomiasis is not only an important human disease, but also causes significant mortality among cattle (23). African trypanosomes are extracellular hemoflagellates. The disease is difficult to treat chemotherapeutically and vaccination has not succeeded due to antigenic variation. African trypanosomes express a variant specific surface glycoprotein that changes during the course of infection, altering the antigenicity of the trypanosomes as the disease progresses (24). In addition, the African trypanosomes appear to induce a generalized immunosuppression in the host (24). Therefore, it was of interest to determine the possible effects of interferon on resistance to this infection.

Production of interferon after infection of animals with a variety of different African trypanosomes has been reported by several groups for many years (5,8). Bancroft and associates first suggested that interferon produced in response to T. brucei infection of mice was a combination of interferons-α/β and -γ (8). In our laboratories, we explored interferon production to a greater extent, with the results providing evidence for a two-tier interferon-α/β and -γ defense against infection with Trypanosoma brucei rhodesiense (25). Mouse strains that were susceptible to infection (C3HeB/FeJ), intermediately resistant to infection (BALB/cJ and CBA/J), and relatively resistant to infection (B10.BR/-SgSnJ) were infected with clone LouTat 1 of T. b. rhodesiense (25). Susceptible strains of mice made little to no detectable interferon. Intermediately resistant mice produced moderate levels of interferon 8-12 days after infection, which coincided with remission of the first wave of parasitemia. The intermediately resistant mice occasionally produced low levels of interferon 4 days post-infection, at the time of commencement of the first wave of parasitemia. All interferon produced by the intermediately resistant strains of mice was characterized as interferon-α/β (25). The resistant B10.BR mouse strain produced two distinct peaks of interferon, one at four days post-infection, and one at 8-12 days post-infection. The first peak was made up of primarily interferon-α/β, and the second peak was primarily interferon-γ (25).

The study described above suggests that both interferon-α/β and interferon-γ were produced only in response to T. b. rhodesiense-infection of strains of mice that were resistant. In addition, the production of interferon-γ coincided with control of parasitemia and production of antibody in the resistant strain of mice (25). In other studies, we were able to show that the production of interferon in response to T. b. rhodesiense was not due to the effects of the variant specific surface antigens, but rather to a common internal factor shared by more than one clone of trypanosome (26). Also, the production of interferon-γ appeared to be due to true antigenic stimulation and not to mitogenic activity of trypanosome antigens, since trypanosomal antigens did not appear to cause mitogenesis of lymphoid cells (26). Therefore, interferon production would escape the complication of immune responses to the trypanosome caused by the constant shift in variant surface glycoprotein expression.

Further studies are required to determine whether interferon plays a role in resistance to primary T. b. rhodesiense infections or whether production of interferon occurs in resistant strains just as an indication of the animal not being debilitated as a result of infection. Whatever the role of interferon is in resistance to primary infections with African trypanosomes, evidence exists for a role for interferon in protection from secondary viral infections (27). Hosts infected with T. b. rhodesiense become immunosuppressed and debilitated as the course of infection progresses, and much of the morbidity and mortality may be caused by secondary infections. In our studies, mice that were resistant to T. b. rhodesiense and which produced interferon were resistant to infection with encephalomyocarditis virus (27). When interferon was not induced, protection was decreased. Therefore, interferon may play a role in protecting immunocompromised infected animals from developing secondary viral infections.

LEISHMAINA DONOVANI

Spcies of Leishmainia can cause visceral and cutaneous disease in humans (28). An early report by Herman and Baron (3) indicated that induction of interferon resulted in inhibition of growth of Leishmania donovani within cells. This could have been due to activation of killing by phagocytic cells by the interferon that was induced.

These studies have been expanded more recently to show that interferon-γ could enhance killing of intracellular Leishmania donovani by stimulating the activity of human mononuclear phagocytic cells (29). However, individuals with active visceral leishmaniasis had cells that were incapable of producing interferon-γ or interleukin-2 (30). In this fashion, the immunosuppression caused by visceral leishmaniasis could result in compromised production of interferon-γ. Interferon, a possibly important defense mechanism to activate cells to kill leishmania, would then not be able to protect the host from the diseases. The establishment for a role for interferon in the natural course of defenses against leishmania will require further study. In addition, the interaction of interferon-γ with other lymphokine-like defense factors against leishmania will also require more experimentation (31).

PLASMODIUM

Several species of Plasmodium are responsible for malaria throughout the world. Over a twenty-year period, there have been several reports of induction of interferon in animals infected with plasmodia (2,32). It has been postulated that the induction of interferon in this case may be due to the mitogenic activity of malarial antigens on host lymphoid cells (33). In addition, treatment of animals with interferon can result in some protection against plasmodia infections (34). These results suggest that interferon could play some role in resistance to malarial infections.

A recent finding was described by two different groups (6,7). They were able to detect circulating interferon in individuals with malaria. These data suggest that similar interferon induction occurs after Plasmodium infection both in experimental animal models and in human disease. Again, since plasmodia appear to induce interferon as a result of mitogenic activity, further experiments must be carried out to definitively determine the role of interferon in natural malarial infections.

TOXOPLASMA GONDII

Toxoplasma gondii causes toxoplasmosis in humans, and is a threat in cases of in utero transmission to fetuses. There has been one early (1) report of induction of an interferon-like substance by Toxoplasma gondii. In addition, a recent report indicated that administration of interferon-γ to mice resulted in increased antibody production and survival when the mice were infected with T. gondii (35).

CONCLUSIONS

Several protozoan parasites appear to share a common property in terms of induction of interferon in their mammalian hosts (1-8,14). In addition, treatment of animals with exogenous interferon or interferon inducers appear to be able to alter the course of several different protozoan infections (3,15,18). Interferon, therefore, can be induced and may play a significant role in host defenses against these organisms.

However, the question remains to be answered whether interferon plays some role in resistance in the natural course of a parasitic infection. It is certainly conceivable that interferon produced during a protozoan infection may affect the course of secondary viral infections. Since many protozoan infections are immunosuppressive, the interferon induced by the protozoa might be of great value to the host in warding off other, perhaps more rapidly fatal, infections.

On the other hand, the data presently available make it difficult to determine if the interferon produced during protozoan infections actually affects the course of natural infcetion. The interferon could either affect the parasites directly, or modulate other host immune responses to the parasites. Definitive proof of a primary role for interferon in resistance to protozoan infections remains to be provided and will require much further experimentation.

ACKNOWLEDGEMENTS

Studies performed in the authors' laboaratories were funded in part by US NASA Award NCC 2-213, and USPHS grants AI-14048 and AI-22441. Cheryl L. Gould was a NASA Space Biology Research Associate. Additional funds were provided from NIH BRSG grant RR-05375 administered by the University of Louisville.

REFERENCES

1. Freshman, M.M., T.C. Merigan, J.S. Remington, and I.E. Brownlee: In vitro and in vivo antiviral action of an interferon-like substance induced by Toxoplasma gondii. Proc Soc Exp Biol Med 123:862, 1966.
2. Huang, K.-Y., W.W. Schultz and F.B. Gordon: Interferon induced by Plasmodium berghei. Science 162:123, 1968.
3. Herman, R., and S. Baron: Effects of interferon inducers on the intracellular growth of the protozoan parasite Leishmania donovani. Nature 226:168, 1970.
4. Rytel, M.W., and P.D. Marsden: Induction of an interferon-like inhibitor by Trypanosoma cruzi in mice. Amer J Trop Med Hyg 19:928, 1970.
5. Talas, M., and E.T. Glaz: Type I interferon induced in mice by infection with Trypanosoma equiperdum. J Infect Dis 139:595, 1979.
6. Rhodes-Feuillete, A., P. Druilhe, M. Canivet, M. Gentilini, and J. Peries: Presence d'interferon circulant dans le serum de malades infectes par Plasmodium falciparum. C R Acad Sci Paris t293 Serie III: 635, 1981.
7. Ojo-Amaize, E.A., L.S. Salimonu, A.I.O Williams, A.O. Akinwolere, R. Shabo, G.V. Alm, and H. Wigzell: Positive correlation between degree of parasitemia, interferon titers and natural killer cell activity in Plasmodium falciparum-infected children. J Immunol 127:2296, 1981.
8. Bancroft, G.J., C.J. Sutton, A.G. Morris, and B.A. Askonas: Production of interferons during experimental African trypanosomiasis. Clin Exp Immunol 52:135, 1983.
9. Isaacs, A., and J. Lindenmann: Virus interference. I. The interferon. Proc Roy Soc Ser B 147:258, 1957.
10. Gresser, I: Commentary on the varied biologic effects of interferon. Cell Immunol 34:406, 1977.
11. Sonnenfeld, G: Modulation of immunity by interferon. Lymphokine Rep 1:113, 1980.
12. Romaña, C: Enfermedad de Chagas. Lopez Libreros Editores, S.R.L., Buenos Aires, 1963.
13. Kierszenbaum, F: The chemotherapy of Trypanosoma cruzi infections (Chagas' Disease). In: Parasitic Diseases, Vol. 2 The Chemotherapy, J. M. Mansfield, ed. Marcel Dekker, New York, pp.133-163, 1984.
14. G. Sonnenfeld and F. Kierszenbaum: Increased serum levels of an interferon-like activity during the acute period of infection with dif-

ferent strains of Trypanosoma cruzi. Am J Trop Med Hyg 30:1189, 1981.
15. Kierszenbaum, F., and G. Sonnenfeld: Characterization of the antiviral activity produced during Trypanosoma cruzi infection and protective effect of exogenous interferon against experimental Chagas' disease. J Parasitol 68:194, 1982.
16. James, S.L., T.L. Kipnis, A. Sher, and R. Hoff: Enhanced resistance to acute infection with Trypanosoma cruzi in mice treated with an interferon inducer. Infect Immun 35:588, 1982.
17. Quan, P.C., B. Rager-Zisman, M. Wittner, and H. Tanowitz: Interferon and natural killer cells in murine Chagas' disease. J Parasitol 69:1164, 1983.
18. Kierszenbaum, F., and G. Sonnenfeld: Interferon inhibits cell infection by Trypanosoma cruzi in vitro. J Immunol 132:905, 1984.
19. Plata, F., J. Wietzerbin, F. Garcia-Pons, E. Falcoff, and H. Eisen: Synergistic protection by specific antibodies and interferon against infection by Trypanosoma cruzi in vitro. Eur J Immunol 14:930, 1984.
20. Wirth, J.J., F. Kierszenbaum, G. Sonnenfeld, and A. Zlotnik: Enhancing effects of gamma interferon on phagocytic cell association with and killing of Trypanosoma cruzi. Infect Immun 49:61, 1985.
21. Nathan, C.F., H.W. Murray, M.E. Weibe, and B.Y. Rubin: Identification of interferon-γ as the lymphokine that activates human macrophage oxidative metabolism and antimicrobial activity. J Exp Med 158:670, 1983.
22. Hatcher, F.M., and R.E. Kuhn: Destruction of Trypanosoma cruzi by natural killer cells. Science 218:295, 1982.
23. Meshnick, S.R.: The chemotherapy of African trypanosomiasis. In: Parasitic Diseases, Vol. 2 The Chemotherapy, J.M. Mansfield, ed., Marcel Dekker, New York, pp. 165-200, 1984.
24. Mansfield, J.M.: Immunology and immunopathology of African trypanosomiasis. In: Parasitic Diseases, Vol. 1 The Immunology, J.M. Mansfield ed., Marcel Dekker, New York, pp. 167-226, 1981.
25. DeGee, A.L.W., G. Sonnenfeld, and J.M. Mansfield: Genetics of resistance to the African trypanosomes V. Qualitative and quantitative differences in interferon production among susceptible and resistant mouse strains. J Immunol 134:2723, 1985.
26. DeGee, A.L.W., G. Sonnenfeld, and J.M. Mansfield: Submitted, 1986.
27. Gould, C.L., A.L.W. DeGee, J.M. Mansfield, and G. Sonnenfeld: Submitted, 1986.
28. Marr, J.J.: The chemotherapy of leishmaniasis. In: Parasitic Diseases, Vol. 2 The Chemotherapy, J.M. Mansfield, ed., Marcel Dekker, New York, pp. 201-228, 1984.
29. Murray, H.W., B.Y. Rubin and C.D. Rothermel: Killing of intracellular Leishmania donovani by lymphokine-stimulated human mononuclear phagocytes. Evidence that interferon-γ is the activating lymphokine. J Clin Invest 72:1506, 1983.
30. Carvahlo, E.M., R. Badaro, S.G. Reed, T.C. Jones, and W.D. Johnson: Absence of gamma-interferon and interleukin-2 production during active visceral leishmaniasis. J Clin Invest 76:2066, 1985.
31. Hoover, D.L., D.S. Finbloom, R.M. Crawford, C.A. Nacy, M. Gilbrerth and M.S. Meltzer. A lymphokine distinct from interferon-γ that activates human monocytes to kill Leishmania donovani in vitro. J Immunol 136: 1329, 1986.
32. Sauveger, F., and B. Fauconnier. The protective effect of endogenous interferon in mouse malaria as demonstrated by the use of anti-interferon globulins. Biomedicine 29:184, 1978.

33. Ojo-Amaize, A.E., J. Vilcek, A.H. Cochrane and R.S. Nussenzweig: Plasmodium berghei sporozoites are mitogenic for murine T cells, induce interferon and activate natural killer cells. J Immunol 133:1005, 1984.
34. Jahiel, R.I., J. Vilcek, and R.S. Nussenzweig: Exogenous interferon protects mice against Plasmodium berghei malaria. Nature 227:1350, 1970.
35. McCabe, R.E., B.J. Luft, and J.S. Remington: Effect of murine interferon-gamma on murine toxoplasmosis. J Infect Dis 150:196, 1984.

V. Molecular Mechanisms of Interferon Action

37. 2′,5′-Oligo(A) Pathway of Interferon Action

Corrado Baglioni

Department of Biological Sciences, State University of New York at Albany, Albany, NY 12222

INTRODUCTION

The elucidation of the structure of 2-5A (1) and the finding that a nuclease (RNase L) is activated by 2-5A (2,3) led to the discovery of the 2-5A pathway of IFN action. Binding of IFN to specific receptors on the cell surface induces transcription of the mRNA for 2-5A synthetase (4). The level of this enzymatic activity present in IFN-treated cells is directly correlated with the extent of protection against an RNA virus, such as EMCV (5). This suggests that the 2-5A pathway is involved in blocking the replication of specific viruses (6) and several experiments have conclusively proven that this pathway plays a major role among the antiviral mechanisms activated by IFN. The different experimental approaches used to study the 2-5A pathway in cell extracts and in virus-infected cells will be reviewed here.

STUDIES IN CELL-FREE SYSTEMS

The 2-5A synthetase is activated when bound to double-stranded RNA (dsRNA) containing more than 30 base-pairs (7). Since dsRNA of this size is only found in virus-infected cells, the 2-5A synthetase is presumably inactive in the cytoplasm of uninfected cells. 2-5A is synthesized in large amounts when high concentrations of ATP, the substrate of the synthetase, and of Mg^{2+} are added to extract of IFN-treated cells (8). 5'-tri- and diphosphate 2-5A activate RNase L by binding to this enzyme; when 2-5A dissociates from RNase L, this enzyme reverts to an inactive state (9). The binding affinity of 2-5A is very high, since 0.3 nM 2-5A activates 50% of the human RNase L (10). This indicates that very small concentrations of 2-5A can cause extensive RNA degradation.

The RNase L cleaves indiscriminately viral and cellular mRNA (2-3). Furthermore, even rRNA in intact ribosomes can be cleaved at a few sites (11). Preferential cleavages at UA, UG and UU sequences yield oligonucleotides terminating with a 3'-phosphate (12-13). This lack of substrate specificity makes difficult to understand how RNase L can specifically cleave viral RNA in IFN-treated cells, but a mechanism accounting for discrimination between viral and host mRNA has been discovered (14):

i) 2-5A synthetase binds to and is activated by dsRNA in replicative complexes of RNA viruses; ii) RNase L is activated by 2-5A in a transient and localized way because of the rapid degradation of these oligonucleotides; iii) nascent viral RNA synthesized by the replicative complexes is specifically cleaved by RNase L. The localized cleavage by RNase L was demonstrated in experiments with isolated replicative intermediates of EMCV and with ribonucleotides containing a double-stranded region (14). The preferential cleavage of nascent viral mRNA by RNase L has been shown in transcription reactions containing purified reovirions (15). Addition of cell extract prepared from IFN-treated HeLa cells greatly reduces the yield of reovirus mRNA, but neither mRNA added to the reactions nor rRNA in ribosomes added with cell extract is appreciably cleaved (15). The yield of reovirus mRNA can be restored to the levels obtained without addition of cell extract by carrying out transcription in the presence of either the inhibitor of 2-5A synthetase 2'-dATP or of the RNase L inhibitor 3'-methyl-5'-monophosphate 2-5A (15). This finding shows that viral transcripts do not accumulate when the 2-5A pathway is activated and that this pathway functions in a discriminatory way by specifically cleaving nascent viral mRNA.

The 2-5A is rapidly degraded in cell extracts (16) and presumably in intact cells. A 2'-phosphodiesterase cleaves 2-5A (17), but recent experiments have shown that 2-5A is also degraded by a phosphatase which removes 5'-terminal phosphates and produces 2-5A derivatives that can bind to RNase L, but do not activate this enzyme (18). 5'-monophosphate 2-5A is an antagonist of 2-5A (19), since it can bind to RNase L without activating this enzyme (20-21), but it is not clear whether the 2-5A degradation products formed in cell extracts or in intact cells (18) are 5'-monophosphate derivatives without further modifications. A possible biological role for these 2-5A derivatives is to restrict the activity of RNase L in INF-treated virus-infected cells to the sites where 2-5A is continually being synthesized. Therefore, the localized activation of RNase L may also result from the degradation of 2-5A to derivatives that inhibit this enzyme.

2-5A IN CELLS

Williams et al. (22) first isolated 2-5A from IFN-treated L cells infected with EMCV. 2-5A concentrations in the nM range were subsequently detected in these cells by a sensitive competition binding assay (20). Nanomolar 2-5A concentrations were also detected in IFN-treated HeLa cells infected with reovirus (23) or incubated with dsRNA (21). These findings suggest that the 2-5A pathway is activated by viral structures containing dsRNA. The 2-5A is detected in the cytoplasm after 3 h of infection with reovirus, and its concentration increases up to 6 h but decreases afterwards (23). The 2-5A is detected only in cells infected at high multiplicity, although cells infected at low multiplicity are best protected by IFN. It seems likely that in the latter cells 2-5A is produced in amounts sufficient to activate RNase L and confer protection to the cells, but too small to be detected even by a very sensitive as-say. Interestingly, no cleavage of rRNA is detected in IFN-treated cells infected at high multiplicity, suggesting that the RNase L is not indiscriminately activated by 2-5A (23).

2-5A has been found in μM concentrations in cells infected with vaccinia virus that is relatively insensitive to the antiviral effect of IFN (24-25). This 2-5A is produced relatively late in the infectious cycle by 2-5A synthetase activated by dsRNA formed by symmetric transcripts of vaccinia virus. The cleavage of rRNA is delayed relative to 2-5A accumulation, suggesting that RNase L is inactive early in the infection, but 2-5A capable of activating RNase L can be recovered from these cells (24-25). It has been suggested that a viral ATPase and phosphatase may be involved in the inhibition of 2-5A synthesis and in 2-5A inactivation in vaccinia-infected cells (26). μM concentrations of 2-5A derivatives are also detected late in the infection with SV-40 of IFN-treated cells (27). These compounds are neither 5'-tri- nor diphosphate 2-5A and are not degraded by phosphatase; this indicates that they lack exposed phosphate groups. Up to 60 nM 2-5A is present in IFN-treated Chang cells infected with HSV, but little rRNA cleavage is observed in these cells (28). However, 5'-triphosphate 2-5A can be recovered from these cells at greater than nM concentration together with two 2-5A derivatives that inhibit RNase L activation (28). These compounds are resistant to phosphatase digestion and apparently lack exposed phosphate groups (28). These observations suggest that the 2-5A pathway plays an important role only among the antiviral mechanisms that inhibit the replication of RNA viruses, whereas it may be irrelevant in the defense against DNA viruses, which are relatively insensitive to the antiviral activity of IFN.

VARIANTS OF THE 2-5A PATHWAY

Cell variants that lack either 2-5A synthetase or RNase L activity are a useful tool for studying the role of the 2-5A pathway. Such variants have been identified by different investigators, but the results obtained have been difficult to interpret in many cases because of the leakiness of these variants. For example, Meurs et al. (29) reported that VSV RNA synthesis is inhibited in IFN-treated human MRC5 cells that have no detectable 2-5A synthetase activity. However, these cells respond to IFN with a small increase in 2-5A synthetase when treated with high concentrations of IFN (30). This reduced response to IFN is apparently due to a low number of IFN receptors (30). Czarniecki et al. (31) reported that a clone of murine NIH 3T3 cells chronically infected with Moloney leukemia virus are resistant to the antiviral activity of IFN. These cells appear to lack RNase L activity (32), but this activity can be recovered in cell extracts prepared with a protease inhibitor (33). Krause et al. (34) have recently reported that low levels of RNase L are present in actively dividing cells of this NIH 3T3 clone and that this enzymatic activity increases during growth arrest to less than 1/2 of the level found in other murine cells. This level of RNase L is apparently insufficient to inhibit EMCV replication in IFN-treated cells (34). These results point out another possible complication in the interpretation of experiments with cell variants: the RNase L level is increased in some cells by growth inhibition, differentiation and IFN treatment (35-36).

Salzberg et al. (37) reported that VSV and mengovirus replication is not inhibited by IFN in a murine cell variant defective in the induction of

2-5A synthetase. However, the IFN-induced protein kinase was not measured in these cells and the loss of protection from virus infection could not be attributed uniquely to the lack of 2-5A synthetase. Experiments by Sen et al. (38) with RD-114 human sarcoma cells show that treatment with IFN does not impair replication of VSV and EMCV. These cells have a low level of 2-5A synthetase activity and no detectable IFN-induced kinase. These experiments yield inconclusive results, like the early observations by Nilsen at al. (39) on PCC4 murine embryonal carcinoma cells. These cells are inducible for 2-5A synthetase but not for the protein kinase (40) and are protected by treatment with IFN from EMCV and mengo, but not from VSV and Sindbis virus (39). It should be pointed out, however, that the level of 2-5A synthetase induced by IFN in PCC4 cells is lower than that induced in L cells, which are well protected by IFN from all these viruses (39). Therefore, the protection conferred by IFN against specific viruses may require different levels of 2-5A synthetase and RNase L.

LOSS OF 2-5A SYNTHETASE BY PRODUCTION OF ANTISENSE RNA

A novel approach to suppress 2-5A synthetase activity in human cells is based on the production of antisense RNA (41). An expression vector was constructed with part of the human papova BK virus, the neomycin resistance gene under the control of the SV40 promoter and 0.5 kb of 2-5A synthetase cDNA inserted in inverted orientation downstream from the BK virus VP promoter. Osteosarcoma cells transfected with this vector and selected for resistance to the neomycin derivative G418 synthesize RNA complementary to 2-5A synthetase mRNA. These cells lack 2-5A synthetase activity and this enzyme is not inducible by IFN (41). In contrast, the 2-5A synthetase is induced in cells transfected with a control vector without the cDNA insert. Such cells are protected by IFN from the cytopathic effect of all RNA viruses tested, whereas cells lacking 2-5A synthetase are not protected from EMCV, VSV and sindbis virus, but are fully protected from influenza virus. Reovirus RNA synthesis is completely suppressed in IFN-treated cells with inducible 2-5A synthetase, but it is only delayed in cells lacking this enzyme. These findings show that a high level of 2-5A synthetase is required for protection by IFN from all the RNA viruses that replicate in the cytoplasm. Protection from influenza virus infection does not require 2-5A synthetase activity and it is only due to the IFN-induced Mx protein (42). The delay of reovirus RNA synthesis in IFN-treated cells lacking 2-5A synthetase may be caused by other antiviral mechanisms. Such cells are perfectly viable (41) and it seems unlikely, therefore, that the 2-5A pathway performs some essential function in human cells outside of the antiviral state elicited by IFN. It cannot be excluded, however, that very small levels of 2-5A synthetase may perform some as yet unidentified physiological function. The cells that lack 2-5A synthetase replicate at a much faster rate than control or parental cells (unpublished observations) and it seems possible that the 2-5A pathway may be involved in some aspect of the regulation of cell proliferation.

2-5A ANALOGUES INHIBITORS OF RNase L

2-5A analogues that can bind to RNase L without activating this enzyme have been introduced in IFN-treated L cells infected with EMCV with the calcium phosphate coprecipitation technique (43). These analogues partially restore EMCV RNA synthesis and virus yield. These results show that the 2-5A pathway plays some role in the IFN action against EMCV replication.

CONCLUSIONS

The experiments with cells producing antisense RNA complementary to 2-5A mRNA provide the best evidence for the unique role of the 2-5A pathway among the antiviral mechanisms induced by IFN. These cells are not protected by IFN from any cytoplasmic RNA virus. It remains to be established whether these cells are protected from DNA viruses and whether the 2-5A pathway plays any role in the inhibition of cell proliferation by IFN.

REFERENCES

1. Kerr, I.M., and R.E. Brown: pppA2'p5'A2'p5'A: An inhibitor of protein synthesis synthesized with an enzyme fraction from interferon-treated cells. Proc. Natl. Acad. Sci. USA 75:256, 1978.
2. Baglioni, C., M.A. Minks, and P.A. Maroney: Interferon action may be mediated by activation of a nuclease by pppA2'p5'A2'p5'A. Nature 273:684, 1978.
3. Clemens, M.J., and B.R.G. Williams: Inhibition of cell-free protein synthesis by pppA2'p5'A2'p5'A: a novel oligonucleotide synthesized by interferon-treated L cell extracts. Cell 13:565, 1978.
4. Merlin, G., J. Chebath, P. Benech, R. Metz, and M. Revel: Molecular cloning and sequence of partial cDNA for interferon-induced (2'-5')oligo(A) synthetase mRNA from human cells. Proc. Natl. Acad. Sci. USA 80: 4904, 1983.
5. Baglioni, C., P.A. Maroney, and D.K. West: 2'5'oligo(A) polymerase activity and inhibition of viral RNA synthesis in interferon-treated HeLa cells. Biochemistry 18:1765, 1979.
6. Baglioni, C.: Interferon induced enzymatic activities and their role in the antiviral state. Cell 17:255, 1979.
7. Minks, M.A., D.K. West, S. Benvin, and C. Baglioni: Structural requirements of double-stranded RNA for the activation of 2'5'-oligo(A) polymerase and protein kinase of interferon- treated HeLa cells. J. Biol. Chem. 254:10180, 1979.
8. Minks, M.A., S. Benvin, P.A. Maroney, and C. Baglioni: Synthesis of 2'-5'-oligo(A) in extracts of interferon-treated HeLa cells. J. Biol. Chem. 254:5058, 1979.
9. Slattery, E., N. Ghosh, H. Samantha, and P. Lengyel: Interferon, double-stranded RNA, and RNA degradation: Activation of an endoribonuclease by $(2'-5')A_n$. Proc. Natl. Acad. Sci. USA 76:4778, 1979.
10. Nilsen, T.W., D.L. Wood., and C. Baglioni: 2',5'-oligo(A) activated endoribonuclease. Tissue distribution and characterization with a binding assay. J. Biol. Chem. 256:10751, 1981.
11. Wreschner, D.H., T.C. James, R.H. Silverman, and I.M. Kerr: Ribosomal RNA cleavage, nuclease activation and 2-5A $(ppp(A2'p)_nA)$ in interferon-treated cells. Nucleic Acids Res. 9:1571, 1981.

12. Floyd-Smith, G., E. Slattery, and P. Lengyel: Interferon action: RNA cleavage pattern of a (2'-5')oligoadenylate-dependent endonuclease. Science 212:1030, 1981.
13. Wreschner, D.H., J.W. McCauley, J.J. Skehel, and I.M. Kerr: Interferon action-sequence specificity of the $ppp(A2'p)_nA$-dependent ribonuclease. Nature 289:414, 1981.
14. Nilsen, T.W., and C. Baglioni: A mechanism for discrimination between viral and host mRNA in interferon-treated cells. Proc. Natl. Acad. Sci. USA 76:2600, 1979.
15. Baglioni, C., A. De Benedetti, and G.J. Williams: Cleavage of nascent reovirus mRNA by localized activation of the (2'-5')oligo(A) dependent endoribonuclease. J. Virol. 52:865, 1984.
16. Minks, M.A., S. Benvin, P.A. Maroney, and C. Baglioni: Metabolic stability of 2'5'oligo(A) and activity of 2'5'oligo(A)-dependent endonuclease in extracts of interferon-treated and control HeLa cells. Nucleic Acids Res. 6:767, 1979.
17. Schmidt, A., Y. Chernajovsky, L. Shulman, P. Federman, H. Berissi, and M. Revel: An interferon-induced phosphodiesterase degrading (2'-5)o-ligoisoadenylate and the C-C-A terminus of tRNA. Proc. Natl. Acad. Sci. USA 76:4788, 1979.
18. Williams, G.J., A. De Benedetti, and C. Baglioni: Inhibition of 2',5'-oligo(A)-dependent endoribonuclease by 2',5'-oligo(A) degradation products. Virology 151:233, 1986.
19. Torrence, P.F., J. Imai, and M.I. Johnston: 5'-O-monophospho-adenylyl(2'-5')adenylyl(2'-5')adenosine is an antagonist of the action of 5'-O-triphosphoryladenylyl-(2'-5')-adenylyl(2'-5')adenylyl(2'-5')adenosine and double-stranded RNA. Proc. Natl. Acad. Sci. USA 78:5993, 1981.
20. Knight, M., P.J. Cayley, R.H. Silverman, D.H. Wreschner, C.S. Gilbert, R.E. Brown, and I.M. Kerr: Radioimmune, radiobinding and HPLC analysis of 2-5A and related oligonucleotides from intact cells. Nature 288:189, 1980.
21. Nilsen, T.W., P.A. Maroney, and C. Baglioni: Double-stranded RNA causes synthesis of 2',5'-oligo(A) and degradation of messenger RNA in interferon-treated cells. J. Biol. Chem. 256:7806, 1981.
22. Williams, B.R.G., R.R. Golgher, R.E. Brown, C.S. Gilbert, and I.M. Kerr: Natural occurrence of 2-5A in interferon-treated EMC virus-infected L cells. Nature 282:582, 1979.
23. Nilsen, T.W., P.A. Maroney, and C. Baglioni: Synthesis of (2'-5')o-ligoadenylate and activation of an endoribonuclease in interferon-treated HeLa cells infected with reovirus. J. Virol. 42:1039, 1982.
24. Goswami, B.B., and O.K. Sharma: Degradation of rRNA in interferon-treated vaccinia virus-infected cells. J. Biol. Chem. 259:1371, 1984.
25. Rice, A.P., W.K. Roberts, and I.M. Kerr: 2-5A accumulates to high levels in interferon-treated, vaccinia virus-infected cells in the absence of any inhibition of virus replication. J. Virol. 50:220, 1984.
26. Paez, E., and M. Esteban: Nature and mode of action of vaccinia virus products that block activation of the interferon-mediated $ppp(A2'p)_nA$-synthetase. Virology 134:29, 1984.
27. Hersh, C.L., R.E. Brown, W.K. Roberts, E.A. Swyryd, I.M. Kerr, and G.R. Stark: Simian virus 40-infected, interferon-treated cells contain 2',5'-oligoadenylates which do not activate cleavage of RNA. J. Biol. Chem. 259:1731, 1984.
28. Cayley, P.J., J.A. Davies, K.G. McCullagh, and I.M. Kerr: Activa-

tion of the ppp(A2`p)$_n$A system in interferon treated, Herpes simplex virus infected cells and evidence for novel inhibitors of the ppp(A2`p)$_n$A-dependent RNase. Eur. J. Biochem. 143:165, 1984.
29. Meurs, E., A.G. Hovanessian, and L. Montagnier: Interferon-mediated antiviral state in human MRC5 cells in the absence of detectable levels of 2-5A synthetase and protein kinase. J. Interf. Res. 1:219, 1981.
30. Baglioni, C., A.A. Branca, S. D'Alessandro, D. Hossenlopp, and K.C. Chada: Low interferon binding activity of two human cell lines which respond poorly to the antiviral and antiproliferative activity of interferon. Virology 122:202, 1982.
31. Czarniecki, C.W., T. Sreevalsan, R.M. Friedman, and A. Panet: Dissociation of interferon effects on murine leukemia virus and encephalomyocarditis virus replication in mouse cells. J. Virol. 37:827, 1981.
32. Epstein, D.A., C.W. Czarniecki, H. Jacobsen, R.M. Friedman, and A. Panet: A mouse cell line, which is unprotected by interferon against lytic virus infection, lacks ribonuclease F activity. Eur. J. Biochem. 118:9, 1981.
33. Nilsen, T.W., S. McCandless, and C. Baglioni: 2'5'-oligo(A)-activated endonuclease in NIH 3T3 cells chronically infected with Moloney murine leukemia virus. Virology 122:498, 1982.
34. Krause, D., A. Panet, G. Arad, C.W. Dieffenbach, and R.H. Silverman: Independent regulation of ppp(A2'p)$_n$A-dependent RNase in NIH 3T3, clone 1 cells by growth arrest and interferon treatment. J. Biol. Chem. 260:9501, 1985.
35. Jacobsen, H., D. Krause, R.M. Friedman, and R.H. Silverman: Induction of ppp(A)$_n$A-dependent RNase in murine JLS-V9R cells during growth inhibition. Proc. Natl. Acad. Sci. USA 80:4954, 1983.
36. Krause, D., R.H. Silverman, H. Jacobsen, S.A. Leisy, C.W. Dieffenbach, and R.M. Friedman: Regulation of ppp(A2'p)$_n$A-dependent RNase levels during interferon treatment and cell differentiation. Eur. J. Bio-chem. 146:611, 1985.
37. Salzberg, S., D.H. Wreschner, F. Oberman, A. Panet, and M. Bakhanashvili: Isolation and characterization of an interferon-resistant cell line deficient in the induction of (2'-5')oligoadenylate synthetase activity. Mol. Cell. Biol. 3:1759, 1983.
38. Sen, G.C., R.E. Herz, and B.Y. Rubin: Antiviral, anticellular and enzyme-inducing activities of interferons in RD-114 cells. J. Gen. Virol. 64:2213, 1983.
39. Nilsen, T.W., D.L. Wood, and C. Baglioni: Virus-specific effects of interferon in embryonal carcinoma cells. Nature 286:178, 1980.
40. Wood, J.N., and A.G. Hovanessian: Interferon enhances 2-5A synthetase in embryonal carcinoma cells. Nature 282:74, 1979.
41. De Benedetti, A., B.A. Pytel, and C. Baglioni: Loss of 2'-5'-oligo-adenylate synthetase by production of antisense RNA results in lack of protection by interferon from viral infections. Proc. Natl. Acad. Sci. USA submitted for publication.
42. Staheli, P., O. Haller, W. Boll, J. Lindenmann, and C. Weissmann: Mx protein: constitutive expression in 3T3 cells transformed with cloned Mx cDNA confers selective resistance to influenza virus. Cell 44:147, 1986.
43. Watling, D., H.T. Serafinowska, C.B. Reese, and I.M. Kerr: Analogue inhibitor of 2-5A action: effect of the interferon-mediated inhibition of encephalomyocarditis virus replication. EMBO J. 4:431, 1985.

38. The Interferon-Induced Protein P1/eIF-2α Kinase

Charles E. Samuel

Section of Biochemistry and Molecular Biology, Department of Biological Sciences, University of California, Santa Barbara, Santa Barbara, CA 93106

INTRODUCTION

Protein phosphorylation-dephosphorylation is an important mechanism by which the functional activity of proteins can be controlled and, hence, biologic processes regulated. Interferons are a family of regulatory proteins that can profoundly affect a number of biologic functions in animal cells including virus replication. Several studies indicate that protein phosphorylation-dephosphorylation may play an important role in the mechanism by which interferons inhibit the replication of certain types of viruses in certain host cells. In this chapter of The Interferon System, we shall emphasize the literature that has appeared since the previous edition (1) concerning the biochemical and biophysical characterization of the interferon-induced double-stranded RNA-dependent P1/eIF-2α protein kinase, and the possible role that the kinase may play in the antiviral action of interferon.

Protein Phosphorylation in Cell-free Extracts Prepared from Untreated and Interferon-treated Murine and Human Cells

The phosphorylation state of two proteins, P1 and α, is acutely sensitive to interferon (IFN) in many types of animal cells (2-5). Protein P1 is a ribosome-associated protein (4,6); α is the smallest subunit of protein synthesis initiation factor eIF-2 (7). The measurement of protein P_1 and eIF-2α phosphorylation *in vitro* typically involves the analysis by $NaDodSO_4$-polyacrylamide gel electrophoresis of the ^{32}P-labeled products of $[\gamma\text{-}^{32}P]$ATP-mediated protein phosphorylation reactions catalyzed by cell-free extracts or partially purified enzyme preparations (8). As measured by this assay, the phosphorylation of P1 and α is routinely elevated about 5 to 10-fold in cell-free extracts prepared from IFN-treated as compared to untreated cells (1-9). A low but frequently detectable basal level of P1 and eIF-2α phosphorylation is observed with cell-free extracts prepared from untreated cells (1-9). In vitro phosphorylation reactions carried out with [γ-^{32}P]ATP reveal relative changes in the extent of phosphorylation of the substrate P1 and α polypeptides, but they do not reveal what fraction of the total available substrate becomes phosphorylated with ^{32}P as compared to the fraction that remains unphosphorylated. With unlabeled ATP as the phosphate donor, the total extent of phosphorylation in vitro of endogenous substrate polypeptide can be assessed by two-dimensional electrophoresis and immunoblotting with antibodies that recognize both the phosphorylated and dephosphorylated forms of the substrate (10). Using this assay, very little of the α subunit of eIF-2 is phosphorylated in the absence of activated, IFN-induced kinase; by contrast, more than 75% of the total pool of eIF-2α is phosphorylated in vitro when the IFN-induced kinase is activated (10).

The increase in phosphorylation of P1 and eIF-2α observed in cell-free extracts prepared from IFN-treated cells as compared to untreated cells is dependent upon the presence of double-stranded RNA (4,7,11). The enhanced phosphorylation in the presence of double-stranded RNA (dsRNA) appears to be due to the activation of an IFN-induced P1/eIF-2α protein kinase rather than to the inhibition of a phosphoprotein phosphatase. The IFN-induced dsRNA-dependent P1/eIF-2α protein kinase is ribosome-associated (4,9); the yield of P1/eIF-2α protein kinase activity obtained following purification from cells treated with IFN is about 5 to 10 times greater than the yield from an equivalent number of untreated cells (9); and, the increase in dsRNA-dependent protein kinase activity in IFN-treated as compared to untreated cells is blocked by actinomycin D (12). By contrast, the phosphoprotein phosphatase which catalyzes the dephosphorylation of eIF-2α(P) is soluble, is dsRNA-independent, and is present at comparable levels in extracts prepared from untreated as compared to IFN-treated cells (57). The dsRNA requirement for phosphorylation of P1 and eIF-2α in vitro by cell-free extracts is eliminated by prior infection of cells with reovirus virions, but not by infection with defective reovirus top component particles prior to extract preparation (10). The enhanced phosphorylation in vitro of P1 and the α subunit of eIF-2 depends in a similar manner upon the multiplicity of infection when catalyzed by extracts prepared from infected cells (10) or, when catalyzed by extracts prepared from uninfected cells, upon the concentration of exogenously added dsRNA (13).

Both natural and recombinant type I and type II IFNs induce the kinase in murine cells (14,15). However, in human cells, only type I IFNs efficiently induce the kinase (16). For example, natural type I Ms IFN-(L_{929}/NDV) efficiently induces the P1/eIF-2α protein kinase in a manner that correlates with the IFN concentration dependence for the appearance of an antiviral state. Recombinant type I Hu IFN-αA/D (E. coli), type II Ms IFN-γ (E. coli) and type II

Ms IFN-γ (COS) all induce an antiviral state as measured by reduction in VSV plaque formation; for each of these IFNs, the IFN concentration dependence for induction of an antiviral state correlates with that for induction of the protein kinase as measured in cell-free extracts (15). The detailed kinetics of induction (14) and of decay (17) of the protein P1/eIF-2α kinase activity correlate with the kinetics of induction and decay of the antiviral viral state in cells treated with a saturating concentration of either natural or recombinant IFN. In human epithelial cells, only type I IFNs such as Sendai virus-induced natural IFN-α or recombinant IFN-αA efficiently induce the P1/eIF-2α protein kinase (15,16,18). Type II recombinant IFN-γ is a very poor inducer of the P1/α kinase in human epithelial cells (16). Furthermore, neither type I IFN-α or type II IFN-γ detectably induce the P1/eIF-2α protein kinase in human fibroblast cells (15,16,19,20).

The protein P1 and eIF-2α kinase activity measured with cell-free extracts prepared from IFN-treated cells, like the induction of an antiviral state measured with whole cells, is cyclic AMP-independent (21,22). S49 (21) and J774.2 (22) murine cell genetic variants deficient in the synthesis or the action of cyclic AMP develop an antiviral state in response to IFN treatment (21,22). In addition, the phosphorylation of protein P1 is enhanced to a similar level in cell-free extracts prepared from IFN-treated wild-type, IFN-treated adenylate cyclase-deficient and IFN-treated cAMP-dependent protein kinase-deficient S49 cells (21).

Protein Phosphorylation in Untreated and Interferon-treated Whole Cells

The extent of phosphorylation *in vivo* of eIF-2 within untreated and IFN-treated whole cells has been examined by utilizing two-dimensional isoelectric focusing/$NaDodSO_4$ polyacrylamide gel electrophoresis and immunoblotting techniques (10,23). About 5 to 10 percent of the α subunit of eIF-2 is phosphorylated *in vivo* in untreated cells, whereas 25 to 30 percent is phosphorylated within IFN-treated mouse cells upon infection with reovirus (10). The phosphorylation of eIF-2α is also elevated within IFN-treated as compared to untreated HeLa cells upon infection with reovirus (24) or encephalomyocarditis virus (23). Maximal phosphorylation *in vivo* of eIF-2α is dependent upon IFN treatment to induce the kinase, and virus infection to activate the kinase (10,23,24). *In vivo* within infected cells, the activation of the P1/eIF-2α protein kinase may be fulfilled by either virus infection or by dsRNA treatment of IFN-treated cells in culture (10,12,23,24).

Properties of the Purified Double-stranded RNA-dependent Protein Kinase

The double-stranded RNA-dependent protein kinase which catalyzes the phosphorylation of ribosome-associated protein P1 and the α subunit of protein synthesis initiation factor eIF-2 has been purified and characterized from murine cells treated with either natural or recombinant IFN (9,13,26-29), and from untreated cells

(9). Several lines of evidence support the conclusion that IFN treatment induces the synthesis of protein P1 which itself possesses the dsRNA-dependent protein P1/eIF-2α kinase activity. First, the dsRNA-dependent phosphorylation of protein P1 is greatly increased in IFN-treated as compared to untreated cells, and the increase in dsRNA-dependent protein kinase activity is blocked by actinomycin D (9,10,12,13). Furthermore, the phosphorylation of murine protein P1 in the presence of S10 extract prepared from IFN-treated human cells is observed when the combination of human and mouse extracts includes S10 prepared from IFN-treated mouse cells, but is not observed when the combination includes S10 from untreated mouse cells (9). Second, purification studies have failed to separate the dsRNA-dependent P1/eIF-2α protein kinase activity from protein P1 (9,13,26,28,29). However, two reports (25,27) suggest that protein P1 may also be the substrate for a second protein kinase and, upon activation by phosphorylation, P1 itself becomes an active kinase that catalyzes the phosphorylation of eIF-2α. Third, the yield of P1/eIF-2α protein kinase activity obtained following purification from cells treated with IFN is about 5 to 10-times greater than the yield from an equivalent number of untreated cells (9). Fourth, the amount of P1 is also increased by IFN treatment of human U (30) and Daudi (31) cells as measured by Western immunoblot analysis. Fifth, the apparent molecular weight of 62,000 observed for native dsRNA-dependent protein kinase by sedimentation analysis (9) is comparable to the molecular weight of 67,000 observed for denatured phosphorylated protein P1 by $NaDodSO_4$ polyacrylamide gel electrophoresis (6). Sixth, protein P1 contains a nucleotide binding site as established by the direct photoaffinity labeling of P1 by ATP. Furthermore, the photoaffinity labeling of protein P1 is dsRNA-dependent (32). Seventh, the phosphorylation of protein P1 present within purified preparations of kinase is independent of reaction volume, which suggests that protein P1 phosphorylation may be an intramolecular autophosphorylation (9).

The purified dsRNA-dependent protein kinase is highly selective for the α subunit of protein synthesis initiation factor eIF-2 and endogenous protein P1 (9). O-Phosphoserine is the major phosphoester linkage in both protein P1 and eIF-2α; no phosphotyrosine is detectable in P1 (7,13,33). P1/eIF-2α kinase activity is dependent upon Mg++, and the K_m for ATP is 5×10^{-6} M (9). Protein synthesis factors other than the α subunit of eIF-2, for example EF-1, EF-2, eIF-3, eIF-4A, eIF-4B and eIF-5, are not substrates (7,9). Likewise, calf thymus and Drosophila histones H1, calf and rabbit thymus histones H2A, H2B, H3 and H4, casein, phosvitin, and α and β tubulin are not detectable substrates or are very poor substrates for the purified P1/eIF-2α kinase (9,50). The purified P1/eIF-2α protein kinase remains dependent upon dsRNA for activation (9). Two forms of P1 have been identified which differ from each other by their phosphorylation patterns; a major P1 phosphopeptide designated X_{ds} is phosphorylated in the presence of dsRNA but not in the absence of dsRNA (13,33). Adenovirus VAI RNA prevents the activation of the P1/eIF-2α protein kinase by dsRNA, both in crude cell-free extracts (34,35) and also when tested with purified P1 kinase and purified VAI RNA (36). Although adenovirus VAI RNA possesses significant secondary structure, neither it nor tRNA can substitute for dsRNA as an activator of the kinase (34).

Monoclonal (31,51,52) and polyclonal (51) antibodies to the IFN-induced phosphoprotein P1 have been prepared. Rabbit antiserum to human protein P1 recognizes with comparable efficiency both human and mouse P1 (51). Mouse monoclonal antibodies to human P1 efficiently recognize human P1, but with one exception (51) either do not recognize or recognize very poorly P1 from mouse cells (51,52). Immunoprecipitates that contain protein P1 also possess a protein kinase activity that catalyzes the phosphorylation of protein P1 and the α subunit of eIF-2 (31,51).

Possible Relationship between the Interferon-induced Protein P1/eIF-2α Protein Kinase and the Interferon-induced Antiviral State

A wide range of different RNA and DNA viruses are sensitive to the antiviral actions of type I (α, β) and type II (γ) interferons (37,38). Among these, the replication of vesicular stomatitis virus (VSV) is acutely sensitive to IFN in almost every kind of animal cell which responds to this class of regulatory proteins (37). By contrast, adenovirus is comparatively resistent to the antiviral actions of interferon in permissive human cells (34,37). Results of cellular and molecular analyses of the actions of highly purified recombinant human IFN-αA and IFN-γ suggest that these human IFNs differentially regulate the expression of certain cellular genes and induce mechanistically distinct antiviral states in human cells (16,39-43). Furthermore, in the case of type I IFN, the available evidence is consistent with a fundamental role of the P1/eIF-2α protein kinase both in the sensitivity of VSV (16,39-41,44) and in the resistence of adenovirus (34,35) to the antiviral actions of IFN.

The major, and possibly only, effect of recombinant IFN-α on the multiplication of vesicular stomatitis virus in the human amnion U epithelial cell line is translation inhibition (39-41). Primary viral mRNA synthesis catalyzed by parental virions is neither quantitatively nor qualitatively affected by IFN-α treatment when measured by dot-blot or gel-blot techniques with hybridization probes to the N, NS, M and G mRNAs. By contrast, primary viral protein synthesis is significantly inhibited by IFN-αA treatment (39-41). Neither the structural integrity of VSV mRNA as measured by Northern blots or the functional integrity of VSV mRNA as measured by _in vitro_ translation catalyzed by cell-free protein synthesizing systems prepared from untreated cells is significantly affected by IFN-αA (40,41). IFN-γ, in contrast to IFN-αA, does not significantly affect the synthesis of either VSV or reovirus polypeptides in human U cells (43,45). The inhibition of VSV replication in human U cells induced by IFN-αA correlates with the induction of the P1/eIF-2α protein kinase; IFN-γ does not detectably induce the protein kinase in human U cells (16). The antiviral activities of IFN-α and IFN-γ are synergistic for the inhibition of VSV but not for the induction of the P1/eIF-2α protein kinase (16).

Vaccinia virus infection of mouse L fibroblasts impairs the activity of the P1/eIF-2α protein kinase and rescues VSV, at the level of protein synthesis, from the antiviral action of IFN in doubly infected cells in culture (44). Vaccinia infection does not signficantly affect VSV RNA synthesis (44). The above results obtained with whole cells in culture (16,41-44) suggest that the IFN-induced P1/eIF-2α protein kinase may play an important role in the antiviral action of IFN against VSV. Similar conclusions have been reached with cell-free protein synthesizing systems prepared from IFN-treated cells (46,47). The pppA(2'p5'A)$_n$-dependent ribonuclease may not be required, and phosphorylation of P1 and eIF-2α by the p1/eIF-2α protein kinase may indeed be sufficient for the dsRNA-dependent inhibition of viral mRNA translation in cell-free systems derived from IFN-treated cells.

Maximal functional expression of the P1/eIF-2α protein kinase in vivo within infected cells as measured by α phosphorylation is dependent upon activation of the IFN-induced protein P1/eIF-2α (10). Activation of the P1/eIF-2α kinase within intact IFN-treated cells may be accomplished by either virus infection of the cells as has been demonstrated with reovirus (10,24) and EMC virus (23) or by treatment of IFN-treated cells in culture with dsRNA (12). However, the nature of the moiety which, in vivo, fulfills the requirement for activation of the P1/eIF-2α phosphorylation is not known. Presumably in most natural situations of viral infection the activating moiety is a structure more subtle than free dsRNA per se. For example, in the case of reovirus, the dsRNA genome of parental reovirions is only partially uncoated during the replication cycle (48) and progeny genome dsRNA synthesis occurs associated with replicase particles rather than "free" in reovirus-infected cells (49).

Certain viruses such as human adenoviruses are relatively resistent to the antiviral action of type I IFNs (37). In the case of adenovirus, a virus-encoded gene product known as VAI RNA antagonizes the antiviral action of IFN-α by preventing the activation of the IFN-induced P1/eIF-2α protein kinase (34). The adenovirus VA RNAs are small viral RNAs which are synthesized in large amounts at late times after infection. Deletion mutants of adenovirus which do not synthesize the major species of VA RNA, VAI RNA, possess a defect in late viral mRNA translation; this defect has been localized to an early step in the initiation of adenovirus late mRNA translation (54,55). The characteristics of the inhibition of adenovirus translation in VAI RNA deletion mutant-infected human 293 cells (54,55) display some similarity with the characteristics of the inhibition of VSV mRNA translation in IFN-treated human U cells (39-41). In human epithelial 293 cells possessing inducible P1/eIF-2α protein kinase, the adenovirus mutant lacking VAI RNA multiplies poorly relative to the parental virus which synthesizes VAI RNA. By contrast, the VAI-mutant multiplies nearly as well as wild-type virus in human fibroblast cells which do not contain detectable dsRNA-dependent, IFN-inducible P1/eIF-2α protein kinase (56). The P1/eIF-2α protein kinase is activated and the function of eIF-2 is impaired in extracts prepared from VAI deletion mutant-infected cells (53,56). By contrast, the P1/eIF-2α kinase is not activated and eIF-2 function is not impaired in cells infected with wild-type adenovirus which synthesizes large amounts of VA RNA (56). Mixing experiments have revealed that the purified VAI RNA inhibits the activation by dsRNA of purified dsRNA-dependent P1/eIF-2α protein kinase (36). The growth of the adenovirus deletion mutant which is unable to produce VAI RNA is inhibited by IFN, while the growth of wild-type adenovirus which produces large amounts of VAI RNA is not affected by IFN (34). Thus, the available evidence is consistent with the possibility that the insensitivity of adenovirus to IFN may be due to the ability of the adenovirus VAI RNA to inhibit the activation of the IFN-induced P1/eIF-2α protein kinase.

ACKNOWLEDGMENTS

The work described in this chapter was supported in part by Research Grants from the National Institutes of Health and the American Cancer Society.

REFERENCES

1. Samuel, C. E. Texas Reports Biol. Med. 41:463-470, 1982.
2. Lebleu, B., G. C. Sen, S. Shaila, B. Cabrer, and P.Lengyel. Proc. Natl. Acad. Sci. USA 73:3107-3111, 1976.
3. Roberts, W. K., A. G. Hovanessian, R. E. Brown, M. J. Clemens, and I. M. Kerr. Nature (London) 264:477-480, 1976.
4. Samuel, C. E., D. A. Farris, and D. A. Eppstein. Virology 83:56 -71, 1977.
5. Zilberstein, A., P. Federman, L. Shulman, and M. Revel. FEBS Lett. 68:119-124, 1976.
6. Samuel, C. E. Virology 93:281-285, 1979.
7. Samuel, C. E. Proc. Natl. Acad. Sci. USA 76:600-604, 1979.
8. Samuel, C. E. Meth. Enzymol. 79:168-178, 1981.
9. Berry, M. J., G. S. Knutson, S. R. Lasky, S. M. Munemitsu, and C. E. Samuel. J. Biol. Chem. 260:11240-11247, 1985.
10. Samuel, C. E., R. Duncan, G. S. Knutson, and J. W. B. Hershey. J. Biol. Chem. 259:13451-13457, 1984.
11. Minks, M. A., D. K. West, S. Benvin, and C. Baglioni. J. Biol. Chem. 254:10180-10183, 1979.
12. Gupta, S. L. J. Virol. 29:301-311, 1979.
13. Lasky, S. R., B. L. Jacobs, and C. E. Samuel. J. Biol. Chem. 257:11087-11093, 1982.
14. Samuel, C. E., and G. S. Knutson. J. Biol. Chem. 257:11789-11795, 1982.
15. Samuel, C. E. In The Biology of the Interferon System, 1985. Elsevier Sci. Publ., in press, 1986.
16. Samuel, C. E., and G. S. Knutson. Virology 130:474-484, 1983.
17. Samuel, C. E., and G. S. Knutson. J. Biol. Chem. 257:11796-11801, 1982.
18. Samuel, C. E., and G. S. Knutson. Virology 114:302-306, 1981.
19. Samuel, C. E., G. S. Knutson, and P. S. Masters. J. Interferon Res. 2:563-574.
20. Holmes, S. L., and S. L. Gupta. Arch. Virol. 72:137-142, 1982.
21. Atwater, J. A., and C. E. Samuel. Virology 123:206-211, 1982.

22. Schneck, J., B. Rager-Zisman, O. M. Rosen, and B. R. Bloom. Proc. Natl. Acad. Sci. USA 79:1879-1883, 1982.
23. Rice, A. P., R. Duncan, J. W. B. Hershey, and I. M. Kerr. J. Virol. 54:894-898, 1985.
24. Nilsen, T. W., P. A. Maroney, and C. Baglioni. J. Biol. Chem. 257:14593-14596, 1982.
25. Ohtsuki, K., M. Nakamura, T. Koike, N. Ishida, and S. Baron. Nature 287:65-67, 1980.
26. Hovanessian, A. G, and I. M. Kerr. Eur. J. Biochem. 93:515-526, 1979.
27. Galabru, J., and A. G. Hovanessian. Cell 43:685-694, 1985.
28. Kimchi, A., A. Zilberstein, A. Schmidt, L. Shulman, and M. Revel. J. Biol. Chem. 254:9846-9853, 1979.
29. Sen, G. C., H. Taira, and P. Lengyel. J. Biol. Chem. 253:5915-5921, 1978.
30. Berry, M. J., G. K. Knutson, and C. E. Samuel. Unpublished observations, 1985.
31. Laurent, A. G., B. Krust, J. Galabru, J. Svab, and A. G. Hovanessian. Proc. Natl. Acad. Sci. USA 82:4341-4345, 1985.
32. Bischoff, J. R., and C. E. Samuel. J. Biol. Chem. 260:8237-8239, 1985.
33. Krust, B., L. Galabru, and A. G. Hovanessian. J. Biol. Chem. 259:8494-8498, 1984.
34. Kitajewski, J., R. J. Schneider, B. Safer, S. M. Munemitsu, C. E. Samuel, B. Thimmappaya, and T. Shenk. Cell 45:195-200, 1986.
35. O'Malley, R. P., T. M. Mariano, J. Siekierka, and M. B. Mathews. Cell 44:391-400, 1986.
36. Munemitsu, S. M., M. J. Berry, J. Kitajewski, T. Shenk, and C. E. Samuel. UCLA Symp. Interferons as Cell Growth Inhibitors and Antitumor Factors. A. R. Liss, Inc., in press, 1986.
37. Stewart, W. E. The Interferon System. Springer-Verlag, 1979.
38. Pfeffer, L. M. Mechanisms of Interferons Actions. Chemical Rubber Co. Press, Cleveland, in press, 1986.
39. Masters, P. S., and C. E. Samuel. J. Biol. Chem. 258:12019-12025, 1983.
40. Masters, P. S., and C. E. Samuel. J. Biol. Chem. 258:12026-12033, 1983.
41. Masters, P. S., and C. E. Samuel. Biochem. Biophys. Res. Commun. 119:326-334, 1984.
42. Ulker, N., and C. E. Samuel. J. Biol. Chem. 260:4319-4323, 1985.
43. Ulker, N., and C. E. Samuel. J. Biol. Chem. 260:4324-4330, 1985.
44. Whitaker-Dowling, P., and J. S. Youngner. Virology 131:128-136, 1983.
45. Samuel, C. E., N. Ulker, G. S. Knutson, X. Zhang and P. S. Masters. In The Biology of the Interferon System, 1984. Elsevier Sci. Publ., pp. 131-140, 1985.
46. Miyamoto, N. G., and C. E. Samuel. Virology 107:461-475, 1980.
47. Miyamoto, N. G., B. L. Jacobs, and C. E. Samuel. J. Biol. Chem. 258:15232-15237, 1983.

48. Silverstein, S. C., and S. Dales. J. Cell Biol 36:197-230, 1968.
49. Morgan, E. M., and H. J. Zweerink. Virology 68:455-466, 1975.
50. Samuel, C. E., G. S. Knutson, M. J. Berry, J. A. Atwater, and S. R. Lasky. Meth. Enzymol. 119:499-516, 1986.
51. Berry, M. J., and C. E. Samuel. Biochem. Biophys. Res. Commun. 133:168-175, 1985.
52. Penn, L. J. Z., and B. R. G. Williams. Proc. Natl. Acad. Sci. USA 82:4959-4963, 1985.
53. Siekierka, J., T. M. Mariano, P. A. Reichel, and M. B. Mathews. Proc. Natl. Acad. Sci. USA 82:1959-1963, 1985.
54. Thimmappaya, B., C. Weinberger, R. J. Schneider, and T. Shenk. Cell 31:543-551, 1982.
55. Schneider, R. J., C. Weinberger, and T. Shenk. Cell 37:291-298, 1984.
56. Schneider, R. J., B. Safer, S. M. Munemitsu, C. E. Samuel, and T. Shenk. Proc. Natl. Acad. Sci. USA 82:4321-4325, 1985.
57. Samuel, C. E., and G. S. Knutson. J. Interferon Res. 2:441-445, 1982.

39. 2′-Phosphodiesterase Degrading IFN-Induced (2′-5′) Oligo A: Possible Role in IFN Action and Cell Growth Control

M. Revel

Department of Virology, Weizmann Institute of Science, Rehovot, Israel

INTRODUCTION

Control of (2'-5') oligo-adenylate nucleotide metabolism is one of the biochemical pathway characteristic of interferons (IFN) action (1-3). This control operates mainly on the synthesis of these nucleotides by the (2'-5') oligo A synthetase (OASE) system. Cloning of OASE cDNA has shown that IFN activates cellular OASE gene expression (4,5) at the transcriptional level (Williams, B.R.G., private commun.), and has revealed the aminoacid sequences of two forms of the enzyme of 40 and 46 Kda (6). Unexpectedly, the OASE turns out to be a multienzyme system comprising four proteins of 40, 46, 67 and 100 Kda (7), which are differentially expressed in various human cells, are found in different intracellular compartments (cytosol, ribosomes, nuclei and cell membranes) and have different requirements for activation by double-stranded (ds) RNA (7). In addition to induction of these various OASEs, the metabolism and action of (2'-5') oligo A is further controlled by the amount of the (2'-5') A-activated latent ribonuclease (1-3,8) and the stability of the (2'-5') A oligonucleotides (9). This review focuses on the specific 2'-phosphodiesterase which degrades (2'-5') oligo A.

PROPERTIES OF THE 2'-PHOSPHODIESTERASE

An enzyme which degrades ppp(A2'p)$_n$A oligonucleotides into 5'-AMP and one ATP, was first purified from mouse L cells and reticulocytes (10,11). The name 2'-phosphodiesterase (2'-PD) given to this enzyme, indicates that it cleaves the 2'-bond of (2'-5') oligo A and has a higher activity on most (2'-5') dinucleotides than on their (3'-5') isomers (11). The enzyme can, however, cleave also 3'-bonds and was found to remove the -CpCpA 3'-terminus of transfer RNA, without causing further degradation to these tRNAs (11). The enzyme has no endonucleolytic activity and requires a free 2' or 3' hydroxyl group; it neither degrades 2',3'-phosphorylated oligonucleotides nor oligodeoxynucleotides (11). This property has been used to produce (2'-5') oligo A analogs with increased stability in cell extracts by substituting the 2',3'-OH with a variety of blocking groups (12) or simply oxydizing with periodate and cleaving the terminal ribose with borohydrate (13).

Purified 2'-PD from mouse reticulocytes appears as a 35-40,000 dalton protein (11). Poorly purified preparations can be contaminated by an endonuclease and by the (2'-5') oligo A-activated nuclease (10,11). Assay of the 2'-PD is best carried out using synthetic A2'p5'A dinucleotides (11,14) and it should be verified that 5'-phosphorylated cleavage products are formed. One unit of 2'-PD is defined as the hydrolysis of 1 nanomol A2'p5'A per hour at 37°C. One should not rely on the decreased activity of ppp(A2'p)$_n$A to inhibit protein synthesis or bind to the RNase (15), as a measure of 2'-PD activity because other enzymes (such as phosphatases removing the 5'-phosphates) also destroy the biological activity of (2'-5') oligo A (13,16). Recent work suggests (9) that the loss of the 5'-phosphates of ppp(A2'p)$_n$A may occur in cells and lead to the inhibition of the latent RNase (16), thereby contributing to localize the RNase activation to some cell compartments.

2'-PD activity was found in mouse L cells (11,17) and HeLa cells (18), in lymphocytes (19) and in various organs (20). It is even found in human serum, where its activity is inhibited by EDTA (20,21).

VARIATIONS IN 2'-PHOSPHODIESTERASE ACTIVITY IN CELLS

A) Interferon-treated cells

The levels of 2'-PD can vary markedly between cell types. Goren et al. (22) found that human diploid fibroblasts strain FS11 had no detectable 2'-PD activity. On the other hand, Burkitt lymphoma Daudi cells had 120 units of 2'-PD activity per mg protein in their 10,000 xg crude extracts prepared with Nonidet P-40. Treatment of these Daudi cells with 5-10,000 U/ml of pure rIFN-α_2 for 24 hours, resulted in a 100% increase in 2'-PD activity (22). In the same experiments, the (2'-5') oligo A synthetase rose 4-5 fold. However, at 2,000 U/ml IFN there was no increase in 2'-PD, while 20 U/ml IFN was sufficient to induce the synthetase. The increase in 2'-PD, therefore, requires higher IFN concentrations than those needed for antiviral and antigrowth effects in these cells (22).

Mouse L cells have also a relatively high constitutive level of 2'-PD and a 2-4 fold increase in 2'-PD activity was observed after 8 hours exposure of these cells to a few hundred units of mouse IFN (11,23). However, such increases in 2'-PD were not observed in a number of other human cell lines (24,25). This situation is similar to what is seen for the (2'-5') oligo A-activated RNase, which is not increased by IFN in a variety of cells (2,3) but does rise after IFN treatment in certain cell lines (8).

In cells in which the 2'-PD is elevated after IFN, this enzyme may contribute to the inhibition of protein synthesis, in addition to the activation of the (2'-5') A-dependent RNase and of the protein kinase (3). Addition of purified 2'-PD to cell-free extracts, inhibits mRNA translation in vitro (11). The inhibition was reversed by adding excess amounts of tRNA, and 2'-PD appears to act by degrading the -CCA terminus of tRNAs in the extracts. This could explain the deficiency in some of the minor tRNA species needed to translate specific leucine codons, which was observed in cell-free extracts of IFN-treated cells (26,27). Such tRNA deficiency was clearly seen with mouse L cells treated by high concentrations of IFN, but may not be apparent in all cells. When it occurs, the tRNA deficiency would inhibit polypeptide chain elongation, adding a further block to the initiation defect caused by the eIF-2 protein kinase and to the ribosome damage caused by the RNase (3). By itself, the 2'-PD would probably not be sufficient to cause a strong inhibition of protein synthesis in the cells.

It may appear paradoxical that the 2'-PD should rise at all in IFN-treated cells, as it would counteract the (2'-5') oligo A synthetase action. However, the 2'-PD may protect cells against overaccumulation of (2'-5') oligo A and excessive activation of the RNase; with the phosphatases, it may also contribute to the localized action of the RNase, suggested to be the basis for its selective action on viral mRNA translation (9,28,29). Indeed, the 2'-PD can be found associated with the RNase, and prevent its activation by (2'-5') oligo A (10).

B) Cell Growth-Related Variations in 2'-Phosphodiesterase

An increase in 2'-PD was observed in Concanavalin A-stimulated lymphocytes as compared to lymphocytes maintained without mitogen (19,29). This 4-6 fold increase measured by the degradation of synthetic (2'-5') ApA in crude extracts or partially purified fractions, was sufficient to inhibit the (2'-5') oligo A synthetase activity in these stimulated lymphocyte extracts (30). This result prompted us to examine other cells in growth and quiescence. Growing cultures of uninfected African Green Monkey kidney cells BSC-1, showed relatively high levels of 2'-PD (40 units/mg protein). When the cells were maintained 10 days in confluence, the 2'-PD decreased 3-fold whereas the synthetase increased 2-fold (19). When non-confluent BSC-1 cultures were starved 3 days for serum, there was a 4-fold decrease in 2'-PD activity with a 2.5 fold increase in synthetase. Furthermore, addition of 10% fetal calf serum to these starved cultures, restored the high 2'-PD levels seen in growing cultures (19). Thus, the ratio of OASE to 2'-PD varied by a factor of 10 according to the growth status of the BSC-1 cells, being high during growth-arrest and low during exponential proliferation.

In a more recent study, Severin and coll. (31) showed that upon serum starvation of NIH 3T3 cells, the 2'-PD level decreased by 80% within 5 days (Fig. 1). The OASE level started to increase after 5 days of serum-starvation and concomitantly the 2'-PD level rose again. These changes are profound but slower than the drop in thymidine incorporation, or the increase in cAMP-dependent protein kinase which occurs in these cells (Fig. 1). The same group proposed that 2'-PD activity may be inhibited by cAMP-dependent phosphorylation of a 18 Kda inhibitor of 2'-PD (32).

Studies in synchronized mouse embryo fibroblasts suggest that both (2'-5') oligo A synthetase and 2'-PD are cell-cycle regulated enzymes (33). In these experiments, tertiary cultures of fresh embryo cells were seeded so as to undergo a synchronous cell division without using blocking drugs and with minimal changes in serum concentrations. The synthetase, which was low in G_1 and beginning of S-phase, rose sharply just before DNA synthesis began to decline at the end of the S-phase (Fig. 2). This OASE induction is very strong and similar to that seen when exogenous IFN is added to G_1 cells. OASE level dropped again when the cells entered G_2. In contrast, the 2'-DP activity was higher in G_1 cells, decreased before the S-phase and increased again when the cells had gone through M and entered a second G_1 phase (Fig. 2). A plot of the OASE over 2'-PD ratio (Fig. 2 lower panel) shows that this ratio is lowest in the first G_1, then increases and drops back to the lowest level at the start of the second G_1 after 48 hours. In this system, OASE induction at the end of the S-phase is regulated at the mRNA level (34), but there is no information on how the 2'-PD levels are regulated.

A MODEL FOR THE VARIATIONS IN (2'-5') OLIGO SYNTHESIS AND DEGRADATION DURING CELL GROWTH

The variations in the synthetase and 2'-PD in cells undergoing growth-transitions can be fitted in a model which would predict correlations between the levels of(2'-5') oligo A and the growth state of the cell. This model differentiates between normal cell cycling on the one hand, and G_0-growth arrest on the other (Fig. 3). This distinction is justified since IFN addition to exponentially growing cells usually only slows down growth causing elongation of all parts of the cell-cycle, while in G_0-arrested cells which are stimulated to reenter the growth cycle by serum or growth-factors, IFN can fully block mitogenesis (35,36). According to the model, normal cycling would be accompanied by an increase in the synthesis of (2'-5') oligo A when the cells move from G_1 toward S, first because of a decrease in 2'-PD in late G_1 and then because of the rise in OASE at the end of the S-phase, possibly corresponding to the arrest of DNA synthesis. OASE drops again in G_2-M, but we propose that it is the increase in 2'-PD degradative activity occurring when cells reenter G_1 (Fig. 2), which correlates with continued cycling of the cells in the presence of growth factors. In contrast, in the absence of serum or growth factors, there is instead a marked drop in 2'-PD, which could lead to accumulation of (2'-5') oligo A despite the low OASE levels. When cells have been serum-starved for several days, OASE increases while 2'-PD is low, leading to accumulation of (2'-5') oligo A nucleotides. Readdition of growth-factors to G_0-arrested cells, increases the 2'-PD (19) reducing (2'-5') oligo A in correlation with the return of the cells to G_1 and with the resumption of growth.

The model in Fig. 3, takes into account the variations in the enzymes of the (2'-5') A metabolism, which have been experimentally observed during the growth-transitions studies reviewed above. The presumed changes in the level of (2'-5') A nucleotides have unfortunately not been measured in these systems, mainly because of the low levels of these nucleotides present in uninfected cells and the problems of ascertaining that one detects ppp(A2'p)$_n$A and not other nucleotides (37). It is clear that besides the OASE and 2'-PD levels, phosphatases (9,13) and other factors such as ATP (38) or ds RNA, can influence (2'-5') A levels. Indeed, (2'-5') A nucleotides are more readily detected in virus-infected cells, presumably because of OASE activation by viral ds RNA (39). However, (2'-5') A is likely to be made in uninfected cells, since RNA from uninfected cells is capable of activating the (2'-5') oligo A synthetase in vitro (29) and furthermore, some OASE subforms do not require high ds RNA (7).

Undoubtedly, the model is very schematic and does not imply that these enzyme variations are the cause of the growth transitions; the model, nevertheless, provides a logical basis for a number of experimental observations on the (2'-5') A system in growth. Changes in the level of (2'-5') oligo A nucleotides were observed in rat liver stimulated to grow by partial hepatectomy (40). The concentration of these nucleotides, measured by radio binding to the RNase and by HPLC, decreased in parallel to the decrease in OASE, reaching a minimum 20 hours after partial hepatectomy when DNA synthesis was high. This was followed by an increase in OASE and nucleotide levels at 36 hours when DNA synthesis declined. Since adult liver cells do not divide, the decrease in (2'-5') A could correspond to the exit of cells from G_o and entry in G_1, as predicted by the model. The reincrease at 36 hours could correspond to the end of the first S-phase of the proliferative liver regeneration. In other studies, elevated levels of (2'-5') A cores were seen during the S-phase (33,41). Experiments in which (2'-5') oligo A was exogenously introduced into cells support the notion that variations in these nucleotides may affect cell mitogenesis. Introduced by $CaPO_4$ precipitation, ppp(A2'p)$_n$A inhibit protein and DNA synthesis (42). The use of cores which can penetrate unpermeabilized cells, has shown antimitogenic effects of A2'pA2'pA in stimulated-lymphocytes (30) and fibroblasts (36) mimicking the effects of IFN itself on the entry of cells into S-phase. The effect of the cores seems genuine to the (2'-5') isomers with a free 5'OH (36) and, despite the higher concentration needed (micromolar instead of nanomolar for ppp(A2'p)$_n$A in vitro), cannot be explained by degradation into AMP (36,43). NIH clone 1 cells, lacking the (2'-5') A-dependent RNase (8), were resistant to the antimitogenic action of the cores (36). Nevertheless, rephosphorylation of the cores was not shown and their action may rather be competition against 2'-PD activity (11). Although activation of the RNase is the only known function of (2'-5') oligo A, it is not excluded that other mechanisms are at play. The recent finding that ppp(A2'p)$_n$A could be introduced in intact cells when conjugated to polylysine (44) and the possibility to synthesize enzymatically large quantities of the nucleotides by using the (2'-5') oligo A synthetase produced by genetic engineering (6), may help answer some of these questions.

In conclusion, the growth-related variations in 2'-phosphodiesterase activity support a role for this enzyme in cell growth regulation. Of particular interest is the serum-stimulation of 2'-PD activity which may be the result of growth-factor action. IFNs appear in many respects as antagonists of growth-factors (35,36) and participate in growth-arrest and terminal differentiation where the (2'-5') oligo A synthetase is markedly increased (3,45). As discussed here, the 2'-PD controlled by both growth-stimulants and IFN, may be a fine-tuning mechanism for (2'-5') A metabolism, and may yet turn out to be instrumental for the antiviral and cell growth-regulatory effects of IFNs.

REFERENCES

1. Williams, B.R.G., and I.M, Kerr: The 2-5A (pppA2'p5'A2'p5'A) system in interferon-treated and control cells. Trends in Biochem Sci 5:138, 1980.
2. Lengyel, P: Biochemistry of Interferons and their actions. Ann Rev Biochem 51:251, 1982.
3. Revel, M: The Interferon System in Man: Nature of the Interferon Molecules and Mode of Action. In:Antiviral Drugs and Interferons: The Molecular Basis of their Activity, Y. Becker, ed. Martinus Nijhoff, Boston, pp. 358-434, 1984.
4. Merlin, G, J. Chebath, P. Benech, R. Metz, and M. Revel: Molecular cloning and sequence of partial cDNA for interferon-induced (2'-5') oligo (A) synthetase mRNA from human cells. Proc Natl Acad Sci USA 80: 4904, 1983.
5. Benech, P, G. Merlin, M. Revel, and J. Chebath: 3'-end structure of the human (2'-5') oligo A synthetase gene: prediction of two distinct proteins with cell type-specific expression. Nucl Acids Res 13: 1267, 1985.
6. Benech, P., Y. Mory, M. Revel, and J. Chebath: Structure of two forms of the interferon-induced (2'-5') oligo A synthetase of human cells based on cDNA and gene sequences. EMBO J 4:2249, 1985.
7. Chebath, J., P. Benech, A. Hovanessian, J. Galabru, and M. Revel: Four different forms of interferon-induced (2'-5') oligo A synthetase identified by immunoblotting in human cells. J Biol Chem in press, 1986.
8. Krause, D., A. Panet, G. Arad, C.W. Dieffenbach, and R.H. Silverman: Independent regulation of ppp(A2'p)$_n$A-dependent RNase in NIH 3T3, clone 1 cells by growth arrest and interferon treatment. J Biol Chem 260:9501, 1985.
9. Baglioni, C., and G.J. Williams: Role of degradation products of 2-5A in the localized cleavage of viral RNA. In: The 2-5A System: Molecular and Clinical Aspects of the Interferon Regulated Pathway, B.R.G. Williams and R.H. Silverman, eds. Alan R. Liss, New York, pp. 275-283, 1985.
10. Schmidt, A., A. Zilberstein, L, Shulman, P. Federman, H. Berissi, and M. Revel: Interferon action: Isolation of nuclease F, a translation inhibitor activated by interferon-induced (2'-5') oligo-isoadenylate. FEBS Lett 95:257, 1978.
11. Schmidt, A., Y. Chernajovsky, L. Shulman, P. Federman, H. Berissi, and M. Revel: An interferon-induced phosphodiesterase degrading (2'-5') oligoisoadenylate and the C-C-A terminus of tRNA. Proc Natl Acad Sci USA 76: 4788, 1979.
12. Imai, J., M,I, Johnston, and P. Torrence: Chemical modification potentiates the biological activities of 2-5A and its congeners. J Biol Chem 257:12739, 1982.
13. Bayard, B., C. Bisbal, M. Shilhol, J, Cnockaert, G. Huez, and B. Lebleu: Increased stability and antiviral activity of 2'-O-phosphoglyceryl derivatives of (2'-5') oligo (adenylate). Roles of phosphodiesterases and phosphatases in (2'-5') oligo (adenylate) catabolism. Eur J Biochem 142:291, 1984.
14. Revel, M., D. Wallach, G. Merlin, A. Schattner, A. Schmidt, and A. Kimchi: Interferon-induced enzymes: Microassays and their applications: Purification and assay of (2'-5') oligoadenylate synthetase and

assay of 2'-phosphodiesterase. Meth Enzymol 79:149, 1981.
15. Knight, M,, P.J. Cayley, R.H. Silverman, D. Wreschner, C.S. Gilbert, R.E. Brown, and I.M. Kerr: Radioimmune, radiobinding, and HPLC analysis of 2-5A and related oligonucleotides from intact cells. Nature 288:189, 1980.
16. Torrence, P.F., J. Imai, and M.I. Johnston: 5-O-monophosphoryl adenylyl (2'-5') adenylyl (2'-5') adenosine is an atagonist of the action of 5'-O-triphosphoryl adenylyl (2'-5') adenylyl (2'-5') adenosine and double-stranded RNA. Proc Natl Acad Sci USA 78:5993,1981.
17. Williams, B.R.G., I.M. Kerr, C.S. Gilbert, C.N. White, and L.A. Ball: Synthesis and breakdown of pppA2'p5'A2'p5'A and transient inhibition of protein synthesis in extracts from interferon-treated and control cells. Eur J Biochem 92:455, 1978.
18. Minks, M.A., S. Benvin, P.A. Maroney, and C. Baglioni: Metabolic stability of 2,5' oligo(A) and activity of 2,5'-oligo(A)-dependent endonuclease in extracts of interferon-treated and control HeLa cells. J Biol Chem 6:767, 1979.
19. Kimchi, A., H. Shure, and M. Revel: Antimitogenic function of interferon-induced (2'-5') oligo(adenylate) and growth-related variations in enzymes that synthesize and degrade this oligonucleotide. Eur J Biochem 114:5, 1981.
20. Krishnan, I, and C. Baglioni: 2'-5' oligo(A) polymerase activity in serum of mice infected with EMC virus or treated with interferon. Nature 285:485, 1980.
21. Sawai, H., K. Ishibashi, M. Itoh, and S. Watanabe: 2'-5'-oligoadenylate and 2'-5'-oligoadenylate phosphodiesterase in human plasma. Biochem Biophys Res Comm 125:1061, 1984.
22. Goren, T., A. Kapitkovsky, A. Kimchi, and M. Rubinstein: High and low potency interferon-α subtypes induce (2'-5') oligoadenylate synthetase with similar efficiency. Virology 130:273, 1983.
23. Kimchi, A., L. Shulman, A. Schmidt, Y. Chernajovsky, A. Fradin, and M. Revel: Kinetics of the induction of three translation-regulatory enzymes by interferon. Proc Natl Acad Sci USA 76:3208, 1979.
24. Verhaegen-Lewalle, M, and J. Content: Phosphodiesterase activity in human cell lines treated or untreated with human interferon. Eur J Biochem 126:639, 1982.
25. Chapekar, M.S, and R.I. Glazer: Cell viability and the (2'-5') oligo(A)-RNase L pathway in human colon carcinoma cells treated with human interferons and double stranded RNA. In: The 2-5A System. B.R.G. Williams and R.H. Silverman, eds. Alan R. Liss, New York, pp.377-384, 1985.
26. Zilberstein, A., B. Dudock, H. Berissi, and M. Revel: Control of messenger RNA translation by minor species of leucyl-transfer RNA in extracts from interferon-treated L cells. J Mol Biol 108:43, 1976.
27. Keith, G., M.L. Gangloff, R. Falcoff, and G. Dirheimer: Incubation of beef $tRNA^{Leu}$ in interferon-treated cells lysates leads to a partial removal of the 3' terminal sequence. Comptes Rendus Acad Sci Paris. 293:795, 1982.
28. Nilsen, T.W, and C. Baglioni: A mechanism for discrimination between viral and host mRNA in interferon-treated cells. Proc Natl Acad Sci USA 76:2600, 1979.
29. Revel, M., A. Kimchi, L. Shulman, A. Fradin, R. Shuster, Yakobson, E, Chernajovsky, Y, A. Schmidt, H. Shure, and R. Bendori: Role of interferon-induced enzymes in the antiviral and antimitogenic effects of

interferon. Ann New York Acad Sci 350:459, 1980.
30. Kimchi, A., H. Shure, and M. Revel: Regulation of lymphocyte mitogenesis by (2'-5') oligo-isoadenylate. Nature 282:849, 1979.
31. Itkes, A.V., O.N. Kartasheva, V.L. Tunitskaya, K.T. Turpaev, C.A. Kafiani, and E.S. Severin: Activities of cAMP-dependent protein kinase and enzymes of 2'-5'-oligoadenylate metabolism in NIH 3T3 cells deepening into the resting state. Exptl Cell Res 157:335, 1985.
32. Itkes, A.V., O.N. Kartasheva, C.A. Kafiani, and E.S. Severin: Inhibition of 2'-phosphodiesterase by cAMP-dependent protein kinase. Involvement of phosphorylation of protein inhibitor. FEBS Lett 176: 65, 1984.
33. Wells, V, and L. Mallucci: Expression of the 2-5A system during the cell cycle. Exptl Cell Res 159:27, 1985.
34. Mallucci, L., J. Chebath, M. Revel, Wells, V, and P. Benech: Interferon and 2-5A synthetase gene expression during the cell cycle. In: The Interferon System, F. Dianzani and G.B. Rossi, eds. Serono Symposia, Vol. 24, Raven Press, pp. 165-170, 1985.
35. Taylor-Papadimitriou, J: Effects of interferon on cell growth and function. In: Interferon 2, I. Gresser, ed. Acad. Press, New York, pp. 13-46, 1980.
36. Kimchi, A., H. Shure, Y. Lapidot, S. Rapoport, A. Panet, and M. Revel: Antimitogenic effects of interferon and (2'-5')-oligoadenylate in synchronized 3T3 fibroblasts. FEBS Lett 134:212, 1981.
37. Brown, R.E, and I.M.Kerr: (p)pp(A2'p)$_n$A is rare in normal mouse tissues while (A2'p)$_n$A but not (p)pp(A2'p)$_n$A appears to be present in E. coli . In: The 2-5A System, B.R.G. Williams, and R.H. Silverman, eds. Alan R. Liss, pp. 3-10, 1985.
38. Paez, E, and M. Esteban: Nature and mode of action of vaccinia virus products that block activation of the interferon-mediated ppp(A2'p)$_n$A synthetase. Virology 134:29, 1984.
39. Silverman, R.H., J.P. Cayley, M. Knight, C.S. Gilbert, and I.M. Kerr: Control of the ppp(A2'p)$_n$A system in HeLa cells: effects of interferon and virus infection. Eur J Biochem 124:131, 1982.
40. Etienne-Smekens, M., P. Vandenbussche, J. Content, and J.E. Dumont: (2'-5') oligoadenylate in rat liver: Modulation after partial hepatectomy. Proc Natl Acad Sci USA 80:4609, 1983.
41. Samuel, D, and H. Cailla: Evolution of intracellular 2.5A during a cell cycle. Antiviral Res ABSTR 1, No 2: p. 83, 1983.
42. Hovanessian, A, and J.N. Wood: Anticellular and antiviral effects of pppA(2'p5'A)$_n$. Virology 101:81, 1980.
43. Schryver, B.B., V. Marsh, M.A. Van der Pas, and D.A. Epstein: 2-5A analogs as mechanistic probes of the 2-5A system. In: The 2-5A System. B.R.G. Williams, and R.H. Silverman, eds. Alan R. Liss, pp. 81-88, 1985.
44. Bayard, B., C. Bisbal, and B. Lebleu: Activation of ribonuclease L by (2'-5')(A)$_4$-Poly(L-lysine) conjugates in intact cells. Biochemistry 25:3730, 1986.
45. Resnitzky, D., A. Yarden, D. Zipori, and A. Kimchi . A: Autocrine β-related interferon controls c-myc suppression and growth-arrest during hematopoietic cell differentiation. Cell 46:31, 1986.

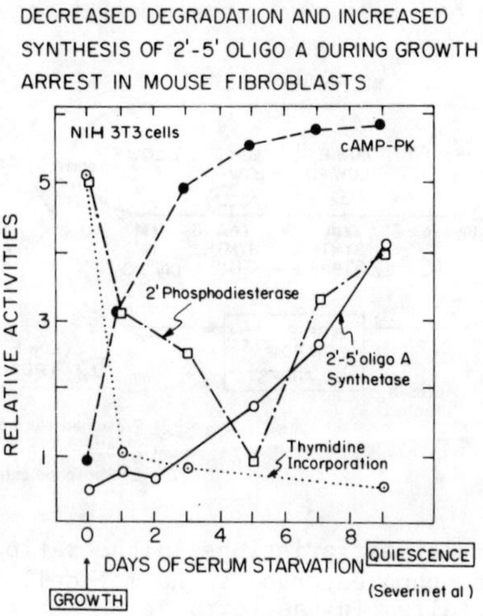

Figure 1. Changes in (2'-5') oligo A synthetase and 2'-phosphodiesterase during transition from growth to quiescence. Data adapted from (31).

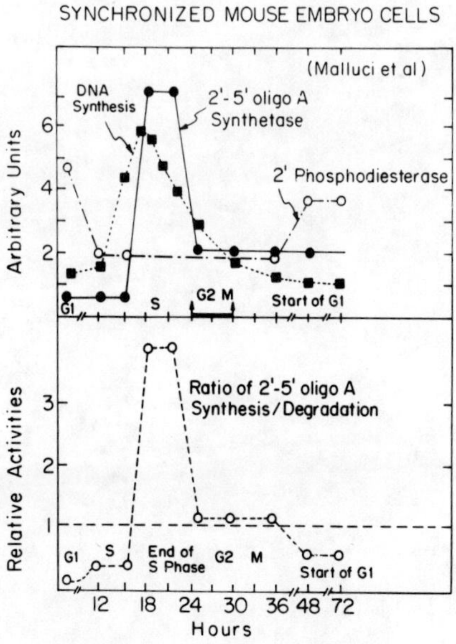

Figure 2. Changes in (2'-5') oligo A synthetase and 2'-phosphodiesterase during cell cycle. Data adapted from (33).

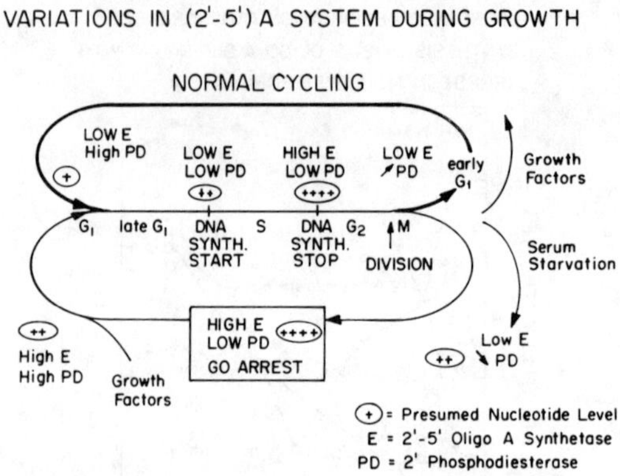

Figure 3. Model correlating variations in the ratio of (2'-5') oligo A synthetase over 2'-phosphodiesterase in normal cell cycling and in G_o-growth arrest. Detailed in the text.

40. MX Protein Pathway of Interferon Action

J. Lindemann and O. Haller

Institute for Immunology and Virology, University of Zurich, Gloriastrasse 30, CH-8028, Zurich, Switzerland

Many years ago a mouse strain was observed which proved resistant to large doses of influenza virus that were lethal to ordinary laboratory mice (1, 2). Screening of numerous inbred strains revealed only one further example of this type of resistance, so that today two such strains are known, A2G and SL (3, and Haller, personal communication). This resistance was inherited as a dominant trait governed by a single autosomal locus, called Mx (4), localized to chromosome 16 (5). Congenic lines could be established by crossing Mx into current laboratory mouse strains such as BALB/c and C57BL/6; each backcross generation was challenged with a suitable dose of influenza virus, which killed off all Mx-negative animals but allowed the Mx carriers to survive. After 10 to 20 backcross generations, congenic resistant animals can be assumed to differ from their susceptible counterparts by but a small fraction of their genome surrounding the Mx locus.

In attempting to explain this resistance phenomenon, several approaches were tried which turned out to be blind alleys. Things began to clear up when it was discovered that treatment of resistant animals with a potent antiserum directed at mouse type 1 interferon (generously provided by Ion Gresser) rendered them fully susceptible (6). When comparing the pattern of interferon-induced proteins, an additional spot was observed in extracts of Mx bearing cells. The presence of this spot correlated with the resistant phenotype (7). It was concluded that interferon induced a protein, Mx protein, which in some way was involved in the antiviral state. This concept was reinforced by the observation that type 2 interferon (gamma) failed to induce Mx protein and failed to protect against influenza virus (8).

How does Mx protein contribute to the antiviral state? Is it antivirally active against influenza virus on its own, or only in collaboration with other interferon-induced proteins? And what is the mechanism of its action? To answer these and related questions it was deemed necessary to clone first Mx cDNA and later the whole Mx gene. Cloning of cDNA, done with the help of Charles Weissmann's laboratory, took advantage of the fact that Mx mRNA was only expected to be present in extracts from interferon-induced Mx positive cells, but not in non-induced extracts or in induced extracts from Mx-negative cells (9). In vitro translation could be conveniently monitored with antibodies to Mx protein, whose preparation was facilitated by the presence of congenic strains: extracts from interferon-treated, Mx-positive cells, when injected into congenic, Mx-negative animals induced polyclonal antibodies directed at the Mx protein; monoclonal antibodies were later also obtained (10).

The protein derived from the Mx cDNA sequence consists of 631 amino acids and has a molecular weight of 72'000. Natural Mx protein and the product of transfected Mx cDNA accumulates in the cell nucleus (11), possibly guided by a stretch of carboxy-proximal basic amino acids (9). Transfected to Mx-negative cells under control of the SV40 early promoter, its constitutive expression as judged by immunofluorescence is variable. Those cells that express Mx protein at a level comparable to naturally Mx-positive, interferon-treated cells prove nonpermissive for influenza virus replication (9). Thus it would appear that Mx protein alone, without cooperation from other interferon-induced proteins, has an inhibitory action on influenza virus.

Microinjection into Mx-negative mouse cells of polyadenylated Mx mRNA synthesized in vitro leads to the production of Mx protein, to its accumulation in the nucleus, and to resistance against influenza virus (Arnheiter and Noteborn, personal communication). Microinjection of antibodies to Mx protein into interferon-induced rat cells neutralizes the antiviral effect against influenza virus (Arnheiter, personal communication).

Transfection across species barriers, with the ultimate aim of creating transgenic animals resistant to influenza virus, seems a reasonable endeavour, since heavy economic losses caused by influenza among domestic animals occur.

Proteins analogous to the mouse Mx protein as judged by cross-reactivity with antibodies and by nucleic acid hybridization are present in the rat and in man (12). These proteins are also induced by type 1 and not by type 2 interferons, and their molecular weights range between 65 and 80 kD. However, the human Mx analogue does not accumulate in the nucleus (12).

Paradoxically, it is the allele which is rare in laboratory mice which seems to represent the wild type. Amongst the many Mx-negative strains, two types of deletions have been noticed (9). In wild mice, the Mx allele is present, but its exact frequency has not yet been established (Haller, personal communication). It is difficult to see what advantage, if any, is conferred by either allele at the Mx locus. No naturally occurring orthomyxovirus infections in mice are known. In man, where influenza virus pandemics might represent powerful selective forces, one would expect an almost universal distribution of an allele favouring survival. If indeed the human Mx equivalent has antiviral activity in man, a search among the rare fatalities in otherwise healthy persons during an influenza epidemic might reveal instances of deletions at the corresponding human locus.

The self-limiting character of influenza virus lesions in Mx-positive mice allows a visualization of the defense mechanisms in action. Thus, a hepatotropic influenza virus variant which, in Mx-negative animals, produces a fulminant generalized liver necrosis, induces only small necrotic foci in Mx-positive mice (13). By immunofluorescence, it can be shown that these foci contain viral antigen in the center, and that cells surrounding each focus contain Mx protein in their nucleus. The sequence of events which this suggests is the following: First, the virus gains a foothold in some cells within the liver. It starts replicating, but at the same time it induces an outcrop of interferon type 1. This impinges on interferon receptors of adjacent cells, thereby inducing the formation of Mx protein. Armed in this manner, the cells surrounding the initial lesion successfully resist virus spread (Juelke and Haller, personal communication). In Mx-negative mice, the first steps are the same, interferon is produced, an antiviral state does form, but one lacking in the ingredient which is essential in protecting against influenza virus, namely the Mx protein. The cells surrounding the lesion remain inadequately armed, and virus spread follows unchecked.

As far as the mechanism of action is concerned, it has been suggested that the block occurs at the level of translation (14) or of transcription (15). The latter seems more likely (Ellen Meier, personal communication). With the possibility of preparing large amounts of Mx protein by genetic engineering, it should become possible to gain insights into the manner in which Mx protein interacts with viral synthesis. The specificity of Mx, which only addresses orthomyxoviruses, might also shed light on the unique replication strategy of this virus group.

The antiviral states induced by interferon are obviously complex. Deficiency in one out of many interferon-induced proteins, Mx protein, renders the antiviral state incapable of dealing successfully with attack by one group of closely related viruses, orthomyxoviruses. Other defects in interferon-induced proteins are known (16), but a corresponding defect in the ensuing antiviral state (if indeed there is one) has not yet been identified. The Mx case is particularly fortunate in that the biologically relevant observation (virus resistance) came first, and the explanation, or at least the beginnings of an explanation in molecular terms, came later. To go the same path in reverse will be much more difficult.

A final irony can be seen in the fact that, had not an accident in the breeding of A2G mice (originally intended to be a mere extension of strain A) introduced a wild type allele into this colony, the whole Mx saga would still be waiting to be discovered.

SUMMARY

Synthesis of the gene product of the wild Mx allele of the mouse, Mx protein, is under strict control by type 1 interferons. Mx protein seems to inhibit influenza virus development, thus accounting for the high degree of resistance to orthomyxoviruses in mice carrying the Mx allele.

ACKNOWLEDGEMENTS

We thank all collaborators who, at one time or another, spent time and energy in what must have seemed to be a quixotic enterprise.

REFERENCES

1. Lindenmann, J.: Resistance of mice to mouse-adapted influenza virus. Virology 16:203, 1962.
2. Lindenmann, J., C.A. Lane and D. Hobson: The resistance of A2G mice to myxoviruses. J Immunol 90:942, 1963.

3. Lindenmann, J., and P. Klein: Furtheer studies on the resistance of mice to myxoviruses. Arch Virol 19:1. 1966.
4. Lindenmann, J.: Inheritance of resistance to influenza virus in mice. Proc Soc Exp Biol Med 116:506, 1964.
5. Staeheli, P., D. Pravtcheva, L.-G. Lundin, M. Acklin, F. Ruddle, J. Lindenmann, and O. Haller: Interferon-regulated influenza virus resistance gene Mx is localized on mouse chromosome 16. Virology 58:967, 1986.
6. Haller, O., H. Arnheiter, I. Gresser, and J. Lindenmann: Genetically determined, interferon-dependent resistance to influenza virus in mice. J Exp Med 149:601, 1979.
7. Horisberger, M.A., P. Staeheli, and O. Haller: Interferon induces a unique protein in mouse cells bearing a gene for resistance to influenza virus. Proc Nat Acad Sci USA 80:1910, 1983.
8. Staeheli, P., M.A. Horisberger, and Haller: Mx-dependent resistance to influenza virus is induced by mouse interferons alpha and beta but not gamme. Virology 132:456, 1984.
9. Staeheli, P., O. Haller, W. Boll, J. Lindenmann, and C. Weissmann: Mx protein: Constitutive expression in 3T3 cells transformed with cloned Mx cDNA confers selective resistance to influenza virus. Cell 44:147, 1986.
10. Staeheli, P., P. Dreiding, O. Haller, and J. Lindenmann: Polyclonal and monoclonal antibodies to the interferon-inducible protein Mx of influenza virus-resistant mice. J Biol Chem 260:1821, 1985.
11. Dreiding, P., P. Staeheli, and O. Haller: Interferon-induced protein Mx accumulates in nuclei of mouse cells expressing resistance to influenza viruses. Virology 140:192, 1985.
12. Staeheli, P., J. Faeh, C. Mortier, and O. Haller: Interferon-induced homologs to mouse Mx protein in humans and rats. In: The Biology of the Interferon System, W.E. Stewart II and H. Schellekens eds. Elsevier Science Publishers, pp. 115-118, 1986.
13. Haller, O.: A mouse hepatotropic variant of influenza virus. Arch Virol 49:99, 1975.
14. Meyer, T., and Horisberger, M.A.: Combined action of mouse alpha and beta interferons in influenza virus-infected macrophages carrying the resistance gene Mx. J Virol 49:709, 1984.
15. Krug, R.M., M. Shaw, B. Brioni, G. Shapiro, and O. Haller: Inhibition of influenza virus messenger RNA synthesis in cells expressing the interferon-induced Mx gene product. J Virol 56:201, 1985.
16. Staeheli, P., M. Prochazka, P.A. Steigmeier, and O. Haller: Genetic control of interferon action: mouse strain distribution and inheritance of an induced protein with guanylate-binding property. Virology 137:135, 1984.

41. Anti-interferon Effects of Viruses

Patricia Whitaker-Dowling and Julius S. Youngner

Department of Microbiology, Biochemistry, and Molecular Biology, School of Medicine, University of Pittsburgh, Pittsburgh, PA 15261

INTRODUCTION

Although interferon (IFN) is a powerful antiviral agent, there are several instances in which IFN is ineffective in restricting viral growth. In some of these instances it has been found that certain viruses can actively block the antiviral state and inhibit the IFN-induced enzymes which are believed to play a role in the restriction of viral growth. The anti-interferon effect of viruses was first reported in 1972 by Youngner et al. (1) who demonstrated that vaccinia virus is insensitive to IFN in rabbit kidney cells and is able to rescue vesicular stomatitis virus (VSV) from IFN-mediated restriction. When this phenomenon was examined in other cell lines, it was found that vaccinia also is able to rescue VSV from the inhibitory effects of IFN in rabbit cornea cells and mouse L cells. In primary chick embryo cells, where vaccinia itself is inhibited by IFN, the DNA virus is unable to rescue VSV (2). Studies with actinomycin D, hydroxyurea and UV-irradiation showed that the rescue of VSV from inhibition by IFN requires the first two hours of vaccinia gene expression (3).

RECENT ADVANCES

In order to determine how vaccinia can overcome the antiviral activity of IFN, the effect of vaccinia coinfection on the VSV replicative cycle in IFN-treated L cells was examined (4). Vaccinia has no effect on VSV penetration (unpublished observation), primary transcription, or on the amount of functional VSV mRNA in the IFN-treated cells. However, vaccinia has a dramatic stimulatory effect on VSV protein synthesis (4).

The vaccinia-mediated rescue of VSV at the level of translation correlates with the ability of vaccinia to inhibit the IFN-induced, dsRNA-dependent kinase, as assayed in vitro (4). A specific kinase inhibitory factor (SKIF) produced by vaccinia that inhibits only the IFN-induced, dsRNA-dependent protein kinase is detected in extracts from IFN-treated vaccinia infected L and HeLa cells (4,5,6,7). The phosphorylation of both the P1 protein and the alpha subunit of eIF-2 is blocked by SKIF (5,7), but the phosphorylation of other cell proteins is unaffected. SKIF activity is also demonstrable when extracts from vaccinia-infected cells are mixed with extracts from IFN-treated cells (7). SKIF is detected as early as 90 minutes after infection with vaccinia (7) and requires RNA and protein synthesis but not DNA synthesis for its production (5). The kinase inhibitory activity is non-dialyzable and is sensitive to heat as well as to extremes of pH. SKIF is not phenol extractable and is unaffected by treatment with ribonucleases (7). The inhibition of the kinase is lost upon dilution of SKIF (by greater than 20-fold) and the SKIF inhibition can be overcome by increasing the amount of dsRNA in the reaction but not by increasing the relative amount of the IFN-induced kinase. The vaccinia-induced inhibitor appears to interact with the dsRNA in a stoichiometric rather than a catalytic manner and extracts from vaccinia-infected cells do not contain increased amounts of dsRNase (8). SKIF does not appear to be a phosphatase (5), or a protease and the inhibitory action of SKIF is reversible (5,7).

The vaccinia-mediated rescue function is not detectable in all cell lines in which vaccinia is insensitive to IFN. A particularly interesting situation exists with two strains of the same rabbit kidney cell line, RK-13. In both of these cell strains vaccinia growth is refractory to the effects of IFN. However, the two cell strains differ in the level at which VSV growth is restricted following IFN treatment. In the cell strain in which IFN treatment blocks VSV at the level of translation, coinfection with vaccinia can completely overcome the IFN-mediated inhibition of VSV growth. This is similar to the situation observed in L cells. In the cell strain in which VSV growth is blocked prior to or at the point of accumulation of primary transcripts, vaccinia is unable to rescue VSV growth (9).

The ability of vaccinia to rescue other viruses from the inhibitory effects of IFN is not limited to rhabdoviruses but has been extended to picornaviruses, such as polio, mengo and encephalomyocarditis (EMC) virus (6,10,11). The rescue of EMC growth in IFN-treated L cells by vaccinia is correlated with a stimulation of EMC RNA and protein synthesis, and an inhibition of the IFN-induced protein kinase (10,11). However, coinfection with vaccinia has no effect on the EMC-induced activation of the 2-5A system as detected by the degradation of rRNA in IFN-treated, EMC-infected cells (11). As has been observed with VSV (3), the EMC genome is relatively stable in IFN-treated L cells since the ability of EMC to be rescued by vaccinia is not lost rapidly following EMC infection (11).

Vaccinia has also been implicated in an inhibition of the 2-5A synthetase-RNase L pathway. Rice and Kerr (12) found that although 2-5A accumulates to high in vivo levels during vaccinia infection of HeLa or L cells, the characteristic cleavage of rRNA expected at these 2-5A levels does not occur. However, both the 2-5A and the 2-5A-dependent RNase are functional when examined in vitro. Paez and Esteban determined that the 2-5A synthetase activity from IFN-treated, vaccinia-infected cells as measured in vitro is partially impaired (6) and it has been suggested that this inhibition may be due to viral-mediated enzymes: an ATPase which blocks the 2-5A synthetase by destroying its substrate and a phosphatase which could dephosphorylate (and thus inactivate) the 2-5A (13). However, the role of these enzymes in the intact cell has not been evaluated and the data of Rice and Kerr indicate that accumulation of functional 2-5A in these cells is not affected by vaccinia infection. Esteban et. al. (14) have suggested that the ability of vaccinia to overcome the effects of IFN and the 2-5A pathway in L cells depends upon cell growth conditions; they find that vaccinia is insensitive to IFN in monolayer cultures but sensitive in IFN-treated suspension cultures of L cells. It is of interest to note that Pacha and Condit have described a ts mutant of vaccinia, which at the non-permissive temperature is blocked at the level of late protein synthesis. This protein synthesis block is coupled with extensive degradation of rRNA (15).

The Herpes family of viruses can also inhibit the activity of the 2-5A pathway in a manner similar to that observed with vaccinia. Cayley et al. (16) compared the 2-5A levels found in IFN-treated Chang cells following infection with EMC, herpes simplex 1 or herpes simplex 2. Although similar levels of 2-5A were detected in cells infected with all three viruses, only low levels of 2-5A-specific rRNA degradation were measured in cells infected with the herpes viruses. This careful study detected 2-5A related compounds in herpes infected cell extracts which were capable of inhibiting the activation of RNase L by authentic 2-5A (16). It should be added that another herpes virus (pseudorabies) has been shown to overcome the antiviral state and rescue VSV growth in IFN-treated cells (8).

In the absence of exogenous IFN treatment, other viruses have been reported to inhibit enzyme activities similar or identical to those associated with the antiviral state induced by IFN. The 2-5A-dependent RNase activity is inhibited by EMC infection in HeLa, L or Ehrlich ascites tumor cells (18). The EMC-induced inhibitor which blocks the nuclease activity apparently affects the ability of the protein to bind the 2-5A molecules. However, the EMC-mediated effect on the nuclease is lost if the cells are treated with IFN (17,18).

Coinfection of untreated L cells with vaccinia and VSV increases VSV yield by 10-fold. This stimulation results from the vaccinia-mediated inhibition of the VSV-directed damage to the host translational machinery. It has been postulated that vaccinia blocks the VSV-mediated inactivation of eIF-2 by inhibition of the dsRNA-dependent kinase present at low constitutive levels in untreated cells (19).

Subsequent to the reports concerning vaccinia, other viruses have been reported to inhibit a dsRNA-dependent kinase. In adenovirus infected cells, it has been shown that the VA1 RNA is needed for the production of the late adeno proteins. Cell-free systems prepared from adeno $VA1^-$ mutant infected cells have identified a dominant inhibitor that causes a defect in the initiation of protein synthesis which can be overcome by the addition of eIF-2 or eIF-2B (20). The dominant inhibitor has been correlated with the phosphorylation of the same proteins (P1 and eIF-2α) that are substrates for the IFN-induced, dsRNA-dependent kinase (21,22). It is thought that this kinase activity is inhibited by the VA1 RNA in cells infected by wild-type adenovirus. The activation of the dsRNA-dependent kinase has been correlated with the defect in the VA1⁻ mutant since this mutant can grow to near normal levels in a cell line (GM2767) which is deficient in the kinase (22). In addition, the growth of the VA1⁻ mutant is inhibited by IFN (an 8-fold inhibition by 1000 units/ml IFN), whereas the wild-type virus is unaffected by IFN (23). Further, *in vitro* assays have demonstrated the ability of VA1 RNA to inhibit the dsRNA activation of the IFN-induced kinase, while other small RNAs such as 5S RNA showed only partial inhibition when used at higher concentrations (23).

Since influenza can grow in cells infected with the adeno VA1⁻ mutant (24), it has been suggested that influenza virus can also inhibit the activity of the same kinase inhibited by wild-type adenovirus. The phosphorylation of exogenously added eIF-2 is detected in extracts of cells infected with adeno VA1⁻ mutant but is much reduced in extracts of cells doubly infected with influenza and the VA1⁻ mutant (25).

DISCUSSION

It is not surprising that some viruses have evolved mechanisms of overcoming the antiviral state induced by IFN. Nor is it surprising that the most potent and complex of these anti-IFN effects are produced by large dsDNA viruses of the Pox and Herpes families which have more genetic flexibility and excess genome capacity for such auxiliary functions. From the data so far available, it appears that the mechanisms of inhibition of the IFN-induced enzymes may vary depending upon the virus group. For example, in the case of adenovirus, a small viral RNA seems to be responsible for the inhibition of the kinase, whereas in the vaccinia system there is no evidence for the involvement of a viral RNA. However, it is important to point out that in both the case of adenovirus and influenza, when the kinase activity is measured by the methods usually used for the IFN-induced kinase, namely, in extracts from IFN-treated cells in the presence of dsRNA, neither virus has any effect on the kinase activity. Therefore, it is not clear that these reports of inhibition by adeno- and the influenza viruses are dealing with the same eIF-2 kinase as the one induced by IFN.

Attention has been focused for the last decade on two enzyme systems that are thought to be responsible for the stringent translational block induced by IFN: the 2-5A synthetase and protein kinase pathways. Although there is evidence that both of these systems can regulate protein synthesis *in vitro*, conclusive proof of their *in vivo* relevance is lacking. The study of the anti-IFN activity of viruses such as vaccinia has provided a strong correlation between the ability of the virus to overcome the antiviral state and to inhibit the dsRNA-dependent enzymes thought to be responsible for the antiviral state. Further investigation into the mechanism of the anti-IFN effects of viruses will provide valuable information for the understanding of the interferon system.

ACKNOWLEDGEMENTS

This work was supported by research grant AI-06264 from the National Institute of Allergy and Infectious Diseases.

REFERENCES

1. Youngner, J., H. Thacore, and M. Kelly: Sensitivity of ribonucleic acid and deoxyribonucleic acid viruses to different species of interferon in cell cultures. J. Virol.10:171, 1972.
2. Thacore, H., and J. Youngner: Rescue of vesicular stomatitis virus from interferon-induced resistance by superinfection with vaccinia virus I. Rescue in cell cultures from different species. Virology 56:505, 1973.
3. Thacore, H., and J. Youngner: Rescue of vesicular stomatitis virus from interferon-induced resistance by superinfection with vaccinia virus II. Effect of UV-inactivated vaccinia and metabolic inhibitors. Virology 56:512, 1973.
4. Whitaker-Dowling, P., and J. Youngner: Vaccinia rescue of VSV from interferon-induced resistance: Reversal of translation block and inhibition of protein kinase activity. Virology 131:128, 1983.
5. Rice, A., and I. Kerr: Interferon-mediated, double-stranded RNA-dependent protein kinase is inhibited in extracts from vaccinia virus-infected cells. J. Virol. 50:229, 1984.
6. Paez, E., and M. Esteban: Resistance of vaccinia virus to interferon is related to an interference phenomenon between the virus and the interferon system. Virology 134:12, 1984.
7. Whitaker-Dowling, P., and J. Youngner: Characterization of a specific kinase inhibitory factor produced by vaccinia virus which inhibits the interferon-induced protein kinase. Virology 137:171, 1984.
8. Whitaker-Dowling, P., and J. Youngner: Vaccinia virus overcomes the antiviral effect of interferon and inhibits the interferon-induced protein kinase. In: The Biology of the Interferon System 1984, H. Kirchner, and H. Schellekens, eds. Elsevier Press, pp. 347-353, 1985.
9. Whitaker-Dowling, P., and J. Youngner: Interferon restricts VSV growth by different mechanisms in two strains of a rabbit kidney cell line. In: The Biology of the Interferon System 1985, H. Schellekens, and W. Stewart, eds. Elsevier Press (in press).
10. Whitaker-Dowling, P., R. Jagus, and J. Youngner: Vaccinia-mediated inhibition of interferon action: Rescue of picornaviruses. In: The Interferon System, F. Dianzani, and G. B. Rossi, eds. Raven Press, pp. 177-181, 1985.
11. Whitaker-Dowling, P., and J. Youngner: Vaccinia-mediated rescue of encephalomyocarditis virus from the inhibitory effects of interferon. Virology (in press).
12. Rice, A., W. Roberts, and I. Kerr: 2-5A accumulates to high levels in interferon-treated, vaccinia virus-infected cells in the absence of any inhibition of virus replication. J. Virol. 50:220, 1984.
13. Paez, E., and M. Esteban: Nature and mode of action of vaccinia virus products that block activation of the interferon-mediated ppp(A2'p)nA-synthetase. Virology 134:29, 1984.
14. Esteban, M., J. Benavente, and E. Paez: Mode of sensitivity and resistance of vaccinia virus replication to interferon. J. gen. Virol. 67:801, 1986.
15. Pacha, R., and R. Condit: Characterization of a temperature-sensitive mutant of vaccinia virus reveals a novel function which prevents virus-induced breakdown of RNA. J. Virol. 56:395, 1985.

16. Cayley, P., J. Davies, K. McCullagh, and I Kerr: Activation of the ppp(A2'p)nA system in interferon-treated, Herpes simplex virus-infected cells and evidence for novel inhibitors of the ppp(A2'p)nA-dependent RNase. Eur. J. Biochem. 143:165, 1984.
17. Cayley, J., M. Knight, and I. Kerr: Virus-mediated inhibition of the ppp(A2'p)nA system and its prevention by interferon. B.B.R.C. 104:376, 1982.
18. Silverman, R., P. Cayley, M. Knight, C. Gilbert, and I. Kerr: Control of the ppp(A2'p)nA system in HeLa cells, effect of interferon and virus infection. Eur. J. Biochem. 124:131, 1982.
19. Whitaker-Dowling, P., R. Jagus, and J. Youngner: Effect of vaccinia on protein synthesis in mouse L cells infected with vesicular stomatitis virus. In: The Biology of Negative Stranded Viruses, D. Kolakofsky, and B. Mahy, eds. Academic Press (in press).
20. Reichel, P., W. Merrick, J. Siekierka, and M. Matthews: Regulation of a protein synthesis initiation factor by adenovirus-associated RNA1. Nature 313:196, 1985.
21. Siekierka, J., T. Mariano, P. Reichel, and M. Matthews: Translational control by adenovirus: Lack of virus-associated RNA1 during adenovirus infection results in phosphorylation of initiation factor eIF-2 and inhibition of protein synthesis. Proc. Natl. Acad. Sci. 82:1959, 1985.
22. Schneider, R., B. Safer, S. Munemitsu, C. Samuel, and T. Shenk: Adenovirus VA1 RNA prevents phosphorylation of the eukaryotic initiation factor 2 α subunit subsequent to infection. Proc. Natl. Acad. Sci. 82:4321, 1985.
23. Kitajewski, J., R. Schneider, B. Safer, S. Munemitsu, C. Samuel, B. Thinnappaya, and T. Shenk: Adenovirus VA1 RNA antagonizes the antiviral action of interferon by preventing activation of the interferon-induced eIF-2α kinase. Cell 45:195, 1986.
24. Katze, M., Y. Chen, and R. Krug: Nuclear-cytoplasmic transport and VA1 RNA-independent translation of influenza viral messenger RNAs in late adenovirus-infected cells. Cell 37:483, 1984.
25. Katze, M., B. Detjen, B. Safer, and R. Krug: Translational control by influenza virus: Suppression of the kinase that phosphorylates the α subunit of initiation factor eIF-2 and selective translation of influenza mRNAs. Mol. Cell. Biol. 6:1741, 1986.

42. Interferons and Oncogenes

E. Knight, Jr., and G. J. Jonak

Central Research and Development Department, E. I. DuPont DeNemours and Co., Wilmington, DE 19898

INTRODUCTION

Interferons and oncogenes have been implicated in the regulation of cellular functions. In 1962 preparations of mouse IFN were shown to inhibit the growth of mouse cells (1). Subsequently IFN was shown to prevent DNA tumor virus-induced transformation of cells (2) and to induce phenotypic reversion in murine sarcoma virus-transformed mouse fibroblasts (3). More recently the cellular oncogenes have been implicated in the regulation of cell growth, development, differentiation and the capacity to transform normal cells into neoplastic cells. The research on oncogenes has provided much information concerning the regulation of cellular genes. Since IFNs can regulate the expression of certain genes and affect the growth of cells it became obvious to ask if IFN can regulate the expression of certain oncogenes. In this report we review only the effect of IFN on the expression of the RNA of the c-myc oncogene. In this proceedings IFN-induced reversion in oncogene transformed cells is also reviewed (4). For a more extensive review of the effect of IFN on the expression of oncogenes the reader should consult reference 5. The effect of IFN on viral oncogenes has not been included since an excellent review on that topic recently appeared (6). Cellular oncogenes are genes that share sequence homology with the oncogenes of the transforming RNA tumor viruses and have the capacity to confer the transformed phenotype on normal cells in transfection assays (see ref. 7,8,9 for review).

EFFECT OF IFN ON C-MYC RNA

The avian, human and mouse c-myc genes are the cellular homologs of the avian myelocytomatosis virus oncogene, v-myc. The expression of the c-myc gene as mRNA and protein is relatively constant in proliferating cells (10,11) but its expression appears to be very low in non-proliferating cells (12). A rapid accumulation of c-myc RNA has been observed after stimulation of non-proliferating cells with specific mitogens or growth promoting agents (see ref. 13 for review). However, cells whose growth had ceased because of induced differentiation (14,15,16) showed a reduction in c-myc expression. Because of these observations it has been speculated that the c-myc gene may be involved in the regulation of cell proliferation. Subsequently it was shown that IFN inhbited the PDGF-mediated stimulation of c-*myc* RNA in Balb/C 3T3 cells (17). Another laboratory, however, reported that the steady state level of c-*myc* RNA in PDGF-induced Balb/C 3T3 cells was slightly increased when the cells were pretreated with IFN for 48 hr (18).

Three groups have investigated the effect of IFN on the steady state level of c-*myc* RNA in human Daudi cells and have reported a substantial reduction in the c-*myc* RNA after IFN treatment (16,19,20). All three groups suggested that the reduction in c-*myc* RNA might be a requirement for the subsequent IFN-induced cessation of cell growth. The reduction in RNA appears to be mediated by a post-transcriptional event(s) since c-*myc* RNA transcription was unaffected even after 24 hr of IFN treatment (20,21). A post-transcriptional mechanism for regulation was also supported by the observation that the IFN causes a 67-80% reduction in the half life of the c-*myc* RNA (20). In contrast, another group reported that the transcription of the c-*myc* RNA was inhibited by IFN treatment of Daudi cells (16) and that c-*myc* mRNA half life was only slightly reduced. These different results may reflect differences in methodology or different control mechanisms in various Daudi cell lines. An IFN-caused cessation in cell growth mediated by c-*myc* was further supported when it was shown that IFN caused no reduction in the steady state level of c-*myc* RNA in Namalva, Raji, Manca and BL67 cells whose growth is not inhibited by IFN (16,22,23). This correlation, however, is not always obvious. IFN-γ inhibits the growth of HeLa cells but actually stimulates 3 fold the level of c-*myc* RNA (24). In Daudi cells that reverted to IFN sensitivity from an IFN-resistant phenotype, the inhibition of cell growth was not preceded by a significant reduction in the c-*myc* RNA (25). These results indicate that if there is a connection between the expression of the c-*myc* gene and the IFN-mediated inhibition of cell growth it involves more than a reduction in the level of c-*myc* RNA.

CONCLUSION

It has been shown in some cells that IFN treatment causes a decrease in the steady state level of c-*myc* RNA which precedes the cessation of cell growth. However, in other cells IFN treatment causes a cessation in cell growth but no accompanying reduction in the level of c-*myc* RNA. Thus no general correlation between IFN-induced cessation of cell growth and the reduction in c-*myc* RNA can be made at this time. Furthermore there is no rigorous proof at present that the expression of the c-*myc* oncogene is involved in the regulation of cell growth. Further investigation on the effect of IFNs on the expression of c-*myc* RNA is warranted however and may lead to a better understanding of the molecular mechanisms by which IFNs regulate cellular genes. Clearly we have just begun to explore the effect of IFNs on the regulation of oncogenes and future research is likely to reveal complexity rather than simplicity. Research should be expanded to include the protein products of the c-*myc* mRNA since they may be directly involved in the regulation of cell growth.

ACKNOWLEDGEMENTS

We acknowledge the collaboration of our colleagues E. D. Anton and B. Friedland for research on IFN and its effect on the c-myc oncogene. We thank J. Hassel for assistance in the preparation of the manuscript.

REFERENCES

1. Paucker, K., K. Cantell, and W. Henle Virology 17:324, 1962.
2. Todaro, G.J. and H. Green J Virol 1:115, 1967.
3. Chany, C. and M. Vignal J Gen Virol 7:203, 1970.
4. Friedman, R.M. (1986) these proceedings.
5. Jonak, G.J. and E. Knight, Jr. (1986) Interferon and the Regulation of Oncogenes in Interferon 7, ed. I. Gresser, Academic Press.
6. Clemens, M.J. and M.A. McNurlan Biochem J 226:345, 1985.
7. Bishop, J.M. Ann Rev Biochem 52:301, 1983.
8. Cooper, G.M. and M.-A. Lane Biochim Biophys Acta 738:9, 1984.
9. Weinberg, R.A. Science 230:770, 1985.
10. Hann, S.R., C.B. Thompson and R.N. Eisenman Nature (London) 314:366, 1985.
11. Thompson, C.B., P.B. Challoner, P.E. Neiman and M. Groudine Nature (London) 314:363, 1985.
12. Kelly, K., B.H. Cochran, C.D. Stiles, and P. Leder Cell 35:603, 1983.
13. Kelly, K. and U. Siebenlist J Clinical Immunol 5:65, 1985.
14. Reitsma, P.H., P.G. Rothberg, S.M. Astrin, J. Trial, Z. Bar-Shavit, A. Hall, S.L. Teitelbaum and A.J. Kahn Nature (London) 306:492, 1983.
15. Dony, C., M. Kessel and P. Gruss Nature (London) 317:636, 1985.
16. Einat, M., D. Resnitzky and A. Kimchi Nature (London) 313:597, 1985.
17. Einat, M., D. Resnitzky and A. Kimchi Proc Natl Acad Sci USA 82: 7608, 1985.
18. Tominaga, S. and P. Lengyel J Biol Chem 260:1975, 1985.
19. Jonak, G.J. and E. Knight, Jr. Proc Natl Acad Sci USA 81:1747, 1984.
20. Dani, C., N. Mechti, M. Piechaczyk, B. Lebleu, P. Jeanteur and J.M. Blanchard Proc Natl Acad Sci USA 82:4896, 1985.
21. Knight, Jr., Jr., E.D. Anton, D. Fahey, B.K. Friedland and G. Jonak Proc Natl Acad Sci USA 82:1151, 1985a.
22. Jonak, G.J., E.D. Anton. B.K. Friedland, Y.-S. Cheng and E. Knight, Jr. in The Biology of the Interferon System 1984. H. Kirchner and H. Schellekens, editors, Elsevier Science Publishers, 205, 1985.
23. Salehzada, T., J.M. Blanchard, N. Mechti, M. Piechaczyk, C. Dani, P. Jeanteur and B. Lebleu Proceedings of the Sixth International Symposium of the Research Institute: The 2-5A System, B.R.G.Williams and R.H. Silverman, eds. Alan Liss, Inc., New York, in press, 1985.
24. Kelly, J.M., C.S. Gilbert, G.S. Stark and I.M. Kerr Eur J Biochem 153:367, 1985.
25. Dron, M.,Modjtahedi, O. Brison and M.G. Tovey Cell Mol Biology 6:1374, 1985.

43. Interferon-Induced Reversion in Oncogene-Transformed Cells

Robert M. Friedman

Department of Pathology, Uniformed Services University of the Health Sciences, F. Edward Hebert School of Medicine, Bethesda, MD 20814-4799

There are several reports that interferons (IFNS) can reverse the transformed and tumorigenic phenotype of cell lines in vitro. Prolonged IFN treatment was associated with reversion of Moloney murine sarcoma virus-transformed Balb/c (1,2) and several other mouse cell lines (3). Mouse IFNα/β treatment was associated with complete reversion of C3H10T1/2 cells transformed by x-irradiation. Only partial or no reversion at all was found in the same cell line transformed by methylcholanthrene or SV_{40} respectively (4,5).

Treatment of Rous sarcoma virus-transformed rat cells resulted in both reduced synthesis of the product of src, $pp60^{src}$, and decreased expression of the transformed phenotype (6). We have been studying an LTR-activated c-Ha-ras1-transformed mouse cell line, RS485. Prolonged IFN treatment of RS485 cultures resulted in reversion of 1 to 15% of the cells. These revertants were then cloned to yield several lines of morphological revertant cells that did not form colonies in soft agar or tumors in nude mice. Biochemical study of revertants indicated the persistence of the transforming ras DNA, but a 4 to 8-fold reduction in the Ha-ras mRNA and the Ha-ras encoded p21 protein (7).

When the interferon treatment was stopped, a small portion (0.1 to 0.01%) of the cells retransformed, but the great majority and their progeny remained nontransformed. The latter were termed persisting revertants (PRs). The former were cloned to give rise to a series of retransformants that had levels of p21 and p21mRNA equivalent to those of the parental RS485 tumor cells. The PRs lines had several interesting properties.

The opinions or assertions contained herein are the private views of the authors and should not be construed as official or necessarily reflecting the views of the Uniformed Services University of the Health Sciences or the Department of Defense.

Persisting Revertants. PRs retained the morphological and biological properties of non-transformed cells in that they exhibited contact inhibition of growth, and did not form colonies in soft agar, or tumors in nude mice; however, the level of ras mRNA and p21 in PRs was comparable to that in transformed RS485 cells. In addition, the PRs resisted transformation by transforming DNA (the mutant EJ/T24 ras), and by many, but not all of those transforming retroviruses tested. The exception to the latter was Moloney murine sarcoma virus carrying the oncogene mos which could retransform PRs (8). In two previous studies spontaneous (9) or mutagen-induced revertants (10) also resisted transformation by various oncogenes (oncs). Both of latter were not associated with IFN treatment, but these findings taken together with ours suggested that revertants of oncogene-transformed cells may have unexpected properties with respect their resistance to transforming substances.

One other aspect of our studies, which may help to elucidate the special properties of PRs, is that they can be rapidly re-transformed by treatment with 5-azacytidine (5-Aza) an agent that inhibits methylation of DNA. Methylation of DNA is associated with inhibition of its expression, so that 5-Aza often activates specific genes (11). That 5-Aza treatment results in retransformation of PRs suggested that long term incubation with IFN may result in inactivation of a specific gene locus associated with transformation. The product of this locus may be a co-factor, such as a growth factor or an onc, that must act in concert with ras or other oncs to result in cell transformation. Alternatively, the PR status could be the result of the activation by IFN treatment of an onc suppressor factor with activity directed against the expression of several oncogenes.

ACKNOWLEDGEMENTS

I wish to thank Rose Mary Mazzaglia for help in preparing this manuscript. This study was supported by NCI grant R01 CA37351.

REFERENCES

1. Chany, C., and M. Vignal: Effect of prolonged interferon treatment on mouse embryonic fibroblasts transformed by murine sarcoma virus. J Gen Virol 7:203, 1970.
2. Bourgeade, M.-F., S. Rousset, D. Paulin, and C. Chany: Reorganization of the cytoskeleton by interferon in MSV-transformed cells. J Interferon Res 1:323, 1981.
3. Hicks, N.J., A. G. Morris, and D. C. Burke: Partial reversion of the transformed phenotype of murine sarcoma virus-transformed cells in the presence of interferon: a possible mechanism for the anti-tumor effect of interferon. J Cell Sci 49:225, 1981.
4. Brouty-Boye, D., and I. Gresser: Reversibility of the transformed and neoplastic phenotype. I. Progressive reversion of the phenotype of X-ray-transformed C3H10T1/2 cells under prolonged treatment with interferon. Int J Cancer 28:165, 1981.

5. Brouty-Boye, D., Y.-E. Cheng, L. B. Chen: Association of phenotypic reversion of transformed cells induced by interferon with morphological and biochemical changes in the cytoskeleton. Cancer Res 41:4174, 1981.
6. Lin, S.L., E. A. Garber, E. Wang, L. A. Caliguiri, H. Schellekens, A. R. Goldberg, and I. Tamm: Reduced synthesis of $pp60^{src}$ and expression of the transformation-related phenotype in interferon-treated Rous sarcoma virus-transformed rat cells. Molec Cell Biol 3:1656, 1983.
7. Samid. D., E. H. Chang, and R. M. Friedman: Biochemical correlates of phenotypic reversion in interferon-treated mouse cells transformed by a human oncogene. Biochem Biophys Res Commun 119:21, 1984.
8. Samid, D., D. Flessate, and R. M. Friedman: Persistent reversion of ras-transformed cells following interferon treatment: Retransformation by 5 azacytidine, but not by specific oncogenes. Mss submitted for publication, 1986.
9. Norton, J.D., F. Cook, P. C. Roberts, J. P. Clewley, and R. J. Avery: Expression of Kirsten murine sarcoma virus in transformed monoproducer and revertant NIH/3T3 cells: Evidence for cell-mediated resistance to a viral oncogene in phenotypic reversion. J Virol 50:439, 1984.
10. Noda, M., Z. Selinger, E. M. Scolnick, and R. H. Bassin: Flat revertants isolated from Kirsten sarcoma virus-transformed cells are resistant to the action of specific oncogenes. Proc Natl Acad Sci USA 80:5602, 1983.
11. Ruggs, A.D., and P. A. Jones: 5-methylcytosine, gene regulation, and cancer. Adv Cancer Res 40:1, 1983.

[illegible] Chang [illegible] treated [illegible]
6. [illegible] J. R. [illegible] K. [illegible]
7. [illegible] and [illegible]
[illegible]
8. [illegible] Serology [illegible]
9. [illegible] after [illegible] treated with [illegible] cells [illegible]
10. [illegible] cells [illegible]
11. [illegible] cancer. [illegible]

VI. Clinical Use

44. Pharmacokinetics and Toxicities of Interferons

Jorge R. Quesada

Department of Clinical Immunology and Biological Therapy, University of Texas Cancer Center M. D. Anderson Hospital and Tumor Institute, Houston, TX 77030

INTRODUCTION

The purification and eventual production of interferons by molecular cloning in the past 5 years have been necessary steps to a better understanding of the pharmacokinetic properties and toxicities associated with its administration in humans. The availability of some recombinant DNA-produced alpha interferons has permitted treatment of a large number of patients as well as testing of diverse methods of administration and a broad range of doses and treatment schemes. The objective of this chapter is to describe some of the pharmacologic properties and to review the side effects and toxicities associated with administration of interferons in man.

ALPHA INTERFERONS

Partially purified and recombinant alpha interferons are readily absorbed following intramuscular, intraperitoneal or subcutaneous administration. Peak serum concentrations are reached within six to eight hrs. and clearance occurs in approximately 24 hs. IFNα seemingly moves freely from the blood into the extravascular compartments but does not cross the blood-brain barrier well (1).

Administration of low doses of natural IFNα [1-9 million units (MU)] by i.m. or s.c. injection in cancer patients induce fever which coincides approximately with the peak serum levels. The febrile reaction is accompanied by chills, myalgias, headaches and less frequently by arthtralgias and nausea. Most symptoms are easily ameliorated with aspirin, acetaminophen or steroids (2).

The purity of recombinant IFNα (rIFNα) has permitted the use of radioimmunometric or ELISA methods in addition to the bioassay that measures antiviral activity. Gutterman et al. (3) have shown that the mean maximum concentration (Cmax) and the area under the curve (AUC) values increased proportionally with rIFNα administered by i.m. injection. The time of the maximum serum concentration observed (tmax) increased with increasing doses varying from 4.6 hs at 3 MU to 6.1 hs at 72 MU. The half life of rIFNα ranged from 6 to 8 hs regardless of the dose. Fig. 1 depicts the mean serum interferon titers after i.m. administration in doses ranging from 3 to 50 million units. The patient population in this study included patients with multiple myeloma, breast cancer and lymphoma (4).

Quesada and Gutterman (4) have shown that clearance at doses above 36 MU was slowed down with serum interferon titers up to 150 u/ml at 24 hs. IFNα serum concentration measured at 4-6 wks intervals showed that the peak IFNα level was significantly higher ($p = 0.02$) on repeated examination. Sherwin et al. (6) pointed out that with daily administration the levels of serum IFN at 24 hs increased with time. These data suggest a steady-state accumulation of rIFNα.

Patients who are administered rIFNα in doses from 50-120 MU may experience a sharp febrile response with severe rigors, nausea, vomiting, severe myalgias and intense headaches, resulting in exhaustion. In most patients who receive IFN daily, the febrile response and accompanying symptoms usually decrease in intensity, eventually disappearing within 7-10 days. This is followed by the onset of fatigue (weakness, tiredness, lack of desire to participate in normal activities, mental laziness, or absence of motivation). Fatigue is the most common dose-limiting toxic effect of IFNs. Most patients receiving > 20 MU/day will require a dose reduction or discontinuation of treatment, but there is a great range of individual variation in tolerance. In most patients, adaptation occurs at low doses (3-10 MU) permitting continuous treatment for prolonged periods. With intermittent schedules of administration (2-3 times per week), tolerance is better.

With high doses of interferons, significant neurologic abnormalities have become apparent. Somnolence, lethargy, confusion and overall mental and motor slowing may occur. Electroencephalograms tracings are consistent with a diffuse encephalopathy. These toxicities are reversible within days if treatment is discontinued. Behavioral changes also occur at low doses (3 MU/d) consisting of loss of incentive, interest, and verbal and motor spontaneity. Few patients complain of paresthesias, suggestive of a mild sensory-motor neuropathy.

Hematologic effects are very common and appear promptly after administration of IFNs. There is a decrease in the leukocyte, granulocyte and lymphocyte counts which promptly recover when IFN is held. Bone marrow findings are consistent with a reversible block in the release of cells but no arrest in maturation of any cell line (2). Interferon-induced leukopenia has not been associated with an increased incidence of infections in cancer patients with normal pretreatment blood counts. Other toxicities include normocytic normochronic anemia and thrombocytopenia.

Gastrointestinal (GI) toxicity consists of anorexia, nausea, vomiting, and diarrhea. In general, the higher the dose, the more frequent the occurrence of GI symptoms. Elevation of transaminase levels is observed in approximately 25%-30% of patients, but may be as high as 80% in patients receiving doses of ≥ 50 MU (5). The most common renal toxicity is proteinuria which affects 15%-20% of patients. Acute renal failure and nephrotic syndrome have been reported (2).

Kidneys seem to be the main organ of catabolism of IFNα. Bocci et al. (1) have shown that IFNα passes in large amounts into the glomerular filtrate and is subsequently degraded by the tubules, resulting in minimal urinary excretion. The pharmacokinetics of either rIFNα or IFNα are not altered significantly in chronic renal failure (2).

There is very limited pharmacologic information regarding i.v. administration in humans. Because of the ready absorption by other methods of administration, this route has not been favored in human studies. Bocci has, however, summarized results of i.v. injections in other species indicating the very steep decay of plasma concentrations (1).

BETA AND GAMMA INTERFERONS

In contrast to alpha IFNs, serum levels of natural IFNβ

or IFNγ are negligible following i.m. or s.c. administration, although i.v. kinetics are similar to IFNα. Despite the absence of measurable serum titer, Quesada et al. (7) have shown evidence of biologic activities, including antitumor effects in patients with breast cancer. Similarly, no detectable serum levels were found after i.m. injections of natural IFNγ (8). This particular behavior may be related to the molecular properties of these IFNs. Binding of their carbohydrate moities to tissue or local catabolism following i.m. injection have been proposed to explain these pharmacologic data.

Clearance after i.v. bolus administration is similar among the different IFNs. However, in contrast to IFNα, granulocytopenia occurred only when IFNγ was administered over 6 to 24 infusion, confirming that the pharmacologic behavior is related to the biologic effects elicited (8). Similar findings were obtained subsequently using rIFNγ (9). The half life of rIFNγ by the i.v. route was 25-35 min and its clearance pattern fitted a one compartment mathematical model, whereas i.m. rIFNγ had a half life of 227-462 min and was compatible with a two-compartment model (9). The clinical side effects and toxicities of IFNγ are similar to those described for IFNα. The severity of the constitutional symptoms by continuous infusion was dose limiting at doses 10 times lower than those seen by the i.m. route. Fever with IFNγ is more protracted, headaches are more frequent and severe and abnormalities of liver function tests may also be more severe than with comparable doses of IFNα (10). Distinctly, IFNγ produces hypertryglyceridemia (9,10).

Antibodies to IFN

Development of neutralizing antibodies to partially pure IFNα or IFNβ occurs in less than 1% of patients whereas the incidence of antibodies to recombinant IFNα varies from 0 to 10% in several studies. A higher incidence (38%) has been observed in patients with renal cell carcinoma (2). Clinically, the development of antibodies to rIFNαA may coincide with an improvement in IFN-induced toxicities. Serum IFN levels after injection are greatly reduced or absent when antibodies are present (3,4).

Non-neutralizing antibodies have been reported in patients receiving recombinant IFNβ. Antibodies to IFNγ have not been detected or reported so far.

No adverse clinical effects have been related to these antibodies. However, in some responsive patients, tumor relapses have occurred coincidentally with the development of neutralizing antibodies, suggesting that the antibodies may abrogate the biologic effects of IFNs in vivo (2,3,4).

CONCLUSIONS

Increasing knowledge of the pharmacokinetic properties of the different IFNs has allowed better design of clinical studies in humans. The toxicities associated to most frequent, prolonged exposure and to the administration of high doses of IFNs has been identified and described. Because future trends will include the combination of these different species of IFNs as well as the combinations of IFNs with other biologic agents, application of this knowledge will be fundamental to the design of such combination studies.

ACKNOWLEDGEMENTS

We wish to thank Linda Reckeweg for the preparation of this chapter.

REFERENCES

1. Bocci V: Distribution, catabolism and pharmacokinetics of interferons. In Finter N.B. and Oldham R.K. eds: Interferon: In vivo and clinical studies. Elsevier Science Pub. 1985, pp. 47.

2. Quesada JR, Talpaz M, Rios A, Kurzrock R, and Gutterman JU: Clinical toxicity of interferons in cancer patients: A Review. J Clin Oncology 4:234, 1986.

3. Gutterman JU, Fine S, Quesada JR, Horning SJ, Levine JF, Alexanian R, Bernhardt L, Kramer M, Spiegel H, Colburn W, Trown P, Merigan T, and Dziewanowski Z: Recombinant leukocyte A interferon: pharmacokinetics single-dose tolerance, and biologic effects in cancer patients. Ann Int Med 96:549, 1982.

4. Quesada JR, Hawkins M, Horning S, Alexanian R, Borden E, Merigan T, Adams F, and Gutterman JU: A collaborative phase I-II study of recombinant DNA-produced leukocyte interferon (Clone A) in metastatic breast cancer, malignant lymphoma, and multiple myeloma. Am J Med 77:427-432, 1984.

5. Quesada JR and Gutterman JU: Clinical study of recombinant DNA-produced leukocyte interferon (Clone A) in an intermittent schedule in cancer patients. JNCI 70:1041, 1983.

6. Sherwin SA, Knost JA, Fein S, et al.: A multiple-dose phase I trial of recombinant leukocyte A interferon in cancer patients. JAMA 248:2461, 1982.

7. Quesada JR, Gutterman JU, and Hersh EM: Clinical and immunological study of beta interferon by intramuscular route in patients with metastatic breast cancer. J Interferon Res 2:593, 1982.

8. Gutterman JU, Rosenblum MG, Rios A, Fritsche A, and Quesada JR: Pharmacokinetic study of partially pure γ-interferon in cancer patients. Cancer Res 44:4164, 1984.

9. Kurzrock R, Rosenblum MG, Sherwin SA, Rios A, Talpaz M, Quesada JR, and Gutterman JU: Pharmacokinetics, single-dose tolerance, and biological activity of recombinant γ-interferon in cancer patients. Cancer Res 45:2866, 1985.

10. Quesada JR, Kurzrock R, Sherwin SA, and Gutterman JU: Phase II studies of recombinant human interferon gamma in metastatic renal cell carcinoma. J Biol Resp Modif (in press).

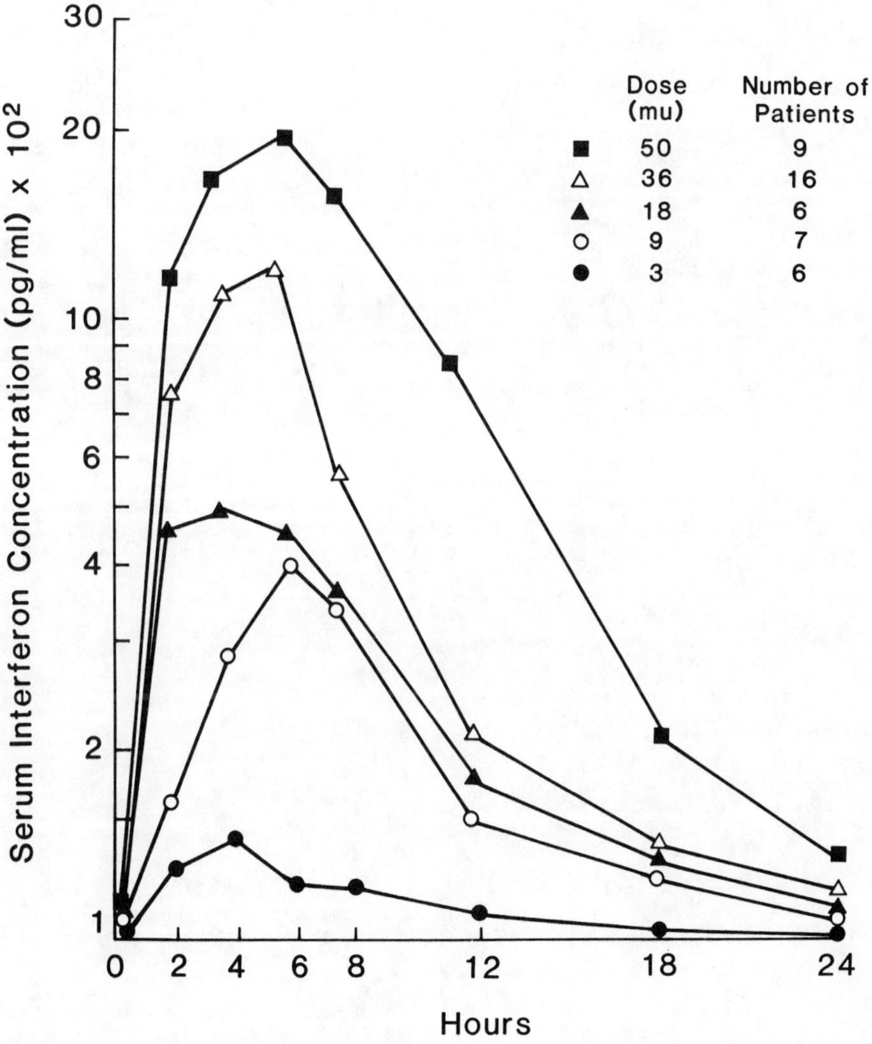

Fig. 1. Median serum concentration of rIFNα measured by enzyme immunoassay, in patients with advanced cancer.

45. Biological Response Modification in Man: Measurement of Interferon-Induced Proteins

E. Borden, D. Paulnock, G. Spear, G. Byrne, J. Merritt, R. Brown

Departments of Human Oncology and Medical Microbiology, University of Wisconsin, Madison, WI 53792

Interferons (IFNs) are prototypic biological response modifiers. Using preclinical studies as guides, it has been possible to identify in treated patients many of the biochemical and cellular effects which have been defined in vitro. Immune effector cell function is modulated (1,2). Proteins of identified function induced include those with 2-5 oligoadenylate synthetase activity (2-5A synthetase), protein kinase, those of the major histocompatibility complex (MHC), and indolamine 2-3 dioxygenase (IDO) Quantitation of an IFN-specific protein response may be a more accurate reflection of biological effectiveness in tissues than measurement of drug serum levels of drug. In this paper, we will focus on protein changes induced in vivo by human IFN. Proteins will be discussed in turn with a presentation of both literature review and specific examples.

MHC Proteins

The protein, first identified as increased in patients receiving IFN, was β_2 microglobulin, a molecule associated with cell surface MHC proteins (3). In vitro, both increased mRNA and augmented protein expression, had been defined (4,5). IFNα at doses of 10×10^6 units resulted in increased serum β_2 microglobulin (3). With continued daily administration of IFNα intramuscularly (i.m.), β_2 microglobulin remained increased over the baseline (6). Of the 8 patients evaluated, increases occurred in all (6).

With IFNγ administration, increases in β_2 microglobulin were almost universal. Of 8 patients assessed 24 hrs after continuous intravenous (i.v.) administration, increases occurred in all (7). Of measurements after i.m. IFNγ, 2- to 5-fold enhancement was found in serum β_2 microglobulin in 17/20 specimens obtained after 2 weeks of daily injections (8). The response was quite sensitive; an i.m. dose of 0.01 mg/M^2 resulted in an increase (8).

All non-erythroid cells normally express β_2 microglobulin. It has not yet been determined which cells result in the increase in serum β_2

microglobulin. Increases in β2 microglobulin on peripheral mononuclear cells (PMC) were identified after IFNαA i.m. (9). Enhancement was found after 24 hrs with return to baseline by 72 hrs after a dose (9). By cell sorting analysis, this increase was associated with a small lymphocyte fraction. One additional cell type which has been defined as having increased β2 microglobulin is the monocyte. We have identified augmented β2 microglobulin expression on monocytes after $IFN\beta_{ser}$ (G.T. Spear *et al.*, submitted). Essentially all monocytes expressed β2 microglobulin prior to treatment. However, the intensity of antigen expression was modestly but almost always ($p<.02$, sign test, two sided) increased when measured 48 hrs later (Figure 1). We have also identified increased β2 microglobulin on monocytes after IFNγ (D. Paulnock *et al.*, manuscript in preparation).

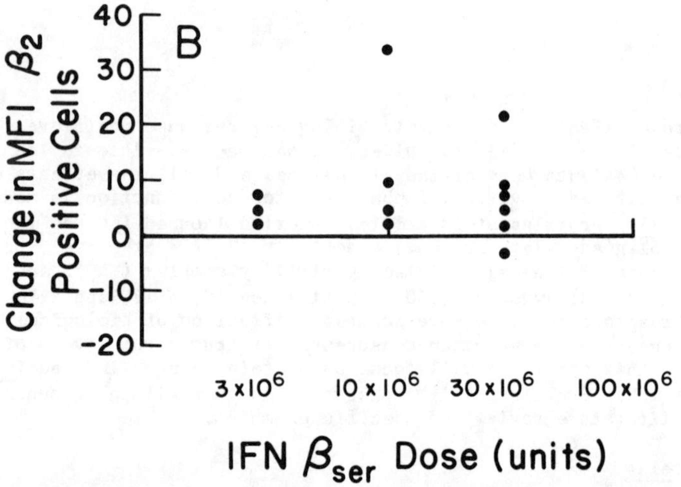

Figure 1. Change in fluorescent intensity of monocytes stained for β2 microglobulin after $IFN\beta_{ser}$. After i.v. injections of $IFN\beta_{ser}$, at 48 hrs peripheral mononuclear cells were collected, isolated on Ficoll-hypaque gradients, stained with anti-β2 microglobulin and fluoresceinated anti-mouse IgG (Becton-Dickinson, Mountain View, CA). Mean fluorescent intensity (MFI) quantitated in the monocyte fraction by fluorescent-activated cell sorter. Each point represents the change in a single patient from baseline before $IFN\beta_{ser}$.

Since β2 microglobulin is filtered at the glomerulus, urine β2 microglobulin has also been evaluated (10). Significant increases in urine β2 microglobulin were confirmed after IFNα2. Increases in another urine protein, albumin, were not observed in the same samples (10).

Specificity of the increase in β2 microglobulin has been demonstrated by parallel measurements in normal individuals and in cancer patients. No significant changes occurred in small lymphocyte or serum β2 microglobulin in two serial evaluations at a 24 hr interval of 10 healthy controls (11). In cancer patients starting cytotoxic chemotherapy, measurements were undertaken at times corresponding to assessments of patients receiving IFNα (6). No β2 microglobulin increase could be identified.

Despite demonstration of induction of MHC-specific mRNA and protein by IFN in vitro (4,5), other components of the MHC have not been frequently assessed in vivo. Enhanced HLA Class I protein expression on peripheral lymphocytes has been identified 24 hrs after $50x10^6$ units i.m. of IFNαA (11). No corresponding increase occurred in a group of normal individuals not receiving IFN (11). Augmentation in HLA Class II components on monocytes occurred within 48 hrs after initiation of $IFN\beta_{ser}$, $3-30x10^6$ units i.v. (G.T. Spear et al., submitted). Both HLA-DR and HLA-DQ component proteins were significantly enhanced. At doses $\geq 10x10^6$ units, increases in the percent of monocytes positive for HLA-DR were identified in almost all patients (Figure 2). At this dose, the number of monocytes expressing identifiable HLA-DR protein increased significantly (p=.02, sign test, two sided). The increase in HLA-DQ was even more marked with an almost 20% average increase occurring in the number of monocytes expressing this protein. No corresponding increase in a non-specific monocyte marker protein, LeuM3, occurred. Since increase in these MHC Class II components on monocyte-macrophages has been associated with augmented immune responsiveness, such increases may be pivotal in mediating biological effects on IFN. Increase in MHC Class II components has also been documented after IFNγ. After 8d and 15d (but not 3d) of daily i.m. injections, a significantly increased number of peripheral mononuclear cells expressed Class II protein (8). After i.v. administration, enhanced expression of monocyte HLA-DR and DQ proteins were documented. Peak increases occurred within 24 hrs and remained increased for 24-72 hrs (D. Paulnock et al., in preparation).

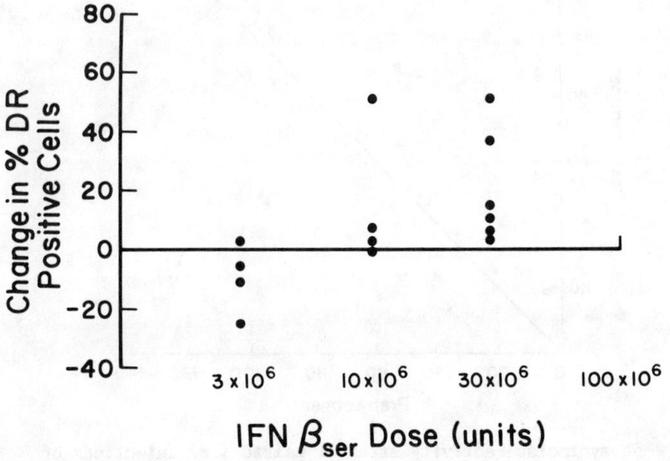

Figure 2. Change in percent of monocytes positive for HLA-DR according to $IFN\beta_{ser}$ dose. Methods are similar to Figure 1 except use of anti-HLA-DR.

2-5A Synthetase

While the exact role of the 2-5A synthetase system in the biologic activity of IFN is not yet clear, increase in 2-5A synthetase activity has been a sensitive indicator of in vitro treatment with IFN. PMC exhibit relatively low but consistent levels of 2-5A synthetase (12). After i.m. injections of IFNα, activity in PMC rose approximately 2 to 10 fold (13). Although the dose required for maximum stimulation of any particular individual varied, overall increased responses occurred with increased dose of IFNα (13). Above doses of $1x10^6$ units, increase in enzyme activity 24 hrs after IFNα was highly significant. IFNα did not, however, regularly produce 2-5A synthetase increase over pretreatment levels in patients with AIDS (14). These patients frequently had increased 2-5A synthetase in PMC prior to exogenous IFN and none of the AIDS patients tested (n=11) had a normal increase after incubation of PMC with IFNα in vitro (14). Serum pharmacokinetics are markedly altered by changing the route of IFN from i.m. to i.v. Yet the 2-5A synthetase response was equivalent when the same dose of IFNα was administered either i.m. or i.v. to six patients. $IFN\beta_{ser}$, given by the i.m. route, resulted in only sporadic and minimal IFN levels in serum (15). Yet, in all patients tested, 2-5A synthetase was increased at 24 hrs when compared with basal levels in PMC from the same patients (Figure 3). Thus, induction and maintenance of a biological response to IFN has been identified in the absence of serum IFN, a pharmacodynamic finding of some significance in the design of clinical therapeutic programs.

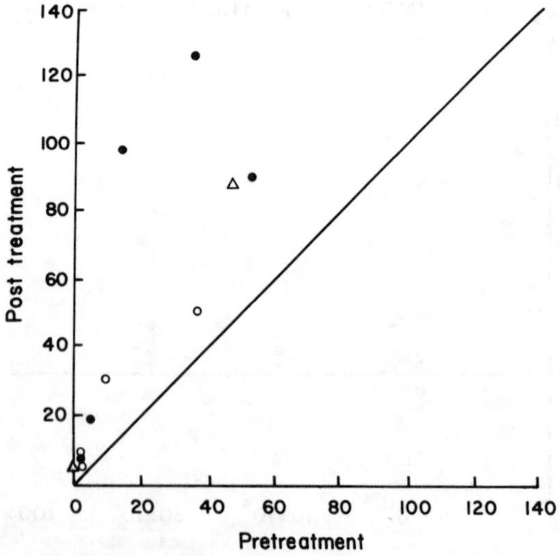

Figure 3. 2-5A synthetase activity after 11 paired i.m. injections of $IFN\beta_{ser}$. Samples obtained at 1×10^6 (○), 10×10^6 (Δ) and 60×10^6 units (●). Frequency of increase $p<.01$ (sign test, two sided). Analysis performed on extracts from peripheral mononuclear cells (12).

More than 20 separate genes and several synthetic hybrid genes for IFN exist. Since the gene products of these loci differ in biological effects, it has been difficult to choose which IFN to develop for clinical trials. Two IFNs α, differing in antiviral potency _in vitro_, were assessed in a Phase I clinical trial (16). When assessed at equal weight doses, an equivalent stimulation of 2-5A synthetase in PMC resulted (16). Thus, measurement of IFN-induced proteins can perhaps serve as a point of reference for comparison of different IFNs.

Indolamine-2,3-Dioxygenase

When human lung fibroblasts were treated with various concentrations of IFNγ, they were found to degrade the essential amino acid tryptophan in a dose and time-dependent manner (17). Similarly, human bladder carcinoma cells were induced to catabolize tryptophan after incubation with IFNγ, but no activity was observed in untreated cells or cells treated with either $IFN\beta_{ser}$ or IFNα. When tryptophan plasma levels were measured in patients who had received i.v. injections of IFNγ as part of a Phase I clinical trial, decreased tryptophan levels were observed when compared to pretreatment values or values obtained from individuals who had received i.v. injections of huIFNα (17). Urine samples from patients who received IFNγ had elevated kynurenine levels when compared to pretreatment levels (17). This result has been confirmed in measurement of kynurenine in urine of subsequent patients receiving IFNγ (Figure 4). Tryptophan degradation was thus induced _in vitro_ and _in vivo_ in response to exogenous IFNγ.

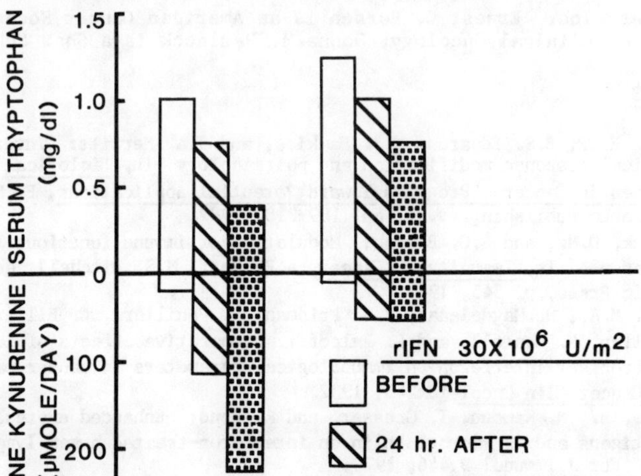

Figure 4. Serum tryptophan and urine kynurenine levels in two patients prior to and then 24 hours and 48 hours after an i.v. dose of 30 x 10^6 units/m^2 of recombinant IFN γ. Serum tryptophan was measured by fluorometric analyis and urine kynurenine was assayed by colorimetric methods (17).

CONCLUSIONS

IFNs are the first biological response modifiers prepared by recombinant DNA technology to impact on treatment of human disease. Underlying therapeutic effects are the selective modulation of gene expression, influence on immune effector cell activity, and altered mitotic and cytological function. Based upon alterations in biological parameters, results of current Phase I and Phase II trials have begun to suggest some possible dose and schedule alterations and allow beginning analysis of structure function relationships. Ultimately, however, for optimal clinical use, studies must better define correlation between biological effects and therapeutic outcome. Definition of which biological effect is most critical will result from Phase III clinical trials.

Use of IFN in conjunction with other therapeutic modalities is just beginning to be probed. Such studies involve an almost infinite number of variables of schedule, route, and timing of IFN administration. Optimal therapeutic use will thus depend even more critically on judicious studies of biological response modification. These will almost certainly include quantitation of changes in the IFN-induced proteins, which have been selectively increased by IFN *in vitro* and in man.

ACKNOWLEDGEMENTS

Studies described in this article were conducted with support from the National Institutes of Health (NO1-CM-07434, CA 21115) and Triton Biosciences, Inc. Ernest C. Borden is an American Cancer Society Professor of Clinical Oncology; Donna M. Paulnock is a Shaw Scholar.

REFERENCES

1. Borden, E.C., B.S. Edwards, M.J. Hawkins, and J.A. Merritt: Interferons: biological response modification and pharmacology. In, *Biological Responses in Cancer: Progress Toward Potential Applications*, E. Mihich, ed., Plenum Publishing, v. 1, pp. 169-218, 1982.
2. Paulnock, D.M., and E.C. Borden: Modulation of immune functions by interferons. In, *Immunity to Cancer*, A.E. Reif, M.S. Mitchell, eds., Academic Press, p. 545, 1985.
3. Lucero, M.A., H. Magdelenat, W.H. Fridman, P. Pouillart, C. Billardon, A. Billiau, K. Cantell, and E. Falcoff: Comparative effects of leukocyte and fibroblast interferon on immunological parameters in cancer patients. *Eur J Cancer Clin Oncol* 18:243, 1982.
4. Fellous, M., M. Kamoun, I. Gresser, and R. Bond: Enhanced expression of HLA-antigens and β2 microglobulin on interferon-treated human lymphoid cells. *Eur J Immunol* 9:446, 1979.
5. Fellous, M., U. Nir, D. Wallach, G. Merlin, and M. Rubinstein: Interferon-dependent induction of mRNA for the major histocompatibility antigens in human fibroblasts and lymphoblastoid cells. *Proc Natl Acad Sci* 79:3082, 1982.
6. Borden, E.C., J.F. Holland, T.L. Dao, J.U. Gutterman, L. Wiener, Y-C. Chang, and J. Patel: Leukocyte-derived interferon (α) in human breast carcinoma. The American Cancer Society Phase II Trial. *Ann Int Med* 97:1, 1982.

7. Gutterman, J.U., M.G. Rosenblum, A. Rios, H.A. Fritsche, and J.R. Quesada: Pharmacokinetic study of partially pure γ-interferon in cancer patients. Cancer Res 44:4164, 1984.
8. Kurzrock, R., J.R. Quesada, M. Talpaz, E.M. Hersh, J.M. Reuben, S.A. Sherwin, and J.U. Gutterman: Phase I study of multiple dose intramuscularly administered recombinant gamma interferon. Cancer Treat Rep, in press, 1986.
9. Horning, S.J., J.F. Levine, R.A. Miller, S.A. Rosenberg, and T.C. Merigan: Clinical and immunologic effects of recombinant leukocyte A interferon in eight patients with advanced cancer. JAMA 247:1718, 1982.
10. Sumpio, B.E., M.S. Ernstoff, and J.M. Kirkwood: Urinary excretion of interferon, albumin, and β_2-microglobulin during interferon treatment. Cancer Res 44:3599, 1984.
11. Nissen, M.H., T. Plesner, J.K. Larsen, B.K. Olesen, and P. Ernst: Enhanced expression in vivo of HLA-ABC antigens and β_2-microglobulin on human lymphoid cells induced by human interferon-α in patients with lung cancer. Enhanced expression of class I major histocompatibility antigens prior to treatment. Clin Exp Immunol 59:327, 1985.
12. Merritt, J.A., E.C. Borden, and L.A. Ball: Measurement of 2',5'-oligoadenylate synthetase in patients receiving interferon-alpha. J Ifn Res 5:191, 1985.
13. Merritt, J.A., L.A. Ball, K.M. Sielaff, D.M. Meltzer, and E.C. Borden: Modulation of 2',5'-oligoadenylate synthetase in patients treated with alpha-interferon: effects of dose, schedule and route of administration. J Ifn Res 6:189, 1986.
14. Preble, O.T., A.H. Rook, R. Steis, R.H. Silverman, D. Krause, G.V. Quinnan, H. Masur, J. Jacob, D. Longo, and E.P. Gelmann: Interferon-induced 2'-5' oligoadenylate synthetase during interferon-α therapy in homosexual men with Kaposi's sarcoma: marked deficiency in biochemical response to interferon in patients with acquired immunodeficiency syndrome. J Infect Dis 152:457, 1985.
15. Hawkins, M.J., S. Horning, M. Konrad, S. Anderson, K. Sielaff, S. Rosno, J. Schiesel, T. Davis, D. DeMets, T. Merigan, and E. Borden: Phase I evaluation of a synthetic mutant of interferon β. Cancer Res 45:5914, 1985.
16. Hawkins, M.J., E.C. Borden, J.A. Merritt, B.S. Edwards, L.A. Ball, E. Grossbard, and K.J. Simon: Comparison of the biologic effects of two recombinant human interferons alpha (rA and rD) in humans. J Clin Oncol 2:221, 1984.
17. Byrne, G.I., L.K. Lehmann, J.G. Kirschbaum, E.C. Borden, C.M. Lee, and R.R. Brown: Induction of tryptophan degradation in vitro and in vivo: a gamma interferon-stimulated activity. J Ifn Res, in press, 1986.

46. Interferon for Respiratory Virus Infections in Man

S. B. Greenberg and R. B. Couch

Departments of Medicine, Microbiology, and Immunology, Baylor College of Medicine, Houston, TX 77030

INTRODUCTION

Volunteer challenge experiments and field trials using intranasal administration of crude preparations of human leukocyte interferon (HuIFN) showed variable efficacy against several respiratory viral infections (2,10,24,31,39,41). No significant side effects were reported. Included in these studies were volunteer challenge experiments which demonstrated that HuIFN was effective in reducing rhinovirus infection and illness (10,11,26,38).

Because of the variable effectiveness and apparent large dose requirement of HuIFN in these early studies, a number of factors were evaluated which could have accounted for the results (3,9,12,13,14,25). These studies indicated that human nasal epithelial cells (NECs) could be made antiviral, although the magnitude of the antiviral state and the slope of the dose response curve were lower in these cells compared to standard human foreskin fibroblasts. In addition, when parainfluenza virus type 3 and coxsackie A21 virus were compared with vesicular stomatitis virus (the standard virus for NEC studies), a reduced level of inhibition by HuIFN in NECs was found (13). Alternatively, previous studies had shown that inhaled particles in the nose were rapidly removed over a 20-30 minute period (1). Johnson et al (25) and Merigan et al (26) found a rapid decline in recoverable HuIFN following intranasal application. Thus, these combined studies using HuIFN for acute respiratory disease suggested that it could be effective for prevention of viral infection and disease, especially when caused by a rhinovirus.

Because of the inherent difficulties in providing HuIFN, alternative sources for human use were needed. IFN-α from stimulation of lymphoblastoid cells with virus was one proposed source; this material was shown to be effective in volunteer studies against a rhinovirus challenge (30). However, the availability of IFN from *Escherichia coli* using recombinant DNA techniques in the early 1980's provided the major stimulus to reevaluation of IFN for acute respiratory virus infections.

CLINICAL STUDIES WITH RECOMBINANT INTERFERON (rIFN)

Recent studies performed with rIFN in volunteers have clearly demonstrated significant antiviral activity for rhinoviruses (Table 1). Samo et al (32,33) showed a significant reduction in illness frequency when either 2.4 or 10 X 10^6 units of rIFN was sprayed intranasally before and for three days following challenge with rhinovirus type 13. No significant reduction in infection rate was observed in these same volunteers. Scott et al (36), Hayden and Gwaltney (16), and Phillpotts et al (29) using a similar schedule found an anti-illness effect with higher daily doses of rIFN, but a significantly reduced infection rate in the IFN treated volunteers was also seen. Turner et al (4) has reported an anti-illness effect but no anti-viral effect of intranasally administered rIFN on coronavirus infection in volunteers. More recently, a dose of rIFN-β given as 6 X 10^6 units/day intranasally for four days was shown to reduce symptom scores and virus isolation frequency among volunteers challenged with a rhinovirus (23). Other volunteer studies, using IFN prophylaxis and influenza virus challenge, have demonstrated some modest effect on illness reduction but variable reduction in infection frequency (5,34). Thus, these studies using rIFN-α for prophylaxis of virus infection confirmed the effectiveness of HuIFN for rhinovirus, provided dose response data for infection and illness, and suggested that coronavirus and influenza virus infections may also be preventable.

In therapeutic studies, Hayden and Gwaltney (15) recently reported some reduction in duration of virus shedding in volunteers inoculated with rhinovirus and a minimal reduction in illness. The dose of rIFN-α that was used in these experiments was approximately 20 X 10^6 units a day for four days beginning 24 hours after virus inoculation. Higgins et al (22) performed a similar study using approximately 35 X 10^6 units a day for four days after challenge with coronavirus 229E. These investigators recorded more significant reduction in illness frequency and decrease in virus shedding among volunteers who had received the rIFN-α after virus challenge.

Several recent studies have examined the prophylactic effect of exogenous rIFN-α against natural respiratory viral infection. rIFN-α was given intranasally in a double-blind, placebo-controlled study in healthy working adults (7,18,20). The frequency of tracheobronchitis symptoms was lower in those who received 10 X 10^6 units of rIFNα compared to placebo. Although the overall rate of illness was significantly higher in the IFN-α recipients during the second and third weeks of treatment, a significant reduction in rhinovirus related illness was demonstrated in the rIFN-α treated adults. Local side reactions occurred in 40 rIFN-α recipients compared with 3 placebo recipients during the third week and included nasal obstruction, blood-tinged nasal mucus, and superficial mucosal ulcerations.

Recently published studies have demonstrated a dose-dependent increase in local reactions in volunteers sprayed with rIFN-α. Samo et al reported local side reactions that included nasal stuffiness, blood tinged mucus, and occurrence of mucosal erosions (32,33). These local reactions ranged from 5% of volunteers who had received 0.7 X 10^6

units daily to 25% of those who had received 10 X 10^6 units daily. All local side reactions in these studies as well as those reported during prophylaxis studies of natural infection disappeared after discontinuation of therapy. Similar local reactions had been observed earlier by Scott et al (35,37), and have recently been reported in a field trial of 2.5 X 10^6 units of rIFN against natural infection (28). To define further the pathogenesis of these local changes, Hayden et al (19) performed sequential nasal biopsies in volunteers given rIFN-α and demonstrated an influx of mononuclear cells that had characteristics of T-lymphocytes within a few days after the onset of spraying. Followup nasal biopsies after discontinuation of the rIFN showed a return to normal appearance. Whether the in vitro cellular infiltration demonstrated after intranasal administration of rIFN completely explains the in vivo local reactions remains to be clarified; several volunteers who were found to have the cellular infiltration did not have local symptoms.

Two studies have been reported in abstract form on the administration of intranasal rIFN-α in both asthmatic adult and pediatric patients. These are the only reported studies to look at the potential use of rIFN-α in a high-risk population such as those with chronic pulmonary disease. In the study by Geha et al(8), children received a dose of 2 X 10^6 units a day for approximately four weeks. The number of days with asthmatic symptoms was significantly less in the rIFN-α group compared with placebo; this was especially true in asthmatic children under the age of 12. In the study by Michaels et al (27) there were no significant difference in frequency of colds or positive viral cultures in the rIFN-α treated patients. Most of the virus isolates in this study were rhinovirus; so, no significant anti-rhinoviral effect was demonstrated. In both studies, the rIFN-α was well tolerated with only mild nasal irritation occurring.

Rhinoviruses are thought to be spread primarily within families. Three recently published studies have defined the prophylactic efficacy of rIFN-α in a family setting (6,17,21). In an abstract report, 1.5 X 10^6 units of rIFN given to contacts of sick family members was associated with a slight reduction in illness and no apparent effect on infection (21). Little specific data relating to virus isolation and serology was given in this abstract. In two large family studies, significant reduction in rhinovirus related illness and infection was observed in those family members taking intranasal rIFN-α after exposure to a family member with an acute upper respiratory illness (6,17). Both Douglas et al (17) and Hayden et al (2) found similar results in the double-blind placebo-controlled studies employing 5 X 10^6 units of rIFN-α for 7 days. Although a significant anti-rhinoviral effect was demonstrated, no protection was found against influenza viruses, parainfluenza viruses or coronaviruses. In addition, local side reactions were present in increased numbers in the rIFN-α treated subjects compared with the placebo controls.

CONCLUSIONS

With the introduction of rIFN, several recent studies have defined the potential use of this antiviral agent in respiratory virus infections. The confirmation of the rhinovirus volunteer challenge studies by recent field trial results demonstrates the usefulness of this model for testing the in vivo efficacy of various doses and preparations of rIFN. The recently published post-exposure family contact studies have documented the ability of an antiviral agent, specifically rIFN, to interrupt the transmission of a rhinovirus infection within the epidemiologic unit of the family. Although both the field trials and tolerance studies have defined the extent of rIFN's local side reactions and the excellent anti-rhinoviral activity, reduction of these local reactions and/or broadening of the in vivo antiviral effect will determine its eventual utility for acute respiratory infections.

REFERENCES

1. Aoki, F.Y., and J. Crawley: Distribution and removal of human serum albumin-technetium 99 instilled intranasally by drops and spray. Br J Clin Pharmacol 3:869, 1976.
2. Arnaudova, V.: Treatment and prevention of acute respiratory virus infections in children with leukocytic interferon. Rev Roum Med-Virol 27:83, 1976.
3. Came P.E., T.W. Schafer, and G.H. Silver: Sensitivity of rhinoviruses to human leukocyte and fibroblast interferons. J Infect Dis (Suppl.) 133:A136, 1976.
4. Davies, H.W, G.M. Scott, J.A. Robinson, P.G. Higgins, R. Wootton, and D.A.J. Tyrrell: Comparative intranasal pharmacokinetics of interferon using two spray systems. J Interferon Res 3:443, 1983.
5. Dolin, R., R. Betts, J. Treanor, S. Erb, S.K. Roth, and R.C. Reichman: Intranasally administered rIFN-α as prophylaxis against experimentally induced influenza in man. In: Proceedings of the 13th International Congress of Chemotherapy, abstract, SE-4. 7/1-7, 1983.
6. Douglas, R.M., B. W. Moore, H.B. Miles, L.M. Davis, N.M.H. Graham, P. Ryan, D.A. Worswick, and J.K. Albrecht: Prophylactic efficacy of intranasal alpha interferon against rhinovirus infections in the family setting. N Engl J Med 314:65, 1986.
7. Farr, B.M., J.M. Gwaltney, K.F. Adams, and F.G. Hayden: Intranasal interferon-α2 for prevention of natural rhinovirus colds. Antimicrob Agents Chemother. 26:31, 1984.
8. Geha, R., J. Maguire, K. McIntosh, and C. Meschievitz: A trial of intranasal alpha interferon in asthmatic children. [Abstract] J Allergy Clin Immunol 77(suppl 1):160, 1986.
9. Greenberg, S.B, M.W. Harmon, P.E. Johnson, and R.B Couch: Antiviral activity of intranasally applied human leukocyte interferon. Antimicrob Agents Chemother 14:596, 1978.
10. Greenberg, S.B. and M.W. Harmon: Clinical use of interferons: Localized application in viral diseases. In: Interferons and Their Application, Handbook of Experimental Pharmacology, P.E. Came and W.A. Carter, eds. Springer-Verlag, Vol 71, pp 433, 1984.
11. Greenberg, S.B., M.W. Harmon, R.B, Couch, P.E. Johnson, S.Z.Wilson, C.C. Dacso, K. Bloom, and J. Quarles: Prophylactic effect of low doses of human leukocyte interferon against infection with rhinovirus. J Infect Dis 145:542, 1982.
12. Harmon, M.W., S.B. Greenberg, and R.B. Couch: Effect of human nasal secretions on the antiviral activity of human fibroblast and leukocyte interferon. Proc Soc Exp Biol Med 142:598, 1976.

13. Harmon, M.W., S.B. Greenberg, P.E. Johnson, and R.B. Couch: Human nasal epithelial cell culture system: Evaluation of response to human interferons. Infect Immun 16:480, 1977.
14. Harmon, M.W., S.B. Greenberg, and P.E. Johnson: Rapid onset of the interferon-induced antiviral state in human nasal epithelial and foreskin fibroblast cells. Proc Soc Exp Biol Med 164:146, 1980.
15. Hayden, F.G and J.M. Gwaltney: Intranasal interferon-α2 treatment of experimental rhinoviral colds. J Infect Dis 150:174, 1984.
16. Hayden, F.G. and J.M. Gwaltney: Intranasal interferon α2 for prevention of rhinovirus infection and illness. J Infect Dis 148: 543, 1983.
17. Hayden, F.G., J.K. Albrecht, D.L. Kaiser, and J.M. Gwaltney,Jr: Prevention of natural colds by contact prophylaxis with intranasal $alpha_2$-interferon. N Engl J Med 314:71, 1986.
18. Hayden, F.G., J.M. Gwaltney, Jr, and M.E. Johns: Prophylactic efficacy and tolerance of low-dose intranasal interferon-alpha, in natural respiratory viral infections. Antiviral Res 5:111, 1985.
19. Hayden, F.G., S.E. Mills, and M.E. Johns: Human tolerance and histopathologic effects of long-term administration of intranasal interferon-α2. J Infect Dis 148:914, 1983.
20. Hayden, F.G., J.M. Gwaltney, Jr. amd M.E. Johns: Prophylactic efficacy and tolerance of low-dose intranasal $interferon-alpha_2$ in natural respiratory viral infections. Antiviral Res 5:111, 1985.
21. Herzog, Ch., R. Berger, M. Fernex, K. Friesecke, L. Havas, M. Just, U.C. Dubach: Intranasal interferon (rIFN- A) for contact prophylaxis against common cold: A randomized, double-blind placebo controlled study. In: The Biology of the Interferon System 1984, H. Kirchker and H. Schellekins, Elsevier Science Publishers B.V. p 581, 1985.
22. Higgins, P.G., R.J. Phillpotts, G.M. Scott, J. Wallace, L.L. Bernhardt, D.A.J. Tyrrell: Intranasal interferon as protection against experimental respiratory coronavirus infection in volunteers. Antimicrob Agents Chemother 24:713, 1983.
23. Higgins, P.G., W. Al-Nakib, J. Willman, and D.A.J. Tyrrell: Interferon-β_{ser} as prophylaxis against experimental rhinovirus infection in volunteers. J Interferon Res 6:153, 1986.
24. Isomura, S., T. Icgujawa, M. Miyazu, H. Naruse, M. Shibata, J. Imanishi, A. Matsuo, T. Kishida, and T. Karaki. The preventive effect of human interferon-alpha on influenza infection; modification of clinical manifestations of influenza in children in a closed community. Biken Journal 25:131, 1982.
25. Johnson, P. E., S. B. Greenberg, M.W. Harmon, B.R. Alford, and R.B. Couch: Recovery of applied human leukocyte interferon from the nasal mucosa of chimpanzees and humans. J Clin Microbiol 4:106, 1976.
26. Merigan, T.C., S.E. Reed, T.S. Hall, and D.A.J. Tyrrell: Inhibition of respiratory virus infection by locally applied interferon. Lancet 1(7803):563, 1973.
27. Michaels, D., H. Foy, H. Krouse, C. Meschievitz, and J. Albrecht: Intranasal interferon prophylaxis of viral infections in adult and pediatric asthmatic patients. [Abstract]. J Allergy and Clin Immunol 77(suppl 1):160, 1986.
28. Monto, A.S, T.C. Shope, S.A. Schwartz, and J.K. Albrecht: Intranasal Interferon-α2b for seasonal prophylaxis of respiratory infection. J Infect Dis 154:128, 1986.
29. Phillpotts, R.J., G.M. Scott, P.G. Higgins, J. Wallace, D.A.J.

Tyrrell, and C.L. Gauci: An effective dosage regimen for prophylaxis against rhinovirus infection by intranasal administration of HuIFN-α_2. Antiviral Res 3:121-136, 1983.

30. Phillpotts, R. J., P.G. Higgins, J.S. Willman, D.A.J. Tyrrell, D.S. Freestone, and W.M. Shepherd: Intranasal lymphoblastoid interferon ("Wellferon") prophylaxis against rhinovirus and influenza virus in volunteers. J Interferon Res 4:535, 1984.

31. Saito, H., H. Takenaka, S. Yoshida, T. Tsubokawa, A. Ogata, F. and J. Imanishi: Prevention from naturally acquired viral respiratory infection by interferon nasal spray. Rhinology 23:291, 1985.

32. Samo, T.C., S.B. Greenberg, J.M. Palmer, R.B. Couch, M.W. Harmon, and P.E. Johnson: Intranasally applied recombinant leukocyte A interferon in normal volunteers. II. Determination of minimal effective and tolerable dose. J Infect Dis 150:181, 1984.

33. Samo, T.C., S.B. Greenberg, R.B. Couch, J. Quarles, P.E. Johnson, S. Hook, and M.W. Harmon: Efficacy and tolerance of intranasally applied recombinant leukocyte A interferon in normal volunteers. J Infect Dis 148:535, 1983.

34. Schiff, G., Personal communication.

35. Scott, G.M, W.E. Stewart, D.A.J. Tyrrell, K. Cantell, T. Cartwright, and V.G. Edy: Skin reactions to interferon inoculations are reduced but not abolished by purification. J Interferon Res 1:79, 1980.

36. Scott, G.M., J. Wallace, J. Greiner, R.J. Phillpotts, C.L. Gauci, and D.A.J. Tyrrell: Prevention of rhinovirus colds by human interferon alpha-2 from Escherichia coli. Lancet 2(8291):186, 1982.

37. Scott, G.M., J. Wallace, D.A.J. Tyrrell, K. Cantell, D.S. Secher, and W.E. Steward II: Interim report on studies on "toxic" effects of human leucocyte-derived interferon-alpha (HuIFN-a). J Interferon Res 2:127, 1982.

38. Scott, G.M., R.J. Phillpotts, J. Wallace, D.S. Secher, K. Cantell, and D.A.J. Tyrrell: Purified interferon as protection against rhinovirus infection. Brit Med J 284:1822, 1982.

39. Scott, G.M., S. Reed, T. Cartwright, and D. Tyrrell: Failure of human fibroblast interferon to protect against rhinovirus infection. Arch Gesamte Virusforsch 65:135, 1980.

40. Turner, R.B., A. Felton, K. Kosak, D.K. Kelsey, and C.K. Meschievitz: Prevention of experimental coronavirus colds with intranasal α-2b interferon. J. Infect Dis, 1986, in press.

41. Yunde, H., M. Gusliang, W. Shuhua, L. Yuying, and L. Hantang: Effect of radix astragali seu hedysari on the interferon system. Chinese Med J 94:35, 1981.

Table 1. Prevention and Treatment of Respiratory Viral Infections by Exogenous rIFN-α

	Challenge Virus	rIFN-α (daily dose)	Duration of rIFN-α (days)	Reduction in Illness/Infection[a]
Volunteer Challenge Experiments				
Prophylaxis Studies				
Samo et al (33)	Rhinovirus 13	0.7×10^6	4	-/-
Samo et al (32,33)	Rhinovirus 13	2.4 or 10×10^6	4	+/-
Phillpotts et al (29)	Rhinovirus 9/14	12×10^6	4	+/+
Scott et al (36)	Rhinovirus 9	22×10^6	4	+/+
Hayden and Gwaltney (16)	Rhinovirus 14	40×10^6	4	+/+
Dolin et al (5)	Influenzavirus A	10×10^6	7	±/+
Schiff et al (34)	Influenzavirus A	10×10^6	4	±/-
Turner et al (40)	Coronavirus 229E	2×10^6	15	+/-
Therapeutic Studies				
Hayden and Gwaltney (15)	Rhinovirus 14	20×10^6	4	-/+
Higgins et al (22)	Coronavirus 229E	35×10^6	4	+/+
Natural Infection Studies				
Pre-exposure Prophylaxis				
Farr et al (7)		10×10^6	28	+/+[b]
Monto et al (28)		2.5 or 3×10^6	28	±/+[b]
Geha et al (8)		2×10^6	28	±/-
Michaels et al (27)		1 or 2×10^6	28	-/-
Post-exposure Prophylaxis				
Herzog et al (21)		1.5×10^6	5	±/-
Douglas et al (6)		5×10^6	7	+/+[b]
Hayden et al (17)		5×10^6	7	+/+[b]

[a](+) = significant reduction in rate, (-) = no significant reduction in rate, (±) = reduced rate, not significant. [b]Significant antiviral effect only against rhinovirus

47. Interferon Use during Hepatitis Virus Infections

Mario Rizzetto[a], Giovanni C. Actis[a], and Luigi Barbara[b]

[a]Division of Gastroenterology, Ospedale Molinette, Turin, Italy; [b]Clinica Medica, Policlinico Sant'Orsola, Bologna, Italy

In the developed world chronic viral liver disease is caused essentially by the Hepatitis B Virus (HBV) and a number of yet unidentified agents called non A, non B hepatitis viruses.Thus only type B hepatitis lends itself to rational antiviral therapy, as the HBV is the sole viral agent of progressive liver disease characterized to-date.
The prospects for treatment of HBV hepatitis have improved in the last few years with the progress in our understanding of the pathobiology of this virus and the development of effective antiviral drugs.

Chronic HB surface antigen (HBsAg)positive hepatitis can be divided in subgroups corresponding to temporal phases of the infection(1).The early phase, characterized by replication of the mature , infectious virion (the Dane particle) is diagnosed on the presence of the HBe antigen(HBeAg), HBV genome (HBV-DNA) and specific DNA polymerase (DNAp) in serum and on the presence of the HB core antigen (HBcAg) in the liver.The late phase, characterized by integration of the viral into the host genome is diagnosed by the finding of antibody to HBeAg(anti-HBe) in serum and the lack of serum and liver markers of the HBV nucleocapsid. Antiviral agents can act on the replicating virion but cannot interfere with the intranuclear assembly of the integrated genome.Thus only HBsAg carriers with active HBV infection are candidate to antiviral therapy , while in principle those with inactive infections are not. Recently , however , it has been recognized that the anti-HBe, the conventional hallmark of inactive HBV infection is not "per se" sufficient to warrant absence of HBV virions ,HBV-DNA being detectable by molecular hybridization techniques in a proportion of patients with this antibody(2).Finally , the discovery of the Hepatitis Delta Virus (HDV),a defective RNA virus dependent on the HBV(3),has disclosed that the finding of the HBsAg does not mean that HBV is the cause of the underlying hepatitis ; a proportion of chronic HBsAg hepatitides are caused by the pathogenic effect of this agent,whose biological properties are different from the HBV.The diagnosis and monitorage of active HDV infection has been

made possible by the development of molecular hybridization assays(4)for the detection of the RNA genome of HDV in serum; indirectly,viral synthesis is also shown by expression of the HD antigen (HD Ag)in liver , detectable in immunohistochemistry(3).As HDV disease is often accompanied by an inactive anti-HBe positive HBV infection , it may mask under an apparently untreatable condition ; recent evidence suggests instead that the HDV may be sensitive to antivirals .
Antivirals used in clinical trials are either synthetic or belong to the interferon (IFN) family. While synthetic antivirals are difficult to handle because of common and severe toxic side-effects, IFN is the agent that has been most extensively investigated and the one holding the best promise of therapeutic benefit.

IFN Production and action in HBV hepatitis

In serum of subjects free of productive viral infections, IFN should be undetectable, in contrast to acute viral illnesses where its concentration increases thousandfolds. This tenet was challenged by early studies that failed to detect substantial IFN increases in symptomatic viral hepatitis (5), gaining to HBV the label of "poor IFN inducer". These studies have been contradicted by a recent report (6) that patients with self-limited viral hepatitis circulate high levels of IFN; their lymphocytes are in an antiviral state, and, as a clinical counterpart, those dying of fulminant hepatitis fail to respond with a IFN flare. The reasons for the discrepancy with previous studies are uncertain, but the timing of the blood samples assayed for IFN and the distinction of acute from chronic hepatitis seems to be critical. A recent work (7) has shown that levels of 2',5' oligoadenylate synthetase are deficient in chronic hepatitis as opposed to acute disease and healthy carriers. These findings would add consistency to the original assumption of a defective IFN activation in some forms of HBV infection, thus providing a rational background to the present trend of limiting IFN therapy to forms of chronic and fulminant viral hepatitis. Theoretically, exogenous IFN can act on HBV replication through two leading pathways. First, by a direct antiviral action it might activate cell endonucleases to break down the nascent viral genomes, the target being the HBV DNA-RNA hybrids. Secondly, the antiviral activity could be mediated by the immunomodulatory effects. The drug might increase the display of MHC class I antigens on the virus-bearing hepatocytes rendering them a suitable target for T cell specific killing, and/or it might help virus demise through NK cell function activation. The available data indicate that HBV patients are biologically capable to utilize exogenous IFN, both in terms of receptor affinity and density(8). Nonetheless, IFN administration quickly induces resistance , as shown by decreased cell binding (8) and NK activation in-vitro (9) in hepatitis patients under IFN treatment.

IFN in the treatment of chronic HBV hepatitis

IFN was first used as a therapeutic agent for viral hepatitis in the mid-seventies.In 1976 Greenberg and co-workers (co.) in Stanford (10)and Desmyter and co. in Leuven (11) reported a significant depression of HB virion synthesis , respectively in 4 patients and 1 patient and two chimpanzees given leukocyte and fibroblast IFN.Treatment induced a fall of DNAp activity in serum but the nucleocapsidic marker returned rapidly to pre-treatment levels following short courses of therapy.
In the same year a distinct but again transient antiviral effect was also obtained in chimpanzees by Purcell and co.(12) using a different strategy, i.e. the induction of endogenous IFN by the IFN inducer polyriboinosinic-polyribocytidylic acid. These studies were seminal in establishing the therapeutic potential of IFN but unfortunately the scarcity of IFN hampered at the time large-scale studies and a number of trials performed around the turn of the seventies produced variable and conflicting results. Scullard and co.(13) reported the elimination of HB virion markers in 37% of the 32 patients entered in the Stanford antiviral study by 1981. Of the 16 patients given IFN alone, 4 (25%) had a permanent inhibition of DNAp. In the responders there was an improvement of symptoms and histological findings compared to non-responders(14).Reports from Europe were less favourable. Human leukocyte IFN, given by Weimar and co.in Holland(15) for a total of 165 million units (mu)in a randomized controlled 6-weeks study had no effect on indices of HBV infection apart from a drop of DNAp in the first week. Likewise , Kingham and co. in England (16) and Muller and co. in Germany (17)observed a fall of DNAp while on treatment but no significant long-term response,respectively in any of two and in 7 of 8 patients given fibroblast IFN at a total dose of 140-800 mu for 2 weeks-6 months. The discrepancy between the American and the European studies might in part be explained by the different total dose of IFN used (higher on average in the US series) and by differences in the potency of the crude preparations of IFN available at the time , the fibroblast-derived being apparently less effective than the leukocyte IFN because of greater instability in body fluids(18).However, the critical point in evaluating the efficacy of IFN was the design of the study , whether controlled or not, as spontaneous loss of HB virion markers can occur yearly in up to 30% of the HBeAg-positive carriers of HBsAg (19,20). The US study was uncontrolled, but the late analysis of the Dutch series (21) revealed that the loss of HBvirion markers in 2 of the 10 treated patients was matched by the spontaneous loss of DNAp and HBeAg in 4 of 10 untreated controls. At the beginning of this decade , the advent of recombinant technology and progress in the purification of lymphoblastoid IFN (ly-IFN), a mixture of alfa-interferons produced by stimulation of a human lymphoblastoid cell line by the Sendai Virus, have made available for clinical use large amounts of byosynthetic and natural IFNs of standardized potency. A number of investigations were performed to establish the optimal

protocol of treatment. Omata and co. (22) have given twice daily for 28 days doses of recombinant alpha-interferon (rIFN) increasing from 36 mu to 100 mu. Despite the usual immediate repression of nucleocapsidic markers of HBV, none of the patients given IFN alone became negative for HBeAg and the DNAp activity rebounded promptly once IFN was discontinued. The transient suppressive effect on HBV was independent of the amount of IFN administered, low doses of 36 mu inhibiting to the same extent as high doses. Similar results were obtained by Dooley and co. (23). Nine patients receiving one to four courses of rIFN thrice weekly for 2 weeks at doses varying from 18 to 100 mu, exhibited a temporary treatment-associated fall of DNAp irrespective of the quantity of IFN; lower doses were much better tolerated though having the same antiviral effect of greater doses.
Lok and co. (24) have likewise shown that intermittent treatment was as effective as daily injections but again better tolerated: a decrease of HBV-DNA and DNAp was seen in each of 11 patients given thrice weekly for 12 weeks 10 mu per meter squared body surface of ly-IFN, followed by a delayed permanent loss of HBeAg in 4 and of HBsAg in 2.
This experience has established the general principles upon which the current therapeutic trials are structured, namely the use of relatively low doses of IFN given intermittently but for prolonged periods of time. Available data from studies with the new generation of interferons, either completed or in progress, are reported in table 1 (ref. 25-33).

Table 1 IFN therapy of chronic HBV hepatitis

Author, ref.	IFN type	IFN total dose (mu)	type of treatment	duration of treat.	duration of follow-up	n°responders/ n°treated (%)
Porres, 25	r	2500/5000	int.	6 m	12 m	9/12 75%
Buschenfelde, 26	r	800/1250	int.	12 w	-	6/8 75%
Barbara, 27	ly	420 m^2	int.	6 m	6-33 m	11/18 61%
Scully, 28	ly	200/400	int.	12 w	9 m	19/34 56%
Dusheiko, 29	r	342/1500	int.	9 w	9-24 m	6/14 43%
Trepo, 30	r	70/240 m^2	int.	4 m	-	4/10 40%
Lok, 31	r	72/720	int.	12-24 w	mean 7.5 m	5/23 22%
Anderson, 32	ly	70/210	daily	28 days	12 m	2/14 14%
Alexander, 33	ly	800 m^2	int.	6 m	6-18 m	2/15 13%

r=recombinant
ly=lymphoblastoid
mu= million units

int.=intermittent
m =months
w = weeks

The rate of therapeutic response, defined as a permanent loss of HB virion markers (maintained throughout the follow-up) varies widely, from 14% to 75%, reflecting differences in the selection of patients , in treatment schedules and , above all , in the duration of the follow-up period; because the HBV can rebound several months after termination of therapy, the rate of success tends to be overestimated in studies with shorter follow-up periods . A few consistent points emerge nevertheless from the sum of data. It appears that the optimal dose of IFN is between 5 and 10 mu given intermittently twice or thrice weekly; this regimen produces a distinct antiviral effect but minimizes toxicity. It also appears that treatment must be prolonged for at least 12 weeks to induce a clinical benefit . With this protocol clearance of HB virions is heralded by a flare of aminotransferases activity sometimes during the third month of therapy . An unanswered question is whether more prolonged treatment could result in a higher rate of response; the study of Porres and co.(25) and our preliminary data (Barbara and co.,27) suggest that a 6 months course might be more effective than a 3 months course, though tolerated equally well. Major side effects are uncommon with these regimens, bone marrow suppression ranking as the most frequent. Relatively minor complaints are instead common. During the first weeks of therapy they include fever, chills, myalgia, headache and nausea. Late side effects occurring also after stopping IFN, include anorexia, fatigue, weight and hair loss ; all are reversible.

Unfortunately , controlled studies with appropriate long-term follow-up periods still face the hard statistical fact that the percentage of IFN responders is not significantly increased compared to spontaneous HBV remissions. This has led to a search for the individual factors that might influence the response rate to the antiviral(34). The analysis has shown that Chinese are less prone to respond than Caucasians, that the sexual habit (hetero- or homosexual) is irrelevant , that being a woman or a short term carrier of HBsAg or having elevated pre-treatment values of aminotransferases increases the likelihood of seroconversion to anti-HBe.

A second approach to improve the therapeutic yield is the combination of IFN with another antiviral, in order to obtain a synergistic effect on HBV. Based on the postulate that steroids withdrawal may render the individual more susceptible to antiviral therapy , presumably by enhancing the immune response of the patient, Omata and co.(22) have pre-treated with a short course of prednisone 5 HBeAg carriers of HBsAg. Following the abrupt withdrawal of the steroid, they have given IFN obtaining the loss of HB virion markers in 3 (60%) of the patients.

Muller and co.(35) have combined cycles of adenine arabinoside with beta-IFN obtaining only transient declines of serum HBsAg and DNAp. They have also given to 4 patients the two antivirals after a steroid pulse; this cocktail has resulted in marked neurotoxicity that forced the interruption of treatment in each patient.

A less drastic approach has been adopted by Schalm and co. (36), who combined simultaneous therapy by IFN and acyclovir, a non-toxic virustatic agent .This protocol has induced clearance of HBV markers in 3 of 5 patients (60%) a significantly higher rate than either IFN or acyclovir alone.

IFN in the treatment of chronic HDV hepatitis

A therapeutic benefit of IFN on HDV disease has been suggested by three pilot studies , one controlled in Italy and two uncontrolled in the US and UK. In these studies the dose of IFN has been adjusted according to the guidelines from the experience with HBV disease. The three studies (table 2) have shown a distinct inhibitory effect of IFN on the indices of HDV replication (HDV-RNA in serum and HD Ag in liver) but a rebound of viral replication and disease activity has been the rule after termination of therapy.

Table 2 IFN therapy of chronic HDV hepatitis

author,ref	IFN type	IFN schedule (mu)	duration of therapy	n°patients treated	results
Rosina,37	r	5/m^2 inter	12 weeks	11	transient HDV/biochemical remission in 7 patients, permanent in 1
Hoofnagle,38	r	5 inter.*	4 months	5	transient HDV/biochemical remission in 3 patients; two of them treated for another 12 months,no benefit
Thomas,39	ly	2.5-10 /m^2 inter.*	12 weeks	5	permanent HDV improvement in 3 patients, transient in 1

r = recombinant , ly = lymphoblastoid,inter.=intermittent
* = first week induction with daily injections

Rosina and co.(37)have obtained the clearance of HDV and amelioration of liver enzymes in 7 of the 8 patients circulating HDV-RNA before therapy. In all but one of the patients the HDV and biochemical parameters have returned to pre-therapy levels after stopping IFN. Hoofnagle and co.(38) noted a marked amelioration in 3 of 5 patients treated for 4 months;two responders werefurther treated for another 12 months without relapsing. However, liver enzymes became elevated in both patients 8 and 10 months after stopping IFN and liver biopsies showed a return of HDV and severe hepatitis.Thomas and co.(39) have obtained a virologic improvement in 3 patients , that was not accompanied by improvement in liver disease. The sum of data suggests that IFN represses replication of HDV and may improve the clinical state. Trials are in progress to determine the benefit of more prolonged courses of IFN in this disease.

References

1. Schafritz D.A., and S.J. Hadziyannis: Hepatitis B Virus DNA in liver and serum, viral antigens, and antibodies, virus replication and liver disease activity in patients with persistent Hepatitis B Virus infection. In Advances in Hepatitis Research, F.V. Chisari ed, Masson U.S.A., pp. 80-90, 1984.

2. Bonino F., F. Rosina, M. Rizzetto, R. Rizzi, E. Chiaberge, R. Tardanico, F. Callea, G. Verme: Chronic hepatitis in HBsAg carriers with serum HBV-DNA and anti-HBe. Gastroenterology, 90:1268, 1986.

3. Rizzetto M., G. Verme, Gerin J.L., Purcell R.H.: Hepatitis Delta Virus Disease. In: Progress in Liver Disease, vol. VIII, Popper H., and Schaffner F. eds, Grune and Stratton, New York, pp. 417-431, 1986.

4. Denniston K.J., B.H. Hoyer, A. Smedile, F.V. Wells, J. Nelson, and J.L. Gerin: Cloned fragment of the Hepatitis Delta Virus RNA genome: sequence and diagnostic application. Science, 232:837, 1986.

5. Hill D.A., J.H. Walsh, and R.H. Purcell: Failure to demonstrate circulating IFN during incubation period and acute stage of transfusion-associated hepatitis. Proc. Soc. Exp. Bio. Med. 136:853, 1971.

6. Levin S. and T. Hahn: Inteferon system in acute viral hepatitis. Lancet, 1:592, 1982.

7. Poitrine A., S. Chousterman, M. Chousterman, S. Naveau, M.N. Thang and J.C. Chaput: Lack of in-vivo activation of the Interferon system in HBsAg positive chronic active hepatitis. Hepatology, 5:171, 1985.

8. Dooley J.S., J. Vergalla and J.H. Hoofnagle: Specific binding of human alpha Interferon to high affinity cell specific binding sites on peripheral blood mononuclear cells: Changes during treatment. Hepatology, 4:1063, 1984.

9. Actis G.C., E. Maran, G. Saracco, P. Bellando, F. Rosina, M. Rizzetto: Delta Hepatitis: modulation of natural killer (NK) activity in vivo and in vitro during therapy with recombinant leukocyte A Interferon. J. Hepatol. 2 (suppl.):S179, 1985.

10. Greenberg H.B., R.B. Pollard, L.I. Lutwick, P.B. Gregory, W.S. Robinson and T.C. Merigan: Effect of human leukocyte interferon on hepatitis B Virus infection in patients with chronic active hepatitis. New. Engl. J. Med. 295:517, 1976.

11. Desmyter J., J. De Groote, V.J. Desmet, A. Billiau, M.B. Ray, A.F. Bradburne, V.G. Edy, P. De Somer: Administration of human fibroblast interferon in chronic hepatitis-B infection. Lancet, ii, 645, 1976.

12. Purcell R.H., W.T. London, V.S. McAuliffe, A.E. Palmer, P.H. Kaplan, J.L. Gerin, J. Wagner, H. Popper, E. Lvovsky, D.C. Wong: Modification of chronic hepatitis B infection in chimpanzees by administration of an interferon inducer. Lancet, ii:757, 1956.

13. Scullard G.H., R.B. Pollard, J.L. Smith, S.L,. Sacks, P.B. Gregory, W.S. Robinson and T.C. Merigan: Antiviral treatment of chronic hepatitis B Virus infection I. Changes in Viral Markers with interferon combined with Adenine Arabinoside. J. Infect. Dis. 143:772, 1981.

14. Scullard G.H., L.L. Andres, H.B. Greenberg, J.L. Smith, V.K. Sawheney, E.A. Neal, A.S. Mahal, H. Popper, T.C. Merigan, W.S. Robinson and P.B. Gregory: Antiviral treatment of chronic hepatitis B Virus infection: improvement in liver disease with interferon and adenine arabinoside. Hepatology, 1:228, 1981.

15. Weimar W., F.J.P. ten Kate, N. Masurel, R.A. Heijtink, S.W. Schalm, H. Schellekens: Double-blind study of leukocyte interferon administration in chronic HBsAg positive hepatitis. Lancet, ii,336, 1980.

16. Kingham J.G.C., N.K. Ganguly, Z.D. Shaari, R. Mendelson, M.J. McGuire, S.J. Holgate, T. Cartwright, G.M. Scott, B.M. Richards and R. Wright: Treatment of HBsAg positive chronic active hepatitis with human fibroblast interferon. Gut, 19:91, 1978.

17. Muller R., F. Deinhardt, H.P. Hofschneider: Long term treatment with human fibroblast interferon in chronic hepatitis B: preliminary data of a controlled trial. In Viral Hepatitis, W. Szmuness, H.J. Alter and J.E. Maynard, eds, Franklin Inst. Press, Philadelphia 1982, pp. 648-649.

18. Weimar W. and Schellekens H.: Differential effects of human leukocyte interferon in HBsAg positive chronic active hepatitis. Eur. J. Clin. Invest. 9:151, 1979.

19. Realdi E., A. Alberti, R. Rugge: Seroconversion from hepatitis B e antigen to anti-HBe in chronic hepatitis B virus infection. Gastroenterology, 79:195, 1980.

20. Hoofnagle J.H., G.M. Dusheiko, L.B. Seeff, A. Jones, J. Waggoner and Z. Buskell-Bales: Seroconversion from Hepatitis B e antigen to antibody in chronic type B hepatitis. Ann. Intern. Med. 94:744, 1981.

21. Schalm S.W., R.A. Heijtink: Spontaneous disappearance of viral replication and liver cell inflammation in HBsAg positive chronic active hepatitis. Results of placebo versus interferon trial. Hepatology, 2:791, 1982.

22. Omata M., F. Imazeki, O. Yokosuka, O. Ito, K. Ughiumi, J. Mori and F. Okuda: Recombinant leukocyte alpha Interferon treatment in patients with chronic hepatitis B infection. Gastroenterology, 88.870, 1985.

23. Dooley J.S., G.L. Davis, M. Peters, J.G. Waggoner, Z. Goodman and J.H. Hoofnagle: Pilot study of recombinant human alpha interferon for chronic type B hepatitis. Gastroenterology, 90:150, 1986.

24. Lok A.S.F., I.V.D. Weller, S.P. Karayiannis, D. Brown, M.J.F. Fowler, J. Monjardino, H.C. Thomas and S. Sherlock: Thrice weekly lymphoblastoid interferon is effective in inhibiting hepatitis B Virus replication. Liver, 4:45, 1984.

25. Porres J.C., V. Carreño , I. Moza, J. Gutier, J.A. Quiroga, J. Bartolomé, J. Cortes, C. Hernandez Guio: Changes of viral markers and liver histology in patients treated during six months with recombinant interferon. J. Hepatol., supplement 2, 1985, 312.

26. Meyer Zum Buschenfelde K.H., G. Hess: Treatment of HBsAg positive chronic hepatitis with recombinant leucocyte alpha A interferon. J. Hepatol., in press.

27. Barbara L., G. Mazzella, M. Baraldini, G. Gasbarrini, F. Giungi, M. Malavolti, L. Mastroroberto, F. Miglio, E. Roda, E. Raise G. Saracco and M. Rizzetto: A ramdomised controlled trial with human lymphoblastoid interferon vs no treatment in chronic B virus infection. Preliminary results. J. Hepatol., in press.

28. Scully L.J., R. Shein, A.S.F. Lok, P. Karayannis, H.C. Thomas: Lymphoblastoid interferon therapy of chronic hepatitis B virus infection: Different racial response. J. Hepatol., supplement 2, 1985, 328.

29. Dusheiko G., A. Dibisceglie, S. Bowyer, E. Sachs, M. Ritchie, B. Schoub, M. Kew: Recombinant Leukocyte Interferon Treatment of Chronic Hepatitis B. Hepatology 5; 556, 1985.

30. Trepo C., D. Ouzan, T. Fontanges, M. Chevallier, P. Chossegros, F. Degos, P. Chevalier, O. Hantz: Therapeutic activity of vidarabin, acyclovir and beta-interferon on HBV C.A.H. J. Hepatol., in press.

31. Lok A.S.F., C.L. Lai, P.C. Wu: Spontaneous and interferon induced HBe antigen to antibody seroconversion in chronic hepatitis B virus infection in Hong-Kong chinese. J. Hepatol., in press.

32. Anderson M.G., T.J. Harrison, A.J. Zuckerman, J.C. Coleman, I.M. Murray Lyon: A controlled trial of Lymphoblastoid interferon (Wellferon) in chronic active hepatitis B. J. Hepatol., in press.

33. Alexander G.J.M., E.A. Fagan, A.L.W.F. Eddleston, R. Williams: A controlled trial of lymphoblastoid interferon in chronic HBV infection: a preliminary report. J. Hepatol., in press.

34. Alexander G., R. Williams: Antiviral treatment in chronic infection with hepatitis B virus. B. Med. J., 292; 915, 1986.

35. Muller R., H. Klein, M. Gebel, H.U. Lautz, R. Brunkhorst, G. Niehoff, F.W. Schmidt: Antiviral procedures in patients with chronic active hepatitis B (CAHB): Data of four randomized controlled studies. J. Hepatol., in press.

36. Schalm S.W., R.A. Heytink, H.R. van Buuren, R.A. de Man: Acyclovir enhances the antiviral effect of interferon in chronic hepatitis B. Lancet 2, 358, 1985.

37. F. Rosina, G. Saracco, M. Rizzetto: Alpha 2 recombinant interferon in the treatment of chronic hepatitis delta virus (HDV) hepatitis. In: The Hepatitis Delta Virus (HDV) and its infection. Eds. M. Rizzetto, J.L. Gerin, R.H. Purcell, Alan R. Liss, New York. Progress in Clinical and Biological Research, in press.

38. Hoofnagle J., K. Mullen, M. Peters, M. Avigan, Y. Park, J. Waggoner, J. Gerin, B. Hoyer, A. Smedile: Treatment of chronic delta hepatitis with recombinant human alpha interferon. In: The Hepatitis Delta Virus (HDV) and its infection. Eds. M. Rizzetto, J.L. Gerin, R.H. Purcell, Alan R. Liss, New York. Progress in Clinical and Biological Research, in press.

39. Thomas H.C., P. Farci, R. Shein, P. Karayannis, A. Smedile, L. Caruso, J.L. Gerin et al.: Inhibition of Hepatitis Delta Virus (HDV) replication by Lymphoblastoid human alpha interferon. In: The Hepatitis Delta Virus (HDV) and its infection. Eds. M. Rizzetto, J.L. Gerin, R.H. Purcell, Alan R. Liss, New York. Progress in Clinical and Biological Research, in press.

48. Interferon Use during Other Virus Infections

T. Cesario, S. Yousefi, G. Carandang, and J. Tilles

Department of Medicine, University of California Irvine Medical Center, 101 City Drive South, Orange, CA 92668

INTRODUCTION

Many of the clinical applications for human interferon (IFN) in the treatment of virus infections have already been covered in the chapters devoted to respiratory viruses, herpesviruses and hepatitis viruses; however, therapeutic trials using human IFN have been undertaken in a variety of diseases either known to be, or presumed to be caused by viruses. We will review the results of these various trials in the following chapter. We have chosen to organize this discussion by disease category.

CONGENITAL RUBELLA

Larsson, et al. (1), reported the use of leukocyte IFN to treat a fourteen month old infant with the congenital rubella syndrome. Administration of 3 million units daily was associated with improvement of skin lesions and disappearance of viremia but persistance of viruria.

MARBURG VIRUS INFECTION

An anonymous author reported in 1977 that a patient with infection due to Marburg virus had been treated with IFN (2). While viremia ceased and the patient recovered, it was impossible to be sure of the role that IFN played in the patients improvement.

RABIES

Five human cases of rabies were reported to have been treated with human leukocyte IFN by Merigan, et al. (3). All cases were given both intrathecal and intramuscular IFN. The dosage range varied from one million units per day IM to 20 million units per day by the same route. Intrathecal doses varied from one half to five million units per day. None of the patients survived and rabies virus was detected at death in all patients either by flourescent staining or other means. Thus, it appeared the IFN conferred no beneficial effects for these individuals.

SUBACUTE SCLEROSING PANENCEPHALITIS

Several reports have appeared in the literature detailing the administration of IFN to patients with subacute sclerosing panencephalitie (SSPE). Both fibroblast and leukocyte IFNs were given. In neither the original report of Behan (4), or the subsequent reports of Bartram, et al. (5), or Bye, et al. (6) could significant benefits be observed. In these trials IFN was given by the intrathecal route as well as by systemic administration. In the most extensive of these trials, that of Bye, et al. (6), IFN dosage was gradually increased from 10 to 40 million units/m , but only three doses were given each patient via the intravenous route. Six additional doses of one million units/m were also given intrathecally.

HUMAN PAPILLOMA VIRUS INFECTION

A number of reports have suggested the IFN therapy might be useful in the treatment of papilloma virus infections. Perhaps the earliest study regarding this subject was that of Haglund, et al. (7). In this initial report human leukocyte IFN in a dose of 3 million units thrice weekly was administered to seven patients suffering from juvenile laryngeal papillomatosis. Analysis of this data suggested that therapeutic benefit might have been obtained from this regimen. Subsequent reports by Goepfert, et al. (8) reported similar success in the treatment of fourteen additional patients with this same problem. Using a dose of 2 million units/m^2 per day, these authors reported that seven of fourteen patients had some response to IFN and two patients had a complete response. In the most recent report, Saito, et al. (9) utilized IFN alpha in conjunction with laser surgery and again reported efficacy. Unfortunately none of these studies have been controlled and therefore have not provided definitive proof of the benefifs of IFN in this setting.

More recently, Einhorn, et al. (10) have reported the case of a woman with severe condylomata acuminata who was treated with IFN alpha (3 million units IM, daily for four weeks and then the same dose thrice weekly). This woman who had failed previous therapeutic regimens, appeared to respond to the IFN. In this same article the authors mention the use of IFN in the treatment of plantar warts but do not provide any details.

Schonfeld, et al. (11) have also reported the use of intramuscular IFN beta in the treatment of condylomata acuminata. In the open part of their study, they treated 22 patients with two million units of IFN daily for ten consecutive days and found that 9 of 11 patients so treated responded with regression of the lesions as compared to 2 of 11 in the control group.

Vance, et al. (12) have recently found that clearing of condylomata acminata occurred in 53% of the cases where lesions were injected with 1 million units of IFN as a single dose. These same authors could establish no efficacy for the recombinant alpha 2 IFN used in this study in the treatment of verruca plantaris.

VIRAL INFECTIONS OF THE EY"

While several publications have reported the effects of IFN in the treatment ocular herpes infections, we will discuss the use of IFN here only for those infections caused by viruses other than herpes. In the last edition of this review, Romano, et al. (13) discussed their studies of the effects of human fibroblast derived IFN for the treatment adeno virus epidemic keratoconjunctivitis. In that study, beta IFN was instilled into the eye in droplet form. One half million units was given six to eight times a day. The use of IFN appearred to shorten the length of the disease, provide relief for the patient and diminish the incidence of complications when compared to the control group.

Subsequently, Adams, et al. (14), have reported their studies of the use of alpha-2 IFN for adenoviral conjunctivitis. The IFN used in this study was administered in a dose of 830,000 units by eye drop four times per day. No significant benefit to the inflammed eye was reported but a preventative effect on infection in the opposite eye may have occurred. This study included a much smaller number of patients than the earlier one.

Stansfield, et al. (15) also reported their experience with the use of leukocyte derived IFN (50,000 units) two times per day. Since the numbers of patients was very small, it was not possible to demonstrate a significant differnce between treated and control groups, but a significant decrease in the spread of infection to other members of the household was observed.

ACQUIRED IMMUNE DEFICIFNCY SYNDROME

Since a large number of immunological defects have been reported to occur in the acquired immune deficiency syndrome (AIDS), several groups of investigators have examined the competance of the IFN system in individuals with this condition. Defects have thus been demonstrated in the ability of patients with AIDS to produce both IFN alpha and IFN gamma. Lopez, et al. (16) have shown that mononuclear cells from patients with AIDS when challenged with fibroblasts infected with Herpes simplex virus Type I, produced significantly less IFN alpha than did normal controls. Furthermore, Murray, et al. (17) have shown that cells from patients with AIDS in 13 of 14 cases failed to produce IFN gamma when stimulated with specific microbial antigens. In addition, Eyster, et al. (18) have reported the presence of acid labile IFN alpha in the blood of patients with this syndrome and Ikossi-O'Connor, et al. (19) described the presence of a serum IFN inactivator in these patients.

Because of the reported deficiencies in the ability to generate IFN as reported above, because of the viral etiology of this disease and because of the antiproliferative potential of IFN, a number of investigators have treated patients with AIDS and Kaposi's sarcoma using a variety of IFN preparations. Frederick, et al. (20), administered human lymphoblastoid IFN to nineteen patients with Kaposi's sarcomas and AIDS. The patients received either 7.5 or 15 million units per m^2 of body surface intramuscularly. The lower dose group received therapy for 28 days and the higher dose group for 20 days. There were two partial improvements in tumors in these patients but no significant effect on coexistant viral infections. Of the immunological parameters assessed in this investigation, only HLA unrestricted cytotoxicity increased in 4 of 8 patients studied.

Krown, et al. (21) treated their patients with 36 to 54 million units of IFN alpha per day and indicated that 50% of their patients overall had some response as regards the neoplastic disease. These authors were unable to find a specific immunological factor that explained the improvements observed but did comment that in some patients the lymphocyte proliferative responses to PHA improved. More recently this group has updated their results (22) and indicated that 38% of the patients treated with the higher dose responded while 17% treated initially with a lower dose improved.

Volberding, et al. (23) treated a group of patients with Kaposi's and AIDS with IFN alpha. Using a low dose regimen (one million units/m^2 body surface area five days per week for two months) three of five patients responded, but using five times this dose, he had a response rate of 40%.

Finally, Gelmann, et al. (24) reported on the treatment of thirty patients with AIDS and Kaposi's sarcoma. These authors used lymphoblastoid IFN in doses ranging 7.5 million to 25 million units/m^2 of body surface per day. The highest dosage regimen proved toxic. Only 23% of their patients had any type of response. No effect on concurrent viral infection could be demonstrated.

Thus, we can conclude from these studies that a limited number of patients with Kaposi's sarcoma and AIDS will respond to IFN therapy; however, the available studies would indicate that complete responses (dissappearance of the tumor) could be expected in less than a quarter of the patients even in the most optomistic of the studies.

A major as yet unanswered question regards the ability of IFN preparations to effect the culturing of the human immune deficiency virus from the blood of afflicted individuals. It is of considerable interest that Ho, et al. (25) reported that recombinant IFN alpha suppressed the replication of this virus in vitro.

REFERENCES

1. Larsson, A., M. Forsgren, S. Hard, H. Strander, K. Cantell: Administration of interferon to an infant with congenital rubella syndrome involving persistant viremia and cutaneous vasculitis Acta Pediat Scand 65:105,1976.
2. Anonymous: Interferon options. Br Med Jour 1:64,1977.
3. Merigan, T, G. Baer, W. Winkler, K. Bernard, C. Gilbert, C. Chany, R. Veronesi, and the Collaborative Group: Human leukocyte interferon administration to patients with symptomatic and suspected rabies. Annals of Neurology 16:82,1984.
4. Behan, P.: Interferon in the treatment of subacute sclerosing panencephalitis. Lancet 1:1059,1981.
5. Bartram, C., J. Henke, J. Treuner, M. Basler, A. Esch, and W. Mortier: Subacute panencephalitis in a brother and sister: Therapeutic trial of fibroblast interferon. Eur J Pediatr 138: 187, 1982.
6. Bye, A., F. Balkwill, D. Brigden, and J. Wilson: Use of interferon in the management of patients with subacute sclrosing panencephalitis. Developmental Medicine and Child Neurology 27: 170, 1985.
7. Haglund, S., P. Lundquist, K. Cantell, and H. Strander: Interferon therapy in juvenile laryngeal papillomatosis. Arch Otolaryngology 107:327 1981.
8. Goepfert, H., J. Gutterman, W. Dichtel, R. Sessions, A. Cangir, M. and Sulek: Leukocyte interferon in patients with laryngeal papillomatosis. Ann Otol Rhino Laryngol 91: 431, 1982.
9. Saito, R., R. Date, K. Uno, S. Ueda, M. Quijano, and Y. Ogura: Treatment of juvenile laryngeal papilloma with a combination of laser surgery and interferon. Auris Nasus Larynx (Tokyo) 12:117 1985.
10. Einhorn, N., P. Ling, and H. Strander: Systemic interferon alpha treatment of human condylomata acuminata. Acta Obstet Gynecol Scand 62: 287, 1983.
11. Schonfeld, A., A. Schattner, M. Crespi, H. Levavi, J. Shoham, S. Nitke, D. Wallach, T. Hahn, O. Yarder, T. Doener, and M. Revel: Intramuscular human injections in the treatment of condylomata acuminata. Lancet 1:1038, 1984.
12.Vance, J., Bart, B., Hansen, R., Reichman, R., McEwem, C., Hatch, K., Berman, B.,and Tanner, J.: Intralesional recombinant alpha 2 interferon for the treatment of patients with condylomata acuminatum or verruca plantaris Arch Dermatol 122:272 1986
13. Romano, A., E. Ladizensky, D. Guarari-Rotman, and M. Revel: Clinical effect of human fibroblast-derived (beta) interferon in treatment of adeno- virus epidemic keratoconjunctivitis and its comlpications. Texas Reports on Biology and Medicine 41:599,1981.
14. Adams, C., E. Cohen, J. Albrecht, and P. Laibson: Interferon treatment of adenoviral conjunctivitis. Am Journ of Opthalmology 98: 432 1984.
15. Stansfield, S, W. de la Pena, S. Koenig, A. Espaillat Cabral, H. Kaufman, M. Hatch, J. Hierholzer, and L. Schonberger: Human leukocyte interferon in the treatment and prophylaxis of acute hemorrhagic conjunctivitis. Journ of Infect Dis 149:822, 1984.

16. Lopez C., P. Fitzgerald, F. Siegal, S. Landesman, J. Gold, and S. Krown: Deficiency of interferon alpha generating capacity is associated with susceptibility to opportunistic infections in patients with AIDS. Ann N.Y. Acad Science 417: 39, 1984.
17. Murray, H., B. Rubin, H. Masur, H. and R. Roberts: Impaired production of lymphokines and immune (gamma) interferon in the acquired immune deficiency syndrome. NEJM 310:883, 1984.
18. Eyster, M., J. Goedert, M. Poon, O. Preble: Acid labile alpha interferon: A possible preclinical marker for the acquired immune deficiency syndrome in hemophilia. NEJM 309:583,1983.
19. Ikossi-O'Connor, J. Ambrus, T. West, M. Lillie, H. Milgrom, and K. Chaddha: Interferon and interferon inactivators in patients with acquired immune deficiency syndrome and Kaposi's sarcoma. Research Communications in Chemical Pathoilogy and Pharmacology 45:271, 1984.
20. Frederick, W., J. Epstein, E. Gelman, A. Rook, G. Armstrong, J. Djeu, L. Jackson, J. Manischewitz, J. Enterline, J. Jacob, H. Masur, and G. Quinnan: Viral infections and cell mediated immunity in immunodeficient homosexual men with Kaposi's sarcoma treated with lymphoblastoid interferon. Journ of Infect Dis 152: 162, 1985.
21. Krown, S. F. Real, M. Krim, Cu nigham-Rundles, B. Koziner, P. Myskowski, B. Safai, and H. Oettgen: Recombinant leukocyte interferon in Kaposi's sarcoma. Ann N.Y. Acad Science 417:431, 1984.
22. Krown, S., F. Real, S. Vadhan-Raj, S. Cunningham-Rundles, M. Grim, G. Wong, and H. Oettgen: Kaposi's sarcoma and the acquired immune deficiency syndrome. Cancer 57:1662, 1986.
23. Volberding, P., R. Valero, J. Rothman, and G. Gee: Alpha interferon therapy of Kaposi's sarcoma in AIDS. Ann N.Y. Acad Science 417:439 1984.
24. Gelmann, E., O. Preble, R. Steis, H. Lane, A. Rook, M. Wesley, J. Jacob, A. Fauci, H. Masur, and D. Longo: Human lymphoblastoid interferon treatment of Kaposi's sarcoma in the acquired immune deficiency syndrome: Clinical response and prognostic parameters. Am Journ Med 78:737, 1985.
25. Ho, D., T. Rota, J. Kaplan, K. Hartschorn, C. Andrews, R. Schooley, and M. Hirsch: Recombinant human interferon alpha A suppresses HTLV III replication in vitro. Lancet 1:602, 1985.

49. Role of Interferons in Ocular Viral Disease

Marilyn P. Langford[a] *and G. John Stanton*[b]

[a]Departments of Ophthalmology and Microbiology and Immunology, Louisiana State University Medical Center, Shreveport, LA 71130; Department of Microbiology, University of Texas Medical Branch, Galveston, TX 77550

INTRODUCTION

It has been suggested that interferon (IFN) and antibody could work together in vivo to protect against viral infection (1) and the combination of IFN and antibody has been considered in treatment of some diseases (2,3). However, the importance of naturally produced IFNs and of antibody in prevention of clinical disease is not well documented. Classically, the primary importance of IFN as a host defense in viral resistance comes from studies showing that IFN reduced virus yields in infected cells and inhibits infection of other cells, that IFN appears early during virus infection in vivo, that application of IFN can prevent virus infection (4), that deletion of IFN increases severity of disease and changes the pathogenesis of viral disease (5), and that agamma-and hypogammaglobulinemic patients recover from most viral infections (6). It is generally accepted that circulating antibody plays the primary role in inhibiting viremia during primary infection and in resistance to reinfection (9, 14-16) since antibody specifically neutralizes the infectivity of a specific virus, passively administered antibody can prevent virus infection (clinical disease) in normal and immunocompromised individuals (6-8), and resistance to establishment of clinical infection can be correlated to the presence of antibody (9-13).

The idea that antibody appears too late relative to the IFN response to be of primary importance during the first (initial) infection (14) is probably the reason why the importance of the combined effects of IFN and antibody has not been investigated. However, detectable local and systemic antibody responses can be detected 3 days post immunization (9,17, 18) suggesting that low (undetectable) levels of antibody could be produced during the first 3 days of infection at a time when IFNβ and/or IFNα is present in many viral infections (14).

*Corresponding author

This paper reviews our reported studies and present data that indicates the importance of the combined effects of endogenous IFNs and antibodies in protection of tissue culture and animals from systemic and ocular infections.

INHIBITORY EFFECT OF IFN AND ANTIBODY IN VITRO

The addition of virus specific antibody and IFNs to cultures preinfected with enterovirus 70 (EV70), coxsackievirus A24 (CA24), adenovirus type 3 (adeno 3) and herpes simplex virus (HSV) resulted in a greater reduction (10 to 10,000 fold) of virus yields than could be accounted for if their antiviral activities were additive. This synergistic effect was demonstrable with different IFNs (α,β, and γ), in different cells and with different concentrations of antibody and IFNs (19).

Interestingly, the synergistic action of IFNγ and antibody was greater against HSV, whereas IFNα and antibody were more effective against CA24, EV70, echovirus 5, echovirus 33, coxsackievirus B, poliovirus, adeno 3, adeno 7, Sindbis virus, and vesicular stomatitis virus (19). This suggests that the synergistic effect may depend upon the time required for establishment of the antiviral state (AVS) (IFNγ requires longer time to establish its AVS) and/or upon some qualitative difference in the AVS induced by the different IFNs. Most important, these results indicated that different IFNs and virus-specific neutralizing antibody can act to synergistically inhibit a number of different viruses.

The effect of endogenous IFN on the protective effect of antibody to CA24 and HSV in infected cultures was deleted by addition of antibody to IFN to determine the absolute effect of antibody on inhibiting virus yields (19). The studies indicated that antibody to IFNβ decreased the protective effect of antibody to CA24 by 99.9% but did not increase virus yields in virus control. Similar results were obtained with actinomycin D inhibition of IFN production. In comparison, the addition of antibody to IFNβ to HSV-infected cells treated with antibody to HSV did not effect the decreases in virus yields due to antibody; most likely because HSV does not induce IFNβ and is relatively insensitive to IFN. However, under conditions of natural infection, IFNs are produced that could act with antibody to inhibit HSV (1). These results indicated that maximal protection by antibody may depend upon IFN and suggested the importance of endogenous IFN in the natural protective effect of antibody against viral infections.

NATURAL OCCURRENCE OF IFN AND ANTIBODY EARLY DURING INFECTION IN VIVO

The significance of synergism during a primary infection was suggested by the simultaneous presence of IFNβ and an early appearing virus specific, neutralizing activity (ENA) caused by either CA20 or EV70 in tears of patients with acute hemorrhagic conjunctivitis (AHC) 24 h after infection (20, 21, 22). However, simultaneous presence of two factors does not prove that they are acting together. Thus studies were done to determine if ENA and IFN could act together to synergistically inhibit virus. Pooled tears (collected 0-3 d post onset of AHC) containing 10 units of ENA to EV70 or CA24 and 50 units of IFNs were used alone or in combination to treat EV70 and CA24 infected cells. The results indicate that the combined effects of ENAs and IFNβ on inhibition of virus yields were 100-fold more than the sum of the effects of ENA and IFNβ alone for both CA24 and EV70. These studies strongly suggest that during primary infection, local neutralizing activity in tears and endogenous IFN can act synergistically to inhibit AHC viruses. Thus, the natural combination of ENA and IFN was felt to be an important host defense against AHC.

EFFECT OF IFN AND ANTIBODY IN VIVO AGAINST HSV INFECTION

Our in vitro studies indicated that endogenous IFN is important to the protective effect of antibody against some viruses (19, 21). Thus, we wanted to determine if endogenously produced IFNs were important to passive antibody treatment of mice infected intraperitonally with HSV. Three to four week-old female ICR mice (15-20g) were injected with various combinations of antibody to mouse IFNα/β , antibody to mouse IFNγ and antibody to HSV, two hours prior to being inoculated with $10^{3.0}$ plaque forming units of HSV. The results of these studies are presented in Table 1. Deletion of the endogenous IFNα/β and IFNγ responses with specific antisera significantly enhanced the infection, as indicated by an increase in mortality from 73% and 36% in control groups to 90 to 100% in IFN depleted groups. Treatment with antibody (256 units/mouse) protected HSV infected mice (mortalities of 9 and 0%). Interestingly, antibody alone could not protect mice receiving antibody to mouse IFNα/β (64 and 45% mortalities) or mice receiving antibody to mouse IFNγ alone. In one of two experiments antibody to HSV protected mice receiving antibodies to IFNα/β and IFNγ. These studies show that depletion of IFN reduces the protective effect of antibody in vivo. These results support our in vitro findings that endogenous IFN enhanced the protective effect of anti-CA24 antibody and our suggestions that HSV could be inducing IFNs in vivo (19). These studies are highly significant in that they show for the first time that the combination of endogenous IFN and antibody may play a defensive role in protection against systemic HSV infection.

Other investigators have shown that treatment of mice with anti-IFN globulin could exacerbate numerous virus infections including herpes simplex infection (5). Since ocular models of HSV infection were not used, the role of endogenously produced IFNs in controlling HSV infection of the eye remained obscure. Our studies (Table 2) clearly show that treatment of mice with either anti-IFNα/β or anti-IFNγ significantly enhances mortality in ocularly infected mice. (The data are representative of three experiments.) The results obtained following treatment with anti-IFNα/β were not surprising since this IFN type has been detected in tears and blood of mice infected with HSV. However, it is surprising that antibodies to IFNγ exacerbated the infection. These results suggest that IFNγ plays an important

TABLE 1. Effect of antibody and endogenous IFN on mouse HSV infection.

Treatment: Antibody to HSV	Antibody to IFNα/β	Antibody to IFNγ	Number of Mice in: Expt. A	Expt. B	% Mortality Expt. A	Expt. B	$\overline{X}$ day of death Expt. A	Expt. B
−	−	−	11	11	73	36	10.4	13.3
+	−	−	11	11	9	0	11.0	−
−	+	−	10	11	90	100	8.3	8.1
+	−	+	11	11	91	91	8.9	10.0
−	+	+	11	11	100	100	8.4	8.2
+	+	−	11	11	64	45	9.0	9.6
+	−	+	11	11	54	0	9.1	−
+	+	+	11	11	91	45	9.0	10.0

[a]Mice received 0.4ml of ascites fluid containing 8000 U/ml of anti-HSV antibody.
[b]Mice received 0.4ml of pooled rabbit antiserum to mouse IFNα/β (6000 units/ml).
[c]Mice received 0.4ml of pooled rabbit antiserum to mouse IFNγ (3200 units/ml).
[d]Mice received 0.4 ml of pooled normal rabbit serum.

Table 2. Anti-interferons enhance mortality in mice infected ocularly with HSV-1 (F-strain).

Treatment	Mortality: # Mice Dead / Total Mice	Percent
Normal rabbit serum (NRS)	2/8	25
Anti-MoIFN α/β	7/8	88
Anti-MoIFN γ	8/8	100

Four to five week old ICR female mice were inoculated ip with NRS (1.5 mls total volume), rabbit anti-IFNγ (1.5 mls, 4,500 U/mouse), or rabbit anti-IFNα/β (4.5 mls, 15,000 U/mouse). One ml was given 20 h pre and 0.5 ml at the time of ocular challenge with HSV-1, F strain (1600 pfu/mouse). At the time of infection, the mice were etherized, eyes scarafied with a 30g needle, and 5 ul of virus dropped onto each eye. Mortality was checked daily for a total of 14 days.

protective role in primary ocular HSV infection in vivo.

Initially, the possible mechanism(s) for the synergistic effect of antibody (ENA) and IFNs at the surface of the eye were thought to be related to the ability of neutralizing activity to retard extracellular spread of virus and to reduce the multiplicity of infection, thus allowing more time for IFN to protect uninfected cells, thereby making low levels of neutralizing activity protective. Any differences in magnitude of the protective effect were thought to be related to the ability of the antibody (or ENA) to neutralize virus, the sensitivity of virus and cells to the IFN type, and the ability of virus to induce endogenous IFN. However, the observation that endogenous IFNs increased the protective effect of antibody in vitro and in vivo suggests the existence of other mechanisms. Recently, we have shown that IFNγ is necessary for IgM response against surface antigens of sheep red blood cells and others have shown that IFNγ is needed for stimulation of immune regulatory cells (24-25). Taken together, our studies suggest that IFN γ may effect the early immune responses of the eye induced by HSV infection.

In additional studies (undertaken to determine whether IFNγ induction was an important early host defense) we found that treatment of mice with anti-IFNγ prior to HSV ocular infection increased mortality and viral levels at both the site of inoculation and in the brain. Anti-IFNs given within the first 48h of ocular HSV infection proved to greatly increase the severity of the disease (27). Since neither IFN α/β nor IFN γ were capable of protecting alone, these studies suggested that synergistic antiviral activity of IFNα/βandIFNγ (28), or IFNs and antibody and/or different IFN mediated host-defense mechanisms (1,29) may function to protect against HSV. Whatever mechanism(s) is (are) involved, they at least have an effect on early virus replication in the eye, since a highly significantly and reproducible difference in virus levels was found as early as 2h post inoculation of antibody to IFNs (27).

SUMMARY

Our studies suggest that, in some virus infections, combinations of even low (undetectable) levels of antibody (ENA) and IFNs which occur early at the site of infection could be largely responsible for the rapid decrease in virus and prevention of clinical disease. In addition, we demonstrate the importance of IFNγ dependent, as well as IFNα/βdependent, host factors in resistance to primary ocular HSV infections.

ACKNOWLEDGEMENTS

The authors thank Martha Guin for assistance in preparation of the manuscript. This study was supported in part by PHS Grants from the NIAID (Al 23789) and from the NEI (EY 017015).

REFERENCES

1. Stanton, G.J., M.P. Langford, D.A. Weigent, J.E. Blalock and S. Baron: Amplification of the interferon system that may influence infections of the eye. In: A. Suran, I. Gery and R.B. Nussenblat (eds.) Proceeding Immunology of the Eye; Workshop III Sp Supp. Immunology Abstracts p. 443-457, 1981.
2. de la Pena, N.C., A. Diaz, A. Damel, E. Bal, L. Puricelli, J. Ejden, E.S. de Lustig: Combined therapy of human interferon (HI) and secretory immunoglobulin (S-IgA) in the treatment of human herpetic keratitis. Biomedicine 28:104, 1978.
3. Worthington, M. and S. Baron: Effect of polyriboinosinic-polyribocytidylic acid and antibody on infection of immunosuppressed mice with vaccinia virus. J Inf Dis 128:308, 1973.
4. Baron, S. The interferon system. American Society for Microbiology 45:358, 1979.
5. Gresser, I., M.G. Tovey, C. Maury and M.T. Bandu: Role of interferon in the pathogenesis of virus diseases in mice as demonstrated by the use of anti-interferon serum: II. Studies with herpes simplex, moloney sarcoma, vesicular stomatitis, newcastle disease, and influenza viruses. J Exp Med 144:1316, 1976.
6. Baron,S.: Mechanism of recovery from viral infection. Advanc Vir Res 10:39, 1963.
7. Fulginiti, V.A., C.H. Kempe, W.E. Hathaway, D.S. Pearlman, O.S. Sieber, J.J. Eller, J.J. Foyner and A. Robinson: Progressive vaccinia in immunologically deficient individuals. In: D. Bergsman (ed.). Immunologic Deficiency Disease in Man Birth Defects Original Articles Series. The National Foundation, New York. p. 129-151, 1968.
8. Allen, J.C. (ed.): Infection and the Compromised Host The Williams and Wilkins Co., Baltimore. p. 1-28, 1976.
9. Ogra, P.L., A. Morag and M.L. Tiku. Humoral immune response to viral infections. In: A.L. Notkins (ed.). Viral Immunology and Immunopathology . Academic Press, New York. p. 57-77, 1975.
10. Frazekas de St. S. Groth, and M. Donnelly: Studies in experimental immunology of influenza: IV. The protective value of active immunization. Aust J Exp Biol Med Sci 28:61, 1950.
11. Barnett, E.V., J.P. Nasou, J.P. Utz and S. Baron: Antibodies to enteroviruses in hypogammaglobulinemic patients. New Eng J Med 262:11, 1960.
12. Morgan, I.M.: Level of serum antibody associated with intra-cerebral immunity in monkeys vaccinated with lansing Poliomyelitis virus. J Immunol 62:301, 1949.
13. Tomasi, T.B., Jr: The immune system of secretions. In: A.G. Oster and L. Weiss (eds.). Foundations of Immunology Series. Prentice-Hall, Inc., New Jersey. p. 109-134, 1976.
14. Fenner, F. Immune mechanisms in viral infections. In F.L. Horsfall, Jr., and I.Tamm (eds.). Viral and Rickettsial Infections of Man .J.B. Lippincott Co., Philadelphia. p.356, 1965.
15. Subrahmanyan, T.P.: A study on the possible basis of age-dependent resistance of mice to poxvirus disease. Aust J Exp Biol Med Sci 46:251, 1968.
16. Schell, K.: Studies on the innate resistance of mice to infection

with mouse pox: I. Resistance and antibody production. Aust J Exp Biol Med Sci 38:271, 1960.
17. Koshland, M.E. and W. Burrows: Quantitative studies of the relationship between fecal and serum antibody. J Immunol 65:93, 1950.
18. Uhr, J.W. and M.S. Finkelstein: The kinetics of antibody formation. Progr Allergy 10:37, 1967.
19. Langford, M.P., A.L. Villarreal, and G.J. Stanton: Antibody and interferon act synergistically to inhibit enterovirus, adenovirus, and herpes simplex virus infection. Infect Immun 41:214, 1983.
20. Langford, M.P., M. Yin-Murphy, Y.M. Ho, J.C. Barber, S. Baron and G.J. Stanton: Human fibroblast interferon in tears of patients with picornavirus epidemic conjunctivitis. Infect Immun 29:995, 1980.
21. Langford, M.P., G.J. Stanton, J.C. Barber and S. Baron: Early-appearing antiviral activity in human tears during a case of picornavirus epidemic conjunctivitis. J Inf Dis 139(6):653-658, 1979.
22. Langford, M.P., J.C. Barber, V.E.F. Sklar, S.W. Clark, P.A. Patriarca, I.M. Onarato, M. Yin-Murphy and G.J. Stanton: Virus specific, early appearing neutralizing activity and interferon in tears of patients with acute hemorrhagic conjunctivitis. Curr Eye Res 4: 233, 1985.
23. Langford, M.P., D.A. Weigent, T.S.Chen, H.M. Johnson and G.J. Stanton: Antibodies to the C-terminus of mouse interferon gamma (MoIFN) neutralizes the immuno-regulatory and antiviral activities of MoIFN γ. J Interferon Res (in press).
24. Brunswick, M. and P.Lake: Obligatory role of gamma interferon in T cell-replacing factor-dependent, antigen-specific murine B cell responses. J Exp Med 161:953, 1985.
25. Steeg, P.S., R.N. Moore, H.M. Johnson and J.J. Oppenheim: Regulation of murine macrophage Ia antigen expression by a lymphokine with immune interferon activity. J Exp Med 156: 1780, 1982.
26. Sidman, C.L., J.D. Marshall, L.D. Shultz, P.W. Gray and H.M. Johnson: Interferon is one of several direct B cell-maturing lymphokines. Nature 309:801, 1984.
27. Stanton, G.J., C. Jordan, A. Hart, H. Heard, M.P. Langford, S. Baron: Non-detectable levels of interferon gamma is a critical host defense during the first days of herpes simplex virus infection. (submitted for publication).
28. Fleischmann, W.R., L.A. Schwarz and C.M. Fleischmann: Requirements for IFN gamma in potentiation of interferon's antiviral and anticellular activities: Identity of mouse and human systems. J Interferon Res 4:265, 1984.
29. Weigent,D.A., M.P. Langford, W.R. Fleischmann and G.J. Stanton: Potentiation of lymphocyte natural killing by mixtures of alpha and beta interferon with recombinant gamma interferon. Infect Immun 40:35, 1983.

50. Clinical Trials with Interferon in Japan

J. Imanishi[a] *and T. Kishida*[b]

[a]Department of Microbiology, Kyoto Prefectural University of Medicine, Kawaramachi-Hirokoji, Kamikyo-ku, Kyoto 602, Japan; [b]Institut Pasteur de Kyoto, Kyoto, Japan

INTRODUCTION

Japan is one of the countries where clinical trials with interferon (IFN) have been carried on actively. The Japanese Government is ahead of the governments of other countries in approving the production of an IFN : the Ministry of Health and Welfare has recently given a new drug approval of human fibroblast IFN (HuIFN-β) to Toray Industries, Co. Ltd. Some Japanese pharmaceutical companies have submitted of recombinant human leukocyte IFN (rHuIFN-αA or rHuIFN-α 2) and natural HuIFN-α (nHuIFN-α) for a new drug approval, and more than 10 Japanese companies are involved in clinical trials with IFN. Furthermore, about 10 Japanese companies are carrying on clinical trials with HuIFN-γ, although none of the companies have yet obtained a new drug approval from the Japanese Ministry of Health and Welfare (Table 1).
The characteristics of clinical trials in Japan are : 1. Many companies join in the trials. All types of IFN (natural and recombinant HuIFN-α, -β and -γ) are used for the clinical trials. 2. The first new drug approval given by the Ministry of Health and Welfare authorized the use only for the therapy of glioblastoma and malignant melanoma in skin, but not for the therapy of hepatitis B virus infection or other viral infections.

CLINICAL TRIALS WITH HuIFN-α AND HuIFN-β

The study on the clinical trials with HuIFN-α and HuIFN-β is highly advanced in Japan, making available a huge number of well analyzed data on the clinical trials.

Dosage, route and duration of the administration and phar-

macokinetics. Dosages of the IFN are different according to the kind of IFN. Natural HuIFN-α or -β is administered at doses of 3 - 20 X 10^6 IU, but mainly at 3 - 10 X 10^6 IU; recombinant HuIFN-αA, at doses of 3 - 100 X 10^6 IU, mainly at 3 - 20 X 10^6 IU.
Japanese patients tolerate a single dosage of 200 X 10^6 IU/ml of HuIFN-αA, but in some cases of continuous administration of HuIFN-α or -β, the administration has to be stopped because of some side effects.
HuIFN-α is mainly administered intramuscularly, while HuIFN-β is administered through an intravenous injection because no or low IFN activity is detected in the serum of the patients when HuIFN-β is injected intramuscularly. In particular diseases, other routes of the administration are employed. For example, in the case of viral infection of eye, IFN was dropped onto eyes, while with the tumor, warts and viral infection in skin, intralesional injection is employed. In the case of brain tumor, IFN is locally injected via Ommaya's reservoir into the dead space created by the resection of tumor. With hepatoma, IFN is administered by the continuous intra-arterial infusion.
In most cases to which clinical trials are applied, IFN is administered every day for 4-100 weeks. In parts of the cases, IFN is administered 1 to 3 times a week.
The pharmacokinetics of all kinds of HuIFNs are well studied. They are different according to the routes of administration, but not different according to the kinds of HuIFNs.
When HuIFN-β is intravenously injected at a dose of 12 X 10^6 IU, IFN activity is detected in the serum immediately after the injection and reaches its peak within half an hour (1). When HuIFN-α A is intramuscularly injected at a dose of 100 X 10^6 IU, the peak of IFN activity (2,060 IU/ml) is detected in the serum 4.68 h after the injection (2).

Side effects. There is hardly any difference in side effects between Japan and other countries.
Main side effects are shown in Table 2.
Usually, there is no correlation between the dosage and the degree of side effects. The kind and the degree of the side effect differ from individual to individual.

Clinical effect. The application of recombinant and natural HuIFN-α and -β has been reported for over 1,000 persons, about whom its clinical effects have been evaluated.

a. Brain tumors and other neuronal tumors. Natural HuIFN-α, recombinant HuIFN-α2 and natural HuIFN-β were used for the treatment of the brain tumor.
Hirakawa and his study group (3) reported that 4 out of 25 patients (16.0%) with brain tumors (23 glioblastomas and 2 malignant gliomas) treated with HuIFN-α via Ommaya's reservoir showed a complete or partial remission (glioblastoma :

3/23, malignant glioma : 1/2).
Similar results were found in 54 patients treated with natural HuIFN-β by another study group (4).
The intramuscular injection of recombinant HuIFN-α2 also showed similar results (5). Of 35 patients with brain tumor, 7 patients (20%) showed a complete or partial remission.
Thus, it was concluded that the administration of HuIFN-α and -β were effective against brain tumors, especially against glioblastoma, medulloblastoma and other gliomas.
Neuroblastoma is the most frequent malignant tumor in childhood, and its prognosis is very poor, especially in stage III and stage IV, in which mortalities for 2 years are 7 and 1 % in children older than 2, repectively.
Sawada et al noticed a partial effect of HuIFN-α on neuroblastoma in stage III (4 cases), but no effect in stage IV (4 cases) (6).

b. Warts and malignant tumors in skins. Natural HuIFN-β was used for the treatment of common and juvenile warts in a double-blind trials (7). Sixty-four patients with bilateral common warts of the extremities were treated with intralesional injection of either HuIFN-β or placebo. More than 81% of the IFN-treated warts were cured or responded to the therapy, whereas only 17% responded to the placebo. There was a significant difference in effectiveness against warts between HuIFN-β and placebo-treated groups.
The same study group also treated 37 patients with the juvenile warts with HuIFN-β. The warts in 17 patients were cured and those in 3 was improved. Cure rate was 54.1% (8).
HuIFN-β was also intratumorally injected into metastatic malignant melanoma and other malignant tumors (9). A significant clinical improvement was found, the improvement rate being about 50%. When the patients with metastatic carcinoma of the skin were treated with HuIFN-β, the improvement rate was 42.9%.
Thus, it was concluded that the local administration of HuIFN was effective against malignant lymphoma, malignant melanoma and other skin tumors.

c. Urogenital tumors. In Japan, the disease to which HuIFN-α is applied most frequently is renal cell carcinoma. A total of 136 cases treated with HuIFN were reported by Japanese study groups : 26 (19.1%) patients showed a complete remission (4; 2.9%) or partial remission (22; 16.2%). All kinds of HuIFN were intramuscularly injected and there is no difference in the effectiveness between recombinant and natural HuIFN-α.
Other urogenital tumors including urothelial carcinoma, prostatic carcinoma and testicular carcinoma were subjected to the treatment with recombinant HuIFN-α. A partial remission was noted in 1 of 9 patients with urothelial carci-

noma, but no remission was noted in any other patients (10).

d. Hematological malignant diseases. Several kinds of HuIFNs were employed in the treatment of adult T cell leukemia (ATL), other leukemias, multiple myeloma and lymphomas. Natural HuIFN-α induced a complete remission in the patients with ATL, partial remission (16.7%) in the patients with multiple myeloma, and a partial remission (15.4%) in the patients with non-Hodgkin lymphomas. Furthermore, hematological remission was shown in 4 of 5 patients in the chronic phase of chronic myelogenous leukemia by the treatment with HuIFN-α (11).
Thus, hematological malignant diseases are also relatively susceptible to the therapy by HuIFN.

e. Other malignant tumors. In general, malignant tumors of gastrointestinal tracts and gynecologic organ are not sensitive to HuIFN, because over 110 patients treated with HuIFN did not show any response (2, 3).
The efficacy rate was also very low (3%) for about 80 patients with bone and soft tissue cancer have been treated with HuIFN.
Head and neck cancer did not respond to IFN therapy, either.

g. Hepatitis B virus (HBV) infections. In Japan, several study groups tried to treat the patients with HBV infection with natural HuIFN-α and HuIFN-β. Suzuki and his members of HuIFN-β research group reported the effect of HuIFN-β on HBe Ag-positive chronic active hepatitis (CAH)(14), and a final evaluation was given to 72 out of 86. HBV-associated DNA polymerase (DNAP) activity decreased during the treatment with HuIFN-β in almost all the cases.
Suzuki et al also tried to treat DNAP-positive CAH with natural HuIFN-α (15), which was intramuscularly injected at a total dose of 19×10^6 IU in 10 cases. The result showed that DNAP became negative in 4 cases during the administration.
Thus, HuIFN-α and -β are useful for the treatment of HBV infection, although their effects are partial and transient. In future, the combination therapy with other antiviral agents should be considered in order to obtain a complete remission in more cases.

h. Viral infection in eye. It is already reported that natural HuIFN-α can be significantly effective against adenovirus-induced epidemic keratoconjunctivitis (EKC). Kitano and his study group compared the effectiveness of HuIFN-β against herpetic keratitis with that of iododeoxyuridine (IDU) (16). HuIFN-β was dropped onto the eyes of 30 patients, while IDU solution was applied to 25. The efficacy rate was 93.3% in the IFN-treated group, and 88.0%

in the IDU-treated group. There was no significant difference between the two groups.

CLINICAL TRIALS WITH HUIFN-γ.

There are few reports about the clinical trials with HuIFN-γ At present, several study group are carrying on trials of phase I to II study. Adachi et al reported on the phase I and II study of recombinant HuIFN-γ. In the phase I study, 7 patients received 2 - 64 X 10^6 U/ml by 1-hour intravenous infusion. The pharmacokinetics of HuIFN-γ were almost the same as those of HuIFN-α or HuIFN-β. Among the side effects were fever with chills, anorexia, nause, vomiting, elevation of serum GOT, leukopenia, and neurotoxic syndrome such as heavy fatigue with somnolence or lethargy (17). Clinical effects are not yet mentioned.

REFERENCES

1. Koyama, Y. : Pharmacokinetics and clinical trials of HuIFN-β in malignant tumors. In. Proceedings of the International Symposium on Interferons, T. Kishida, eds. ISIFN, pp. 189-195, 1983.
2. Taguchi, T. : Phase I study of recombinant human interferon αA (Ro22-8181) in patients with malignant tumors. Jpn J Cancer Chemother 12:456, 1985.
3. Hirakawa, K. : Clinical phase II study of HuIFN-α (MOR-22) in brain tumor. personal communication
4. Nagai, M. : Clinical trials of human fibroblast interferon (HuIFN-β) on malignant brain tumors. J Jpn Soc Cancer Ther 18:60, 1983.
5. Kitamura, K. : Phase II study of interferon-α 2 (Sch 30500) for brain tumors. Clin Med Drug (Rinsho Iyaku) 1:43, 1985.
6. Sawada T., T. Sugimoto, T. Itoi, T. Matsumura, T. Kusunoki, T. Kishida, O. Watanabe, and F. Besso : Clinical use of alpha-interferon in neuroblastoma. In. Proceeding of the International Symposium on Interferons, T. Kishida, eds. ISIFN, pp. 217-222, 1983.
7. Niimura, M. : Intralesional human fibroblast interferon in common warts. J Dermatol 10:217, 1983.
8. Niimura, M. : Therapy of juvenile verruca plana by HuIFN-β. Nishinihon J Dermatol 45:59, 1983.
9. Ishihara, K. : Clinical trials of human fibroblast interferon (HuIFN-β) in the treatment of malignant tumors of the skin. J Jpn Soc Cancer Ther 18:41, 1983.
10. Yoshimoto, J., T. Tsushima, Y. Matsumura, H. Ohmori, N. Saito, H. Tanaka, T. Asahi, K. Ohkita, T. Takahashi, K. Namba, N. Ishito, T. Josen, and H. Kamada : Phase II study or recombinant human leukocyte A interferon on urogenital cancer patients. Jpn J Cancer Chemother 12:465, 1985.
11. Koyama, S., M. Ohnishi, M. Urushiyama, H. Hirosawa, K. Kishi, M. Takahashi, Y. Moriyama, and A. Shibata : Effects

of interferon on chronic myelogenous leukemia. Progress in Med. (Igaku no Ayumi) 132:880, 1985.
12. Sekiya, S., H. Iwasawa, H. Ishige, and H. Takamizawa : Clinical trials of interferon to gynecologic cancers. Acta Obst Gynaecol Jpn 37:1241, 1985.
13. Kasamatsu, T. K. Ohmi, S. Takeuchi, H. Takamizawa, M. Matsuzawa, T. Kawana, K. Ueda, H. Kubo, Y. Tsumuji, Y. Kawashima, and M. Sugase : Clinical study of recombinant interferon alpha-2 (Sch 30500) in advanced gynecological cancers. Jpn J Cancer Chemother 12:1656, 1985.
14. Suzuki, H. : Effect of human fibroblast interferon (HuIFN-β) on HBe antigen positive chronic active hepatitis. In. Proceedings of the International Symposium on Interferons, T. Kishida, eds. ISIFN, pp. 259-266, 1983.
15. Suzuki H., F. Ichida, S. Furuta, T. Hirasawa, S. Iino, A. Ohbayashi, T. Takino, S. Yamamoto, N. Hattori, K. Ito, M. Yano, M. Mayumi, K. Nishioka, and T. Oda : Human IFN-α and -β therapies of HBV-associated DNA polymerase positive chronic active hepatitis and its comparison. Acta Hepatol Jpn 24:955, 1983.
16. Kitano, S., et al : Clinical effect of HuIFN-β on herpetic keratitis, compared with the effect of IDU. Jpn Rev Clin Ophthalmol 77:1777, 1983.
17. Adachi, K., M. Ogawa, N. Usui, J. Inagaki, N. Horikoshi, K. Inoue, H. Nakada, A. Tada, H. Yamazaki, and T. Mukaiyama : A phase I - II study of recombinant interferon gamma. Jpn J Cancer Chemother 12:1331, 1985.

Table 1. The present state of development of HuIFN in Japan (as of April 1986)

IFN	Name of Company	stage
α, natural	Fuso P.C.	phase I - II
α, natural	Hayashibara Biochem., Ohtsuka P.C., Mochida P.C.	submitting
α, natural	Green Cross	submitting
α, natural	Sumitomo P.C.	submitting
α, recombinant	Essex Nippon, Yamanouchi P.C.	submitting
α, recombinant	Nippon Roche, Takeda P.C.	submitting
α, recombinant	Toyo Jozo	preclinical
β, natural	Toray Ind, Daiichi P.C.	phase IV
β, natural	Ajinomoto	preclinical
β, natural	Green Cross	phase I
β, natural	Mochida P.C.	phase III
β, natural	Sunstar	phase I
β, recombinant	Kyowa Hakko, Toray Ind.	phase II
β, recombinant	Mitsui Toatsu Chem.	preclinical
γ, natural	Hayashibara Biochem.	preclinical
γ, recombinant	Meiji Seika	phase II
γ, recombinant	Asahi Kasei Chem.	preclinical
γ, recombinant	Daiichi P.C., Toray Ind.	phase II
γ, recombinant	Kanebo	?
γ, recombinant	Kyowa Hakko	phase II
γ, recombinant	Nippon Roche, Takeda P.C.	phase II
γ, recombinant	Searle	phase II
γ, recombinant	Suntory	phase II

Table 2. Side effects of HuIFN found in Japanese patients

1. fever, chills
2. fatigue
3. nausea, vomiting, anorexia, diarrhea
4. numbness
5. dizziness
6. skin eruption, itching
7. headache
8. arthralgia, lumbago
9. epigastralgia
10. tachycardia, hypotension
11. insomnia, convulsion
12. leukopenia, lymphocytopenia
    granulocytopenia, thrombocytopenia
13. elevation in GOT, GPT, LDH
14. elavation in creatinine, proteinurea

51. Clinical Studies with Polynucleotides

Hilton B. Levy

National Institute of Allergy and Infectious Diseases, NIH, Frederick Cancer Research Facility, Frederick, MD 21701-1013

INTRODUCTION

Compounds that will cause animals or tissue culture cells to synthesize interferon have been under study for many years. The original impetus for their development was the fact that it was, until recently, very difficult to obtain enough interferon to do a clinical test of the antiviral efficacy of interferon, even in mice, let alone humans. The development of DNA recombinant techniques for preparation of interferon has, to a large extent, overcome this problem although interferon continues to be expensive and is not available in unlimited amounts even now. In addition, the interferons, particularly the alpha interferons, exist in many different molecular forms, each the expression of a different gene. These different interferons have somewhat different biological activities from each other, possibly affecting different components of the effector cell population that responds to the interferon system. It appears reasonable to think that the interferon population induced by the synthetic inducers will resemble the natural mixture that is produced under physiological conditions, and which may therefore express all the biological properties of the mixture. Moreover, data developed over the past several years have shown that the interferon system is closely linked to the immune system, and that interferon and its inducers modify many immune parameters, both in vitro and in vivo. The relevance of these observations to the present chapter is that interferon and its inducers do not always bring about identical alterations. That is to say, in a number of tests, even though the inducer leads to the production of large quantities of interferon, the modulation of the immune parameter brought about by the inducer may be different, both quantitatively and qualitatively, from that brought about by interferon.

A number of inducers have been developed, of which the most intensive studied are the double stranded RNAs or polynucleotides. Four of these have been tested clinically--polyadenylic-polyuridylic acid (polyA.polyU), polyinosinic-polycytidylic acid (polyI.polyC), a complex of polylysine, carboxymethylcellulose with polyI.polyC (polyICLC), and a complex of modified polyI.polyC called Ampligen, in which base mis-matching is deliberately introduced. The purpose of this review is to summarize data obtained with these compounds in the clinical setting. Some relevant material of a non-clinical nature will also be presented.

PRE-CLINICAL STUDIES

Early data, presented in ref. (1), reported the following: polyA. polyU, and polyI.polyC both induced augmentation of the production by mice of antibodies to several antigens. A single injection in mice causes a marked increase in the proportion of T cells in the spleen, within 3 days after the injection. PolyA.polyU induces only very slight levels of serum interferon in mice, while polyI.polyC leads to the production of very high levels, so that there is strong disassociation of interferon production and immune enhancement.

Both polyI.polyC and polyA.polyU cause strong inhibition of growth of some rodent tumors(1); Ampligen also has antitumor activity in mice but at a lower level of effectiveness.(3)

PolyI.polyC was tested in two clinical trials in cancer patients. Only low levels of interferon were induced, and there was no antitumor action noted. Toxicities were very mild but, because of the lack of effect, these studies were not pursued. Subsequent work revealed that there is present in primate serum a much higher concentration of enzyme activity that inactivates polyI.polyC than there is in rodents, and it is thought that the lack of effectiveness of polyI.polyC in primates is attributable to its ease of hydrolysis by primate serum.

Chemical Characteristics of the Polynucleotide Inducers

The complex polyICLC was developed in an attempt to make a derivative of polyI.polyC that would be able to resist the hydrolytic action of primate serum. PolyI.polyC forms a complex with poly lysine, but at anything but very low concentrations, it is a gummy precipitate. However, if the poly lysine first is complexed with carboxymethylcellulose and then further complexed with polyI.polyC a soluble material called polyICLC is formed, which is partially resistant to hydrolysis and which can induce the formation of high levels of interferon in primates, including man. Studies with polyICLC preparations in which the molecular weight of the components is changed shows that the ability to induce interferon is a strict function of the ability to resist hydrolysis by primate serum. Previous reviews have described many of the properties of this material.(2) In a subsequent section, we will discuss some of the recent clinical observations made with polyICLC.

Much of the early work with polyA.polyU, including its chemistry, has also been reviewed.(1) PolyA.polyU has been shown to be more readily hydrolized by mouse serum than is polyI.polyC. Ten minutes of incubation of the former with mouse serum leads to extensive inactivation, but has no effect on polyI.polyC. PolyA.polyU also has a lower thermal denaturation temperature than polyI.polyC. Any substitution for either an A in the polyA strand or a U in the polyU strand reduces the effectiveness of the complex as an immune enhancing agent.

Ampligen

This compound is one of several ds.RNAs in which a uridine is substituted at intervals in the polycytidylic acid chain--in this case one U for every 12 Cs. At the point where there is an Uridylic acid molecule a bond does not form with the inosinic acid on the opposing chain, thus rendering the ds.RNA readily susceptible to attack by hydrolytic enzymes. This compound retains some of the ability of polyI.polyC to induce interferon in rodents, and to inhibit virus growth and tumor growth in rodents, but to a significantly lesser extent than the parent compound. It also is significantly less toxic in mice than is polyI.polyC.

CLINICAL STUDIES

There have been a number of clinical trials with the double-stranded RNAs. The best controlled have been adjuvant trials with polyA.polyU when used in human breast cancer in conjunction with surgery; the most varied have been with polyICLC, while the reported trials with Ampligen have been the most limited.

PolyA.PolyU

Based on observations in animal models, a trial of polyA.polyU as an adjuvant in conjunction with surgery was performed at the Institut Gustave-Roussy in Villejuif, France. All patients received standard treatment, which was surgery alone when axillary nodes were negative, or surgery plus cobalt irradiation when they were invaded. Patients were divided into two groups. One received the above treatment plus polyA.polyU, one injection per week of 30 mg. for six weeks. The other received the standard treatment plus a placebo, and served as a control. There were 300 patients, about evenly matched and evenly divided as to number. In 1983, when the mean time of follow up was 87 months, it was found that those patients that had received polyA.polyU had an actuarial survival rate of 71 percent, while the placebo group had a rate of 57 percent, with a p value for the difference being $<.05$. The difference was even greater in that a subgroup of patients where there was evidence of disease in the lymph nodes, 67 percent versus 48 percent, with a p value of <0.02. No interferon was found in the serum of patients receiving polyA.polyU, although there was an increase in the levels of two enzymes associated with the presence of interferon, namely a protein kinase and 2', 5' A synthetase. NK cell activity was also frequently increased in those patients receiving the duplex. The mean percentage of E-rosette forming cells also was increased in those patients. There was extremely little toxicity seen in any of these patients--a mild fever or, occasionally, a mild myalgia.(4)

There have been no reports of studies with polyA.polyU being used as primary therapy, only those in an adjuvant setting.

PolyICLC

There have been a number of small studies with poly ICLC. They will be summarized individually.

Seven patients with multiple myeloma that had become refractory to conventional therapy were treated with polyICLC, by i.v. route, three times weekly, at doses ranging from 1 to 12 mg./m^2. The highest level produced unacceptable levels of toxicity (see below). Table 1 summarizes the clinical responses in these patients. It is clear that there was some efficacy of the drug in this disease. However, it is likely, in light of evidence developed later, that these patients were receiving doses of drug that maximized toxicity and minimized the degree of immune enhancement obtainable.(5)

In an open study in children terminally ill with leukemia, there were no clear-cut remissions. There were seen some antileukemic effects in that bone marrow became free of abnormal cells, but the children died of their disease before it could be determined if normal marrow would have grown back.(6) These children were very sensitive to the side effects of polyICLC.

There is a form of juvenile laryngopapillomatosis that requires frequent surgical intervention (sometimes, up to twice monthly). This illness is reasonably well controlled by the use of polyICLC, 12 mg./m^2, weekly or t.i.w. Table 2 shows the effects of the drug on the frequency of need for surgery in six patients. These children were better able to tolerate the side effects of polyICLC than were the very ill leukemic children, but they also showed significant toxicity at the high drug doses used. Whether lower doses would be as effective has not been determined.(7)

PolyICLC has been examined in patients with polyneuropathy (Guillian-Barre syndrome), and with multiple sclerosis.(8,9) In 12 peripheral neuropathy patients, half have shown objective improvement, ranging from modest to dramatic, while the others have shown none. These patients show an extreme sensitivity to fever. Their muscular weakness is worsened by fever, and so it was with polyICLC, which is a pyrogen. However, by 24-48 hours, they regain their pretreatment strength, and frequently by the third day, there is demonstrable improvement in one or more of the measuring parameters. Similar side effects were seen with the M.S. patients. A group of 10 M.S. patients have been treated with monthly infusions of polyICLC for 10-18 months. All initially stabilized or improved. Three had improvement of the DSS (disability status score), and four of the Ambulatory Index. Four deteriorated after 5, 10, 14, and 17 months. It was concluded that polyICLC can be given safely to these patients and that a controlled trial is warranted.

It was noted that the male M.S. patients made about five times as much interferon in response to a given dose of polyICLC as did the female patients, as shown in Figure 1. Subsequent work showed that this phenomenon was true for Rhesus monkeys and for mice. It was also found in mice that NK cell activation by polyICLC was greater in males than in females. Interestingly, pretreatment of mice with either alpha or gamma interferon instead of polyICLC also resulted in greater NK cell activation in males than in females.

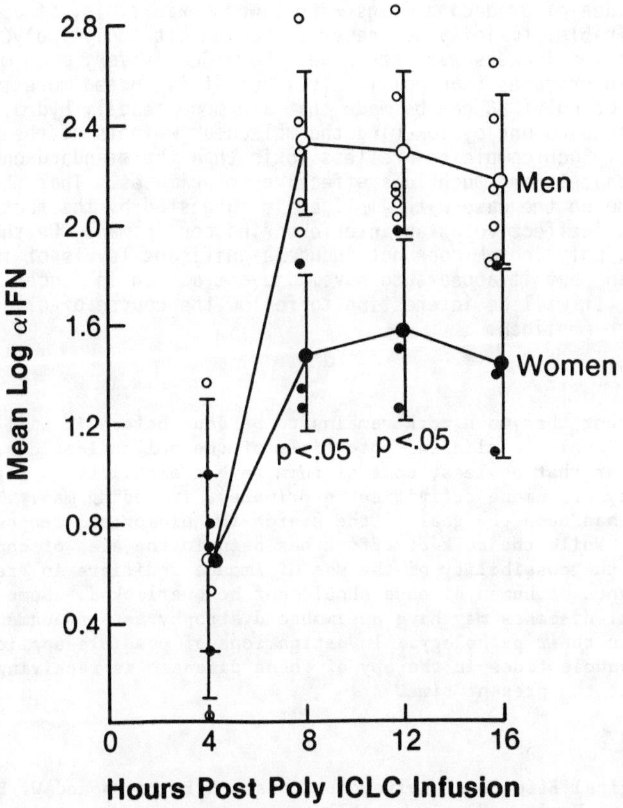

Figure 1. Difference between men and women in interferon production induced by polyICLC.

Ampligen

A totally different approach to the use of ds. RNAs has been proposed by Carter and T'so.(3) These investigators, working on the assumption that polyI.polyC has proven too toxic for use in man, have developed complexes of polyribonucleotides that are more readily hydrolizable than polyI.polyC. The reasoning was that such complexes would be stable just long enough to induce the biologic effects desired and then would be inactivated by hydrolysis. They did this by inserting a molecule of uridylic acid for every 12th molecule instead of cytidylic acid in the polyC chain. The U cannot bond with the I on the opposing chain, thus producing a more readily hydrolizable duplex which they named Ampligen. There clearly is very little toxicity. There was little or no interferon made. A few of the ten patients may have had a slight rise in NK cell activity.(10) The limited amount of data do not permit an evaluation of possible clinical efficacy. Further studies are being contemplated at this time.

While the idea of producing drugs with lower toxicity is, of course, highly desirable, toxicity was never a problem with polyI.polyC. Rather, ineffectiveness was the issue. PolyICLC is very much more effective in primates than polyI.polyC, but it is indeed more toxic. Variations of polyICLC can be made that are more readily hydrolizable than the standard one by lowering the molecular weights of the components. Such complexes are less toxic than the standard one, but unfortunately are much less effective in primates. That this may prove to be the case with Ampligen is suggested by the fact that Ampligen is ineffective as an interferon inducer in man. On the other hand, polyA.polyU does not induce significant levels of interferon in man, but it appears to have adjuvant action in cancer treatment. It will be interesting to follow the course of clinical studies with Ampligen.

CONCLUSIONS

It is apparent that much work remains to be done before it will be possible to evaluate clinical potentials of the polynucleotides. It is also clear that at least some of them have the ability to augment a wide variety of immune activities in primates, including man. This, of course, has been the goal of the search for biological response modifiers. While the bulk of effort has been in the area of cancer treatment, the possibility of the use of immune modifiers in treatment of other types of human disease should not be overlooked. Some of the neurological diseases may have an immune dystrophy as a fundamental component in their pathology. Investigations of possible application of the polynucleotides in therapy of these diseases is receiving some attention at the present time.

BIBLIOGRAPHY

1. Biological Effects of Polynucleotides. R.F. Beers and W. Braun, eds. Springer-Verlag, New York, 1971.
2. Levy, Hilton B.: Utilization of Stabilized Forms of Polynucleotides. In: Polymers in Medicine, E. Chiellini and P. Guisti, eds. Plenum Publishing Corp., New York, 1984.
3. Carter, W.A., J. O'Malley, and M. Beeson: An Integrated Study of the PolyI.PolyC Complex and Its Mismatched Analogues. Molecular Pharmacol 12:440, 1976.
4. Lacour, Jean: Clinical Trials Using Polyadenylic Polyuridylic Acid as an Adjuvant to Surgery in Treating Different Human Tumors. J Biol Resp Mod 4:438, 1985.
5. Voakes, J., B.G.M. Durie, A. Levine, J. Jett, H. Levy, and S. Salmon: AACR Abstracts, 1980.
6. Lampkin, B.C., A.S. Levine, H.B. Levy, W. Krivit, and D. Hammond: Cancer Research 45:5904, 1985.
7. Leventhal, B.G., A.S. Levine, and H.B. Levy: J Pediatrics 99:614, 1981.
8. Engel, W.K., R. Cuneo, and H.B. Levy: Lancet 503, 1978.
9. Bever, C.T., Jr., D.E. McFarlin, and H.B. Levy: J Int Res 4:484, 1985.
10. Carter, W.A., D.R. Strayer, H.R. Hubbell, and I. Brodsky: J Biol Res Mod 4:495, 1985.

TABLE 1. PolyICLC in Patients with Multiple Myeloma

M-Component Type	Comments
kappa light chains	67% decrease in B-J excretion, plus correction of hypercalcemia and disease stabilization with first period of treatment. 44% decrease in B-J excretion when poly (ICLC) restarted 2 months later. Normocalcemic for 5 months.
IgG kappa	M-component decrease from 5.2 gm to 3.9 gm. Improved bone pain and performance status (became ambulatory) for 2-3 months.
IgG lambda	Trial stopped because of toxicity (malignant hypertension).
IgM kappa	Plasmaphoresis requirement decreased from q 14 days to q 28 days.
IgG kappa	Stable disease parameters for 2 months.
lambda light chains	Died one week after initiation of poly (ICLC).
IgG kappa	50% decrease in serum IgG M-component, plus symptomatic benefit.

TABLE 2. Effect of PolyICLC on Frequency of Need for Surgery in Six Patients with Juvenile Laryngo Papilloma

	Age (Years)		Frequency of Surgery	
Patients	at Dx	at Rx	During 9 Months Before Rx	During 6 Months of Rx
1	1.5	4	18	0
2	1.5	3	23	4
3	2	3	8	0
4	2	6	5	1
5	54	61	4	0
6	41	47	3	0

52. Treatment of Virus-Associated Tumors with Interferon (IFN)

B. G. Leventhal

CMSC 804, Johns Hopkins Hospital, Baltimore, MD 21205

INTRODUCTION

The tumors discussed below, both benign and malignant, have all been consistently associated with the presence of a DNA virus. There is no proof that the virus is, in fact, the principal inducer of the malignant process in any of these tumors. This is not intended as an exhaustive review of these tumors but only of the attempts to use interferon for their management.

PAPILLOMAVIRUS ASSOCIATED TUMORS

A number of different types of lesions have been shown to contain papillomavirus DNA either in plasmid form or integrated into cellular DNA. The viruses have been subtyped and found to be not only species but tissue specific (1) (See Table 1).

Most of these diseases have a significant percentage of lesions which undergo spontaneous regression with time. This means that randomized controlled trials are necessary to establish true therapeutic efficacy of IFN.

Skin lesions

Most cutaneous warts are considered to be benign conditions, and for this reason there have not been many therapeutic trials of a material which is not without toxicity. However patients may be willing to undergo therapy because they find the lesions painful and/or unsightly. Vance et al. (2) randomized patients with plantar warts to receive local injection of placebo, 10^5IU or 10^6IU of human recombinant alpha-2 IFN (SCH 30500). A single wart on each patient was injected intralesionally 3 times weekly for 3 weeks. The warts were evaluated before each treatment and up to 9 weeks posttreatment. One hundred patients completed the full 12 week study and there was no difference in response between the 3 groups. Clearing of the treated wart at week 12 occured in 4/30 (13%) of the patients who received 10^6IU of IFN, 7/32 (22%) of those who received 10^5IU and 8/38 (21%) of those who received placebo. Five patients, all in the 10^6IU group withdrew because of adverse symptoms, 2 because of local pain at the injection site and 3 because of systemic flu like symptoms.

Niimura (3) performed a randomized double blind study of cutaneous warts directly injected with either fibroblast interferon or placebo;

81% of interferon and only 17% of placebo treated lesions regressed. An unusual patient with immune abnormalities and severe cutaneous warts was treated by Pazin (4), and responded to direct injection, but not systemic therapy with leukocyte interferon. These authors felt that intralesional therapy was effective, but not a practical way to manage the disease since the response was delayed and required multiple injections.

Genital lesions

Condyloma acuminata

These can occur in the labia, vagina, cervix or prepuce or around the anal sphincter. They are thought to be venereally transmitted and more common in patients with immunodeficiency. They will regress spontaneously in about one third of patients (5), but they are unsightly and uncomfortable and may cause problems during childbirth. They can be removed by cryosurgery, laser therapy or application of agents such as podophyllin or 5 fluoruracil. About 10% of patients will fail to respond to local therapy (6). In one small study (7) 3/4 women appeared to have had regression of their lesions after multiple direct injections of $1\text{-}5\times10^5$ IU of leukocyte IFN (Ultrapure HuIFN alpha). In another large randomized study (2) 91/114 patients with condyloma acuminatum completed local treatment with placebo vs. two doses of alpha IFN. Complete clearing of the treated wart occurred in 4/29 (14%) of patients receiving placebo; 6/32 (19%) of those receiving 10^5 IU of IFN and 16/30 (53%) of those receiving 10^6 IU intralesionally at week 12 after initiation of treatment. The high dose group showed better wart regression than the other two groups ($p<.01$), however there was no significant difference among the three treatment groups for noninjected warts. Systemic administration of lymphoblastoid alpha IFN (5,8) has also been employed for cases resistant to local therapy with other agents. Two sequential protocols were used. In the first one, 17 patients were given IFN i.m. at 5 Mu/M^2 daily for 28 days followed by the same dose thrice weekly for 2 additional weeks. In the second protocol 51 patients were given IFN i.m. at either 1 or 3 Mu/M^2 daily for 2 weeks followed by the same dosage for an additional 4 weeks. The complete response rate for doses of 1 Mu/M^2 was 43%, for 3 Mu/M^2 was 57% and for 5 Mu/M^2 was 69%. Some patients who had only a partial response at the end of the prescribed initial treatment period were continued longer on therapy before a complete response was achieved. All patients given the 5 Mu/M^2 dose had to have the amount reduced because of biologic side effects, while only 5/37 (14%) of those given 3 Mu/M^2 and no patient given 1 Mu/M^2 required a reduction in dosage. The patients in the study given 5 Mu/M^2 were found to have papillomavirus type 6 where analysis was possible (8). Thus systemic alpha IFN in relatively low doses may be efficacious in the treatment of this disease when it is resistant to local therapy, and is probably better tolerated than local injections. In view of this successful therapy in adult patients, systemic IFN was used in two prepubertal girls with condyloma,who probably acquired the disease via sexual abuse. Complete response occurred in both after a six week course of therapy (9). There has also been complete regression of lesions in 9/11 patients treated with intramuscular IFN (10), although a second study could not be reproduce these results (11).

Penile condylomata

Local injection of penile lesions with doses ranging from 10^5-10^6U of alpha IFN resulted in complete regression of lesions in 3/6 patients (7). Thus one suspects that the response rate of penile lesions overall will be about the same as that of vaginal/vulvar lesions. Gross et al. (11) describe one patient whose lesions changed from the typical histology of benign flat condylomas to those of squamous carcinoma in situ during therapy. They found integrated HPV 16 DNA in the malignant lesions from this patient, and suggest that future clinical studies of papillomavirus associated lesions treated with IFN should include analysis of papillomavirus type, since IFN may not control infection with the types with a higher malignant potential.

Cervical Intraepithelial neoplasia (CIN)

This diagnosis includes lesions of lower grade classified as moderate to severe dysplasia (CIN I and II) and CIN III (carcinoma in situ). Choo et al. (12) have treated 12 patients with varying grades of this disease with IFN, 2 x 10^6U twice weekly by perilesional injections under colposcopic guidance. Treatment continued until the colposcopically recognized lesion completely regressed and exfoliation of dyskaryotic cells ceased, and then for an additional 3-4 weeks. Five patients, all with CIN III were treated with IFN . Although they appeared to have a rapid initial response, only 2 achieved a complete regression and the other three were treated with cryosurgery. Two patients, both with CIN III were given lymphoblastoid IFN and both achieved complete remission, although disease recurred in one and was treated with hysterectomy. Two patients with CIN II were treated with leucocyte IFN and both achieved complete regression. Three patients with CIN III were treated with leucocyte IFN. One did not achieve remission and was treated with cryosurgery. The other two did achieve complete remission, however in one there was a recurrence of invasive carcinoma 9 months later. A preliminary communication (13) notes that a double blind placebo controlled clinical trial of leukocyte IFN gel in patients with CIN III is currently underway.

Recurrent respiratory papillomatosis

This disease, although rare, represents a serious clinical problem because of its tendency to recur and spread throughout the respiratory tract, and because the laryngo-tracheal location presents a potential threat to the airway. These lesions are known to undergo malignant degeneration occasionally, particularly if the patient has been exposed to radiation therapy, but occasional squamous malignancies have been seen in patients who have received no known carcinogen (14). Since the initial report by Haglund et al. (15) of responses in this disease, there have been several uncontrolled studies summarized in Table 2 (15-19). It appears that the majority of patients respond to alpha IFN with at least partial regression. Patients with adult onset may be more responsive than those with juvenile onset, although both are associated with the same virus type (20). It is difficult to quantitate this disease precisely and, therefore, partial responses are difficult to define. In addition, recurrence after a disease free period of a few months occurs in at least half the patients (21). Persistence of virus after IFN treatment in histologically normal appearing areas of epithelium has been demonstrated (22). It may be, therefore that IFN inhibits proliferation of cells but does not eradicate virus in these patients. Two randomized controlled clinical studies are currently underway, one employing lymphoblastoid (23) and one leukocyte (24) IFN. These may help to establish the response rate with greater certainty. It is clear that IFN represents useful adjunctive therapy but cannot be relied upon for total disease control, at least not after treatment lasting only a few months. In contrast, IFN when given i.v. to 3 patients (25,26) caused no response and showed little effect when given i.m. to 2 patients who later responded to alpha IFN (27).

EPSTEIN BARR VIRUS ASSOCIATED MALIGNANCIES

Burkitt lymphoma

One unusual patient with a B cell proliferative disorder which terminated in Burkitt lymphoma failed to respond to IFN (28). One patient (29) had a brief partial response to $50x10^6U/m^2$ administered as part of a phase I trial of recombinant alpha 2 IFN. There are reports of patients with indolent B cell lymphomas and leukemias (e.g. hairy cell leukemia) responding to IFN (30), although virus association with these tumors has not been demonstrated.

Nasopharyngeal carcinoma

Treuner et al (26) treated 4 patients with IFN. One had a complete response, two partial and one did not respond. Two adult patients treated with alpha IFN were described as having "stable" disease (31). Connors et al. (32) treated 13 patients. One who was treated with both alpha and β IFN did not respond. The other 12 were treated with leukocyte IFN. Patients received 10^7U i.m. for 30 days. Two patients had partial resonses, two had minor responses (<50% regression of disease), 2 had stable disease and the remaining 5 showed disease progression. No complete responses were seen, and eventually disease progressed in all patients despite continued therapy. It seems that the role of IFN deserves perhaps further attention in this tumor, but alpha IFN probably does not have sufficient activity to warrant its use as a single agent.

KAPOSI'S SARCOMA

This disease once considered to be a rare and indolent neoplasm occurring primarily in the elderly has, in the 1980s, reached epidemic proportions in patients with the acquired immunodeficiency syndrome (AIDS). Although the AIDS syndrome is related to infection with an RNA virus, it has been suggested that cytomegalovirus may be involved in the etiology of this tumor in these patients. Real et al (37) treated patients in sequential trials with different doses. In the initial protocol 36 patients were entered and treated with $36x10^6U$ recombinant leukocyte A IFN (Roferon). A major response was seen in 38% of these patients, but unacceptable toxicity occurred in 27% of them. These included severe fatigue (6), neutropenia (2), thrombocytopenia (2) and symptomatic hypotension (1). Flu like symptoms and nausea, vomiting, forgetfulness, confusion and depression as well as abnormalities in serum aspartate aminotransferase levels were also seen in many of the patients. Because of this, the next study was conducted at a lower dose ($3x10^6U$). Toxicity at this level was acceptable but only 3% responses were seen in 39 patients. However, 17% of low dose nonresponders responded when the doses were escalated. Only 10% of patients showed unacceptable toxicity with progressive dose escalation up to $36x10^6U$. Responses were seen to both high ($50x10^6U$ i.v.) and low ($1x10^6U$ s.c.) dose in a study by Groopman (34). Thus high dose interferon does appear to be effective for some patients with this disorder, and it would seem prudent to begin at an initial lower dose and escalate as tolerance permits.

INTERFERON TOXICITY

It is obvious that this is not a nontoxic material. It is difficult for adults to tolerate doses of 5 Mu/m^2 or higher for any period of time without experiencing intolerable lassitude and fatigue. Children may tolerate higher doses at least for short periods of time (29). Chills, fever, headache, nausea and myalgias occur at all dosage levels, although they tend to decrease with continued administration of the material. The most common laboratory abnormalities have been changes in liver function tests and leukopenia, with occasional thrombocytopenia. There have been antibodies to interferon reported in a certain percentage of patients, although this does not appear to have interfered with response (P.Weck, personal communication)

ASSAYING THE EFFECT ON THE IMMUNE SYSTEM

The activity of interferon is standardized in units which reflect decreases in viral plaque forming ability in vitro. However, it has been postulated that the activity of interferon in many diseases is related either to its antiproliferative activity or to its effect on the immune system. Since the effects on the immune system are pleiotropic, it is difficult to pick a single one to assay. For some time it has been known that interferon could increase NK activity of leukocytes activated in vitro and that patients with certain malignant conditions might have a lower level of these cells circulating than normal individuals (35). Unfortunately, there is a great variation in the baseline values of NK activity in patients as well as in normal controls, which makes changes in this assay difficult to interpret (36). In fact, a number of patients have had a fall in NK activity after interferon administration. For this reason people have been trying to use biochemical assays such as the change in 2'5'-oligoadenylate synthetase (OAS) levels in lymphocytes to assess the level of interferon activity. In one study of patients with laryngeal papillomatosis it was found that the increase in level of OAS activity was associated with response, which reversed as the treatment was interrupted and the level fell (37). In patients with AIDS and Kaposi's sarcoma, however, the baseline level is often high and rises in levels of OAS were not sufficient to predict a good clinical response (38). Thus the more abnormal the patient's baseline immune status, the more difficult it seems to be to assay the relevant factors which will predict response.

SUMMARY

There appears to be a spectrum of responses to alpha IFN, with the more indolent lesions of condyloma acuminata responding well to relatively low doses of 2 MU/m , often with permanent clearing of lesions, while the somewhat more rapidly growing laryngeal papillomas respond to doses in the 2-5 MU/m , but frequently regrow once treatment is stopped. The highly aggressive lesions of Kaposi's sarcoma respond to doses an order of magnitude higher where toxicity is often prohibitive. IFN is clearly a useful therapy in these conditions, but cannot be used alone for treatment. Its precise role in the overall management of these diseases is not yet fully established, and there is insufficient evidence to assess the clinical utility of IFN beta.

REFERENCES

1. Gissman, L., M. Boshart, M. Durst, et al.: Presence of human papillomavirus in genital tumors. J. Invest. Dermatol.83:26s,1984.
2. Vance, J.C., B.J. Bart, R.C. Hansen, et al.: Intralesional recombinant alpha-2 interferon for the treatment of patients with condyloma acuminatum or verruca plantaris. Arch Dermatol, 122:272, 1986.
3. Niimura, M. Interferon in skin disease. Gan To Kagaku-Ryoho. 11:221, 1984.
4. Pazin, G.J.: Interferon in papilloma virus infections Antiviral Research,(Suppl), 1:251, 1985.
5. Gall, S.A., C.E. Hughes, and K. Trofatter: Interferon for the therapy of condyloma acuminatum. Am J Obstet gynecol, 153:157, 1985.
6. Silva, P.D., J.P. Micha and D.G. Silva: Management of condyloma acuminatum. J Am Acad Dermatol, 13:457, 1985.
7. Geffen, J.R., R.J. Klein, and A.E. Friedman-Kien: Intralesional administration of large doses of human leukeocyte interferon for the treatment of condylomata acuminata. J Inf Dis, 150:612, 1984.
8. Gall, S.A., C.E. Hughes, P. Mounts, et al: Efficacy of human lymphoblastoid interferon in the therapy of resistant condyloma acuminata. Obstet Gynecol, 67:643, 1986.
9. Trofatter, K.F., P.C. Enslich, C.E. Hughes, and S.A.Gall: Human lymphoblastoid interferon (wellferon) in primary therapy of two children with condylomata acuminata. Obstet Gynecol, 67:137, 1986.
10. Schonfield, A., S. Nitke, A. Schattner, et al: Intramuscular human interferon- injections in treatment of condyloma accuminata. Lancet, i:1038, 1984.
11. Gross, G., H. Ikenberg, and L. Gissman: Bowenoid dysplasia in human papillomavirus-16 DNA positive flat condylomas during

interferon- treatment. Lancet, i:1467, 1984.
12. Choo, Y.C., W.H. Seto, C. Hsu, et al: Cervical intraepithelial neoplasia treated by perilesional injection of interferon. Brit J Obset and Gyn, 93:372, 1986.
13. Coleman, D.V.: Evaluation of interferon treatment of cervical intraepithelial neoplasia. Acta Cytologica (Balto.), 292:192, 1985.
14. Solomon, D., R.L. Smith, H.K. Kashima, et al.: Malignant transformation in non-irradiated recurrent respiratory papillomatosis. Report of a case and review of the literature. Laryngoscope, 95:900, 1985.
15. Haglund, S., P. Lundquist, K. Cantell, and H. Strander: Interferon therapy in juvenile laryngeal papillomatosis. Arch Otolaryngol, 107:327, 1981.
16. Goepfert, H., R.B. Sessions, J.U. Gutterman, et al.: Leukocyte interferon in patients with juvenile laryngeal papillomatosis. Ann Otol Rhinol Laryngol, 91:431, 1982.
17. McCabe, B.F. and K.F. Clark: Interferon and laryngeal papillomatosis: the Iowa experience. Ann Otol Rhinol Laryngol, 92:2, 1983.
18. Bomholt, A.: Interferon therapy for laryngeal papillomatosis in adults. Arch Otolaryngol, 109:550, 1983.
19. Zenner, H.P., W. Kley, P. Claros, et al: Recombinant interferon-alpha-2C in laryngeal papillomatosis: preliminary results of a prospective multicentre trial. Oncology, 42(suppl 1):15, 1985.
20. Mounts, P, T.C. Wu, B.G. Leventhal, et al.: Analysis of human papillomavirus type 6 in the respiratory and genital tracts during interferon therapy. In: Papillomaviruses: Molecular and clinical aspects, P.M. Howley and T.R. Broker, eds. Alan R. Liss, pp. 137-154, 1985.
21. Leventhal, B.G.: Treatment of virus-associated tumors and papillomas with interferons. In: Interferon, Vol. 4: In vivo and clinical studies, N.D. Finter and R.K. Oldham, eds. Elsevier Science Publishers, B.V., p. 325, 1985.
22. Steinberg,E.M., W.C. Topp, P.A. Schneider, and A.L. Abramson: Laryngeal papilloma virus infection during clinical remission. New England J Med, 308:1261, 1983.
23. Kashima, H., B.G. Leventhal, P. Mounts, et al.: Scoring system to access severity and course in recurrent respiratory papillomatosis. Papillomaviruses: Molecular and clinical aspects, P.M. Howley and T.R. Broker, eds. Alan R. Liss, pp. 125-135, 1985.
24. Healy, G.B. and A.L. Trowbridge: Interferon in recurrent respiratory papillomatosis: a multicenter controlled clinical trial. Papillomaviruses: Molecular and clinical aspects, P.M. Howley and T.R. Broker, eds. Alan R. Liss, pp. 181-184, 1985.
25. Gobel, U., W. Arnold, W. Wahn, et al: Comparison of human fibroblast and leukocyte interferon in the treatment of severe laryngeal papillomatosis in children. Eur J Pediatr, 137:175, 1981.
26. Treuner, J., G. Dannecker, K.E. Joester, et al.: Pharmacological aspects of clinical stage I/II trials with human interferon in children. J Interferon Res, 1:373, 1981.
27. Schouten, T.J. and J.H. Bos: Interferon voor de behandeling van juvenile papillomatosis van de larynx. Ned T Geneesk, 124:1650, 1980.

28. Thestrup-Pedersen, K., V. Esmann, S. Bisballe, et al.: Epstein-Barr virus induced lymphoproliferative disorder converting to fatal Burkitt like lymphoma in a boy with interferon inducible chromosomal defect. Lancet, ii:997, 1980.
29. Ochs, J., M. Abromowitch, S. Rudnick, and S.B. Murphy: Phase I-II study of recombinant alpha-2 interferon against advanced leukemia and lymphoma in children. J Clin Oncol, 4:883, 1986.
30. Golomb, H.M., A. Jacobs, A. Fefer, et al.: Alpha-2 interferon therapy of hairy cell leukemia: a multicenter study of 64 patients. J Clin Oncol, 4:900, 1986.
31. Laszlo, J., A.T. Huange, W.D. Brenckman, et al.: Phase I study of pharmacological and immunological effects of human lymphoblastoid interferon given to patients with cancer. Cancer Res, 43:4458, 1983.
32. Connors, J.M., W.A. Andiman, C.B. Howarth, et al.: Treatment of nasopharyngeal carcinoma with human leukocyte interferon. J Clin Oncol, 3:813, 1985.
33. Real, F.X., J.F. Oettgen, and S.E. Krown: Kaposi's sarcoma and the acquired immunodeficiency syndrome: treatment with high and low doses of recombinant leukocyte A interferon. J Clin Oncol, 4:544, 1986.
34. Groopman interferon trial in Kaposi's. Ann Intern Med, 100:671, 1984.
35. Seltzer, V., A. Doyle, and A.S. Kadish: Natural cytotoxicity in malignant and premalignant cervical neoplasia and enhancement of cytotoxicity with interferon. Gynecol Oncol, 15:340, 1983.
36. Maluish, A.E. and R.B. Herberman: Assessment of biological responses: what to measure and when. Cancer Treat Rep, 69:1165, 1985.
37. Lodemann, E., B. Kornhuber, V. Gerein, and C. Ilberg: (2'5') Oligo (A) synthetase as a monitor of interferon action in juvenile laryngeal papillomatosis. J Interferon Res, 4:283, 1984.
38. Preble, O.T., A.H. Rook, R. Steis, et al.: Interferon induced 2'-5' oligoadenylate synthetase during interferon-alpha therapy in homosexual men with Kaposi's sarcoma: marked deficiency in biochemical response to interferon in patients with acquired immunodeficiency syndrome. J Inf Dis, 152:457,1985.

TABLE 1. VIRUS SUBTYPES ASSOCIATED WITH SPECIFIC LESIONS (1)

Tissue	virus subtype
Plantar warts	1
Hand warts	2
Malignant lesions, epidermolysis verruciformis	5
Benign papillomas, larynx, genital area	6,11
Premalignant and malignant lesions genital area	16,18

TABLE 2. INTERFERON TREATMENT OF RECURRENT RESPIRATORY PAPILLOMATOSIS

Onset of disease	Patients treated			Reference
	number	complete response	partial response	
Partially purified leukocyte interferon alpha (10^3 u/dose)				
Juvenile	7	2	5	(15)
	12	3	5	(16)
	19	6	11	(17)
adult	2	2		(16)
	8	7		(18)
Purified recombinant alpha 2C (1.5×10^5 u/kg)				
juvenile	15	9	4	(19)
adult	5	2	3	(19)

53. Interferons in Hematological Malignancies

Jorge R. Quesada, Moshe Talpaz, and Jordan U. Gutterman

Department of Clinical Immunology and Biological Therapy, University of Texas Cancer Center M. D. Anderson Hospital and Tumor Institute, Houston, TX 77030

INTRODUCTION

The introduction of interferons for the treatment of human cancer marked a departure from traditional immunotherapy and has become the prototype of new agents now included in the broader concept of biologic response modifiers. The antitumor activity of interferon does not depend solely on the activation or stimulation of the host's immune system but also in other unique properties of these family of proteins, namely potent antiviral and antiproliferative activities. These have now been proven to be effective in the therapy of B cell neoplasms and particularly hairy cell leukemia (HCL) as well as chronic myelocytic leukemia (CML).

The purpose of this review is to discuss the present status of treatment of these hematologic neoplasms with alpha interferons.

HAIRY CELL LEUKEMIA

We began in October 1982 treatment of selected HCL patients with a partially purified preparation of interferon alpha. Our first report included seven patients who received daily doses of partially purified IFNα by intramuscular injection. Three patients had a complete remission and four had a partial remission (1).

The criteria of response defined complete remission (CR) and partial remission (PR) as an absence or more than 50% reduction of hairy cell leukemic infiltrate in both bone marrow aspirates and biopsies respectively; and the recovery of the hematologic indexes (Hemoglobin: >12 gm/dl; granulocytes: >1,500 cells/cc and platelets: >100,000/cc). Subsequently, an additional 15 patients on this study confirmed the activity of IFNα in all stages of HCL (2). It became apparent that IFNα reduced significantly morbidity factors such as transfusion requirements and infections in these patients. The confirmation of these results using purified recombinant IFNα (rIFNα) by our group and other investigators proved that the antileukemic activity resided in the IFN molecule and not that of other contaminants in the partially purified preparation. We have reported recently on the results of 30 patients who received rIFNα (3). In this study, nine complete and 17 partial remissions were documented, for a response rate over 85%. Peripheral blood hematologic indexes improved or normalized in all patients and malignant adenopathy responded in 12 of 13 patients. In that study, 7 patients with splenomegaly (and therefore candidates for splenectomy) volunteered to receive rIFNαA as frontline therapy. All of them showed a rapid reduction in the size of the spleen. The incidence of CR was significantly higher ($p = 0.01$) in previously untreated patients (5 of 7) than in those in whom splenectomy had been performed (4 of 23), presumably because the disease was treated at an earlier stage in untreated patients (3).

Other investigators have reported similar results as shown in Table 1 (1-13). The differences in the rate of response and in the incidence of complete remissions may be related to selection of patients, different treatment schedules and length of treatment. Altogether, these studies have confirmed that interferons alpha are highly effective therapy for all stages of the disease, and the treatment of choice for post-splenectomized patients with progressive cytopenias. IFNα is also an adequate initial treatment for selected untreated patients.

None of our patients have relapsed while receiving IFNα or rIFNα but it is still not known for how long a patient should be treated or the duration of unmaintained remissions. We are addressing these questions by discontinuing treatment with interferon at 2 years, in one study (1,2) and at one year on the other one (3). It has become evident that treatment for less than 6 months is probably insufficient because there are patients who continue to improve beyond this point and remissions have been obtained as late as 10 or 12 months after initiation of treatment.

The toxicity of low doses of alpha IFNs is minor except for unusually sensitive individuals (approximately 5%) in whom moderate to severe fatigue may require reduction from daily to thrice weekly administration. The usual influenza-like symptoms upon first exposure to IFN are well tolerated and short-lived. In the majority of patients, tumor remissions resulted in an improved quality of life, they eliminated the need for transfusing blood products, reduced the incidence of infections, and apparently restored immune deficits in some of the patients (3).

INTERFERONS IN OTHER B-CELL NEOPLASMS

The first clinical reports on the antitumor activity of IFNα in cancer included patients with B-cell non-Hodgkin's lymphomas (NHL) and multiple myeloma (MM) (14,15). The responses obtained in these tumors have been subsequently confirmed by other investigators both with natural and with recombinant purified interferons.

Using alpha interferons for non-Hodgkin's lymphomas (NHL), a response rate, ranging from 25% to 80% (median 50%) has been obtained with diverse doses and schedules in low grade lymphomas, but a lower response rate for tumors of intermediate or high grade lymphomas (16,17).

Preliminary reports seem to indicate that chronic lymphocytic leukemia (CLL) is less sensitive to IFNα than low grade NHL. This has been further confirmed in a larger number of patients using rIFNα (18). Only two of 18 patients achieved a PR (11%). Most of these patients, however, had advanced disease which had been previously treated with a variety of traditional chemotherapeutic agents.

The results obtained in the treatment of MM with IFNα are discussed in detail elsewhere in this volume. We have found that response rate in MM are related to the stage of disease and history of prior chemotherapy. Our data indicate that patients previously treated with chemotherapy (refractory or relapsing) have, in general, a poor response rate (varying from 0 to 28%; median 12%). In contrast, remissions occurred in 50% to 100% of previously untreated patients. In a randomized study conducted at M.D. Anderson Hospital and Wisconsin University, seven of 14 (50%) previously untreated patients achieved a CR or PR, whereas only 2 of 13 (15%) previously treated patients did so (19).

The disparity in the responsiveness among the different B-cell neoplasm is intriguing. This is, conceivably, related to the stage of differentiation. Thus, a more primitive cell of origin (acute leukemia, CLL) seemingly is more resistant to IFNα than those of more mature B cells (HCL, MM). It is noteworthy that hairy cells express plasma cell associated antigens, relating the stage of differentiation of this B-cell disorder closer to multiple myeloma (20).

CHRONIC MYELOCYTIC LEUKEMIA

Following the observations that IFNα induced granulocytopenia in cancer patients and that it exerted an inhibitory effect in the growth of committed myeloid precursors, Talpaz and collaborators initiated a clinical study using IFNα in patients with CML. The initial report involved seven patients treated with partially purified IFNα in doses ranging from 9 to 15 MU daily. Hematologic remission of the disease was obtained in 5 patients including decrease in the size of the spleen in 3 of 3 patients (21). Subsequent experience with partially purified IFNα has confirmed the efficacy of this agent in the treatment of CML. Twenty-four of 27 patients with CML in the benign phase responded to treatment with 20 achieving a complete hematologic remission (CHR) and 4 a partial hematologic remission (PHR) (22). The criteria of response included normalization of peripheral blood counts and cell morphology (CHR) or by a reduction of more than 75% of the leukocyte and platelet count (PHR). IFNα was shown to be extremely effective in controlling CML-associated thrombocytosis, even in the absence of a response in the WBC or the bone marrow. The doses higher than those used in HCL were required to induce remissions in CML (Table 2).

Noteworthy, IFNα induced karyotypic changes in 7 of the responsive patients with a decrease in the percentage of Philadelphia chromosome-positive cells (Phl+) and the induction of mosaicism in the bone marrow. The bone marrow effects and the restoration of normal hematopoiesis are similar to the effects observed in HCL. The elimination of suppressive influences in the bone marrow may be a consequence of the reduction in the malignant clone that led, in turn, to a normal pattern of proliferation and differentiation of residual normal stem cells.

Confirmation of these results with recombinant-DNA derived IFNα has been published (23). Fourteen of 17 patients responded to treatment, including 5 patients who had splenomegaly in whom the spleen returned to normal size. Bone marrow cellularity declined from a median of 92.5% to 57.5% and in 6 patients complete suppression of Philadelphia cells was observed. The proto oncogene c-abl is translocated in Ph' CML from chromosome 9 to chromosome

22. It is juxta posed to the BCR (breakage cluster region) gene on chromosome 22. This event is likely to be intimately associated with either the transformation or the accelerated growth of CML cells. The demonstration of IFNα inhibitory activity of oncogene expression was demonstrated in several models, and it's activity in CML might be the result of a similar effect.

CONCLUSIONS

The unusual sensitivity of these malignancies to IFNα or the mechanisms underlying its antitumor effect have not been elucidated. Because the multiple biologic activities of IFNs is likely that the mechanism of action is multifactorial, including a direct antiproliferative effect, induction of differentiation or enhancement of immune effector cells. Elsewhere in this review each of these IFN activities is dealt with in more detail. We have also speculated in the deficiency of the IFN system in explaining the results obtained in HCL (1). Indeed the prompt and consistent response is reminiscent of the results obtained when a deficient hormone or vitamin is replaced by exogenous products. Preliminary data in our laboratory indicate a deficiency of IFNα production in patients with HCL (unpublished). Finally, the activities of IFN in these hematologic neoplasms may be related to its ability to modulate gene expression including the expression oncogenes or the function of their products.

ACKNOWLEDGEMENT

We wish to acknowledge Linda Reckeweg for the preparation of this chapter.

TABLE I

THERAPY OF HAIRY CELL LEUKEMIA WITH ALPHA INTERFERONS

TYPE	DOSE	NO. PTS	CR	PR	MR	REFERENCE
IFNα	3 MU/d	22	5	13	4	Quesada (1,2)
IFNα	3 MU/d	10	1	6	3	Hagberg (4)
rIFNα	3-12 MU/d	30	9	17	4	Quesada (3)
rIFNα	2 MU/m²/tiw	8	0	7	1	Ratain (5)
rIFNα	2 MU/m²/tiw	14*	0	6	8	Jacobs (6)
rIFNα	2 MU/m²/tiw	8	1	6	0	Hoffmann (7)
rIFNα	2 MU/m²/tiw	14	3	10	1	Flandrin (8)
rIFNα	3 MU/d	17	7	10	0	Thompson (9)
rIFNα	5 MU/d	6	2	3	1	Gastl (10)
rIFNα	3 MU/d	14	1	12	0	Foon (11)
rIFNα	5 MU/d	26	3	15	4	Huber (12)
rIFNαLy	3-6 MU/d	17*	2	13	2	Worman (13)

MU = million units; CR = complete remission; PR = partial remission; MR = minor response.

*criteria of response not specified; results are approximations.

TABLE II

ALPHA INTERFERONS IN CHRONIC MYELOCYTIC LEUKEMIA

IFN	DOSE(MU)	NO. PTS	CHR	PHR	%RESPONSE	INVEST
IFNα	9-15	27	20	4	89	Talpaz
rIFNα	5/m²	17	13	1	82	Talpaz
rIFNα	4/m²	6	6	-	100	Niederle

REFERENCES

1. Quesada JR, Reuben J, Manning JT, Hersh EM, and Gutterman JU: Alpha interferon for induction of remission in hairy cell leukemia. N Engl J Med 310:15, 1984.

2. Quesada JR, Hersh EM and Gutterman JU: Treatment of hairy cell leukemia with alpha interferon. Proc Am Soc Clin Oncol 3:207, 1984 (abstr).

3. Quesada JR, Hersh EM, Manning J, Reuben J, Keating M, Schnipper E, Itri L, and Gutterman JU: Treatment of hairy cell leukemia with recombinant α-interferon. Blood (in press).

4. Hagberg H, Aim G, Bjorkholm M, Glimeluis B, Killander A, Simonsson B, Sundstrom C, Ahre A: Alpha interferon treatment of patients with hairy cell leukaemia. Scand J Haematol 35:66, 1985.

5. Ratain MN, Golomb HM, Vardiman JW, Vokes EE, Jacobs RH and Daly K: Treatment of hairy cell leukemia with recombinant $alpha_2$ interferon. Blood 65:644, 1985.

6. Jacobs AD, Champlin RE, Golde SW: Recombinant α-2 interferon for hairy cell leukemia. Blood 65:1017, 1985.

7. Hofmann V, Scheel A, Schwarzmeier J, Talstad I, Varini M, Kaplan S, Sauter C, and Fehr J: Wirksamkeit von interferon-α2 (E. coli) bei der Haarzell-Leukamie. Schweiz Med Wochenschr 115:235, 1985.

8. Flandrin G, Sigaux F, Castaigne S, Billard C, Aguet M, Boiron M, Falcoff E, and Degos L: Treatment of hairy cell leukemia with recombinant alpha interferon. I. Quantitative study of bone marrow changes during the first months of treatment. Blood 67:817, 1986.

9. Thompson JA, Brady J, Kidd P and Fefer A: Recombinant alpha-2 interferon in the treatment of hairy cell leukemia. Cancer Treat Rep 69:791, 1985.

10. Gastl G, Denz H, Abbrederis C, Huber H, Troppmair J, Wiegele J, Niederwieser D, Flener R, and Huber C:

Treatment with low dose human recombinant interferon-alpha-2 ARG induces complete remission in patients with hairy cell leukemia. Onkologie 8:143, 1985.

11. Foon KA, Maluish AE, Abrams PG, Wrightington S, Stevenson HC, Alarif A, Fer MF, Overton WR, and Poole M, Schnipper E, Jaffe ES, and Herberman RB: Recombinant leukocyte A interferon therapy for advanced hairy cell leukemia. Therapeutic and Immunologic Results. Am J Med 80:351, 1986.

12. Huber C, Flener R, and Gastl G: Interferon-alpha-2C in the treatment of advanced hairy cell leukaemia. Oncology 42:7, 1985.

13. Worman CP, Catovsky D, Bevan PC, Camba L, Joyner M, Green PJ, Williams HJH, Bottomley JM, Gordon-Smith EC, and Cawley JC: Interferon is effective in hairy-cell leukemia. Brit J Haemat 70:759, 1985.

14. Merigan TC, Sikora K, Breeden JH, Levy R, Rosenberg SA: Preliminary observations on the effect of human leukocyte interferon in non-Hodgkin's lymphoma. N Engl J Med 299:1449, 1978.

15. Gutterman JU, Blumenschein GR, Alexanian R, Yap HY, Buzdar AU, Cabanillas F, Hortobagyi GN, Hersh EM, Rasmussen SL, Harmon M, Kramer M, and Peska S: Leukocyte interferon-induced tumor regression in human metastatic breast cancer, multiple myeloma, and malignant lymphoma. Ann Int Med 93:399, 1980.

16. Quesada JR, Hawkins M, Horning S, Alexanian R, Borden E, Merigan T, Adams F, and Gutterman JU: Collaborative phase I-II study of recombinant DNA-produced leukocyte interferon (Clone A) in metastatic breast cancer, malignant lymphoma, and multiple myeloma. Am J Med 77: 427, 1984.

17. Foon KA, Sherwin SA, Abrams PG, Longo DL, Fer MF, Stevenson HC, Ochs JJ, Bottino GC, Schoenberger CS, Zeffren J, Jaffe ES and Oldham RK: Treatment of advanced non-Hodgkin's lymphoma with recombinant leukocyte A interferon. N Engl J Med 311:1148, 1984.

18. Foon KA, Bottino GC, Abrams PG, Fer MF, Longo DL, Schoenberger CS, and Oldham RK: Phase II trial of recombinant leukocyte A interferon in patients with

advanced chronic lymphocytic leukemia. Am J Med 78: 216, 1985.

19. Quesada JR, Alexanian R, Hawkins M, Barlogie B, Borden E, Itri L, and Gutterman JU: Treatment of multiple myeloma with recombinant alpha interferon. Blood 67:275, 1986.

20. Anderson KC, Boyd AW, Fisher DC, Leslie D, Schlossman SF, and Nadler LM: Hairy cell leukemia: a tumor of pre-plasma cells. Blood 65:620, 1985.

21. Talpaz M, McCredie KB, Mavligit GM, and Gutterman JU: Leukocyte interferon-induced myeloid cytoreduction in chronic myelogenous leukemia. Blood 62:689, 1983.

22. Talpaz M, McCredie KB, Kantarjian H, Trujillo J, Keating J, and Gutterman JU: Chronic myelogenous leukemia: hematologic remissions with alpha interferon. Brit J Hematol (in press).

23. Talpaz M, Kantarjian HM, McCredie KB, Trujillo JM, Keating MJ, and Gutterman JU: Hematologic remission and cytogenetic improvement induced by recombinant human interferon $alpha_A$ in chronic myelogenous leukemia. N Engl J Med 314:1065, 1986.

54. The Use of Interferon in the Treatment of Multiple Myeloma

John J. Costanzi and Richard B. Pollard

University of Texas Medical Branch, Galveston, TX 77550

INTRODUCTION

The treatment of multiple myeloma clearly improved with the introduction of phenylalanine mustard almost two decades ago, but subsequent gains in treatment have been only modest (1). Recent interest has focused on four or five-drug induction regimens to improve remission rates and survival, however, almost all patients still relapse or become refractory to treatment within two to three years (2,3). Subsequent salvage therapy in these patients with relapsing or refractory myeloma has not produced high response rates or improved survival (4,5,6,7,8,9,10). The need for new drugs which are active in this disease is clear.

Pre-clinical studies have documented the antiproliferative activity of natural and recombinant interferons against myeloma cell lines (4). Early clinical studies confirmed the activity of interferon in the treatment of some patients with multiple myeloma (12,13,14,15,16). These combined studies totaled 25 patients whose response rate was 25%. While the results of these studies utilizing natural interferon must be regarded as preliminary, interferon therapy has clearly been shown to influence the level of abnormal serum proteins and modify the course of disease in some patients. Results of a multi-institutional Phase II clinical trial utilizing recombinant alpha-2 interferon (INTRON-Schering) in 38 patients with relapsing and refractory multiple myeloma has been reported (17).

This paper will discuss the results of this clinical trial using alpha-2 interferon in relpasing and refractory patients with multiple myeloma. In those patients who do not respond to interferon or who have responded and subsequently relapsed, their response to re-institution of chemotherapy will also be discussed. And then the use of alpha-2 interferon combined with Melphalan and Prednisone in the treatment of 30 previously untreated patients with multiple myeloma will be analyzed.

METHODS

Intron (Schering-Sch 30500) interferon used in this study is a highly purified human alpha-2 interferon produced by recombinant DNA techniques in E. coli (18). Alpha-2 interferon was administered in three different dose schedules (Table 1).

TABLE I: INTERFERON REGIMENS

	EVALUABLE	NUMBER OF RESPONDERS
1. 3-100 x 10^6/IU/m2/d IV three times weekly x 2 weeks, then 10 x 10^6/IU/m2 S.C. three times weekly	18	3
2. 30-50 x 10^6 IU/m6/d I.V. for 5 days every 14 days, x 4 courses, then, 10 x 10^6 IU.m2 S.C. three times weekly x 3 months	7	2
3. 2 x 10^6/m2/d S.C. three times weekly x 3 months, then 10 x 10/m2/d S.C. three times weekly	13	2
TOTAL	38	7

As each schedule had similar toxicity and produced responses at rates not statistically significantly different from each other, results of all studies are combined.

Those patients who relapsed after responding to interferon or who did not respond to the interferon were placed on the following VBAP/VMCP chemotherapy regimen (drugs that they previously received):

VBAP
Vincristine 1 mg IV
BCNU 30 mg/M2 IV
Adriamycin 30 mg/M2 IV
Prednisone 100 mg p.o. q.d. x 4 days
Every 4 weeks for 3 courses

VMCP
Vincristine 1 mg IV
Melphalan 4 mg/M2 p.o. q.d. x 4 days
Cyclophosphamide 100 mg/M2 p.o. q.d. x 4 days
Prednisone 100 mg p.o. q.d. x 4 day
Every 4 weeks for 3 courses

Cooper et al (19) recently published the utilization of Alpha-2 interferon with Melphalan and Prednisone in 30 previously untreated patients. Interferon was administered subcutaneously three times per week during week I and repeated during week II. It was given at five different dose levels: 0.5, 1.0, 2.0, 5.0 and 10.0 x 106 IU/M2. Melphalan (9mg/M2 orally) and prednisone 40mg/M2 orally were administered on days 2-5 of week 2. The melphalan dose was escalated or de-escalated depending on the nadir white blood counts. 5-7 patients were entered on each dose level and there were no dose escalation within patients.

Response criteria utilized were those recommended by the Chronic Myeloma Task Force Study Group (20). A complete response (CR) was defined as the disappearance of serum paraprotein measured by at least 2 serum protein electrophoretic determinations 4 weeks apart and a qualitative immunoelectrophoresis. If present, a decrease in urinary light chain protein (Bence Jones proteins) to 0.1 grams/24 hours was required on 2 determinations, as well as the disappearance of any soft tissue masses. Additional criteria included a return of hematological parameters to normal values. A partial response (PR) was defined as a decrease in the serum paraprotein to 50% or more below the pre-treatment level as measured by at least 2 serum protein electrophoretic determinations 4 weeks apart and if urinary light chains were present, the decrease had to be 50% or more below pretreatment levels based on at least 2 determinations. Bone marrow determinations, although performed, were not required to determine a partial remission. Changes in the serum monoclonal protein or urine monoclonal protein greater than 25% but less than 50% of the pre-study determinations were categorized as minor responses. Subjective and objective toxicity were scored according to criteria established by the World Health Organization (WHO) (21). Actuarial survival curves were compared utilizing generalized Wilcoxon (Breslow) and Savage (Mantel-Cox) statistics (22).

INTERFERON ALONE

Of the 38 evaluable patients there were a total of 7 responders (18%). There was one patient with a complete response and six partial responders. There were variable response rates among patients from different prognostic sub-groups. Among patients who were primary refractory, having never responded to prior therapy, there were 2/19 (10.5%) responses, whereas among patients who had previously responded there were 5/19 responses (26%). Three of six patients who had relapsed while off chemotherapy responded to interferon treatment. The amount of prior treatment also profoundly affected the response rate to interferon. Two of five patients who only received single alkylating agent therapy previously, responded to interferon, where as only three of 25 patients who had failed multiple alkylating agent therapy responded.

Three of the 7 responders continue to respond for greater than one year on continued maintenance therapy. One patient had a partial response for 40 weeks and then converted to a complete response with disappearance of abnormal M-protein and radiographic confirmation of healing lytic bone lesions. This CR now continues greater 170 + weeks. In addition to the 7 patients who had responses by conventional criteria, there were an additional 13 patients who had at least a 25% decrease in their abnormal paraprotein documented on at least one follow-up visit (minor response). Additionally, a number of patients who did not meet response criteria for improvement in abnormal protein did have subjective improvement in bone pain during the course of interferon treatment. Of 29 patients who entered the study with documented bone pain, 18 improved and 10 remained unchanged during the course of treatment. Only one patient had worsening of bone pain during interferon treatment. Responses occurred rom 7-14 weeks after initiation of therapy.

The median survival for non-responders is 6.9 months versus 11.3+ months for responders and 15.4 months for patients who meet minor response criteria. These are statistically significant differences ($p < .05$) for responders and minor responders vs. non-responders. Despite the known limitations of this type of analysis (22), this finding suggests that the attainment of complete plus partial responses and possibly minor responses might give survival benefit.

Interferon therapy was well tolerated in the schedules used with only 4 patients discontinuing therapy due to adverse effects. The hematologic and non-hematologic toxicity was more severe during the induction phase than during the maintenance phase when patients had doses titrated to their maximum tolerated dose. In almost all cases it was possible to titrate individual patient's doses to a tolerable level. The most commonly occurring side effect was a complex of constitutional symptoms characterized as "flu-like" (fever, malaise, anorexia). Some aspects of this flu-like syndrome occurred in over 90% of patients. During induction, 46% of patients reported these symptoms to be moderate to severe, but only 13% had these persistently during maintenance. Other significant non-hematologic toxicities included confusion and somnolence. They were completely reversible upon cessation of interferon therapy. Similarly, elevated hepatic transaminases were observed in 4 patients during IV induction but resolved promptly upon discontinuation of interferon.

These patients received lower doses of interferon during maintenance therapy without subsequent elevation of liver enzymes.

Hematologic toxicity was strongly related to baseline hematologic parameters. Among patients that began with WBC greater than 2000, 54% had nadirs less than 2000. During maintenance, 32% of patients had nadirs that required dose adjustment. Similarly, among patients with baseline platelet counts greater 50,000, 31% had nadirs less 50,000 after interferon therapy. There was no evidence of cumulative hematologic toxicity. Other chemical toxicities were uncommon and all reversible.

The effectiveness of this recombinant alpha-2 interferon in a population of pre-treated relapsing patients suggests that additional trials are warranted to study the effects of alpha-2 interferon in previously untreated patients either as a single agent or in combination with standard alkylating agents or corticosteroids.

CHEMOTHERAPY AFTER INTERFERON

A group of 9 patients had been resistant originally to chemotherapy. Only one of those patients responded to interferon. After these patients were placed on the VBAP/VMCP chemotherapy, 2 noted partial responses, 1 had stable disease and 5 noted increasing disease.

Another 9 patients had originally either responded (7 patients) or had no response without increasing disease (2 patients) and then relapsed on chemotherapy and were placed on interferon. Two of those patients responded to the interferon. When these 9 patients were then placed on the VBAP/VMCP chemotherapy, 6 noted a response, 1 had no response and 2 had increasing disease.

Toxicity was carefully monitored in these patients. Most of the toxicity was mild to moderate and consisted of nausea and reversible leukopenia and thrombocytopenia. The responders had a survival ranging from 8+ to 34+ months with a median of 23 months. The non-responders had a survival range of 4 to 22 months with a median of 7 months.

It can be concluded that a significant proportion of patients who relapsed on their original chemotherapy and subsequent interferon will respond to the reinstitution of the chemotherapy. It may be postulated that in subsequent studies combining interferon and chemotherapy, the interferon should probably be administered before the chemotherapy.

INTERFERON WITH MELPHALAN AND PREDNISONE

Cooper et al (19) followed this lead when they treated 30 untreated patients with multiple myeloma with inteferon followed by melphalan and prednisone. In that study the limiting toxic effects were: a. alpha-2 interferon induced flu-like symptoms and fatigue; b. dose related myelosuppression and; c. dose related compromise in doses of melphalan over time. The maximal tolerated dose of alpha-2 interferon was 5.0 x 10 IU/M2 subcutaneous three times a week; dose de-escalation of interferon should occur depending upon patient tolerance of interferon induced fatigue/flu-like symptoms and myelosuppression. In that study responses were seen in at least as many patients as would be expected with melphalan and prednisone alone. Among 24 evaluable patients, there were 18 (75%) responses with a median duration of 10+ months (range 2-15+). This response rate compares favorably with that reported for melphalan and prednisone alone and suggests that alpha-2 interferon does not antagonize melphlan and prednisone and does not appear likely to worsen the response rate known to occur with melphalan and prednisone alone.

SUMMARY

This trial demonstrates the effectiveness of interferon in the management of patients with relapsing multiple myeloma. Although two thirds of the patient population had received extensive prior treatment, 7/38 patients responded. Three of the 7 responders have had a survival time of greater than 1 year with marked improvement in performance status and one patient has achieved a durable and ongoing complete remission, which is rarely seen with chemotherapy. If the patients are analyzed according to prior treatment, one finds 2/5 responses among patients who had previously received only melphalan and prednisone, compared to 2/8 for those who had received multiple alkylators plus other chemotherapeutic agents.

Of the 19 evaluable patients who were initially refractory to chemotherapy, only 2 responded to interferon. This 10% response rate is minimal and is similar to chemotherapy results whose responses are usually less than 10%. This low response in refractory patients was also noted in earlier interferon trials.
When the resistant patients were placed on the VBAP/VMCP chemotherapy only 2 out of 9 responded. But when the relapsing patients were given the same chemotherapy 6 out of 9 responded and remain so with a median length of response of 23 months. This chemotherapy did not produce any unusual toxicity in this group of patients.

A subsequent study recently published used interferon with melphalan and prednisone in which the chemotherapy was administered after the interferon. The limiting toxicity included dose related myelosuppression and alpha-2 interferon induced flu-like symptoms and fatigue. Responses were seen in at least as many patients as would be expected with melphalan and prednisone alone.

Interferon is an active compound in the treatment of multiple myeloma. It should continue to be studied alone in patients with previously untreated disease and should continue to be utilized with other cytotoxic agents in untreated and previously treated patients.

REFERENCES

1. Bergsagel, D.E., Sprague, C.C., Austin, C. (1962): Evaluation of new chemotherapeutic agents in the treatment of multiple myeloma, IV. (L-phenylalanine mustard NSC 8806). Cancer Chemother. Rep. 21:87.

2. Durie, B.G.M., Salmon, S.E. (1982): The current status and future prospects of treatment for multiple myeloma. Clin. Hematol. 11:181.

3. Bergsagel, D. (1983): Progress in the treatment of plasma cell myeloma. J. Clin. Oncology 1:510.

4. Blade, J., Feliue, Rozman C. (1983): Cross-resistance to alkylating agents in multiple myeloma. Cancer 52(5):786.

5. Bergsagel, D.E., Cowan, D.H., Hasselback, R. (1972): Plasma cell myeloma: Response of melphalan-resistant patients to high-dose intermittent cyclophosphamide. C.M.A. Journal 101:851.

6. White, D., Bersagel, D., Rapp, E.F. (1981): Failure of cyclophosphamide to produce response in melphalan-resistant multiple myeloma. Blood 58 (supplement):11169a, 1981.

7. Bennett, J.M., Silver, R., Ezdinli, E. (1978): Phase II study of adriamycin and bleomycin in patients with multiple myeloma. Cancer Treat. Rep. 62:1367.

8. Cohen, J.H., Bartolucci, A.A. (1972): Hexamethylmelamine and prednisone in the treatment of refractory multiple myeloma. Amer. J. Clin. Oncol. 5:21.

9. Presant, C.A., Klahr, C. (1978): Adriamycin 1,3-bis(2-chloroethyl)-1-nitrosourea (BCNU, NSC #409962) cyclophosphamide plus prednisone (ABC-P) in melphalan-resistant multiple myeloma. Cancer 42:1222.

10. Lake-Lewin,D., Myers, J., Lee, B.J. (1979): Phase II trial of pyrazofurin in patients with multiple myeloma refractory to standard cytotoxic therapy. Can.Treat. Rep. 63:1403.

11. Aapro, M., Alberts, D., Salmon, S. (1983): Cancer Chemo. PHA 10, 161, 1983.

12. Mellstedt, H., Bjorkholm, M., Johansson, B. (1979): Interferon therapy in myelomatosis. Lancet I: 245.

13. Mogensen, K.E., Cantell, K. (1977): Production and

preparation of human leukocyte interferon. J. Pharmacol Exp. Ther. 1:369.

14. Gutterman, J.U., Blumenschein, G.R., Alexanian, R. (1980): Leukocyte interferon - induced tumor regression in human metastatic breast cancer, multiple myeloma, and malignant lymphoma. Ann. Inter. Med. 93:399.

15. Alexanian, R., Gutterman, J., Levy, H. (1982): Interferon treatment for multiple myeloma. Clin. Hematol. 11:211.

16. Mellstedt, H., Aahre, A., Bjorkholm, M.D (1982) Interferon therapy of patients with myeloma. In: Immunotherapy of Human Cancer, Elseview North Holland, Inc Terry/Rosenberg (eds): p.387.

17. Costanzi, J., Cooper, M.R., Scarffe, J.H., Ozer, H., Grubbs, S.S., Ferraresi, R., Pollard, R. and Spiegel, R.J.: Phase II Study of Recombinant Alpha-2 Interferon in Multiple Myeloma. J. Clin. Onc. 3:654, 1985.

18. Struli, M., Nagata, S., Weissman, C. (1980): At least three human type alpha interferon: Structure of alpha-2. Science 209: 1343.

19. Cooper, M.R., Fefer, A., Thompson, J., Case,Jr., D.C., Kempf, R., Sacher, R., Neefe, J., Bickers, J., Scarrfe, J.H., Spiegel, R., and Bonneme. Alpha-2 Interferon/Melphalan/Prednisone in Previously Untreated Patients with Multiple Myeloma: A Phase I-II Tiral. Ca Treat Rep 70:473, 1986.

20. Miller, A.B., Hoogstraten, B., Staquet, M., Winkler, A. (1981): Reporting results of cancer treatment. Cancer 47: 207, 1981.

21. Mantel, N. (1966): Evaluation of survival data and two new rank order statistics arising in its consideration. Cancer Chemother. Rep. 50:163.

22. Anderson, J.R., Cain, K.C., Gelber, R.D. (1983): Analysis of survival by tumor response. Journal of Clinical Oncology 1:710.

55. Interferon: Potential Use in Solid Tumors

E. Bonnem

Clinical Research Division, Schering Corporation, Kenilworth, NJ 07033

INTRODUCTION

The interferons (IFN) represent a novel class of compounds; novel in the sense that against the frame-work of classical oncologic agents, they do not fit into any common schema of alkylator, intercalator or spindle inhibitor. Rather, the interferons appear to affect any number of different levels of a cell's functions, including effects upon oncogene expression, alterations in cell membrane antigens, direct antiproliferative effects and effects upon cell cycling. Indirect effects are primarily those ascribed to immunologic activation NK cell, ADCC, monocyte-macrophage, etc. Whether or not any or all of these functions play a role in the treatment of solid tumors is not known. However, often in oncology, theory lags behind practice. The practitioner's concern is not with IFN's theoretical mechanisms, but rather with its practical application. This review, therefore, will focus upon the role of interferon in the treatment of solid tumors. Much of the focus will be upon the alpha interferons, with mention of clinical trials with beta or gamma when available.

Abbreviations: IFN (Le) - Non-recombinant leucocyte α IFN; IFN-β-SER - Recombinant β-IFN; rIFN-α2A - Recombinant α IFN-2A; rIFN-γ - Recombinant IFN-γ; rIFN-α2b - Recombinant α IFN-2b; nIFN-α - Non-recombinant αIFN

MELANOMA

Advanced melanoma is generally considered to be a refractory disease. Thus, any indication of response to IFN would be interpreted as encouraging. Krown et al. administered IFN(Le) to 43 patients with advanced disease at a dose of 3-9 MU i.m. daily for 42 days. Only one objective response occurred in a patient with skin nodules and this patient developed new nodules while others regressed (1). Retsas et al. reported 17 patients entered into a trial of nIFN-α at a dose of 2.5 MU/m^2 daily for 30 days. One patient was treated with intralesional therapy. Of 17 patients, only one obtained a partial response for melanoma-in-transit, lasting 6 months (2). Twenty-three patients were studied with IFN (rIFN-α2A), 50 x 10^6 MU/m^2 i.m. t.i.d. by Creagan et al. Of 20 evaluable patients, three patients achieved objective evidence of partial response (soft tissue, lung, nodes, and liver by radionuclide scan) lasting 2-3 months (3). In 10 patients treated with rising doses of intralesional rIFN-α2A, no significant responses were obtained (4). An interesting finding was noted by Borgstrom et al. with the observation that when IFN was combined with cimetidine, tumor regression occurred in 4 of 15 patients (3 complete, 1 partial) (5,6). This observation was confirmed in a study by another group of investigators in which 6 of 16 evaluable patients obtained tumor regression (3 partial, 1 minor response) (7). These two studies utilized IFN(Le). Another group utilizing IFN (rIFN-α2b) in combination with cimetidine could not confirm these findings (8). The reason for these discrepant results is not apparent.

As a single agent IFN is of limited value. Nonetheless, it is intriguing to note that regardless of the type of IFN α utilized or the route or dose, that the response rate remains consistently 10-15%, including some complete responses. Complete responses are generally not seen with cytotoxic agents and entice clinicians to explore ways to maximize this outcome. The Eastern Cooperative Oncology group, for instance, is randomizing high risk surgically resected patients to receive rIFN-α2b vs observation. The results of this adjuvant trial will be eagerly awaited.

RENAL CELL CARCINOMA

Like malignant melanoma, renal cell carcinoma (RCC) has a disappointingly low, yet definite, response rate in the range of 10-30%.

The initial trials of IFN(Le) were performed in 37 patients, of which 11 responded (2 complete, 9 partial) for periods lasting 3-12+ months (9). A second trial randomized low dose (1 MU/day x 28 days) vs high dose (10 MU/day x 28 days). Although toxicity was greater at the higher dose, two patients responded, while none responded at the lower dose. Response durations were 3+ and 8+ months (10). Krown et al. administered IFN (rIFN-α2A) to 27 patients with RCC at 50 MU/m^2 i.m. three times per week. Ten were previously untreated. Nineteen patients were evaluable with responses seen in six patients; however, only two qualified as true partial responders (lung, soft tissue, liver). Duration of response was 20 and 32+ weeks. Four patients developed neutralizing antibodies (11). In a second randomized trial with IFN (rIFN-α2A) reported by Quesada et al., patients received either 2 or 20 MU/m^2/day i.m. for 8 weeks. No responses occurred in 15 patients who received the low dose IFN. In contrast, in the high dose group, 12/41 (29%) obtained either complete or partial responses with a median duration of 3 months. Neutralizing antibodies developed in seven responsive and nine non-responsive patients. There was suggestive evidence that the appearance of antibodies may abrogate response.(12) However, a second study at an alternate institution failed to support the findings with regard to antibody development.(13) Thus, although there is a definite trend towards the abrogation of response with the development of antibodies, larger numbers of patients are required to determine the ultimate significance. rIFN-α2b was also tested in a low dose (2 MU/m^2 SQ T.I.W.) vs high dose (30 MU/m^2 IV x 5) in 26 patients. No neutralizing antibodies were detected, although the response rate was a disappointingly low 10%. Responses occurred in both treatment arms.(14)

Thus, as with melanoma, there are many unanswered questions. Is there really a dose response? Does the development of antibodies abrogate the response? Could the impact upon the disease be greater if it were administered post-operatively in patients at high risk for relapse? Future studies are very much needed to better define the role of alpha IFN in renal cell carcinoma.

No published data on IFN-β-SER are available. However, preliminary findings of IFN-γ have been reported. Patients were entered into a Phase I-II trial and received 10-3000 mcg/m^2/day daily. Six of thirty-five (17%) obtained responses.(15) Larger numbers of patients are required to confirm these data.

OVARIAN CANCER

Ovarian carcinoma represents an interesting arena for trials with any of the interferons because it remains confined to the abdominal cavity. This condition permits an intraperitoneal route of administration.

The initial trials were reported with systemic IFN(Le) at a dose of 3 MU daily i.m. Two of 13 previously treated patients obtained a response, although the duration was not reported.(16) Another trial at 1 MU daily i.m. resulted in 1/15 patients obtaining a partial response lasting 7 months.(17) Systemically administered rIFN-γ has also been tried in relapsing patients. Because of the toxicity, some of the 14 patients entered into the trial dropped out before completing treatment. Nevertheless, four patients (one clinical CR 3 PR) responded, suggesting activity for the compound.(18) The most promising trial was with rIFN-α2b administered a 50 MU in 14 previously treated patients. There were four surgically documented complete responses, one partial response and one clinical complete response. The duration of response was 5-14+ months.(19) Preliminary results of IFN-β are available in eight patients treated at a dose of 3 MU units i.p. B.I.W. Although no responses were documented, four patients had disappearance of ascites.(20)

The most logical next step with these encouraging findings would be to combine recombinant α and γ intraperitoneally in advanced disease or to pursue adjuvant trials after initial debulking with either agent alone.

BLADDER CARCINOMA

Carcinoma of the bladder is a heterogeneous disease ranging in its malignant manifestations from a relatively benign papilloma and superficial carcinoma to invasive widespread disease. In general, there have been few well-designed trials of the IFNs in bladder carcinoma. Only scattered reports of efficacy exist, usually with few patients. One report by Hill et al. of IFN(Le) at 3 MU i.m. daily for 3 weeks each month resulted in complete responses in two of four patients with superficial carcinoma. Follow-up in both patients was 12 and 7 months, respectively.(21) One other case of a patient with recurrent bladder papillomatosis was described in a Phase I trial of IFN(Le). A partial response lasting 7+ months was reported but no other details were provided (22). Four patients who were refractory to surgical electrocautery and radiation were given IFN(Le) transurethrally by cystoscope once/day for 21 days at a dose of 2 MU; two of the four patients were given simultaneous parenteral injections. All four patients obtained responses (3 complete, 1 partial) for periods of 3-24+ months (23). Another combined modality protocol examined IFN(Le), 1 MU i.m. q.o.d. for 6 months followed by attempted transurethral resection was reported by Scorticatti et al. All patients appeared to respond to this treatment and many, in comparison to their baseline, had decreased recurrence rates. However, it is difficult to separate the effects of IFN from surgery in this highly select group of patients (24). A Phase I-II trial of rIFN-α2b administered intravesically has been reported in 17 patients. Doses ranged from 50-100 MU T.I.W. for 8 weeks. Complete response occurred in 6/8 with carcinoma-in-situ, 0/8 papillary carcinoma and 1/1 with both histologies.(25) These data, while encouraging, require additional confirmation and comparison to standard agents.

BREAST CARCINOMA

Carcinoma of the breast was one of the earliest targeted diseases for trials of IFN-α and one in which many discrepancies have occurred. It has also been an area of inconclusive results. The original trials utilized IFN(Le) at 3-9 MU i.m. daily. Partial responses occurred in 22% (26). Another trial of IFN (Le) in 17 patients produced partial responses in 41%. Correlates of response included prior responsiveness to chemotherapy or hormonal manipulation and soft tissue predominant disease (26,27). More extensive Phase II testing with both recombinant interferons at various doses/schedules has failed to produce significant responses (29,31,32). Of 44 patients in both trials, only one patient obtained a partial response.

There are several potential explanations for these contradictory results. The ACS trials consisted mainly of previously untreated patients, whereas in the other trials, patients had all failed at least one form of standard cytotoxic or hormonal therapy. The ACS noted that patients who responded tended to be older than non-responders ($p = 0.05$) (30). The IFN (rIFN-α2A) trial was equally weighted by pre- and postmenopausal women. If the ACS's conclusion about menopausal status is correct, statistical variations would have led to an invalid conclusion in the rIFN-α2A study in which only 10 of 19 patients were postmenopausal. Additionally, dose reduction was required in all patients treated on that trial, whereas dose escalation occurred in the ACS trials. Dose reduction could conceivably alter outcome. Finally, the IFN(Le) preparation of IFN represents a general probe of several IFNs of low specific activity, whereas the recombinant IFN represents a trial of a single IFN with high specific activity.

IFNs are known to cause cell surface antigen expression in a variety of cell lines (33,34) including the augmented expression of estrogen-binding protein receptor (ER) in tissue homogenates of breast carcinoma. The clinical significance of this has not yet been fully explored. When viewed in conjunction with the ACS trial in which tumor response tended to occur in an older population, it would suggest the possibility that future trials be limited to postmenopausal or ER-positive tumors. Additionally, this finding would suggest a trial of IFN followed by a hormonal manipulation in an attempt to augment responsiveness to the primary hormonal agent.

KAPOSI'S SARCOMA

The recent epidemic form of Kaposi's sarcoma seen in victims of acquired immunodeficiency syndrome has also been reported to respond to recombinant IFN.

Krown et al. studied rIFN-α2A at a dose of 36-54 MU and reported responses in 5 of 12 (3 complete, 2 partial) patients. Two patients had been previously treated with radiation and another IFN preparation. The median duration of response had not been achieved in the group of responders at the time of reporting. It is interesting to note that NK activity and OKT4/OKT8 ratios improved after IFN therapy, but that these changes did not correlate with response (36,37). This would sugget that the antitumor effects of IFN in Kaposi's sarcoma is a cytotoxic effect rather than immune mediated. Recently, this trial has been reported more completely after expansion to a randomized low dose (3 MU) vs high dose (36 MU). Complete or partial responses were noted in 38% of patients who received the high dose vs 3% of those at the low dose. The median durations were 18 and 10 months, respectively. Prior opportunistic infections correlated negatively with response.(38). A pilot study of rIFN-α2b randomizing 20 patients to receive 1 MU/m^2/s.c. vs. 50 MU/m^2 i.v. 5 days per week on alternate weeks was reported by Volberding et al. Partial responses occurred in four of nine high-dose and one of nine low-dose patients (39). A subsequent study of 20 patients administered 50 MU/m^2 5 days per week on alternate weeks produced responses in 8 of 20 patients (2 complete, 6 partial) (40). Opportunistic infection (OI) appeared to be less prevalent in the responding group of patients, although it remained a problem. More recently Rios et al. reported their experience with nIFN-α at 20 MU/m^2 i.m. daily for 60 days. Twenty patients were entered into the study, of whom eight had obtained a response (4 complete, 4 partial). The median duration of response was 14+ weeks. No comment was made on the incidence of OI (41).

Another trial of nIFN-α randomized between 7.5, 15 or 25 MU/m^2 daily IM. Because of toxicity, all patients actually received between 6 and 15 MU/M^2, thus abrogating the interpretation of dose and response. Three partial responses were obtained. However, as with the rIFN trials, prior history of OI predicted for a poor outcome. Response also correlated with a higher total lymphocyte and OKT-4 positive cells.(42)

To summarize, therefore, all alpha interferons appear active to one degree or another. Predictors of response include non-visceral involvement, absence of B symptoms, a less altered immune defect (higher T4/T8 ratio) and no prior OI. The mechanism of action in this disease is unknown but may include direct antiviral effects against HTLV-III/LAV, direct cytotoxic effects or, as yet undefined, immune augmentation. The future of this disease probably lies in earlier intervention in those patients designated "at risk" to incur the full blown syndrome of AIDS. Gamma IFN, for instance, has been shown to augment monocyte-macrophage function in vitro from patients with AIDS. Whether or not alpha IFN may play a role in viral positive individuals who do not have AIDS is currently being evaluated.

MALIGNANT GLIOMA

Malignant gliomas have recently been added to the list of tumors where the interferons may be active. The initial trials were reported from Japan with both intrathecal and intravenously administered IFN-β at doses ranging from 1 to 10 MU. There were 8 responses (1 CR, 7 PR), although survival was not commented upon.(43) nIFN-α was administered to 17 patients in doses ranging from 10 to 30 MU/m^2 3 x week. Six patients had tumor reductions of 25% or more. Four of six had expired, but the median survival was 511 days.(44)

While these studies are most intriguing, larger numbers of patients with longer follow-up and a comparison to standard therapy (radiation ± IFN) are required in order to determine the impact upon survival.

LUNG/GASTROINTESTINAL MALIGNANCIES

Because of space limitations, it will be sufficient to note that none of the interferons have demonstrated any antitumor activity in lung carcinoma or gastrointestinal malignancies. The reader is referred elsewhere for additional details.(45)

CONCLUSIONS/FUTURE DIRECTIONS

The interferons have been in clinical trials for approximately 8-10 years. They represent one of the first attempts by the medical community to utilize biologics in the treatment of human disease. What have we learned and in what direction does it point us?

First, an unresolved schism exists with respect to dose and antitumor response. *In vitro* stem cell assay work would (for the alpha IFNs) suggest that *higher* doses produce greater anti-proliferative effects in the absence of any immune effector cells. However, *in vitro* results also suggest that high (pharmacologic) doses ablate *most* immune functions which we are currently able to measure. If the interferons act as immune modulatory agents to produce their antineoplastic effects, we should administer less. If immune function has no relationship to antitumor response, we should administer more. The clinic does not answer the question, with the exception of Kaposi's sarcoma and possibly renal cell carcinoma; in these circumstances, the evidence points strongly to a dose/response relationship.

Second, the interferons act slowly. This raises several issues. For instance, a patient's response may be designated "no change" for 2-3 months and suddenly at month four obtain a partial response. In a similar sense, there are also reports of patients in whom rapid progression was halted after the administration of IFN. The patient remains "stable" for long periods, but never obtains a classical response. Does our definition of response need to be altered for the biologics?

Third, and perhaps most provocative, we have come through the last ten years approaching these agents in classical oncologic terms. Perhaps, this is incorrect. While the violin, cello, trumpet, etc. produce individual notes, they sound much different when acting as part of an orchestra. In a similar sense, each of the individual IFNs will, in all probability, never fully express their antineoplastic potential until used (a) together (b) with other lymphokines (c) with monoclonal antibodies (d) with other cytotoxic agents or (e) after *ex vivo* activation of effector cells. Thus, the permutations are myriad and constrain us to recognize that we have only just begun.

REFERENCES

1. Krown SE, Burk M, Kirkwood JM, et al. The American Cancer Society trial of human leukocyte interferon in malignant melanomas: preliminary results. *Antiviral Res* 34; 1981.
2. Retsas S, Priestman TJ, Newton KA, Westbury G. Evaluation of human lymphoblastoid interferon in advanced malignant melanoma. *Cancer* 51:273-6; 1983.
3. Creagan ET, Ahmann DL, Green SJ, et al. Recombinant leukocyte A IFN in disseminated malignant melanoma. *Am Soc Clin Oncol* 2:58; 1983.
4. Abrams PG, Sherwin SA, Ward J, et al. A Phase I trial of recombinant leukocyte interferon administered by intralesional injection. *Am Soc Clin Oncol* 2:48; 1983.
5. Borgstrom S, von Eyben FE, Flodgren P, et al. Human leukocyte interferon and cimetidine for metastatic melanoma. *N Engl J Med* 307:1080-1; 1982.
6. Flodgren P, Borgstrom S, Ingvar C, et al. Metastatic malignant melanoma: regression induced by combined treatment with interferon and cimetidine. *Antiviral Res* 1:36; 1983.

7. Hill NO, Pardue A, Khan A, et al. Interferon and cimetidine for malignant melanoma. N Engl J Med 308:286; 1983.
8. Lipton A. Harvey HA, Simmonds MA, White DS, et al. Lack of enhanced activity of systemic interferon by cimetidine in malignant melanoma. Am Soc Clin Oncol 3:56; 1984.
9. Quesada JR, Gutterman JU, Rios A. Interferons in the treatment metastatic renal cell carcinoma. Antiviral Res 1:35; 1983.
10. Kirkwood JM, Harris JE, Vera R, Sandler S. Randomized trial of two doses of leucocyte interferon in metastatic renal cell carcinoma: the American Cancer Society collaborative trial. Proc Am Assoc Cancer Res 24:146; 1983.
11. Krown SE, Einzig Al, Abramson JD, et al. Treatment of advanced renal cell carcinoma with recombinant leukocyte interferon. Am Soc Clin Oncol 2:58; 1983.
12. Quesada JR, Rios A, Swanson D, et al; Antitumor activity of recombinant derived interferon alpha in metastatic renal cell carcinoma. J Clin Oncol 3:1522-1528; 1985.
13. Figlin RA,deKernion E, Mukamel E, et al; Recombinant leucocyte A interferon antibody development in advanced renal cell carcinoma. Proc Am Soc Clin Onc 1986; 5:222.
14. Kempf RA, Grunberg SM, Daniels JR et al; Recombinant interferon alpha-2 in a phase II study of renal cell carcinoma. Proc Am Soc Clin Onc 3:59; 1984.
15. Garnick MB, Reich SD, Maxwell B, et al; Phase I/II study of recombinant gamma interferon in advanced renal cell carcinoma. TNO Meeting Procedings; Tampa Florida; 139; 1985.
16. Einhorn N, Cantell K, Einhorn S, Strander H. Human leukocyte interferon therapy for advanced ovarian carcinoma. Am J Clin Oncol 5:167-72; 1982.
17. Freedman RS, Gutterman JU, Wharton JT, et al; Leucocyte interferon in patients with epithelial ovarian carcinoma. J Biol Resp Modifiers 2:133-138; 1983.
18. Welander C, Homesley H, Levin E, et al. Phase II trial of the efficacy of human recombinant interferon gamma in recurrent ovarian carcinoma. Proc Am Soc Clin Onc 5:221; 1986.
19. Berek JS, Hacker NF, Lichtenstein A, et al. Intraperitoneal recombinant α interferon for salvage immunotherapy in Stage III epithelial ovarian cancer. Cancer Res 44:4447-4453; 1985.
20. Rimbaldi A, Introna M. Intraperitoneal administration of interferon beta in ovarian cancer patients. Cancer 56:294-301; 1985.
21. Hill HO, Pardue A, Khan A, et al. Clinical trials of human leukocyte interferon in malignancy. Tex Rep Biol Med 41:634-40; 1981.
22. Christophersen IS, Jordal R, Osther K, et al. Interferon therapy in neoplastic disease: a preliminary report. Acta Med Scand 204:471-6; 1978.
23. Ikic D, Maricic Z, Oresic V, et al. Application of human leukocyte interferon in patients with urinary bladder papillomatosis, breast cancer and melanoma. Lancet 1:1022; 1981.
24. Scorticatti CH, de la Pena NC, Bellora OG, et al. Systemic IFN-alpha treatment of multiple bladder papilloma grade I or II patients: pilot study. J Interferon Res 2:339-43; 1982.

25. Torti FM, Shortliffe LD, Williams RD, et al. Superficial bladder cancers are responsive to alpha-2-interferon administered intravesically. Proc Am Soc Clin Onc 3-160; 1984.
26. Borden E, Holland JF, Dao TL. Leukocyte derived interferon (alpha) in human breast carcinoma. The ACS USA Phase II trial. Ann Intern Med 97:1-6; 1982.
27. Gutterman JH, Blumenschein GR, Alexanian R, et al. Leukocyte interferon induced tumor regression in human metastatic breast cancer, multiple myeloma and malignant lymphoma. Ann Intern Med 93:399-406; 1980.
28. Horning SJ, Levine JF, Miller RA. Clinical and immunological effects of recombinant leukocyte A interferon in eight patients with advanced cancer. JAMA 247:1718-22; 1982.
29. Sherwin SA, Mayer D, Ochs JJ, et al. Recombinant leucocyte interferon A in advanced breast cancer: results of a Phase II efficacy trial. Ann Intern Med 98:598-602; 1983.
30. Borden E, Holland JF, Dao TL. Leukocyte derived interferon (alpha) in human breast carcinoma. The ACS USA Phase II trial. Ann Intern Med 97:1-6; 1982.
31. Muss H, Caponera M, Stuart J, et al. Intravenous interferon α_2 in patients with advanced breast cancer; a Phase II study. Am Soc Clin Oncol 2:99; 1983.
32. Silver HKB, Connors J, Salinas FA. A prospective randomized study of dose response with lymphoblastoid interferon. Antiviral Res 1:90; 1983.
33. Hattori T, Pack M, Bougnoux P. Interferon induced differentiation of U937 cells. Comparison with other agents that provide differences of human myeloid or monocyte like cell lines. J Clin Invest 72:237-44; 1983.
34. Perussia B, Dayton ET, Lazarus R, et al. Immune interferon induces the receptor for monomeric IgG, on human monocytic and myeloid cells. J Exp Med 158:1092-113; 1983.
35. Dimitrov NV, Myer C, Einhorn S, et al. Interferon as modifier of estrogen receptors in cancer tissues. Proc Am Assoc Cancer Res 23:240; 1982.
36. Krown SE, Real FX, Cunningham-Rundles S, et al. Kaposi's sarcoma and immunodeficiency in homosexual men: response to recombinant leukocyte A interferon: Third Annual International Congress for Interferon Research, Miami, No. 30; Nov 1-3, 1982.
37. Krown SE, Real FX, Cunningham-Rundles S, et al. Preliminary observations on the effect of recombinant leukocyte A interferon in homosexual men with Kaposi's sarcoma. N Eng J Med 308:1071-6; 1983.
38. Real FX, Oettgen HF and Krown S. Kaposi's sarcoma and the acquired immunodeficiency syndrome. Treatment with high and low doses of recombinant leucocyte A interferon. J Clin Onc 4:544-551; 1986.
39. Volberding P, Moran T, Abrams D, et al. Recombinant alpha interferon therapy of Kaposi's sarcoma in acquired immunodeficiency syndrome. Am Soc Hematol 62:118a; 1983.
40. Volberding P, Gotlieb M, Rothman J, et al. Therapy of Kaposi's sarcoma in acquired immune deficiency syndrome (AIDS) with α-2 recombinant IFN. Am Soc Clin Oncol 2:53; 1983.

41. Rios A, Mansell PW, Newell GR. Treatment of acquired immunodeficiency syndrome related Kaposi's sarcoma with lymphoblastoid interferon. J Clin Onc 3:506-512; 1986.
42. Gelmann EP, Preble OT, Steis R, et al. Human lymphoblastoid interferon treatment of Kaposi's sarcoma in the acquired immunodeficiency syndrome. Am J Med 78:737-741; 1985.
43. Nagai M, Arai T, Kohno S, Iizuka E: Current status of interferon therapy on malignant brain tumor. Dept. of Neurosurgery, Kokkyo Univ. School of Med. Gan No Rinsho (JAPAN) 29 (6) 608-15, ISSN 1983.
44. Malignant Glioma Treatment with interferon. M. Mahaley, M. Urso, R. Whaley, R. Selker, T. Williams, A. Guaspari. Proc Am Soc Clin Onc 4:229; 1985.
45. Bonnem EM and Spiegel RJ. Interferon α: Current status and future promise. J Biol Resp Mod 3:580-598; 1984.

56. Interferon Use for Sarcomas

H. Strander

Department of Oncology (Radiumhemmet), Karolinska Hospital, S-104 01 Stockholm, Sweden

INTRODUCTION

Interferon (IFN) therapy for sarcomas was originally initiated in a Swedish adjuvant osteosarcoma trial in 1971 (1,2,3). The trial was based on the assumption that IFN therapy might be more effective against a small tumor load. Some evidence at the time of the initiation of the trial indicated that sarcomas in man might be caused by viruses. Experience has since that time accumulated both by in vitro and in vivo use of IFN and both by employing animal models and doing clinical trials (1). The early animal work is not considered in this short review since it has been fully discussed elsewhere (4).

INTERFERON TREATMENT OF MURINE SARCOMA CELLS

Inhibition of murine osteosarcoma cell growth in vitro by IFN has been accomplished (5). The inhibition is temperature dependent (6). Dose dependency has been established (7). Such IFN-treated sarcomas have shown different changes like the ones seen in phospholipids (8), the partial reversion of transformed phenotypes (9) and antigenic changes (19). Effects on the cytoskeleton have been observed (11) and mouse sarcomas have shown changes in the 2′-5′A synthetase system after treatment with IFN in vitro (12).

EXPERIMENTAL IN VIVO MODELS

The antitumor action of IFN in vivo has been extensively discussed elsewhere (1,4,13). PDGF is able to enhance the growth of sarcomas and such action is counteracted by IFN (14). Sarcoma growth can be enhanced or inhibited by IFN depending on the way treatment is given (15).

All types of IFNs are able to exert effects on sarcomas (15,17) and this model work has to be taken into consideration in clinical sarcoma trials. IFN probably has an important role to play for in vivo sarcoma development and the immune system is probably involved. Lesional treatment might be optimal but several studies have demonstrated that osteosarcomas can be affected in murine systems by systemic IFN treatment (18,19) although not always so (20).

Sarcomas can be inhibited in rats (21) and rat osteosarcoma models have been developed (22). The results obtained by employing the latter models have been rather negative perhaps due to IFN-inhibitors like sarcolectins (23), antagonists also present in human sarcomas (24).

IFN TREATMENT OF HUMAN SARCOMA CELLS

Human fibro- and osteosarcomas can be affected in vitro by IFNs and these growth inhibitory effects are dose-dependent (25,26,27).

The continuation of IFN and chemotherapy has been used (28) and also monoclonal antibody-directed IFN preparations against osteosarcoma cells have been developed (29).

HUMAN SARCOMAS IN NUDE MICE

The nude mouse system has been used for the treatment of human osteosarcomas (30,31,32). Various IFN preparations inhibit the growth of different human sarcomas grown as xenografts in nude mice. Osteosarcomas have been sensitive to rather high IFN doses. Different tumors have varied in their sensitivity to different human IFNs. Some of the xenografts have retained their basic histologic appearance during IFN treatment. In some tumors, however, the malignant tissue has been replaced by normal appearing bone trabculae and bone marrow cells and mineralization has also occurred. All human osteosarcomas have an aneuploid or tetraploid content which does not change during IFN treatment. Tumors from IFN-treated mice have had the same proportions of cells in S-phase as control tumors.

IFNs IN SARCOMA PATIENTS

Osteosarcoma

The IFN-α adjuvant trial in Stockholm for the treatment of classical osteosarcomas has recently been summarized (1,2,3). In this trial IFN therapy is combined with differentiated surgery (33). The trial has been critisized due to small number of patients and non-randomization (34). There are 4 groups to consider in this adjuvant trial: a concurrent chemotherapy-treated group (adriamycin and/or methotrexate), a concurrent non-adjuvant treated group, a historical control group and an IFN-treated group. The dose of IFN-α has been 3×10^6 U daily i.m. for one month and thereafter 3 times a week for an additional 17 months. Over the last 1.5 years we have given the IFN daily. The 5-year survival is for the IFN-treated group 50%, for the concurrent chemotherapy-treated group 36%, for the concurrent control group 34% and for the historical control group 14%. The prognosis is worse for the historical group based on prognostic factor analysis. The differences between the concurrent groups are not statistically significant.

Several investigators have studied IFN effects on patients with advanced metastatic disease. Japanese experiments in this respect have been rather encouraging (35,36) with 3 partial regressions seen in 5 patients. Caparros et al. (37) were unable to see any effects on 11 osteosarcoma patients and one patient with chondrosarcoma. Kotz et al. (38) treated 8 patients with osteosarcoma but long term results have not been presented.

A large, multicenter cooperative study on osteosarcoma patients has been undertaken in West Germany (39,49). More than a hundred patients were entered and given IFN (β-type) or no IFN in combination with chemotherapy. No IFN effects were registered but it will still be interesting to see the long-term results of this particular trial.

Ewing's sarcoma

No clinical IFN trials on Ewing's sarcoma have been reported. The invasive capacity of Ewing's sarcoma cells in vitro increased, however, probably due to raised collagenase levels (41). We treated one patient with Ewing's sarcoma with IFN-α without registering any effect.

Soft tissue sarcoma

Harris et al. (42,43) treated 20 patients with soft tissue sarcoma with human IFN-β. Patients had previously been treated by other means. One partial response was seen.

Kaposi's sarcoma

Several research groups have treated the Kaposi's sarcoma seen in connection with aids in young homosexual men with IFN. This research area was initiated by the Memorial Sloan-Kettering group (44-51). Several other groups have treated Kaposi patients since (52-75).

To summarize briefly IFN therapy can be effective in this disease and at doses which can be tolerated by most patients. Potentiation of irradiation has been documented. Low dose IFN-α therapy has been without antitumor efficacy. An objective response rate of between 25-60% has been reported by sole IFN treatment. This is comparable to chemotherapy results. Trials have also been performed where IFN has been combined with chemotherapy. Responders have had low rates of opportunistic infections but direct immune stimulation has not been documented. On the other hand no randomized study comparing IFN therapy to other treatments has established whether IFN is able to prolong survival in the treated patients. Favourable factors predicting survival in IFN treated patients have become more and more elucidated. The combination of human α-interferon and vinblastin seems to constitute an interesting approach as opposed to the VP-16/IFN combination which has given negative results.

CONCLUSIONS

Some human sarcomas can undergo regressions by IFN treatment. The experimental background for the evaluation of such treatments is, however, scanty, and it is difficult at present to see how response rates are going to improve with the IFN application techniques presently being used. Since some patients do respond, however, it is considered extremely important that further trials are conducted in this area.

REFERENCES

1. Strander, H.: Interferon treatment of human neoplasia. Adv Cancer Res 46:1, 1986.
2. Strander, H., Aparisi, T., Broström, L-Å., Einhorn, S., Ingimarsson, S., Nilsonne, U. and Söderberg, G.: Adjuvant interferon therapy in primary osteosarcoma. In: Current Concepts of Diagnosis and Treatment of Bone and Soft Tissue Tumors, Springer-Verlag, Berling-Heidelberg, pp. 119-130, 1984.
3. Strander, H., Aparisi, T., Broström, L-Å., Einhorn, S., Ingimarsson, S., Nilsonne, U. and Söderberg, G.: Adjuvant treatment of osteosarcoma with human IFN-α. In: Interferon Research, Clinical Application and Regulatory Consideration. K.C. Zoon, P.D. Noguchi and T-Y. Liu, eds. Elsevier Publ Co, New York-Amsterdam-Oxford, pp. 247-253, 1984.
4. Stewart, II, W.E.: The interferon system, pp. 1-421, Springer-Verlag, New York, 1979.
5. Glasgow, L.A., Crane, J.L. and Kern, E.R.: Antitumor activity of interferon against murine osteogenic sarcoma cells in vitro. J. Nat Ca Inst 60:659, 1978.
6. Delbruck, H.G., Alloncke, M. and Jasmin, C.: Influence of increased temperature on the inhibition of rat osteosarcoma cell. Multiplication in vitro by interferon. Biomedicine Express 33:239, 1980.
7. Degré, M.: Antiviral and cell multiplication inhibitory activities on an interferon sensitive murine sarcoma cell line. Acta Path Microbial Scand B, 88:219, 1980.
8. Chandrabose, B., Pottathil, R. and Cuatrecasas, P.: Changes in fatty acyl chains of phospholipids induced by interferon in mouce sarcoma S.180 cells. Fed Proc 40:1591, 1981.
9. Hicks, N.J., Morris, A.G. and Burke, D.C.: Partial reversion of the transformed phenotype of murine sarcoma virus-transformed cells in the presence of interferon: a possible mechanism for the antitumor effect of interferon. J Cell Sci 49:225, 1981.
10. Wivel, N.A. and Pitha, P.M.: Interferon treatment of murine meth-A sarcoma cells: Effects on the malignant phenotype and expression of tumor-specific and H-2 antigens. Int J Cancer 30:649, 1982.
11. Bourgeade, M.F., Rousset, S., Paulin, D. and Chany, C.: Reorganization of the cytoskeleton by interferon in MSV-transformed cells. J Interferon Res 1:323, 1981.
12. Wreschner, D.H., Bakhanashvili, M. and Salzberg, S.: Effect of interferon on growth properties of cells transformed by murine sarcoma virus. Isr J Med Sci 18:22, 1982.
13. Gresser, I. and Tovey, M.G.: Antitumour effects of interferon. Bioch Bioph Acta 516:231, 1978.
14. Inglot, A.D. and Inglot, O.: Platelet-derived growth factor (PDGF) enhances the growth of Moloney sarcoma virus-induced tumors in mice. Arch Immunal Ther Exp 29:431, 1981.
15. Murasko, D.M., Fresa, K. and Mark, R.: Enhancement or inhibition of tumor growth by interferon: dependence on treatment protocol. Int J Cancer 32:751, 1983.
16. Vengris, V.E., Wivel, N.A., Glasgow, G. and Pitka-Rowe, P.M.:

The effect of purified interferons on transplantable mouse tumors. Proc. Annu Meet Am Assoc Cancer Res 25:241, 1984.
17. Kataoka, T., Oh-hashi, F., Sakurai, Y., Usuki, K. and Ida, N.: Immunity-associated activity of mouse interferon in murine tumor therapy. Cancer Res 44:5661, 1984.
18. Glasgow, L.A. and Kern, E.R.: Effect of interferon administration on pulmonary osteogenic sarcomas in an experimental murine model. J Natl Ca Inst 67:207, 1981.
19. Satomi, H.: The antitumor effect of interferon against murine osteogenic sarcoma. Nippon Seikeigeka Gakkai Zasshi 57:199, 1983.
20. Taylor, G.N., Kern, E.R., Braaten, B., Glasgow, L.A., Wrenn, M.E., Atherton, D.A., Mays, C.W., Charrier, K. and Ayoroa, G.: Failure of interferon to inhibit plutonium-induced osteosarcomas in mice. J Natl Ca Inst 72:1137, 1984.
21. Marquet, R.L., Schellekens, H., Westbroek, D.L. and Jeekel, J.: Effect of treatment with interferon and cyclophosphamide on the growth of a spontaneous liposarcoma in rats. Int J Cancer 31:223, 1983.
22. Jasmin, C., Allouche, M., Jude, J.G., Klein, B., Thiery, J.P., Perdereau, B., Gongora, R., Gongora, G. and Mazabraud, A.: Un modele experimental d' osteosarcome chez le rat. Sem Hop Paris 58:1684, 1982.
23. Jiang, P.H., Chany-Fournier, F., Robert-Galliot, B., Sarragne, M. and Chany, C.: Sarcolectin: An interferon antagonist extracted from hamster sarcomas and normal muscles. Isolation, characterization, and purification. J Biol Chem 258:12361, 1983.
24. Jiang, P.H., Chany-Fournier, F., Sarragne, M., Gregoire, A. and Chany, C.: Detection of an interferon antagonist, sarcolectin, in human sarcomas and muscles. Int J Cancer 34:625, 1984.
25. Strander, H. and Einhorn, S.: Effect of human leukocyte interferon on the growth of human osteogenic sarcoma cells in tissue culture. Intern J Cancer 19:468, 1977.
26. Ito, M. and Buffett, R.F.: Cytocidal effect of purified human fibroblast interferon on tumor cells in vitro. J Natl Ca Inst 66:819, 1981.
27. Vastola, K.A., Diviak, L.F. and O' Malley, J.A.: Activity of gamma interferon against human tumor cell lines. Proc Am Assoc Cancer Res 24:650, 1983.
28. Broström, L.A.: The combined effect of interferon and methotrexate on human osteosarcoma and lymphoma cell lines. Cancer Lett 10:83, 1980.
29. Embleton, M.J.: Monoclonal antibodies to osteogenic sarcoma antigens. Immunol Ser 23:181, 1984.
30. Masuda, S., Fukama, H. and Beppu, Y.: Antitumor effect of human leukocyte interferon on human osteosarcoma transplanted into nude mice. Eur J Cancer Clin Oncol 19:1521, 1983.
31. Brosjö, O., Bauer, H., Broström, L.A., Nilsson, O., Reinholt, F., Strander, H. and Tribukait, B.: Growth inhibiting effects of human leukocyte interferon on human osteosarcoma xenografts in nude mice. 3rd European Conference on Clinical Oncology and Cancer Nursing. June 16-20, 1985. Stockholm, Sweden, p. 79, 1985.
32. Hofmann, F., Groscurth, P., Morant, R., Cserhati, M., Honegger, H.P. and von Hochstetter, A.: Effects of leukocyte interferon (E.Coli) on human bone sarcoma growth in vitro and in the nude

mouse. Eur J Cancer Clin Oncol 21:859, 1985.
33. Nilsonne, U.: Limb-preseving radical surgery for malignant bone tumors. Clin Orthop 191:21, 1984.
34. Bramwell, V.: Current and former osteosarcoma trials. 3rd European Conference on Clinical Oncology and Cancer Nursing. June 16-20, 1985. Stockholm, Sweden. p. 7, 1985.
35. Ito, H., Murakami, K., Yanagawa, T., Ban, S., Sawamura, H., Sakakida, K., Matsuo, A., Imanishi, J. and Kishida, T.: Effect of human leukocyte interferon on the metastatic lung tumor of osteosarcoma. Case Reports. Cancer 46:1562, 1980.
36. Ban, S., Yamagiwa, T., Yanagawa, T., Sakakida, K., Ito, H., Murakami, K., Matsuo, A., Imanishi, J. and Kishida, T.: Effect of human leukocyte interferon on metastatic lung tumor of osteosarcoma and primary lung cancer. In: The clinical Potential of Interferons R. Kono and J. Vilcek, eds. University of Tokyo Press, pp. 223-230, 1982.
37. Caparros, B., Rosen, G. and Cunningham-Rundles, S.. Phase II trial of interferon (IFN) in metastatic osteogenic sarcoma. Proc Am Assoc Cancer Res 23:474, 1982.
38. Kotz, R., Plattner, E., Ramach, W., Flener, R. and Bodo, G.: Vertraglichkeitsprüfung von humanem lymphoblasten-interferon. Kontrollierte studie bei 8 osteosarkom-patienten mit 3-jahres-uberleben. Arzneim Forsch 32:446, 1982.
39. Winkler, K., Beron, G., Kotz, R., Salzer-Kuntschik, M., Beck. J., Beck, W., Brandeis, W., Ebell, W., Erttmann, R., Gobel, U. et al.: Neoadjuvant chemotherapy for osteogenic sarcoma: results of a cooperative German/Austrian study. J Clin Oncol 2:617, 1984.
40. Purfurst, C., Beron, G., Torggler, S., Kotz, R., Salzer-Kuntschik, M. and Winkler, K.: Ergebnisse der studien Coss-77 und Coss-80 fur die adjuvante chemotherapie bei osteosarkom der extremitäten. Klin Pädiatr 197:233, 1985.
41. Siegal, G.P., Thorgeirsson, U.P., Russo, R.G., Wallace, D.M., Liotta, L.A. and Berger, S.L.: Interferon enhancement of the invasive capacity of Ewing sarcoma cells in vitro. Proc Natl Acad Sci USA 79:4064, 1982.
42. Harris, J., Gupta, T.D. and Vogelzang, N.: Fibroblast interferon (HuIFN - Beta) in the therapy of soft tissue sarcoma - The American Cancer Society/Illinois Cancer Council Study. Proc Annu Meet Am Soc Clin Oncol 3:57, 1984.
43. Harris, J.E., Das Gupta, T. and Vogelzang, N.: Treatment of soft tissue sarcoma with fibroblast interferon (HuIFN-Beta)-American Cancer Society/Illinois Cancer Council Study. Final Report. Proc Am Soc Clin Oncol 4:222, 1985.
44. Krown, S.E.: Interferons and other biological response modifiers in the treatment of Kaposi's sarcoma. 19th Annual San Francisco Cancer Symposium, "Cancer and Aids", March 2-4, 1984. San Francisco, CA, p. 9, 1984.
45. Krown, S.E., Real, F.X., Cunningham-Rundles, S., Myskowski, P.L., Koziner, B., Fein, S., Mittelman, A., Oettgen, H.F. and Safai, B.: Kaposi's sarcoma an immunodeficiency in homosexual men: Response to recombinant leukocyte A inteferon (IFLrA). Third Anual Internatinal Congress for Interferon Research, November 1-3, 1982, Miami, Florida University of South Florida, 1982. (Abstract).
46. Krown, S.E., Real, F.X., Cunningham-Rundles, S., Myskowski,

P.L., Koziner, B., Fein, S., Mittelman, A., Oettgen; H.F. and Safai, B.: Preliminary observations on the effects of recombinant leukocyte A interferon in homosexual men with Kaposi's sarcoma. N Engl J Med 308:1071, 1983.
47. Krown, S.E., Real, F.X., Krim, M., Cunningham-Rundles, S., Koziner, B., Myskowski, R.L., Safai, B. and Oettgen, H.F.: Recombinant leukocyte A interferon in Kaposi's sarcoma. Ann NY Acad Sci 437:431, 1984.
48. Krown, S.E., Real, F.X., Krim, M., Cunningham-Rundles, S., Koziner, B., Myskowski, P.L., Safai, B. and Oettgen, H.F.: Interferons and other biological response modifiers in the treatment of Kaposi's sarcoma. Front Radiat Ther Oncol 19:138, 1985.
49. Real, F.X., Krown, S.E., Krim. M., Myskowski, P.L., Safai, B. and Oettgen, H.F.: Treatment of Kaposi's sarcoma (KS) with recombinant leukocyte A interferon (rIFN-Alpha A). Proc Annu Meet Am Soc Clin Oncol 3:55, 1984.
50. Real, F.X., Krown, S.E., Nisce, L.Z. and Oettgen, H.F.: Unexpected toxicity from radiation therapy in two patients with Kaposi's sarcoma receiving interferon. J Biol Response Mod 4:141, 1985.
51. Vadhan-Raj, S., Wong, G., Gnecco, C., Cunningham-Rundles, S., Krim. M., Real, F.X., Oettgen, H.F. and Krown, S.E.: Immunological variables as predictors of prognosis in patients with Kaposi's sarcoma and the acquired immunodefiency syndrome. Cancer Res 46:417, 1986.
52. Volberding, P.: Therapy of Kaposi's sarcoma in aids. Semin Oncol 11:60, 1984.
53. Volberding, P.: Therapy of Kaposi's sarcoma with interferon. AIDS. The Epidemic of Kaposi's sarcoma and Opportunistic Infections. A.E. Friedman-Kien and L.J. Laubenstein, eds. New York, Masson, p. 63-67, 1984.
54. Volberding, P.: Alpha-interferon therapy of Kapsi's sarcoma in aids. J Cell Biochem Suppl 8A:9, 1984.
55. Volberding, P.A.: The problem of Kaposi's sarcoma in aids. Front Radiat Ther Oncol 19:91, 1985.
56. Volberding, P.A. and Mitsuyasu, R.: Recombinant interferon alpha in the treatment of acquired immune deficiency syndrome-related Kaposi's sarcoma. Semin Oncol 12:2, 1985.
57. Volberding, P., Gottlieb, M., Rothman, J., Rudnick, S., Conant, M., Derezin, M., Weinstein, W. and Groopman, J.: Therapy of Kaposi's sarcoma (KS) in acquired immune deficiency (AIDS) with Alpha-2 recombinant interferon (IFN). Proc Am Soc Clin Oncol 2:C-206, 1983.
58. Volberding, P., Valero, R., Rothman, J. and Gee, G.: Alpha interferon therapy of Kaposi's sarcoma in aids. Ann NY Acad Sci 437:439, 1984.
59. Volberding, P.A., Wofsy, C.B. and Abrams, D.I.: Interferon and interleukin-2 therapy of Kaposi's sarcoma. Adv Exp Med Biol 187:151, 1985.
60. Mitsuyasu, R., Volberding, P., Jacobs, A., Champlin, R., Moran, T., Golando, J., Valero, R. and Spiegel, R.: High dose Alpha-2 recombinant interferon (IFN) in the therapy of epidemic Kaposi's sarcoma (KS) in acquired immune deficiency (AIDS). Proc Annu Meet Am Soc Clin Oncol 3:51, 1984.
61. Odajnyk, C. and Muggia, F.M.: Treatment of Kaposi's sarcoma:

overview and analysis by clinical setting. J Clin Oncol 3:1277, 1985.
62. Odajnyk, D., Laubenstein, L., Friedman-Kien, A., Ostreicher, R., Vilcek, J., Rubinstein, P. and Krigel, R.: Therapeutic trial of human gamma-interferon (IFN) in patients with epidemic Kaposi's sarcoma (eKS). Proc Annu Meet Am Soc Clin Oncol 3:61, 1984.
63. Rios, A., Mansell, P., Newell, G., Reuben, J., Whisnant, J., Hersh, E. and Gutterman, J.U.: The use of lymphoblastoid interferon HuIFN Alpha (Ly) in the treatment of acquired immunodefiencey syndrome (AIDS) related Kaposi's sarcoma (KS). Proc Annu Meet Am Soc Clin Oncol 3:63, 1984.
64. Rios, A., Mansell, P.W., Newell, G., Reuben, J., Hersh, E.M. and Gutterman, J.U.: The use of interferon (IFN) in the treatment of acquired immunodeficiency syndrome (AIDS) related Kaposi's sarcoma (KS). International Conference on Acquired Immunodeficiency Syndrome (AIDS). April 14-17, 1985. Atlanta, Georgia, p. 21, 1985.
65. Rios, A., Mansell, P.W., Newell, G.R., Reuben, J.M., Hersh, E.M. and Gutterman, J.U.: Treatment of acquired immunodeficiency syndrome-related Kaposi's sarcoma with lymphoblastoid interferon. J Clin Oncol 3:506, 1985.
66. Rios, A., Mansell, P., Newell, G., Reuben, J., Whisnant, J., Hersh, E.M. and Gutterman, J.U.: The use of lymphoblastoid interferon HuIFN Alpha (Ly) and vinblastine in the treatment of acquired immunodeficiency syndrome (AIDS) related Kaposi's sarcoma (KS). Proc Am Soc Clin Oncol 4:6, 1985.
67. Ikossi-O'Connor, M.G., Ambrus, J.L., West, T., Lillie, M.A., Milgrom, H. and Chadha, K.C.: Interferon and interferon inactivators in patients with acquired immune deficiency syndrome and Kaposi's sarcoma. A preliminary report. Res Commun Chem Pathol Pharmacol 45:271, 1984.
68. Thiele, G., Schuff-Werner, P., Rahlf, G., Mahrle, G. and Ippen, H.: "Klassische form" des Kaposi-sarkoms: Immunologie und interferontherapie. Hautarzt 35:349, 1984.
69. Groopman, J.E., Gottlieb, M.S., Goodman, J., Mitsuyasu, R.T., Conant, M.A., Prince, H., Fahey, J.L., Derezin, M., Weinstein, W.M., Casavante, C. et al.: Recombinant alpha-2 interferon therapy for Kaposi's sarcoma associated with the acquired immunodeficiency syndrome. Ann Intern Med 100:671, 1984.
70. Lonberg, M., Odajnyk, C., Krigel, R., Laubenstein, L., Wernz, J., Green, M. and Muggia, F.: Sequential and simultaneous Alpha-2 interferon (IFN) and VP16 in epidemic Kaposi's sarcoma (eKS). Proc Am Soc Clin Oncol 4:2, 1985.
71. Krigel, R.L., Odajnyk, C.M., Laubenstein, L.J., Ostreicher, R., Wernz, J., Vilcek, J., Rubinstein, P. and Friedman-Kien, A.E.: Therapeutic trial of interferon-gamma in patients with epidemic Kaposi's sarcoma. J Biol Response Mod 4:358, 1985.
72. Preble, O.T., Rook, A.H., Steis, R., Silverman, R.H., Krause, D., Quinnan, G.V., Masur, H., Jacob, J., Longo, D. and Gelmann, E.P.: Interferon-induced 2'-5'oligoadenylate synthetase during interferon-Alpha therapy in homosexual men with Kaposi's sarcoma: Marked deficiency in biochemical response to Interferon in patients with acquired immunodeficiency syndrome. J Infect Dis 152:457, 1985.
73. Frederick. W.R., Epstein, J.S., Gelmann, E.P., Rook, A.H., Armstrong, G.R., Djeu, J.Y., Jackson, L., Manischewitz, J.F., Enterline, J., Jacob, J., et al.: Viral infections and cell-mediated

immunity in immunodeficient homosexual men with Kaposi's sarcoma treated with human lymphoblastoid interferon. J Infect Dis 152:162, 1985.
74. Fischl, M.A., Gorowski, E., Koch, G., Wang, G., Fletcher, M., Lucas, S., et al.: Human lymphoblastoid interferon treatment of Kaposi's sarcoma in association with the acquired immunodeficiency syndrome. International Conference on Acquired Immunodeficiency Syndrome (AIDS). April 14-17, 1985. Atlanta, Georgia, p. 40, 1985.
75. Gelmann, E.P., Preble, O.T., Steis, R., Lane, H.C., Rook, A.H., Wesley, M., Jacob, J., Fauci, A., Masur, H. and Longo, D.: Human lymphoblastoid interferon treatment of Kaposi's sarcoma in the acquired immune deficiency syndrome. Clinical response and prognostic parameters. Am J Med 78:737, 1985.

57. The Use of Interferons in the Treatment of Certain Diseases of the Central Nervous System

L. Jacobs,[a] A. M. Salazar,[b] and J. A. O'Malley[c]

[a]Dent Neurologic Institute, Millard Fillmore Hospital, 3 Gates Circle, Buffalo, NY 14209; [b]Walter Reed Army Medical Center, Vietnam Head Injury Study, Washington, DC 20307; [c]Roswell Park Memorial Institute, Buffalo, NY 14263

Supported in part by Grants from the Baird, James H. Cummings and Bernard B. Hoffman Foundations, and the Delaware North Company of Buffalo, N.Y. and National Institutes of Health (NS19649).

INTRODUCTION

There has been considerable interest in the potential therapeutic efficacy of the interferons (IFNs) in certain central nervous system (CNS) diseases of known or purported viral, dysimmune and neoplastic etiologies. In this communication we will review some recent studies that have been conducted on diseases manifesting each of these etiologies (single, combined) and attempt to show the rationale for administering the IFNs as well as the results of treatment. Space limitations do not permit a review of therapeutic efficacy studies of the IFNs conducted to date on the broad spectrum of neurologic diseases. (See Salazar et al).[1] Studies concerning the four conditions covered in this chapter were, in general, begun or completed subsequent to that review.

Multiple Sclerosis - Multiple sclerosis (MS) is a disease that is usually characterized clinically by exacerbations and remissions of neurologic symptoms and signs that are disseminated anatomically and temporally and pathologically by demyelinating lesions of the CNS. Less frequently the clinical course is progressive without exacerbations and remissions. The rationale for using IFNs in MS is the body of evidence suggesting that the disease is caused by a previous or ongoing viral infection of the CNS of a dysimmune host and the known antiviral and immunomodulatory effects of the IFNs[1].

Interferons may help to clear persistent viral infections by enhancing the expression of major histocompatibility (MHC) antigens at the surface of infected cells thus, exposing them to specific cytotoxic lymphocytes.[1-4] However, this action may risk increasing T cell dependent immunopathology if the infection is widespread.[2] Paradoxically IFNs have also been implicated in helping to establish persistent viral infections in some systems.[5] In addition interferons may act as mediators of T-cell suppressor activity, while in other systems they increase the T4/T8 ratio.[6-8] Variations in suppressor T-cell activity occur during the natural course of MS, decreasing shortly before or during exacerbations and rebounding during remissions.[9,10] These fluctuations may be an essential ingredient of the exacerbation-remission cycle of MS. Autogenous IFN induced naturally by the products of CNS tissue destruction has been postulated to play a role in establishing remission in the later stages of an untreated MS exacerbation.[1] Administration of IFN might help induce remission from exacerbation by reestablishing T-cell suppressor activity and if this effect endures, provide prophylaxis against future exacerbations. Administration of IFN-B (intravenously, intraventricularly) provided both suppressant and prophylactic effects on experimental allergic encephalomyelitis in mice (animal model of MS).[11-13] These protective effects were most marked following intraventricular administration of IFN-B.

Two early trials on small numbers of patients indicated that systemically administered leukocyte interferon (IFN-α) was of no benefit in MS.[14,15] It was suggested that the lack of response was possibly due to the failure of IFN to cross the blood-brain barrier (BBB). It was further suggested that a trial of intrathecally administered IFN was warranted in MS. The first study of intrathecally administered IFN was reported by Jacobs et al in 1981.[16] That preliminary study included 20 patients with definite MS; Ten recipients received 1 x 10^6 IRU of IFN-B by serial lumbar punctures (LPs) performed biweekly for four weeks and then monthly for 5 months and ten controls received the genereally accepted next best therapy (intramuscular adrenocorticotropic hormone) as needed for exacerbations. The recipients showed a significant reduction in exacerbation rates ($P<.01$, t test) when analyzed after 1.5 years and 2.4 years on the study, but the controls showed no change in rates during that period of time. In June, 1982, the original 10 control patients were crossed over and began receiving IT IFN-B according to a schedule that was slightly modified from that of the original 10 recipients (attempting to reduce toxicity).[17,18] The crossover was done after the controls had been on the study for approximately two years without receiving IFN-B and had shown no change in their exacerbation rates. The original 10 recipients continued to be followed by serial neurologic assessments. The last report on these patients was in 1985 during which time the original recipients had been followed for 5.3 years (mean) since beginning the study and the controls had been followed 2.9 years (mean) since the June 1982 crossover.[18] By that time there had been further significant decrease in the exacerbation rates of the recipients during the study compared with before the study ($P < .001$, Wilcoxan matched pairs). Moreover, the control patients' prestudy exacerbation rate, which had not changed during the first two years of the study (before they received IT IFN-B) had been significantly reduced ($P < .03$, Wilcoxan) during the 2.3 years since receiving IT IFN-B.[18] There was a trend for the overall clinical conditions of the patients to be improved after receiving IT IFN-B compared with before treatment, but this was not statistically significant because some patients deteriorated clinically despite the fact that their exacerbations had been reduced or eliminated. The clinical toxic side effects of treatment (headache, low grade fevers, weakness, myalgia) were mild to moderate and cleared completely within 24-48 hours. Cerebrospinal fluid changes, including pleocytosis (mean 329/cu ml) and protein elevation (mean 58/cu ml) were transient with maximum levels being noted during the first month of treatment. The CSF cell counts returned to normal in all of the recipients, but the CSF protein level remained elevated in (mean 46 mg/dL) seven.[17,18]

The initial and follow-up findings of this preliminary study indicated a sustained beneficial effect of IT administered IFN-B (reduced exacerbations) in MS patients for more than 5 years following treatment in the original recipients and approximately 3 years following crossover treatment in the original controls. The beneficial long-term effect of IT administered IFN-B occurred following a six month treatment phase after which retreatment was not necessary. Also, the temporary toxic side effects observed seemed to be acceptable in view of the benefits achieved.

The preliminary study had certain shortcomings including: a) Small number of patients with mixed types of MS, b) Lack of double-blinding and c) Different pre-study exacerbation rates in original recipients and controls. The preliminary study was not blinded because the toxic side effects of IFN-B administration that are not reproduced by innocuous placebo would have readily distinguished recipient from control patients. When we began the preliminary study we did not know how to alleviate those toxic side effects to the point that adequate blinding could be achieved. We later learned of the efficacy of small doses of oral Indomethacin for reducing the toxic side effects of IFN-B administered IT which allowed true double blinding (vida infra).

In 1983 a larger, multicenter study of the efficacy of IT administered IFN-B was begun[19]. This study corrected the preliminary study's shortcomings and should definitively determine whether this treatment is effective in MS as indicated by the preliminary study. Seventy six patients with definite MS, each with aggressive exacerbating-remitting disease were included in the study.[20] The only significant finding of the preliminary study was a reduction in exacerbation rate following IFN-B treatment; therefore exacerbation rate is the major focus of the current study. The patients were randomized to a recipient or control group using a stratification based on prestudy exacerbation rate (less than 2 or 2 or more exacerbations/yr) and then were assessed in terms of exacerbation rates (pre-study vs. on-study) and serial clinical evaluations. The study was blinded by using separate treating and examining physicians, performance of false LPs on controls and administration of small oral doses of Indomethacin to recipients and placebo Indomethacin capsules to controls. The treatment phase differed slightly from the preliminary study in that one rather than two LPs per week were performed for the first four weeks of the study and then one LP per month for the next five months (total LPs with IFN-B administered - 9 rather than 13 as in the preliminary study). The study duration will be 2 years and the final results will be known in July, 1986. However, interim analysis has shown that the IFN-B so administered was well tolerated, the clinical and CSF toxic side effects were less severe than in the preliminary study and the study was successfully double blinded.[20] A critical factor in the successful double blinding was the use of Indomethacin which dramatically reduces the toxic side effects of IFN-B administered IT (possibly through inhibition of prostaglandin E_2 synthesis).[18,20,21] Indomethacin might also have partially accounted for the reduced CSF toxicity observed in the double blinded compared with the preliminary study. The maximal pleocytosis in the double blinded study was only 30% of that observed in the preliminary study; the degree of CSF protein elevation was also reduced (by 20%) compared with the preliminary study.[17,20]

Recently, Knobler and associates completed a study testing systemically administered IFN-α in MS.[22] Twenty-four patients with definite MS received 5 x 10^6 IRU of IFN-α by subcutaneous injections daily for 6 months followed by a washout period. A significant reduction in exacerbation rates was observed in the 15 patients who had strictly exacerbating-remitting disease while they were receiving IFN compared with 2 years prior to the study, but no change was seen in patients with stable or progressive forms of the disease. The benefit observed in those patients may have resulted from passage of IFN from systemic circulation into the CNS through a partial breakdown of the BBB that may occur in MS patients[23] or the systemic immunoenhancing effects of IFN. It will be important to see if those patients experience long-term prophylaxis against repeated exacerbations as has been observed in the patients in the preliminary study of IT administration of IFN-B.[18] Two follow-up articles on those patients reported an increase in immunoglobulin G (IgG) synthesis (systemically, intrathecally), increased T4/T8 ratio, increased natural killer cell (NKC) and the production of antibodies to a protein contaminant in the IFN-α solution following systemic treatment.[24,25]

Johnson and Alter recently conducted a much larger randomized study testing the effect of lower doses (2 x 10^6 IRU) of IFN-α administered subcutaneously in 98 MS patients with strictly exacerbating-remitting disease.[26] No benefit of IFN-α compared with placebo was observed with the lower dose regimen so the effects of systemically administered IFN-α in MS patients may be strongly dose-related.

Most recently, Panitch and associates studied the effects of recombinant gamma IFN (IFN γ) in 18 MS patients with exacerbating-remitting disease.[27] Patients were given low (1-ug), intermediate (30 ug) or high (1,000 ug) doses of IFN γ by intravenous infusion twice weekly. There was a significant increase in exacerbations during treatment compared with before it ($P < .01$). The exacerbations were not dose related nor were they specifically related to IFN-induced alterations in immune function.

These results are contrary to the previously cited observations with IFN-α and B in MS. In certain systems such as murine lymphocytic choriomeningitis (LCM), treatment with IFN worsened the disease possibly by enhancing the expression of MHC antigens at the cell membrane of infected cells and exposing them to the action of specific T-lymphocytes.[2] Gamma IFN was much more potent than IFN-B as an inducer of MHC antigens on virus infected cells.[2-4] The results of the clinical study seem to demonstrate the extreme sensitivity of the CNS in MS to the effects of IFN-γ and the probable role of autogenously produced IFN-γ in the MS exacerbation-remission cycle. While the mechanisms underlying the induction of exacerbations by IFN-γ are speculative, there seem to be no indications for its use in further therapeutic trials in MS. It offers no theoretical or practical advantages over IFN-α or B, and may, in a significant number of patients, potentiate disease activity.[27]

Amyotrophic Lateral Sclerosis - Amyotrophic lateral sclerosis (ALS) is a progressive disease of the CNS in which both upper and lower motor neurons degenerate leading to profound weakness, muscle wasting and death, usually within four years. The basic cause of this disease remains unknown, but a viral etiology has been postulated since its earliest descriptions by Charcot.[1] Several indirect lines of evidence suggest a slow or persistent viral etiology including: a) A delayed, post polio form of ALS exists, b) Other chronic post-infectious conditions (eg postencephalitic parkinsonism) include amyotrophic cases, c) Some cases of Jakob-Creutzfeld disease (proven slow viral etiology) have ALS features, and d) An imperfect murine retrovirus mouse model of ALS has been developed. However conventional virologic techniques have not definitely detected a virus in cases of ALS.

Two early trials of IFN inducers (tilorone, Poly ICLC intravenously) in ALS patients failed to detect any beneficial response.[1,28] Rissanen treated two ALS patients with 3 x 10^6 IRU of IFN-α subcutaneously, again without discernible benefit.[29] However, the known impermeability of the BBB to IFNs prompted other studies in which IFN was administered directly into the cerebrospinal fluid (CSF) containing spaces. Bouche and associates administered IFN-B intrathecally twice per week for the first month and then bimonthly for the next 6 months in 11 patients with ALS.[30] A gradually increasing dosage schedule was used and as much as 5 x 10^6 IRU was administered during one LP. Toxic side effects of fever, headache and myalgia usually lasted 24 hours and then cleared completely. Although the treatments were well tolerated by all patients no clinical benefit was observed during two years of follow-up. Similar negative results have been noted by Salazar, et al (unpublished work) in 6 ALS patients treated with intrathecal IFN-B. In another study Mora and associates administered 1 x 10^6 u of IFN-α by LP once per week for 6 months to 10 ALS patients.[21,31] They observed a marked reduction in toxic side effects of IFN by administration of Indomethacin, 50 mg. orally for 3 doses which increased tolerance of treatment, but no clinical benefit of treatment was observed. More recently, Olarte and Shafer conducted a double-blind crossover trial of oral Levannisole in 59 ALS patients.[32] This substance, a T-cell stimulator, which can be either immunosuppressive or immunomostimulatory had no clinical beneficial effect during 12 months observation.

Subacute Sclerosing Panencephalitis - Subacute sclerosing panencephalitis (SSPE) is a progressive and fatal neurologic disease caused by infection with measles virus producing inflammation, demylination and gliosis of the brain. Symptoms usually appear as subtle behavioral changes at 8 to 10 years of age and usually progress inexorably to coma and death within 1 to 3 years. In 5-10% of the cases symptoms may stabilize or even improve spontaneously. The disease process induces autogenous IFN production by the CNS; high levels of IFN were found in the CSF of 38% of SSPE patients by Joncas and associates.[33] Early studies of the potential therapeutic efficacy of exogenously administered IFNs or their inducers in SSPE were disappointing. Administration of the IFN inducer, pyran copolymer combined with dibromdesoxyuridine resulted in only transient improvement in one of three patients. Guggenheim administered intravenous poly I:C to seven SSPE patients without benefit.[34] However, Chany reported complete recovery in one of three SSPE patients treated early in the disease with combined IFN-isoprinosine compound.[35] In 1981, Behan treated three SSPE patients with 3 x 10^6 IRU of IFN-α intramuscularly daily for 20 - 90 days.[36] One patient also received 12 x 10^6 IRU intrathecally over 3 days. None of the patients seem to benefit clinically from the treatment and it was concluded that partially purified IFN-α was of no value in SSPE.

However, in 1986 there were two reports of substantial benefit of IFN-α administered intraventricularly or intrathecally in SSPE patients. Panitch and associates treated three children with stages II-III SSPE with human IFN-α administered intraventricularly in gradually increasing dosages of 2.5 x 10^5 per week to 1 x 10^6 IRU twice per week over a 6 month period of time.[37] All three improved to varying degrees and for different lengths of time (1.5 - 12 months) after cessation of treatment. Clinical remissions were associated with decreasing titers of measles virus antibody in CSF and reduced rates of intrathecal IgG synthesis. In another 1986 report using lower doses of human IFN-α, Huttenlocher and associates observed sustained but incomplete remission in one SSPE patient for two years following an intrathecal course of 1 x 10^6 IRU every other day for 30 days which was repeated 6 months later.[38] Another patient improved for 6 months after a course of 15 similar intrathecal treatments. Three other SSPE patients in that study showed no benefit following treatment.

Meningeal Metastases - The antineoplastic properties of the IFNs are well recognized. The mechanisms of this effect are not understood; some possibilities include IFN's inhibition of oncogene expression, activation of natural killer cells, increase in histocompatibility antigen expression, modification of growth factors and macrophage stimulation.[39] There have been numerous studies of the efficacy of IFNs against malignancies outside of the CNS which are beyond the scope of this communication. The use of IFNs in the treatment of CNS malignancies has been more limited because of the known impermeability of the BBB to these substances.

However, there have been promising, albeit mixed results in the treatment of neoplastic involvement of the meninges. In 1981, Misset and associates reported treating five patients with acute lymphoid leukemic and one patient with non-Hodgkins' lymphoma meningeal relapse with 1.3 x 10^6 IRU of IFN-B administered intrathecally daily or every other day up to remission or treatment failure (5 to 8 treatments)[40]. This treatment resulted in complete remission lasting 11 months in one patient, but appeared to be of no benefit in the other five patients. The tolerance to treatment was excellent and the side effects observed were temporary and less severe than those that typically follow systemic IFN therapy. In 1984 Slatkin and associates reported the results of administering IFN-α (1 to 4 x 10^6 IRU) intraventricularly weekly to biweekly to two patients with leptomeningeal gliomatosis.[41] Malignant cells cleared from the CSF and symptoms of radiculopathy were reduced for 2 to 11 months after treatment during which time there was no clinical evidence of new meningeal disease. In a 1985 report, Obbens and associates noted clearing of CSF malignant cells following intraventricular administration of IFN-α in four patients with meningeal metastases (primaries - pineal area, lung oat cell, breast, large cell lymphoma).[42] The CSF clearing lasted 6 to 10 weeks while the clinical improvement was less dramatic. The relatively large doses of IFN-α administered intraventricularly in that study (up to 6 x 10^6 IRU per treatment; ave. 13 treatments) were well tolerated and toxic symptoms cleared within 24-48 hours in most patients. Intraventricular and intrathecal administration of IFN- or B was well tolerated in those cancer patients and may hold promise as a treatment of leptomeningeal malignancies. Based upon the preliminary findings, further clinical trials are warranted.

SUMMARY

It is premature to assign a place to the IFNs (alone or in combination with drugs) in the treatment of diseases of the CNS. However, the continued interest in these hormones as therapeutic agents seems to be well founded.

Pathophysiologic data seem to indicate a basic role of autogenous IFN in the exacerbation-remission cycle of MS. Exogenously administered IFN protects mice against EAE, an experimental model of MS. In preliminary studies, both IFN-α and B significantly reduced the exacerbation rates of humans with MS. Interferon-beta administered intrathecally seemed to exert the more powerful antiexacerbation effect and also provided prophylaxis against future exacerbations for more than five years. A large, multicenter, double blinded study assessing the effects of intrathecally administered IFN-B is currently being conducted and will definitively determine whether this treatment is effective in MS. The results of this study will be known in late 1986.

The purported viral etiology of ALS prompted studies of systemically administered IFN inducers and intrathecally administered IFN-α, but no beneficial effect of treatment has been observed in this disease.

Some patients with SSPE seemed to respond to treatment with intrathecal IFN-α, sometimes with apparently permanent remissions. Those showing favorable responses were a distinct minority treated, but trials of IFNs in SSPE should be continued because this disease is almost always fatal when treated with other regimens.

Preliminary studies indicate that intrathecally and intraventricularly administered IFN-α and IFN-B are effective in clearing CSF of malignant cells and reducing symptoms in patients with leptomeningeal metastases. The beneficial effects of IFNs in these patients have always been temporary.

REFERENCES

1. Salazar, AM, Gibbs CJ, Gajudsek DC, et al: Clinical use of interferons: Central nervous system disorders, in Came P, Carter WA (Eds): *Handbook of Experimental Pharmacology*. Berlin, Springer-Verlag, vol 71:472-497, 1983.
2. Jacobson S, Friedman RM, Pfau JC: Interferon induction by lymphocytic choriomeningitis virus correlates with maximum viralence. *J Gen Virol* 57:275, 1981.
3. Bukowski JF, Welsh RM: Interferon enhances the susceptibility of virus infected fibroblasts to cytotoxic T cells. *J Exp Med* 161:257, 1985.
4. Wong GHW, Bartlett PF, Clark-Lewis I, et al: Inducible H-2 and Ia antigens on brain cells. *Nature* (Lond)310, 1984.
5. Sekellick MJ, Marcus PI: The interferon system as a regulator of persistent infection. *Ann N.Y. Acad Sci* 350:545, 1980.
6. Kadish AS, Tansey FA, Yu GSM, et al: Interferon as a mediator of human lymphocyte suppression. *J Exp Med* 151:637, 1980.
7. Onsrud M: Enhancement of suppressor cell generation in human mixed lymphocyte cultures by interferon. *Int Archs Allergy Appl Immun* 67:315, 1982.
8. Aune TM, Pierce CW: Activation of a suppressor T-cell pathway by

intereferon. Proc Nat Acad Sci 79:3808, 1982.
9. Antel JP, Arnason BGW, Medof ME: Suppressor cell functions in multiple sclerosis - correlation with clinical disease activity. Ann Neurol 5:338, 1979.
10. Huddlestone JR, Oldstone MBA: T suppressor (Tg) lymphocytes fluctuate in parallel with changes in the clinical course of patients with multiple sclerosis. J Immunol 123:1615, 1979.
11. Abreu SL: Suppression of experimental allergic encephalomyeolitis by interferon. Immunol Commun 11:1, 1982.
12. Abreu LS, Tondreau J, Levine S, et al: Inhibition of passive localized allergic encephalomyelitis by interferon. Int Arch Allergy Appl Immun 72:30, 1983.
13. Hertz F, Deghenghi R: Effect of rat and beta human interferon on hyperacute experimental allergic encephalomyelitis in rats. Agents and Actions 16:397, 1985.
14. Fog T: Interferon treatment of multiple sclerosis patients: A pilot study, in Boese A (Ed): Search for the Cause of Multiple Sclerosis and Other Chronic Diseases of the Nervous System. Weinheim, Verlag Chemie, 1980, p. 490.
15. Ververken H, Carton H, Billiau A, et al: Intrathecal administration of interferon in MS patients? in Kazrcher S, Loenthal A, Strosberg A (Eds): Humoral Immunity in Neurological Diseases. New York, Plenum Publishing Corp. 1979, p. 625.
16. Jacobs L, O'Malley J, Freeman A, et al: Intrathecal interferon reduces exacerbations of multiple sclerosis. Science 214:1026, 1981.
17. Jacobs L, O'Malley J, Freeman A, et al: Intrathecal interferon in multiple sclerosis. Arch Neurol 39:609, 1982.
18. Jacobs L, O'Malley JA, Freeman A, et al: Intrathecal interferon in the treatment of multiple sclerosis: Patient follow-up. Arch Neurol 42:841, 1985.
19. Jacobs L, O'Malley JA, Freeman A, et al: Intrathecal interferon as treatment of multiple sclerosis: A planned multicenter study. Arch Neurol 40:683, 1983.
20. Jacobs L, Salazar AM, Herndon R, Reese P: Intrathecal interferon in the treatment of multiple sclerosis in, R Smith (Ed): Interferons in the Treatment of Neurologic Disorders, M Dekker Inc., New York, 1986 (In press).
21. Mora JS, Kao KP, Munsat TL: Indomethacin reduces the side effects of intrathecal interferon. N Engl J Med 310:126, 1984.
22. Knobler RL, Panitch HS, Braheny SL, et al: Systemic alpha-interferon therapy of multiple sclerosis. Neurology 34:1273, 1984.
23. Aita JF, Bennett DR, Anderson RE, et al: Cranial CT appearance of acute multiple sclerosis. Neurology 28:251, 1978.
24. Panitch HS, Francis GS, Hooper CJ, et al: Serial immunological studies of multiple sclerosis patients treated systemically with human alpha-interferon. Ann Neurol 18:434, 1985.
25. Rice GPA, Woelfel EL, Talbot PJ, et al: Immunological complications in multiple sclerosis patients receiving interferon. Ann Neurol 18:439, 1985.
26. Johnson KP, Alter M: Personal Communication.
27. Panitch HS, Haley AS, Hirsch RL, et al: A trial of gamma interferon in multiple sclerosis: Clinical results. Neurology 36(Suppl 1):285, 1986.
28. Olson WH, Simons JA, Halaas GW: Therapeutic trial of tilorone in amyotrophic lateral sclerosis: Lack of benefit in a double-blind, placebo-controlled study. Neurology 28:1293, 1978.
29. Rissanen A, Palo J, Myllyla G, et al: Interferon thereapy for amyotrophic

lateral sclerosis. Ann Neurol 7:392, 1980.
30. Bouche P, Hanin B, Castaigne P: Effects of intrathecal interferon therapy in amyotrophic lateral sclerosis. Neurology 36:735, 1986.
31. Mora JS, Munsat TL, Kao KP, et al: Intrathecal administration of natural human alpha interferon in amyotrophic lateral sclerosis. Neurology, 1986 (in press).
32. Olarte MR, Shafer SQ: Levamisole is ineffective in the treatment of amyotrophic lateral sclerosis. Neurology 35:1063, 1985.
33. Joncas JH, Robillard LR, Boureault A, et al: Interferon in serum and cerebrospinal fluid in subacute sclerosing panencephalitis. J Canad Med Assoc 115:309, 1976.
34. Guggenheim MA, Baron S: Clinical studies of an interferon inducer, polyriboinosinic-polyribocytidylic acid (Poli(I) Poly (C)) in children. J Infect Dis 136:50, 1977.
35. Chany C: Discussion in, Perspectives in Virology, Vol XI, New York, Alan Liss Inc., 1981, p. 266.
36. Behan P: Interferon in treatment of subacute sclerosing panencephalitis. Lancet (May 9,):1059, 1981.
37. Panitch HS, Gomez-Plascencia J, Norris FH, et al: Subacute sclerosing panencephalitis: Remission after treatment with intraventricular interferon. Neurology 36:562, 1986.
38. Huttenlocker PR, Picchietti DL, Roos RP, et al: Intrathecal interferon in subacute sclerosing panencephalitis. Ann Neurol 19:303, 1986.
39. Friedman RM: Interferons. New York, Academic Press, 1981.
40. Misset JL, Mathe G, Horoszewicz JS: Intrathecal interferon in meningeal leukemia. N Engl J Med 304:1344, 1981.
41. Slatkin NE, Jaeckle KA, Lukes SA, et al: Treatment of leptomeningeal gliomatosis with human leukocyte interferon: Results in two patients. Neurology 34(Suppl 1):151, 1984.
42. Obbens EAMT, Feum LG, Leavens ME, et al: Phase I clinical trial of intralesional or intraventricular leukocyte interferon for intracranial malignancies. J Neuro-Oncol 3:61, 1985.

Index